W9-AZF-037

CHRONIC COMPLICATIONS OF

# DIABETES

# CHRONIC COMPLICATIONS OF
# DIABETES

EDITED BY

JOHN C. PICKUP MA, BM, DPhil, MRCPath

DIVISION OF CHEMICAL PATHOLOGY
UNITED MEDICAL AND DENTAL SCHOOLS OF
GUY'S AND ST THOMAS'S HOSPITALS
GUY'S HOSPITAL, LONDON

AND

GARETH WILLIAMS MA, MD, FRCP

DEPARTMENT OF MEDICINE
THE UNIVERSITY OF LIVERPOOL
ROYAL LIVERPOOL HOSPITAL, LIVERPOOL

OXFORD
BLACKWELL SCIENTIFIC PUBLICATIONS
LONDON EDINBURGH BOSTON
MELBOURNE PARIS BERLIN VIENNA

To Caroline, Timothy and Kim;
Selma, Matthew, Charlotte and Joshua


Editorial Offices:
Osney Mead, Oxford OX2 0EL
25 John Street, London WC1N 2BL
23 Ainslie Place, Edinburgh EH3 6AJ
238 Main Street, Cambridge
Massachusetts 02142, USA
54 University Street, Carlton
Victoria 3053, Australia

Other Editorial Offices:
Librairie Arnette SA
1, rue de Lille
75007 Paris, France

Blackwell Wissenschafts-Verlag GmbH
Düsseldorfer Str. 38
D-10707 Berlin
Germany

Blackwell MZV
Feldgasse 13
A-1238 Wien
Austria



First published 1994

Set by Setrite Typesetters Ltd, Hong Kong
Printed and bound in Italy
by Vincenzo Bona s.r.l., Turin

DISTRIBUTORS

Marston Book Services Ltd
PO Box 87
Oxford OX2 0DT
(*Orders*: Tel: 0865 791155
Fax: 0865 791927
Telex: 837515)

USA
Blackwell Scientific Publications, Inc.
238 Main Street
Cambridge, MA 02142
(*Orders*: Tel: 800 759–6102
617 876–7000)

Canada
Times Mirror Professional Publishing, Ltd
130 Flaska Drive
Markham, Ontario L6G 1B8
(*Orders*: Tel: 800 268–4178
416 470–6739)

Australia
Blackwell Scientific Publications Pty Ltd
54 University Street
Carlton, Victoria 3053
(*Orders*: Tel: 03 347–5552)

A catalogue record for this title
is available from the British Library

ISBN 0-632-03795-4

Library of Congress
Cataloging-in-Publication Data

Chronic complications of diabetes/edited by
John C. Pickup and Gareth Williams.
p. cm.
Includes bibliographical references
and index.
ISBN 0-632-03795-4
1. Diabetes — Complications.
I. Pickup, John C. II. Williams, Gareth.
[DNLM: 1. Diabetes mellitus — complications.
WK 835 C557 1994]
RC660.C446 1994
616.4'62—dc20
DNLM/DLC
for Library of Congress

# Contents

# List of Contributors

PETER J. BARRY FRCS, FCOphth, *Royal Victoria Eye and Ear Hospital and St Vincent's Hospital, Dublin, Ireland*

D. JOHN BETTERIDGE BSc, MD, PhD, FRCP, *University College and Middlesex School of Medicine, London, UK*

RUDOLF W. BILOUS MD, FRCP, *Diabetes Care Centre, Middlesborough Central Hospital, Middlesborough, UK*

KNUT BORCH-JOHNSEN MD, *Steno Diabetes Center, 2820 Gentofte, Denmark*

MICHAEL BROWNLEE MD, *Alberta Einstein College of Medicine, The Bronx, New York, USA*

RAYMOND BRUCE MB, ChB, *Wynn Institute for Metabolic Research, London, UK*

BASIL F. CLARKE MB, FRCPE, *The Royal Infirmary, Edinburgh, UK*

CAROLINE J. CRACE PhD, *Formerly at Northern General Hospital, Sheffield, UK*

ADRIAN J. CRISP MA, MD, FRCP (UK), *Addenbrooke's Hospital, Cambridge, UK*

TORSTEN DECKERT MD, DMSc, *Steno Memorial Hospital, Gentofte, Denmark*

MICHAEL E. EDMONDS MD, MRCP, *King's College Hospital, London, UK*

DAVID J. EWING MD, FRCP, *The Scottish Office, Home and Health Department, Edinburgh, UK*

ALI V.M. FOSTER BA (Hons), DPodM, SRCh, *King's College Hospital, London, UK*

ANASUYA GRENFELL MA, MD, MRCP, *Jeffrey Kelson Diabetic Centre, Central Middlesex Hospital, Park Royal, London, UK*

KRISTIAN F. HANSSEN MD, *Aker Hospital, Oslo, Norway*

SUSAN E. HALL MD, *Toronto General Hospital, Toronto, Canada*

STEPHEN L. HYER MD, MRCP, *St George's Hospital, London, UK*

ROGER H. JAY MA, MB, BS, MRCP, *University College and Middlesex School of Medicine, London, UK*

HARRY KEEN MD, FRCP, *United Medical and Dental Schools, Guy's Hospital, London, UK*

RONALD R. KLEIN MD, MPH, *University of Wisconsin, Madison, USA*

EVA M. KOHNER MD, FRCP, *Royal Postgraduate Medical School, London, UK*

CATHLEEN J. MULLARKEY MD, *158 Mockingbird Court, Three Bridges, NJ 08887, USA*

JOHN C. PICKUP MA, BM, DPhil, MRCPath, *United Medical and Dental Schools, Guy's Hospital, London, UK*

MASSIMO PORTA MD, PhD, *University of Sassari, Italy*

MARK W. SAVAGE MB, ChB, MRCP, *University of Liverpool, Liverpool, UK*

ANGELA C. SHORE BSc, PhD, *Royal Devon and Exeter Hospital, Exeter, UK*

R. GARY SIBBALD BSc, MD, FRCP(C), ABIM, DAAD, *Women's College Hospital, University of Toronto, Toronto, Canada*

JUDITH M. STEEL MB ChB, FRCPEd, *Edinburgh Royal Infirmary, Edinburgh, UK*

JOHN C. STEVENSON MB, MRCP, *Wynn Institute for Metabolic Research, London, UK*

P.K. THOMAS DSc, MD, FRCP, FRCPath, *Royal Free Hospital School of Medicine, London, UK*

JOHN E. TOOKE MA, MSc, DM, MRCP, *Royal Devon and Exeter Hospital, Exeter, UK*

GIAN CARLO VIBERTI MD, FRCP, *United Medical and Dental Schools, Guy's Hospital Campus, London, UK*

JAMES D. WALKER BSc, MRCP, *St Bartholomew's Hospital, London, UK*

JOHN D. WARD BSc, MD, FRCP, *Royal Hallamshire Hospital, Sheffield, UK*

JACQUELINE N. WILKINSON BSc, SRN, *Northwick Park Hospital, Harrow, UK*

GREG WILKINSON FRCP(Edin), MRCPsych, *The London Hospital Medical College, London, UK*

GARETH WILLIAMS MA, MD, FRCP, *Royal Liverpool Hospital, Liverpool, UK*

R. MALCOLM WILSON DM, MRCP, *Royal Hallamshire Hospital, Sheffield, UK*

# Preface

Everyone concerned with the care of diabetic patients is aware of the immense burden of misery that can be inflicted by the long-term complications of the disease – blindness, renal failure, impotence, a hugely-increased frequency of coronary artery disease, strokes and amputations, and much more. Even though this affects only a proportion of diabetic patients, understanding the causes of this catalogue of catastrophe, identifying the sufferers and those at most risk and developing effective treatments for the complications has rightly become a major preoccupation for diabetologists in recent years.

The chronic complications of diabetes have now assumed a new importance. Although there has been compelling circumstantial evidence for many years that the severity of hyperglycaemia and its duration are intimately linked with long-term tissue damage, definitive proof has been lacking. It has therefore been somewhat an article of faith that efforts to improve glycaemic control will be rewarded with prevention or slowing of retinopathy, nephropathy, neuropathy and other complications.

But now several recent prospective, randomized and controlled studies, culminating in the landmark Diabetes Control and Complications Trial (DCCT) in North America, have at last clearly shown that the institution and maintenance of nearnormoglycaemia will delay the onset or slow the progress of complications, at least in insulin-dependent diabetes. Strict blood glucose control can now join photocoagulation and anti-hypertensive treatment as effective therapies for diabetic microangiopathy. The DCCT and its implications, both within and beyond the remit of the trial are discussed on p. xi, by Professor Harry Keen, who was closely involved in the early design of the DCCT.

With this in mind, most of the time of diabetologists in the coming years is likely to be spent in identifying those at risk of developing complications and in preventing, detecting and treating the complications. We believe, therefore, that the publication of this book is timely. It has been developed from the recently-published *Textbook of Diabetes*, which we were also privileged to edit. Many readers indicated to us that there is a real need for some of the wealth of information in that book to be made available in a shorter text, specifically focused on all aspects of the long-term complications, and suitable for a wide range of health care professionals. The relevant chapters from the parent volume have, therefore, been collected together here and updated as necessary.

The approach taken by the authors is both clinical and scientific. In each system the biochemical and pathophysiological background leads on to a practically-orientated review of clinical features and management. Once again, we are grateful to the authors and publishers for helping us to present this book in the readable and richly-illustrated style which characterized the original *Textbook*. Our grateful thanks are also due to Adrian Walker and Mark Savage for assisting with the otherwise unrewarded task of proof-reading.

JOHN C. PICKUP
GARETH WILLIAMS
*London and Liverpool,*
*November 1993*

# The Diabetes Control and Complications Trial (DCCT): a note added in proof

The publication of the long-awaited results of the Diabetes Control and Complications Trial (DCCT) [1], in late 1993, will have such a profound influence on our understanding of the causes of and treatment approaches to chronic diabetic complications in the next few years that it is mandatory that this volume includes some mention of the study. This note was, therefore, added in proof.

The Diabetes Control and Complications Trial (DCCT) emerged after many years of cogitation in the US as to how finally to establish the scientific link between the level of diabetic control and the risk of angiopathic complications in man. It was clearly impossible to assign people randomly to a 'poor' control group in any clinically-acceptable study. However, it was the evidence of the late 1970s, that quite dramatic and sustainable improvements in average glycaemia and glycated haemoglobin were obtainable from intensified management regimens (e.g. continuous subcutaneous insulin infusion (CSII), multiple daily injections, frequent blood glucose self monitoring), that made such a trial possible. Existing levels of control could, therefore, ethically be compared with the newly-attainable levels of 'super-control' and this was the basis of the 9-year, NIH-based DCCT.

1441 very fully-informed and motivated insulin-dependent diabetic patients aged 13–39 years (about 20% of them 'adolescent') agreed to accept random allocation to experimental (intensified) or standard (conventional) regimens of diabetes care. These regimens differed in their response goals (i.e. glycated haemoglobin values, self-monitoring results) and in the methods used to achieve them. Essentially, patients on intensified management received CSII or three or more insulin injections/day, self-monitored blood glucose levels at least four times daily (and sometimes at night) and maintained close, regular and frequent contacts with their health care professional team. The conventional group continued largely unchanged on one or two injections daily and performed tests as necessary. Participants and health care professionals (HCP) were masked as to key outcomes, though informed to take action if certain ethical threshold values were breached. Though falling short of the goal of $HbA1_C \leq 6.05\%$, the intensive group promptly dropped their mean value of this to 7.0% from about 8.8%, maintaining it there for the trial duration. The conventional group continued virtually unaltered.

One price of intensified control was an increased risk of severe hypoglycaemia, that which required help from another person, which was three times higher than in the conventional group. Interestingly, hypoglycaemia rates in both groups fell by about one half over the duration of the trial, presumably a learning curve for both patient and HCP.

The major complication outcome of the study, the appearance or advance of significant degrees of diabetic retinopathy (sustained three-step advance using the Wisconsin Early Treatment of Diabetic Retinopathy Study [ETDRS] scale) was reduced by approximately half in the intensively-treated group, as were some of the relatively infrequently occurring 'severity indices' such as proliferative retinopathy or laser treatment. Progression to clinical proteinuria and the appearance of 'microalbuminuria' was also reduced to a similar extent. Equally striking was the halving of the emergence of clinical, autonomic and electrophysiological manifestations of diabetic neuropathy. So substantial and consistent were these treatment effects that the study was brought to an end one year ahead of its proposed run.

Apart from the now unequivocal evidence of the value of intensified management, the DCCT has provided an untold wealth of new information on the course of IDDM and its complications. It has also raised acutely in the minds of HCPs and patients the question of how improved control is to be achieved. The DCCT evidence, at least for retinopathy, suggests that any degree of reduction in $HbA_{1C}$ will reduce complications risk (i.e. there was no evidence of a threshold effect) but also that it was very difficult to achieve and maintain the sort of levels that will virtually obviate the complication. Only 5% of intensively-treated patients had an average $HbA_{1C}\%$ $\leq$6.05% for the trial duration, though over 40% managed to achieve this at some point(s) during the trial. Almost predictably, hypoglycaemia risk rose as mean $HbA_{1C}$ fell.

The DCCT results must inevitably reinforce the argument for improved diabetic control, perhaps spilling over to include NIDDM patients, in whom, of course, quite different cost-benefit relationships may apply. How improved glycaemic control is to be achieved clinically is a question that can largely be solved only in the delicate and sometimes prolonged negotiation between individual patients and their HCPs. The point of balance found for each 'best compromise' will depend on many factors — liability to hypoglycaemia, the presence of already advanced complications, infancy and childhood, the availability of resources, and the level of education and training of patients and professionals among them.

HARRY KEEN

## Reference

1 Diabetes Control and Complications Trial Research Group. The effect of intensive treatment of diabetes on the development and progression of long-term complications in insulin-dependent diabetes mellitus. *N Engl J Med* 1993; **329**: 977–86.

# PART 1
# GENERAL MECHANISMS OF DIABETIC COMPLICATIONS

# 1 The Determinants of Microvascular Complications in Diabetes: An Overview

**Summary**

• The 'microvascular' ('microangiopathic' or 'small-vessel') complications of diabetes include retinopathy, nephropathy and neuropathy, even though the contribution of microangiopathy to neuropathy remains uncertain.

• Microvascular complications are specific to diabetes and do not occur without long-standing hyperglycaemia. Other metabolic, environmental and genetic factors are undoubtedly involved in their pathogenesis.

• Both IDDM and NIDDM are susceptible to microvascular complications, although patients with NIDDM are older at presentation and may die of macrovascular disease before microvascular disease is advanced.

• The duration of diabetes and the quality of diabetic control are important determinants of microvascular disease but, because of other individual factors, do not necessarily predict their development in individual patients.

• Different microvascular complications are commonly associated in individual patients, but their prevalence as a function of the duration or severity of diabetes may differ markedly.

• In IDDM, background retinopathy is rare before 5 years of diabetes but its prevalence increases steadily thereafter to affect over 90% of patients after 20 years. After several years of diabetes, the risk of proliferative changes is about 3% of patients per year, with a cumulative total of over 60% after 40 years.

• Diabetic nephropathy affects 20–40% of patients with IDDM, particularly those presenting before puberty and possibly those with an inherited tendency to hypertension. NIDDM patients are also susceptible to nephropathy.

• Over 40% of subjects with IDDM survive for more than 40 years, half of them without developing significant microvascular complications.

The terms 'microvascular' or 'microangiopathic' complications commonly embrace diabetic retinopathy, nephropathy and neuropathy, even though the classification of the latter as a true microvascular complication remains controversial (see Chapter 10). The purpose of this chapter is to outline in general the factors thought to contribute to the development of these complications. The possible pathophysiological mechanisms, are reviewed later (Chapters 2–4) and the specific complications themselves in Chapters 5–17.

Most investigators now agree that diabetic microvascular complications result from the interaction of multiple metabolic, genetic and other factors, of which chronic hyperglycaemia is the most significant. Microvascular complications are common to both IDDM and NIDDM (in which severe complications may occur) and do not develop in the absence of long-standing hyperglycaemia. Epidemiological and long-term clinical studies strongly suggest that hyperglycaemia, or closely associated factors, is of major importance in both the initiation and progression of microvascular disease. Moreover, there is evidence that the various microvascular complications have a common cause. Diabetic patients with incipient nephropathy (persistent microalbuminuria) have 5–10 times the risk of developing proliferative retinopathy than those free from albuminuria; moreover, diabetic nephropathy is almost invariably accompanied by retinopathy. The evolution of the various complications therefore seems to be interrelated.

However, there is immense variability in susceptibility to microvascular disease, which in individual patients cannot be predicted from their glycaemic behaviour. Other factors must therefore be involved. Some of the putative determinants of microvascular disease will now be discussed in more detail.

## Age

IDDM patients whose disease appears before puberty have an increased risk of developing diabetic nephropathy, which is associated with premature death [1], but apparently not with retinopathy in these cases [2].

Many NIDDM patients are relatively old when diabetes appears and some do not survive long enough to develop severe microvascular complications. However, some studies suggest that the frequency of retinopathy in NIDDM is similar to that in IDDM of equivalent duration [3]. There may be qualitative differences in retinopathy between NIDDM and IDDM, in that proliferative retinopathy is rarer and visual loss due to maculopathy is commoner in NIDDM as compared with IDDM. NIDDM patients are by no means 'protected' against nephropathy, even though this is commonly viewed as a complication predominantly of IDDM. About 40% of North American diabetic patients requiring renal dialysis have NIDDM, and nephropathy is particularly common in those ethnic groups (e.g. Asian and Afro-Caribbean populations) in which NIDDM appears at earlier ages [4].

## Sex

Both sexes are vulnerable to diabetic microvascular disease, although there is an unexplained male preponderance of diabetic nephropathy and proliferative retinopathy [5]; there are no systematic glycaemic differences between males and females.

## Duration of diabetes

This is an important determinant of microvascular disease although, as discussed below, the relationship between duration of diabetes and the evolution of the complications is not simple. The issue is further complicated in NIDDM, whose insidious onset may follow several years of subclinical disease; clinically important microvascular complications may be present at diagnosis.

Diabetic treatment can prevent acute metabolic deterioration but does not achieve biochemical normality, resulting in a novel condition including various combinations of hyperglycaemia, hyperketonaemia, hyperlipidaemia and other disturbances. These 'components of diabetic exposure' are interdependent to a certain degree and their levels are generally reflected by the integrated plasma glucose and $HbA_1$ concentrations, the most convenient measures in clinical use.

Each component can be characterized by its intensity, duration and cumulative dose (= mean intensity × duration). Epidemiological studies suggest that specific microvascular complications, although generally interrelated, may be determined by different aspects of exposure to these metabolic abnormalities. Various dose–response curves are theoretically possible. With a linear response, for example, the *incidence* of a complication would rise in proportion to the duration of diabetes, and the *cumulative risk* of the complication would rise considerably faster, in proportion to the square of the duration [6]. Other possible dose–response profiles include an incidence rate which rises to a plateau after a certain cumulative dose, or even one which decreases. In each of these cases, the cumulative risk increases with time, but the relationships between the incidence rate and the duration of diabetes differ markedly. Such divergences are illustrated by the cases of diabetic retinopathy and nephropathy in IDDM.

### *Risk profiles of retinopathy in IDDM*

Figures 1.1 and 1.2 respectively show the incidence rate and cumulative risk of background and proliferative retinopathy in IDDM patients. The first conclusion is that the prevalence of both increases with increasing duration of the disease; indeed, after 20 years, over 95% of IDDM patients have demonstrable retinopathy, although mostly without visual impairment [2]. Background retinopathy is rare before 5 years of diabetes, suggesting that duration is more important than intensity, although the latter presumably must exceed some threshold (Fig. 1.3) [6].

The risk profile for proliferative retinopathy, the principal cause of blindness in IDDM, is strikingly different. Patients become vulnerable after several years of diabetes and the incidence increases

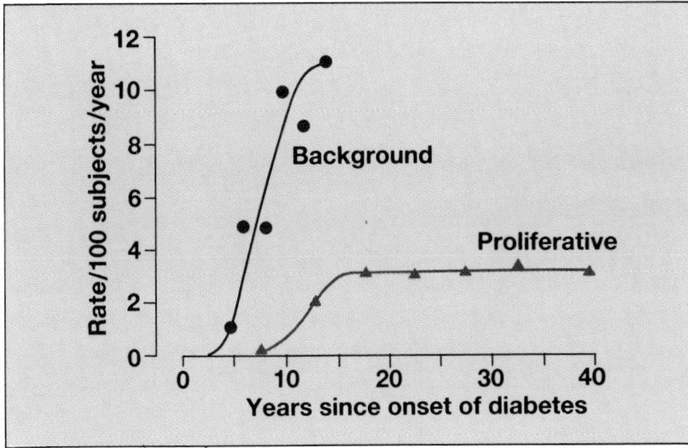


**Fig. 1.1.** Incidence rates of background and of proliferative retinopathy in subjects with IDDM, as a function of the duration of diabetes. (Redrawn from [6] with permission from *The New England Journal of Medicine*.)

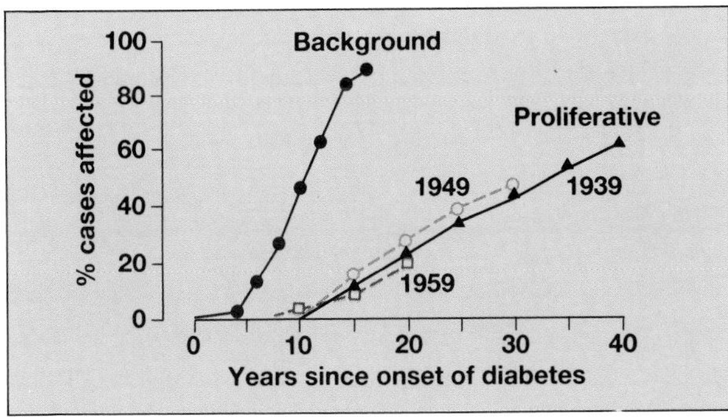


**Fig. 1.2.** Prevalence of background retinopathy and cumulative incidence of proliferative retinopathy in IDDM as a function of the duration of the disease. The data for proliferative retinopathy have been calculated for three cohorts of patients, diagnosed in 1939, 1949 and 1959. (Redrawn from [6] with permission from *The New England Journal of Medicine*.)

rapidly between 10 and 15 years (Fig. 1.1), at a time when background retinopathy has already developed in virtually all patients. Thereafter, the incidence rate remains remarkably constant at about 3% of previously unaffected patients per year, regardless of whether they have been diabetic for 20 or 40 years. The cumulative risk of proliferative retinopathy after 40 years of diabetes is about 62% (Fig. 1.2). The fact that the incidence rate of proliferative retinopathy does not decline even after many years of diabetes suggests that almost all IDDM patients are susceptible to this complication, just as they are to background lesions. However, the constant risk of proliferative retinopathy after 15 years' duration implies a different pathophysiological process. As noted before, a constant risk cannot be explained by dependence on the cumulative exposure to diabetes, as the

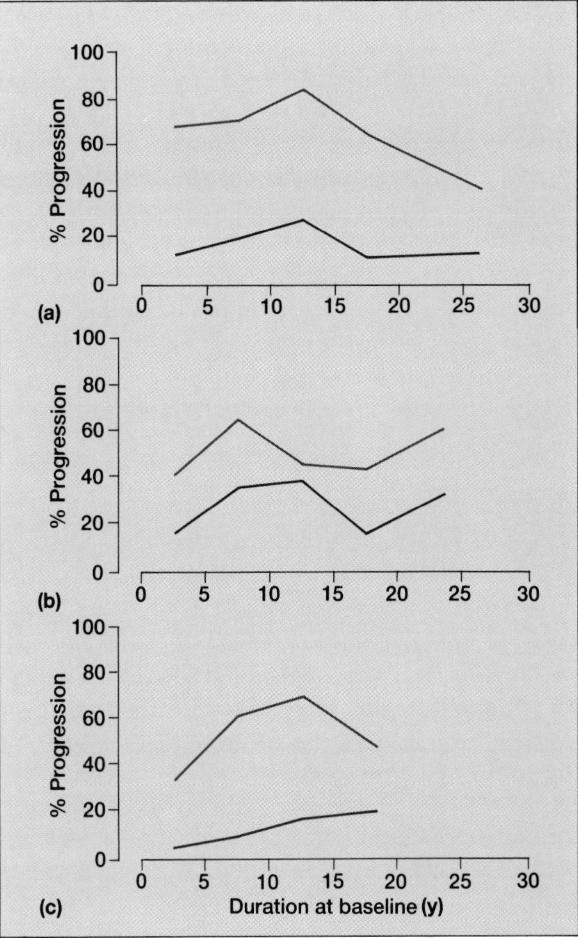


**Fig. 1.3.** 4-year progression of retinopathy by quartiles of glycosylated haemoglobin and duration of diabetes as measured at baseline examination in persons with (a) younger-onset diabetes; (b) older-onset diabetes, taking insulin; and (c) older-onset diabetes, not taking insulin. Red line = lowest quartile $HbA_1$. Blue line = highest quartile $HbA_1$. Note that retinopathy progresses more in the patients in the highest quartile than in the lowest, in each group, although the relationship with the duration of diabetes is variable. (Redrawn from [16] with permission from the *Journal of the American Medical Association*.)

incidence would increase steadily with duration. A more likely cause is some acute effect of the intensity of the exposure, such as the haemodynamic alterations which accompany severe hyperglycaemia [7]. These may contribute to retinal ischaemia and neovascularization in the presence of damaged retinal vessels which are unable to autoregulate blood flow. This hypothesis is consistent with the observation that the risk of proliferative retinopathy is related to the intensity of exposure to diabetes during the several years preceding the onset of this complication.

A final observation is that the risk curves for the development of proliferative retinopathy in cohorts of patients diagnosed in 1939, 1949 and 1959 are virtually superimposable (Fig. 1.2). This implies that any improvements in diabetic management during these decades have not affected the natural history of the complication; fortunately, however, the advent of photocoagulation has revolutionized its prognosis (Chapter 8) and recent evidence, discussed in recent developments at the end of this chapter, strongly indicates that the long-term imposition of improved metabolic control can reduce the risks of serious diabetic retinopathy.

### *Nephropathy*

The pattern is quite different for diabetic nephropathy. After 40 years of diabetes, the cumulative incidence of nephropathy in IDDM patients was 45% of those who developed diabetes in 1939 (Fig. 1.4), but was substantially lower in those diagnosed 20 years later, showing that improved health care or other environmental factors can influence the prevalence of diabetic nephropathy [1, 6]. The frequency rises steeply to a maximum of 21% after 20 years and thereafter falls slowly (Fig. 1.5). This suggests that only a subset of patients are susceptible to diabetic nephropathy. The scarcity of new cases of nephropathy among patients who have had diabetes for many years is due to the fact that this complication has occurred in most of the susceptible persons earlier in the course of diabetes.

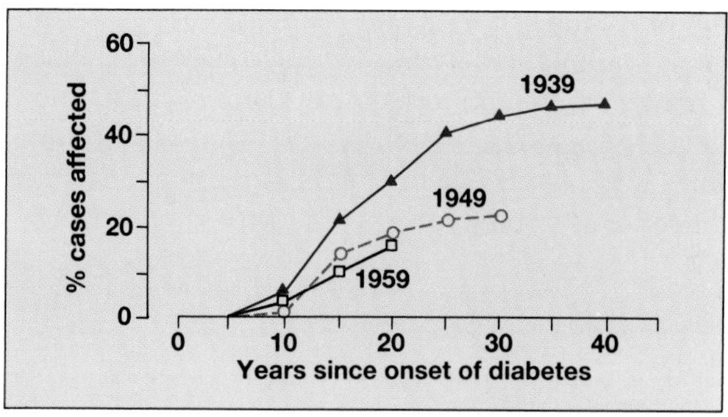


**Fig. 1.4.** Cumulative incidence of nephropathy (persistent proteinuria) according to the duration of IDDM, in separate cohorts of patients diagnosed in 1939, 1949 and 1959. (Redrawn from [6] with permission from *The New England Journal of Medicine*.)

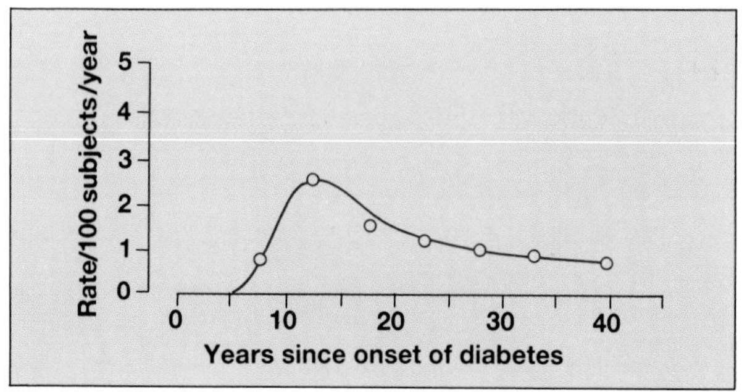


**Fig. 1.5.** Incidence rate of nephropathy (defined as persistent proteinuria) according to the duration of IDDM. (Redrawn from [6] with permission from *The New England Journal of Medicine*.)

## Genetic factors

Little is known about the possible genetic factors which determine microvascular complications, although their role may differ between the various complications and between IDDM and NIDDM. Genetic factors seem unimportant in determining retinopathy in IDDM, in that many co-twins with IDDM of similar duration show marked differences in the extent of retinopathy [8].

Susceptibility to nephropathy has recently been attributed to a genetic predisposition to hypertension, as indicated by a parental history of high blood pressure [10] or abnormally high sodium–lithium countertransport activity in red blood cells [11]; the latter is a marker for essential hypertension which aggregates in affected families. Young adults with 14–18 years of IDDM had a threefold higher risk of nephropathy if one or both parents were hypertensive and the risk increased still further if their glycaemic control was poor [10]. However, this does not appear to be a universal finding and further study is required to clarify the possible role of an inherited tendency to hypertension (see Chapter 14).

Genetic (and/or social) factors may contribute to extended survival of IDDM patients, as the parents of long-term surviving IDDM subjects also tend to live longer than expected [12].

There is no firm evidence concerning the possible role of HLA types in microvascular disease, for example, in patients with neuropathy [9]. This area is particularly difficult to investigate in IDDM patients, a high proportion of whom (over 90% in some populations) possess DR3 and/or DR4 genotypes.

## Hypertension

Hypertension is inextricably linked with the advanced (macroalbuminuric) stage of diabetic nephropathy, but its involvement in the earlier evolution of microalbuminuria is controversial (see Chapter 18). As retinopathy and nephropathy often develop together, it is difficult to ascribe a definite role for hypertension in the pathogenesis of diabetic retinopathy.

### Glycaemic control

As mentioned above, hyperglycaemia is now implicated in the genesis and progression of microvascular complications, although the relationship may be complex and may vary from one complication to another [13].

Epidemiological studies show that the risk of developing microvascular complications is very low when the blood glucose value 2 h after an oral glucose tolerance test is less than about 11 mmol/l [14] (Fig. 1.6). Pirart [15] followed 2795 diabetic subjects — both IDDM and NIDDM — for up to 25 years and concluded that poor long-term glycaemic control was clearly related to a higher prevalence and incidence of neuropathy, nephropathy and particularly severe retinopathy (Fig. 1.7). More recently, a strong correlation between previous $HbA_1$ levels and the development of background and proliferative retinopathy has been shown by Klein *et al*: the risk of developing proliferative retinopathy is 22 times higher in those patients with $HbA_1$ values during the previous 4 years in the highest quartile as compared with those in the lowest quartile of the population [16]. Microalbuminuria, thought to precede overt diabetic nephropathy and a powerful independent predictor of excess cardiovascular mortality [17–20], is associated with higher $HbA_1$ levels than in patients without microalbuminuria (HJ Bangstad *et al.* unpublished observations).

There is therefore convincing evidence that blood glucose levels are important in the evolution of microangiopathy in the diabetic population at large. None the less, not all patients with chronic, severe hyperglycaemia develop severe microangiopathy and, conversely, a few with seemingly good control may develop severe complications. Hyperglycaemia and its associated metabolic abnormalities therefore seem to be necessary but not always sufficient for the development of severe diabetic complications. As mentioned above, the genetic and environmental factors responsible for individual susceptibility remain unknown and, at present, high-risk patients cannot be identified before they develop indications of microangiopathy. There is evidence, however, that patients with microalbuminuria (urinary albumin excretion 30–300 mg/day; see Chapter 13) are at greatly increased risk of developing overt nephropathy and of dying prematurely from macrovascular disease [17–20]. Microalbuminuria presumably reflects widespread damage through the entire vascular bed.

Apart from the adverse effect of sustained hyper-

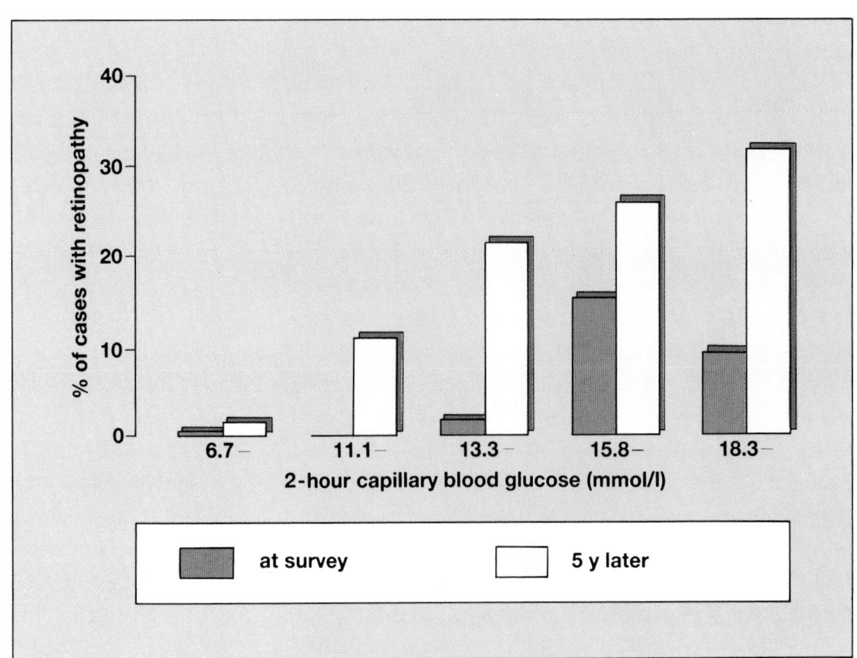


**Fig. 1.6.** Frequency of diabetic retinopathy in diabetic patients and those with impaired glucose tolerance in the Bedford survey, as a function of the 2-h capillary blood glucose value after a 50-g oral glucose load. Histograms show frequency at survey and 5 years later. (Data from [14] with permission from *The Lancet*.)

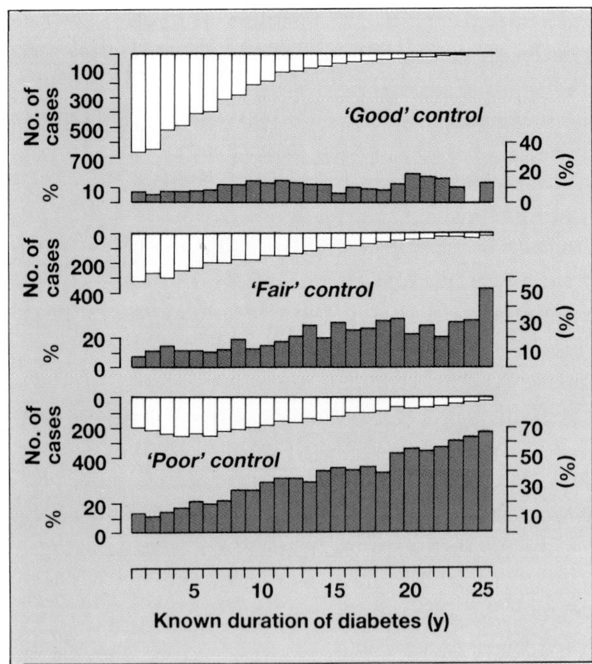


**Fig. 1.7.** Prevalence of diabetic neuropathy (pink) as a function of duration of diabetes (yellow) in patients with 'good', 'fair' and 'poor' control. Clinical and biochemical data were collected annually from 4398 cases, over a 25-year period. (Redrawn from [15].)

glycaemia, large variations in blood glucose levels over extended periods may also contribute to microangiopathy. Recent studies have convincingly shown that rapid improvement in blood glucose control from previously high levels may cause transient deterioration in diabetic retinopathy [21], and may even provoke proliferative changes [22]. An older clinical observation is that imposition of good glycaemic control, especially with insulin treatment, may temporarily aggravate or precipitate diabetic neuropathy (Chapter 11). However, the possible role of *hyper*glycaemia must not be forgotten: large glycaemic falls are only possible if the preceding levels were high. The available evidence suggests that long-term improvements in glycaemic control, which are now feasible with continuous subcutaneous insulin infusion (CSII) or intensified injection regimens, can ameliorate the course of *early* diabetic nephropathy, retinopathy and neuropathy [23–25], and that any worsening in these is only a temporary phenomenon. Indeed, animal studies suggest that by establishing tight metabolic control from the onset of diabetes, it may be possible to prevent the development of microvascular complications [26].

The biochemical mechanisms through which high blood glucose levels might damage the microvasculature are unknown. Theoretical possibilities are dealt with later in this section (Chapter 3), which include a direct toxic effect of glucose itself or of some unidentified associated metabolite; glycation of structural proteins and enzymes; abnormalities of the polyol pathway; and haemodynamic factors, including the hyperperfusion and loss of autoregulation that are caused by hyperglycaemia in many tissues [7].

### Implications for health care

In view of the huge effort expended on diabetic management, it is clearly important to ask whether there is any evidence that the quality of care in any way modifies the course of diabetic microvascular disease. There are encouraging signs that this is so, such as the finding that patients attending a specialized hospital diabetic clinic live significantly longer than those who do not [27], and the recent demonstration that mortality in IDDM has fallen [1]. Furthermore, the optimistic message to our patients is that 42% of IDDM subjects survive for more than 40 years, half of them without developing late diabetic complications [5].

The last few years have therefore witnessed both a great increase in our understanding of microvascular disease and a decline in relative mortality, indicating that improved diabetes care may be rewarded by reducing the terrible impact of the microvascular complications of the disease.

### Recent developments

The view that hyperglycaemia is the central factor in the pathogenesis of diabetic microvascular disease has been strengthened [28]. The Oslo study has shown that after 7–8 years of intensified insulin treatment the rate of progression of background retinopathy is dependent on four factors [29]:

**1** The duration of diabetes at the start of the study;
**2** The degree of retinopathy at the start;
**3** The initial glycosylated haemoglobin; and
**4** The reduction in glycosylated haemoglobin during the study.

The progression of microalbuminuria is also dependent on high blood glucose levels, as assessed by glycosylated haemoglobin [30]. It has been recently shown that microalbuminuria is not only a marker of subsequent development of diabetic nephropathy; it is also an indicator of early diabetic nephropathy as there are already clear morphological changes in the glomerulus at this stage [31]. The progression of peripheral neuropathy is also dependent on mean blood glucose levels, as those with an $HbA_{1c}$ over 9% in the Oslo study had a significant deterioration in nerve conduction velocity over 8 years of the study (unpublished observations).

The Stockholm randomized study ([32] and unpublished) has recently shown that serious retinopathy (defined as diabetic retinopathy needing laser photocoagulation) is more frequent in the control group than in the intensified insulin treated group. This means that those with high glycosylated haemoglobin values ($HbA_{1c}$ >9%) are more prone to develop serious retinopathy.

These data have convincingly shown that the rate of progression of all three microvascular complications (there is increasing evidence that neuropathy is indeed a microvascular complication [33, 34]) is dependent on mean blood glucose levels during the period of observation. The risk of serious progression of microvascular complications is low when the $HbA_{1c}$ is 7.5–8% over several years. It is important that it is not necessary to normalize blood glucose levels completely in order to avoid serious microvascular complications. It appears that there is a *therapeutic window*, with $HbA_{1c}$ values between 7 and 8%, when there is an acceptably low level of hypoglycaemia and low risk of serious microvascular complications. It is probably easier to arrest early nephropathy and neuropathy than retinopathy. The retina has a long memory of antecedent blood glucose levels, so it will perhaps take 4–5 years of good blood glucose control to stop progression of diabetic retinopathy.

KRISTIAN F. HANSSEN

## References


1 Kofoed-Enevoldsen A, Borch-Johnsen K, Kreiner S *et al.* Declining incidence of persistent proteinuria in type 1 (insulin-dependent) diabetic patients in Denmark. *Diabetes* 1987; **36**: 205–9.

2 Klein R, Klein BEK, Moss SE, Davis MD, De Mets DL. The Wisconsin epidemiologic study of diabetic retinopathy. II Prevalence and risk of diabetic retinopathy when age at diagnosis is less than 30 years. *Arch Ophthalmol* 1984; **102**: 520–6.

3 Nathan DM, Singer DE, Godine JE *et al.* Retinopathy in older type II diabetics. Association with glucose control. *Diabetes* 1986; **35**: 797–901.

4 Grenfell A, Watkins PJ. Diabetic nephropathy: Epidemiology, natural history. In: Watkins PJ, ed. *Long Term Complications of Diabetes. Clinics in Endocrinology and Metabolism.* Vol 15. London: WB Saunders, 1986: 783–805.

5 Borch-Johnsen K, Nissen H, Salling N *et al.* The natural history of insulin-dependent diabetes in Denmark: 2. Long-term survival — who and why. *Diabetic Med* 1987; **4**: 211–16.

6 Krolewski AS, Warram JH, Rand LI, Kahn CR. Epidemiologic approach to the etiology of type 1 diabetes mellitus and its complications. *N Engl J Med* 1987; **317**: 1390–8.

7 Zatz R, Brenner BM. Pathogenesis of diabetic microangiopathy; the hemodynamic view. *Am J Med* 1986; **80**: 443–53.

8 Leslie RDG, Pyke DA. Genetics of diabetes. In: Alberti KGMM, Krall LP, eds. *The Diabetes Annual 3.* Amsterdam: Elsevier, 1987.

9 Boulton AJM, Worth RC, Drury J. Genetic and metabolic studies in diabetic neuropathy. *Diabetologia* 1984; **26**: 15–19.

10 Krolewski AS, Caressa N, Warram JH, Laffe LMB, Christlieb AR, Knowler WC, Rand LI. Predisposition to hypertension and susceptibility to renal disease in insulin-dependent diabetes. *N Engl J Med* 1988; **318**: 140–5.

11 Mangili R, Bending JJ, Scott G, Gupta A, Viberti GC. Increased sodium–lithium counter-transport in red blood cells in patients with insulin-dependent diabetes and nephropathy. *N Engl J Med* 1988; **318**: 146–50.

12 Nissen H, Borch-Johnsen K, Nerup J. Long term survival with Type 1 diabetes mellitus — a familial trait? *Diabetologia* 1986; **29**: 576A.

13 Hanssen KF, Dahl-Jørgensen K, Lauritzen T *et al.* Diabetic control and microvascular complications: the near-normoglycemic experience. *Diabetologia* 1986; **29**: 677–84.

14 Jarrett RJ, Keen H. Hyperglycaemia and diabetes mellitus. *Lancet* 1976; **ii**: 1009–12.

15 Pirart J. Diabetes mellitus and its degenerative complications: A prospective study of 4400 patients observed between 1947 and 1973. *Diabetes Care* 1978; **1**: 168–88.

16 Klein R, Klein BEK, Moss SE, Davis MD, De Mets DL. Glycosylated hemoglobin predicts the incidence and progression of diabetic retinopathy. *J Am Med Ass* 1988; **260**: 2864–71.

17 Viberti GC, Jarrett RJ, Mahmud U *et al.* Microalbuminuria as a predictor of clinical diabetic nephropathy in insulin dependent diabetes mellitus. *Lancet* 1982; **ii**: 1430–2.

18 Parving H-H, Oxenbøll B, Svendsen PA, Christiansen JS, Andersen AR. Early detection of patients at risk of developing diabetic nephropathy: A longitudinal study of urinary albumin excretion. *Acta Endocrinol* 1982; **100**: 550–5.

19 Borch-Johnsen K, Andersen PK, Deckert T. The effect of proteinuria on relative mortality in Type 1 (insulin-dependent) diabetes mellitus. *Diabetologia* 1985; **28**: 590–6.

20 Borch-Johnsen K, Kreiner S. Proteinuria: value as predictor of cardiovascular mortality in insulin-dependent diabetes mellitus. *Br Med J* 1987; **294**: 1651–4.

21 Dahl-Jørgensen K, Brinchmann-Hansen O, Hanssen KF *et al.* Rapid tightening of blood glucose control leads to transient deterioration of retinopathy in insulin dependent diabetes mellitus. The Oslo Study. *Br Med J* 1985; **290**: 811–15.

22 Rosenlund E, Haakens K, Brinchmann-Hansen *et al.* Transient proliferative retinopathy during intensified insulin treatment. *Am J Ophthalmol* 1988; **105**: 618–25.

23 Dahl-Jørgensen K, Brinchmann-Hansen O, Hanssen KF *et al.* Effect of near-normoglycaemia for two years on progression of early diabetic retinopathy, nephropathy and

neuropathy. *Br Med J* 1986; **293**: 1195–9.

24 Feldt-Rasmussen B, Mathiesen ER, Deckert T. Effect of two years of strict metabolic control on progression of incipient nephropathy in insulin-dependent diabetes. *Lancet* 1986; **ii**: 1300–4.

25 Deckert T, Feldt-Rasmussen B, Borch-Johnsen K *et al.* Proteinuria, an indicator of malignant angiopathy. In: Andreani D, Crepaldi G, Di Mario U, Pozza G, eds. *Diabetic Complications: Early Diagnosis and Treatment*. Chichester: John Wiley, 1987: 257–61.

26 Engermann RL, Kern TS. Progression of incipient diabetic retinopathy during good glycemic control. *Diabetes* 1987; **36**: 808–12.

27 Borch-Johnsen K, Nissen H, Salling N, Henriksen E, Kreiner S, Deckert T, Nerup J. The natural history of insulin-dependent diabetes mellitus in Denmark: Long term survival with and without late diabetic complications. *Diabetic Med* 1987; **4**: 201–10.

28 Hanssen KF, Bangstad HJ, Brinchmann-Hansen O, Dahl-Jørgensen K. Blood glucose control and diabetic microvascular complications: long term effects of near-normoglycaemia. *Diabetic Med* 1992; **9**: 697–705.

29 Brinchmann-Hansen O, Dahl-Jørgensen K, Sandvik L, Hanssen KF. The effect of seven years of intensified insulin treatment on diabetic retinopathy *Br Med J* 1992; **304**: 19–22.

30 Dahl-Jørgensen K, Bjøro T, Kierulf P, Sandvik L, Hanssen KF. Long-term glycemic control and kidney function in insulin-dependent diabetes mellitus. *Kidney Int* 1992; **41**: 920–3.

31 Bangstad HJ, Østerby R, Dahl-Jørgensen K *et al.* Early glomerulopathy is present in young, insulin-dependent diabetic patients with microalbuminuria. *Diabetologia* 1993, in press.

32 Reichard P, Berglund B, Britz A, Cars I, Nilsson BY, Rosenqvist U. Intensified conventional insulin treatment retards the microvascular complications of insulin-dependent diabetes mellitus (IDDM). The Stockholm Diabetes Intervention study after five years. *J Intern Med* 1991; **230**: 101–8.

33 Malik PA, Newrick PG, Sharma AK *et al.* Microangiopathy in human diabetic neuropathy: Relationship between capillary abnormalities and the severity of neuropathy. *Diabetologia* 1989; **32**: 92–102.

34 Tesfaye S, Harris ND, Wilson RM, Ward JD. Exercise-induced conduction velocity increment: A marker of impaired peripheral nerve blood flow in diabetic neuropathy. *Diabetologia* 1992; **35**: 155–59.

# 2 Pathophysiology of Microvascular Disease: An Overview

**Summary**

• In diabetes, the microvasculature shows both functional and structural abnormalities.
• The structural hallmark of diabetic microangiopathy is thickening of the capillary basement membrane. The main functional abnormalities include increased capillary permeability, blood flow and viscosity, and disturbed platelet function. These changes occur early in the course of diabetes and precede organ failure by many years.
• Many chemical changes in basement membrane composition have been identified in diabetes, including increased Type IV collagen and its glycosylation products, decreased heparan sulphate proteoglycan and increased binding of plasma proteins.
• In patients with poorly controlled diabetes, even of short duration, blood flow is increased in many tissues including skin, retina and kidney in the latter, this is reflected by an elevated glomerular filtration rate.
• Increased capillary permeability is manifested in the retina by leakage of fluorescein and in the kidney by increased urinary losses of albumin which predict eventual renal failure. Both defects probably reflect a generalized vascular abnormality which may also involve the intima of large vessels.
• Platelets from diabetic patients show an exaggerated tendency to aggregate, perhaps mediated by altered prostaglandin metabolism. Plasma and whole blood viscosity are increased whereas red blood cell deformability is decreased in diabetes. These rheological defects, together with the platelet abnormalities, may cause stasis in the microvasculature, leading to increased intravascular pressure and to tissue hypoxia.
• The production by endothelial cells of von Willebrand factor and endothelial-derived relaxing factor (nitric oxide) and other substances may also be abnormal in diabetes and could contribute to microthrombus formation.

Microvascular disease, notably retinopathy and nephropathy, is frequently seen in patients with long-standing IDDM and may affect NIDDM subjects of shorter disease duration. Indeed, microvascular damage is so characteristic of the veteran diabetic patient that it could almost be considered as part of the natural history of the condition.

The abnormalities associated with diabetic microangiopathy are both structural and functional. Structural changes include thickening of the capillary basement membrane throughout the body together with mesangial expansion in the glomerulus, while functional, haemodynamic alterations include increased blood flow, raised intravascular pressure and enhanced vascular leakiness. The relationship between the structural and functional abnormalities, and whether either or both are the cause or consequence of diabetic microangiopathy, are still matters for investigation and debate.

This chapter will review the various pathophysiological mechanisms suggested to play a role in diabetic microvascular disease. The biochemical defects identified are discussed in detail in Chapter 3 and the functional changes of the microcirculation in general in Chapter 4. Specific aspects relating to the causes of retinopathy and nephropathy are described in Chapters 6, 14 and 15.

## Structural changes

The light microscopic appearances of 'hyalinization' (thickening) of the retinal capillaries in diabetic patients were first reported in 1949 [1]. This is now recognized as a characteristic feature of diabetic retinopathy [2, 3]. Subsequently, electron microscopic studies have revealed thickening of the capillary basement membrane (CBM) to be the ultrastructural hallmark of diabetes-induced damage in a wide variety of tissues [4–6].

### *The structure and function of the normal capillary basement membrane*

#### STRUCTURE

On light microscopy, the CBM is an amorphous sheath which encloses the capillary endothelial cells. Electron microscopy reveals a fibrillary structure, with inner and outer clear zones (*lamina lucida (rara) interna* and *externa*) and an intermediate *lamina densa* (Fig. 2.1). The thickness of the CBM correlates with the intracapillary pressure, the thickest membranes being found normally in the capillaries of the leg muscles.

Type IV collagen is the most abundant protein found in the CBM. Other constituents include the proteoglycans heparan, chondroitin and dermatan sulphates, and glycoproteins such as laminin, fibronectin and entactin [7, 8]. The sulphate groups carried by a number of these proteins confer a net anionic charge which is thought to contribute to the charge-dependent permselectivity of the vessels, especially in the glomerular capillaries (see Chapter 14). In the glomerular basement membrane, proteoglycans have a half-life of approximately 1 week; chemical modification resulting in altered charge-permselectivity characteristics can therefore induce functional changes relatively rapidly [9].

#### FUNCTION

The basement membrane acts as a structural support for the vessel wall, preventing overdistension under normal conditions, and forming a scaffolding during endothelial cell repair and regeneration. Although the charge characteristics and porosity of the CBM may partly determine the permeability of the capillary wall, the endothelial cells themselves provide the major barrier limiting permeation of macromolecules in most capillary beds. In the glomerular capillary, the epithelial foot processes also contain heparan sulphate proteoglycans which may contribute to charge-selective permeability.

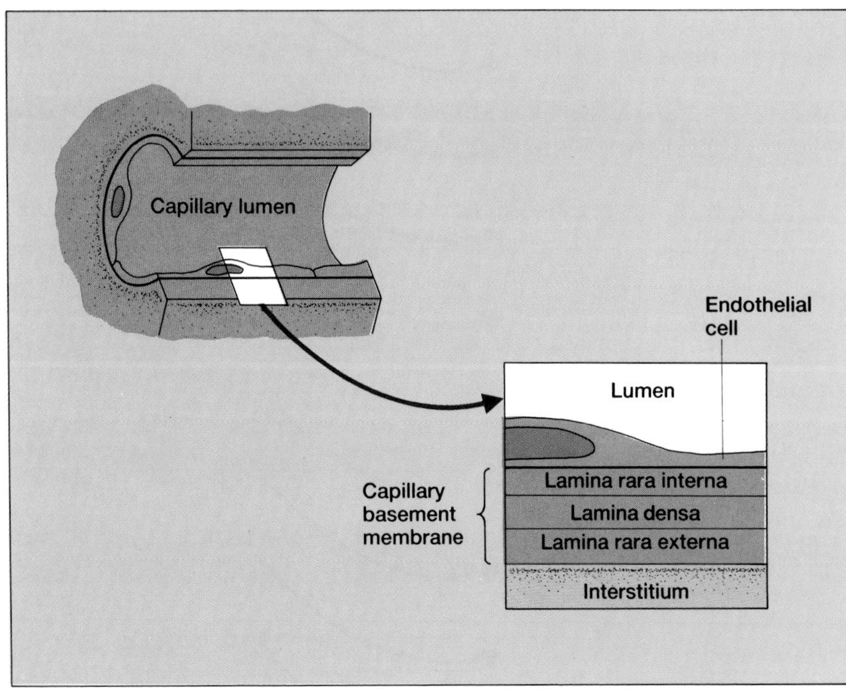


**Fig. 2.1.** Structure of the capillary basement membrane.

### *The capillary basement membrane in diabetes*

Increased thickness of the CBM in diabetic patients has been demonstrated by morphometric techniques in the kidney, retina, skin, skeletal muscle, brain and heart [5, 6, 10–13]. Increased accumulation of basement membrane material in the kidney has also been confirmed by chemical analysis.

Several constituents of the CBM are chemically modified in diabetes (see Table 2.1) [8]. Immunofluorescent techniques have demonstrated increased amounts of a variety of plasma proteins including albumin, IgG, IgM and C3 in glomerular basement membranes and mesangium, renal tubular basement membranes, skeletal muscle sarcolemmal and capillary basement membranes of diabetic animals and humans [14, 15]. It is possible that non-enzymatic glycosylation of basement membrane constituents in diabetes may favour increased binding of plasma proteins (Chapter 3).

## Pathogenesis of the capillary basement membrane changes in diabetes

### *Biochemical changes*

The pathogenesis of diabetic microangiopathy is likely to be multifactorial. Possible biochemical mechanisms are discussed in detail in Chapter 3.

#### HYPERGLYCAEMIA AND PROTEIN KINASE C ACTIVITY

It is not clear whether hyperglycaemia *per se* or hyperglycaemia-induced functional vascular changes initiate or promote diabetic microangiopathy. The late complications of diabetes appear to affect cells and tissues which do not require insulin for glucose uptake. This suggests that hyperglycaemia has an important pathogenic role.

Recently, hyperglycaemia has been shown to cause an increase in cellular protein kinase C activity in cultured bovine retinal, renal and aortic endothelial cells, which results from enhanced *de novo* synthesis of diacylglycerol from glucose [16]. Protein kinase C is involved in a variety of important cellular functions, including signal transduction of responses to hormones, growth factors, neurotransmitters and drugs. In vascular smooth muscle cells, protein kinase C modulates growth rate, DNA synthesis and hormone receptor turnover, in addition to contraction. Protein kinase C may therefore be a multipurpose intracellular mediator whose activity is stimulated by prolonged exposure to hyperglycaemia and which could lead to disturbances.

**Table 2.1** Some chemical changes in capillary basement membrane reported in diabetes (see [8]).

- Increased Type IV collagen and its glycosylation products
- Decreased heparan sulphate proteoglycan and a reduction in its degree of sulphation
- Decreased sialic acid
- Increased hydroxylysine/hydroxylysine-disaccharide units
- Decreased lysine
- Increased or decreased laminin and fibronectin
- Increased plasma protein binding (albumin, IgG, IgM, C3)

#### THE POLYOL PATHWAY

Enhanced polyol pathway activity, with increased metabolism of glucose to sorbitol catalyzed by the rate-limiting enzyme, aldose reductase, has been suggested as a possible mechanism of microvascular disease in diabetes. Inhibition of aldose reductase (Fig. 2.2) by various drugs reduces tissue levels of sorbitol and prevents the development of certain chronic diabetic complications such as cataracts and neuropathy in diabetic animals; aldose reductase inhibitors have also been shown to reduce levels of proteinuria in an animal model of diabetic nephropathy [17–19]. Studies in human diabetic patients are in progress and the results are awaited with interest, although preliminary data do not suggest an obvious beneficial effect (see Chapter 3).

#### NON-ENZYMATIC GLYCOSYLATION

Increased levels of glucose promote synthesis of proteins, including those of the basement mem-

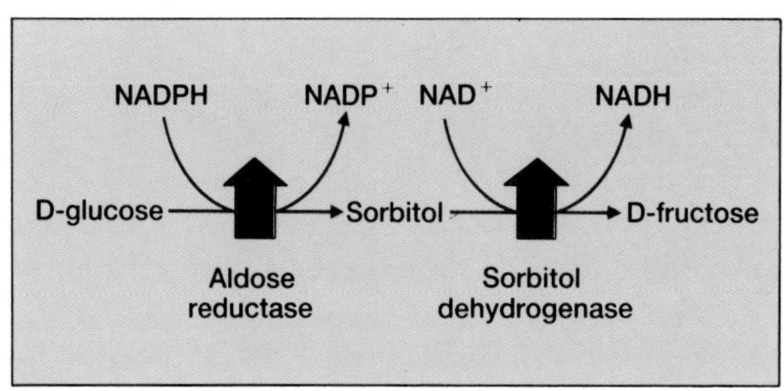


**Fig. 2.2.** The sorbitol (polyol) pathway.

brane, and continued hyperglycaemia leads to increased levels of non-enzymatic glycosylation products in a variety of vascular constituents [20–22].

As described in Chapter 3, cross-linked end-products of non-enzymatic glycosylation may accumulate in various cells and tissues. It has been shown that the administration of aminoguanidine to diabetic rats prevents increased cross-linking of aortic collagen [23, 24]. The effects of such compounds in other diabetic complications, or their possible use in man, are unknown.

### *Functional changes*

#### INCREASED BLOOD FLOW

Increased capillary permeability and haemodynamic disturbances can be demonstrated in subjects with diabetes of short duration, long before any structural tissue or organ damage is evident (see Chapter 4). For example, the glomerular filtration rate (GFR) and the urinary excretion of plasma proteins are abnormally high in a proportion of short-term insulin-dependent patients, especially during periods of poor metabolic control [25–28] (see Chapter 14). Current evidence, based mainly on micropuncture studies in the rat, suggests that the raised GFR ('hyperfiltration') is related to an elevation of both renal plasma flow (RPF) and the transglomerular pressure gradient [29]. Strict metabolic control for 12 months has been shown to normalize glomerular hyperfiltration in IDDM patients, the GFR returning to the previously elevated level if glycaemic control is relaxed [30]. Experience is too limited at present to be able to define precisely the role of glomerular hyperfiltration in the pathophysiology of diabetic nephropathy: prospective and controlled studies of matched cohorts of diabetic patients with and without hyperfiltration have revealed that the GFR fell more quickly in the hyperfiltering group, although there was no evidence of accelerated progression to the later stage of clinical proteinuria in this group [31] (S.L. Jones *et al.*, unpublished observations).

The resting forearm blood flow in newly diagnosed, untreated IDDM patients is almost twice that of non-diabetic controls and is normalized by 1–2 weeks of strict metabolic control [27]. As blood pressure is unchanged, elevated blood flow must indicate a reduction in vascular resistance (i.e. vasodilatation) in the forearm.

Retinal blood flow is increased, mean circulation time in the retina is reduced and retinal vessels are dilated in diabetic subjects [32–34] (see Chapter 6). The possibility that the elevated retinal blood flow and intravascular pressure may be important in the pathogenesis of diabetic retinopathy is supported by the finding of an association between the level of systolic blood pressure and the rate of development of diabetic retinopathy in Pima Indians [35]. Furthermore, patients with a unilateral reduction in retinal blood flow caused, for example, by raised intra-ocular pressure, show slower progression of diabetic retinopathy on the affected side [36].

#### VASCULAR PERMEABILITY

The role of increased glomerular permeability in the pathogenesis of diabetic nephropathy is more clearly established. In both IDDM and NIDDM patients, a subclinical elevation in the albumin excretion rate (AER) is predictive of later clinical proteinuria and organ damage [37–41] (see Chapters 13 and 14). Increased urinary losses of albumin and IgG are thought to originate from the glomerulus, as urinary excretion of $\beta_2$-microglobulin, an indicator of tubular function, is normal in diabetes. Recently, urinary transferrin levels have also been shown to be elevated in some diabetic patients and to be significantly correlated with urinary albumin excretion rates [42].

A strong correlation has been described between glycosylated haemoglobin levels and the urinary excretion rates of albumin and IgG [43]. Although associations do not necessarily imply cause (or effect), these findings suggest that the subclinical elevation of the glomerular filtration of these plasma proteins is, in fact, related to metabolic control. This concept has been further strengthened in recent years by the finding that prolonged correction of hyperglycaemia using various techniques can either lower AER or prevent it from increasing [44–46]. Some more recent observations are discussed in the update to Chapter 1.

Elevations in AER not only predict renal disease but are also associated with proliferative retinopathy and increased cardiovascular mortality [47, 48]. Recently, it has been proposed that an increased AER reflects a more generalized vascular dysfunction which involves capillaries of the glomerulus and retina and the intima of large vessels [49]. In support of this hypothesis, the transcapillary escape rates of albumin and fibrinogen have been shown to be increased in patients with modest elevations of the urinary AER [50, 51]. A genetically-determined alteration of the composition of the extracellular matrix, resulting in loss of heparan sulphate proteoglycan, is proposed as an important mechanism in these processes; although plausible, this concept is supported at present by only a few data (Fig. 2.3).

Retinal capillaries display increased leakage of fluorescein early in the course of diabetes. Using the technique of vitreous fluorophotometry, accumulation of fluorescein in the vitreous after intravenous injection has been demonstrated in young diabetic patients who have either no retinopathy or only mild background changes [52, 53]. Fluorescein leakage is greater in patients with poor metabolic control and is reduced by improved control [54].

### RHEOLOGICAL FACTORS

Abnormal blood viscosity and platelet function have also been proposed as possible causes or mediators of microangiopathy in diabetes. Platelets from diabetic patients show an increased sensitivity to aggregation induced by ADP, adrenaline or collagen, and there is some evidence that this increased sensitivity correlates with certain diabetic complications [55]. Activation of the prostaglandin synthetase system, resulting in either elevated levels of prostaglandins or decreased levels of the vasodilator prostacylin, could underlie altered platelet sensitivity [56, 57]. Furthermore, changes in other rheological properties of blood have been described, including increased plasma and whole blood viscosity and decreased red cell deformability. These defects would act to impede blood flow and hence increase intravascular hydrostatic pressure [58, 59], and could also predispose to sludging of blood in capillaries and therefore to hypoxia and poor nutrition of the tissues.

Endothelial cells produce prostaglandins and endothelial-derived relaxing factor (EDRF; now known to be nitric oxide) which inhibit the adherence of platelets to the vascular wall as well as

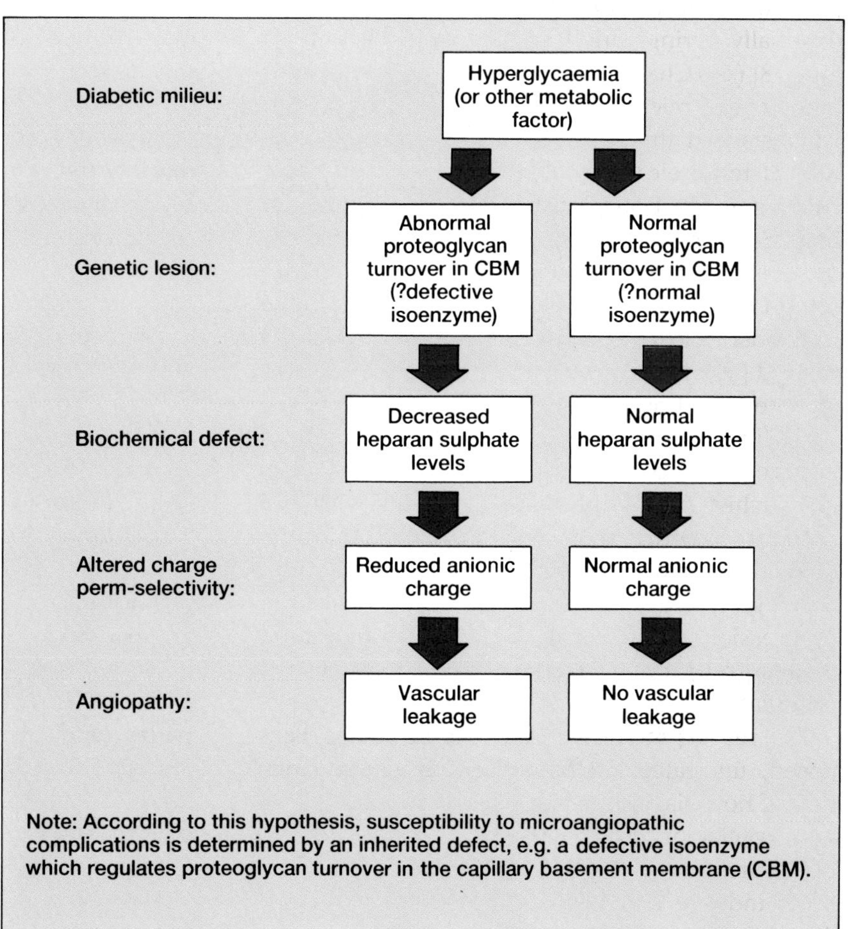


**Fig. 2.3.** Possible basis for susceptibility to microangiopathic complications of diabetes. (Redrawn from [49].)

modulating vascular tone. Studies of human diabetes have produced conflicting evidence of altered levels of these endothelial products, although some recent reports suggest a reduction in EDRF production (for a review of this area, see [60]).

Other endothelial products have been shown to be abnormal in diabetic subjects with evidence of diabetic microangiopathy. The tissue plasminogen activator response to exercise is impaired, whereas levels of von Willebrand factor, a glycoprotein synthesized by endothelial cells and responsible for platelet adhesion to the subendothelium, is increased in diabetic subjects with microalbuminuria or clinical nephropathy [61]. Together, these disturbances would favour an increased tendency to coagulation and a reduced ability to resolve microthrombi in diabetic subjects who have an increased AER.

In view of the cross-sectional nature of these studies, it is not possible to determine whether these changes are of primary importance in the pathogenesis of diabetic microangiopathy or arise as a consequence of this.

## Conclusions

Many metabolic and other factors may therefore contribute to the structural and functional abnormalities which characterize diabetes microangiopathy. Fig. 2.4 shows a possible pathway through which insulin deficiency and hyperglycaemia could lead to abnormalities in the basement membrane and endothelium, and disturbed haemodynamic and rheological properties in diabetes. The end-points of this pathway are the tissue damage and organ failure caused by diabetic microangiopathy.

## Recent developments

### *Cellular toxicity of high glucose concentrations*

Studies since the mid-1980s have highlighted the potential importance of glucose toxicity in the pathogenesis of the vascular complications of diabetes, and there have been several recent advances in this area.

High glucose levels have been found to reduce

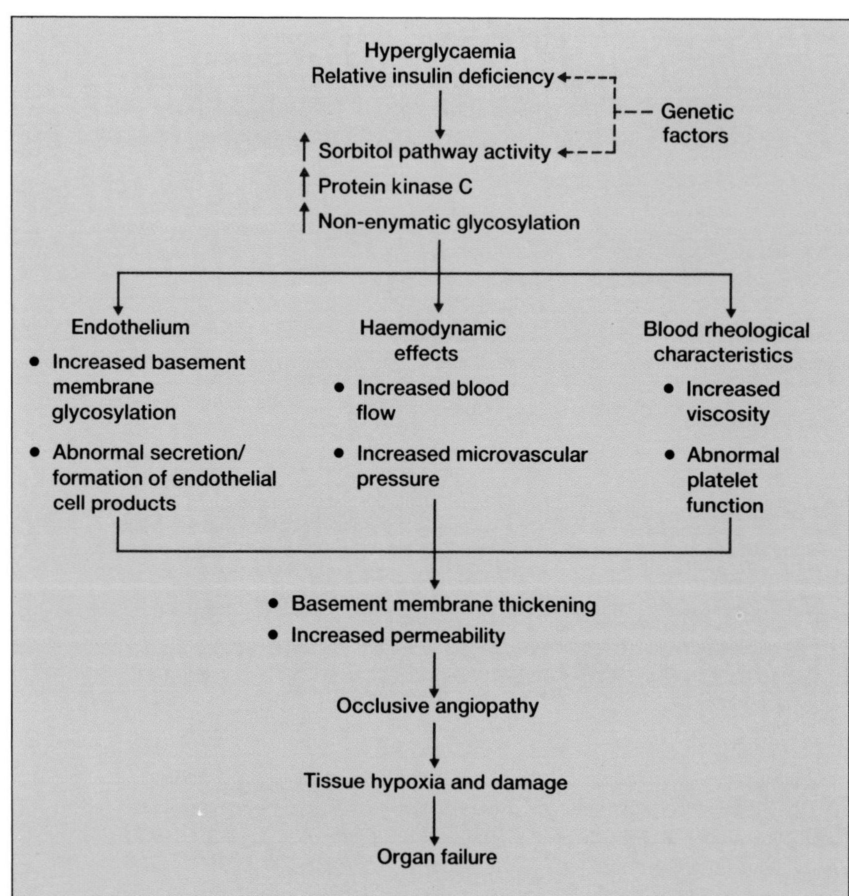


**Fig. 2.4.** A possible pathogenetic pathway of diabetic microangiopathy.

replication of bovine retinal pericytes [62, 63] and, by some authors, to increase cell death in pericytes cultured from Rhesus monkeys [64]. The absolute rate of collagen synthesis is enhanced in pericyte cultures in the presence of high glucose concentrations [65], and there is evidence that chronic exposure to high glucose reduces the ability of retinal pericytes to contract in response to endothelin [66]. These findings, which appear to be independent of enhanced activation of the polyol pathway or of the accumulation of advanced glycosylation end-products (see Chapter 3), suggest a mechanism whereby hyperglycaemia may lead to loss of pericytes and perhaps to impaired autoregulatory function in the retinal microcirculation.

When exposed to high ambient glucose concentrations, endothelial cells derived from different vascular beds display delays in replication [67, 68] and in progressing through the cell cycle [69] and, in some cases, excess cellular death [67]. High glucose levels induce DNA damage in the form of an increased number of breaks in DNA, and also increase DNA repair processes [70, 71]. As well as impairing the replicative response, high glucose concentrations also compromise the migratory capacity of endothelial cells [72]. Prolonged exposure to high glucose increases the synthesis of fibronectin, collagen Type IV and laminin and reduces prostacyclin synthesis [73, 74]. The synthesis and release of tissue plasminogen activator (tPA) and plasminogen activator inhibitor-1 (PAI-1) are augmented in endothelial cells cultured in high glucose concentrations, resulting in a decrease in fibrinolytic activity in the medium [75]. These glucose-induced events would be expected to damage the integrity of the vascular endothelial lining and its capacity to discourage thrombus formation.

Epithelial and mesangial cells of renal origin, cultured in a high-glucose medium, synthesize and accumulate increased amounts of fibronectin, collagen Type IV and I, and laminin [76–79]. These abnormalities of extracellular matrix production are accompanied by decreased cell replication, increased total protein synthesis and an increase in mean cell size, suggesting that high glucose levels may induce cellular hypertrophy [80]. High glucose has also been found to reduce the number of tight-junction complexes in endothelial cells [81], which may provide one explanation for the increased vascular permeability in diabetes.

Some of these glucose-induced disturbances have now been characterized at the molecular level. High glucose levels affect the expression of a number of genes encoding components of the extracellular matrix. Endothelial and mesangial cells cultured in high glucose concentrations exhibit increased levels of mRNA for fibronectin, laminin and collagen Type IV [73, 76–78, 82]; proximal tubule cells show increased levels of collagen IV mRNA [79], while endothelial cells exhibit increased levels of mRNA for tPA and PAI-1 [75]. In several of these processes, it is the rate of gene transcription which appears to be affected [73, 79]. The mechanism by which high glucose concentrations might alter gene expression is not entirely clear but a critical time of cell exposure to high glucose is required, and the effects appear to be independent of either glucose metabolism (L-glucose has the same effect as D-glucose) or of the activation of cAMP or protein kinase C [73, 83]. The effects of high glucose on endothelial cell gene expression are poorly reversible and persist even after the cells have undergone several replications in normal glucose medium. This 'memory' phenomenon appears to be gene-specific [84], suggesting that the structure or regulation of the target gene may be important in the susceptibility to an 'imprinting' effect of high glucose.

High glucose concentrations can therefore alter the biosynthetic programme of vascular cells in directions consistent with the lesions of diabetic vascular disease. Some of these actions occur at the level of gene transcription.

JAMES D. WALKER
GIAN CARLO VIBERTI

## References


1 Ashton N. Vascular changes in diabetes with particular reference to retinal vessels. *Br J Ophthalmol* 1949; **33**: 407–20.
2 Friedenwald JS. A new approach to some old problems of retinal vascular disease. *Am J Ophthalmol* 1949; **32**: 487–98.
3 Friedenwald JS. Diabetic retinopathy. *Am J Ophthalmol* 1950; **33**: 1187–99.
4 Hidayat AA, Fine BS. Diabetic choroidopathy: light and electron microscopic observations of seven cases. *Ophthalmology* 1985; **92**: 512–22.
5 Johnson PC, Brendel K, Meezan E. Human diabetic perineurial cell basement membrane thickening. *Lab Invest* 1981; **44**: 265–70.
6 Johnson PC, Brendel K, Meezan E. Thickened cerebral cortical capillary basement membranes in diabetics. *Arch Pathol Lab Med* 1982; **60**: 214–17.
7 Scott PG. Macromolecular constituents of basement membranes: A review of current knowledge on their structure and function. *Can J Biochem Cell Biol* 1983; **61**: 942–8.
8 Williamson JR, Tilton RG, Chang K, Kilo C. Basement

membrane abnormalities in diabetes mellitus: relationship to clinical microangiopathy. *Diabetes/Metabolism Reviews;* 1988; **4**: 339–70.

9 Cohen MP, Surma ML, Wu VY. *In vivo* biosynthesis and turnover of glomerular basement membrane in diabetic rats. *Am J Physiol* 1982; **242**: F385–9.

10 Østerby R, Hansen R. A quantitative estimate of the peripheral glomerular basement membrane in recent juvenile diabetes. *Diabetologia* 1965; **1**: 97–100.

11 Tilton RG, LaRose LS, Kilo C, Williamson JR. Absence of degenerative changes in retinal and uveal capillary pericytes in diabetic rats. *Invest Ophthalmol Vis Sci* 1986; 27: 716–21.

12 Silver MD, Huckell VF, Lorber M. Basement membranes of small cardiac vessels in patients with diabetes and myxodema: Preliminary observations. *Pathology* 1977; **9**: 213–20.

13 Siperstein MD, Unger RG, Madison LL. Studies of muscle capillary basement membranes in normal subjects, diabetic, and prediabetic patients. *J Clin Invest* 1968; **47**: 1973–99.

14 Mauer SM, Michael AF, Fish AJ, Brown DM. Spontaneous immunoglobulin and complement deposition in glomeruli of diabetic rats. *Lab Invest* 1972; **27**: 488–94.

15 Chavers B, Etzwiler D, Michael AF. Albumin deposition in dermal capillary basement membrane in insulin-dependent diabetes mellitus. A preliminary report. *Diabetes* 1981; **30**: 275–8.

16 Lee T-S, Saltsman A, Ohashi H, King GL. Activation of protein kinase C by elevation of glucose concentration; proposal for a mechanism in the development of diabetic vascular complications. *Proc Natl Acad Sci* 1989; **86**: 5141–5.

17 Robison WG Jr, Kador PF, Akagi Y, Kinoshita JH, Gonzalez R, Dvornik D. Prevention of basement membrane thickening in retinal capillaries by a novel inhibitor of aldose reductase, tolrestat. *Diabetes* 1986; **35**: 295–9.

18 Beyer-Mears A, Cruz E, Edelist T, Varagiannis E. Diminished proteinuria in diabetes mellitus by sorbinil, an aldose reductase inhibitor. *Pharmacology* 1986; **32**: 52–60.

19 Chandler ML, Shannon WA, DeSantis L. Prevention of retinal capillary basement membrane thickening in diabetic rats by aldose reductase inhibitors. *Invest Ophthalmol Vis Sci* 1984; **25**: 159.

20 Li W, Shen S, Khatami M, Rockey JH. Stimulation of retinal capillary pericyte protein and collagen synthesis in culture by high-glucose concentration. *Diabetes* 1984; **33**: 785–9.

21 Li W, Khatami M, Rockey JH. The effects of glucose and an aldose reductase inhibitor on the sorbitol content and collagen synthesis of bovine retinal capillary pericytes in culture. *Exp Eye Res* 1985; **40**: 439–44.

22 Brownlee M, Cerami A, Vlassara H. Advanced glycosylation end products in tissue and the biochemical basis of diabetic complications. *N Engl J Med* 1988; **318**: 1315–21.

23 Brownlee M, Vlassara H, Cerami A. Nonenzymatic glycosylation and the pathogenesis of diabetic complications. *Ann Intern Med* 1984; **101**: 527–37.

24 Brownlee M, Vlassara H, Kooney A, Ulrich P, Cerami A. Aminoguanidine prevents diabetes-induced arterial wall protein cross-linking. *Science* 1986; **232**: 1629–32.

25 Mogensen CE. Kidney function and glomerular permeability to macromolecules in juvenile diabetes. *Dan Med Bull* 1972; **19** (suppl 3): 1–40.

26 Ditzel J, Junker K. Abnormal glomerular filtration rate, renal plasma flow, and protein excretion in recent and short-term diabetics. *Br Med J* 1972; **2**: 13–19.

27 Parving H-H, Noer I, Deckert T *et al*. The effect of metabolic regulation on microvascular permeability to small and large molecules in short-term juvenile diabetics. *Diabetologia* 1976; **12**: 161–166.

28 Christiansen JS, Gammelgaard J, Tronier B *et al*. Kidney function and size in diabetics, before and during initial insulin treatment. *Kidney Int* 1982; **21**: 683–8.

29 Hostetter TH, Troy JL, Brenner BM. Glomerular hemodynamics in experimental diabetes. *Kidney Int* 1981; **19**: 410–15.

30 Wiseman MJ, Saunders AJ, Keen H, Viberti GC. Effect of blood glucose glomerular filtration rate and kidney size in insulin-dependent diabetics. *N Engl J Med* 1985; **312**: 617–21.

31 Lervang HH, Jensen S, Brochner Mortensen J, Ditzel J. Early glomerular hyperfiltration and the development of late nephropathy in Type 1 (insulin-dependent) diabetes mellitus. *Diabetologia* 1988; **31**: 723–9.

32 Kohner EM, Hamilton AM, Saunders SJ *et al*. The retinal blood flow in diabetes. *Diabetologia* 1975; **11**: 27–33.

33 Soeldner JS, Christacopoulos PD, Gleason RE. Mean retinal circulation time as determined by fluorescein angiography in normal, prediabetic and chemical diabetic subjects. *Diabetes* 1976; **25** (suppl 2): 903–8.

34 Skovborg F, Nielsen Aa V, Lauritzen E *et al*. Diameters of the retinal vessels in diabetic and normal subjects. *Diabetes* 1969; **18**: 292–8.

35 Knowler WC, Bennett PH, Ballintine EJ. Increased incidence of retinopathy in diabetics with elevated blood pressure. *N Engl J Med* 1980; **302**: 645–50.

36 Behrendt T, Duane TD. Unilateral complications in diabetic retinopathy. *Trans Am Acad Ophthalmol Otol* 1970; **74**: 28–32.

37 Viberti GC, Hill RD, Jarrett RD, Argyropoulos A, Mahmud U, Keen H. Microalbuminuria as a predictor of clinical nephropathy in insulin-dependent diabetes mellitus. *Lancet* 1982; **i**: 1430–2.

38 Mogensen CE, Christensen CK. Predicting diabetic nephropathy in insulin-dependent patients. *N Engl J Med* 1984; **311**: 89–93.

39 Jarrett RJ, Viberti GC, Argyropoulos A *et al*. Microalbuminuria predicts mortality in non-insulin dependent diabetics. *Diabetic Med* 1984; **1**: 17–19.

40 Mogenesen CE. Microalbuminuria predicts clinical proteinuria and early mortality in maturity-onset diabetes. *N Engl J Med* 1984; **310**: 356–60.

41 Mathiesen ER, Oxenbøll K, Johansen PAa, Svendsen PA, Deckert T. Incipient nephropathy in Type 1 (insulin-dependent) diabetes. *Diabetologia* 1984; **26**: 406–10.

42 O'Donnell MJ, Martin P, Florkowski CM, Toop MJ, Chapman C, Barnett AH. Transferrinuria and tubular proteinuria in Type 1 (insulin-dependent) diabetes mellitus. *Diabetic Med* 1988; **5**: 15A.

43 Viberti GC, Mackintosh D, Bilous RW, Pickup JC, Keen H. Proteinuria in diabetes mellitus: role of spontaneous and experimental variation of glycaemia. *Kidney Int* 1982; **21**: 714–20.

44 The Kroc Collaborative Study Group. Blood glucose control and the evolution of diabetic retinopathy and albuminuria. *N Engl J Med* 1984; **311**: 365–72.

45 Feldt-Rasmussen B, Mathiesen E, Deckert T. Effect of two years of strict metabolic control on progression of incipient nephropathy in insulin-dependent diabetics. *Lancet* 1986; **ii**: 1300–4.

46 Dahl-Jørgensen K, Hanssen KF, Kierfulf P, Bjoro T, Sandvik L, Aageraes O. Reduction of urinary albumin excretion after 4 years of continuous subcutaneous insulin infusion in insulin-dependent diabetes mellitus; the Oslo study. *Acta Endocrinol* 1988; **117**: 19–25.

47 Kofoed-Envoldsen A, Jensen T, Borch-Johnsen K, Deckert T.

Incidence of retinopathy in Type 1 (insulin-dependent) diabetes; associations with clinical nephropathy. *J Diab Complic* 1987; **3**: 96–9.
48 Borch-Johnsen K, Kreiner S. Proteinuria: a predictor of cardiovascular mortality in insulin-dependent diabetes-mellitus. *Br Med J* 1987; **294**: 1651–4.
49 Deckert T, Feldt-Rasmussen B, Borch-Johnsen K, Jensen T, Kokoed-Envoldsen A. Albuminuria reflects widespread vascular damage; the Steno hypothesis. *Diabetologia* 1989; **32**: 219–26.
50 Feldt-Rasmussen B. Increased transcapillary escape rate of albumin in Type 1 (insulin-dependent) diabetic patients with microalbuminuria. *Diabetologia* 1986; **29**: 282–6.
51 O'Hare JA, Twoney BM, Ferriss JB *et al*. Metabolic control, hypertension and microvascular complications independently affect transcapillary escape of albumin in diabetes. *Diabetologia* 1982; **22**: 391–2.
52 Cunha-Vaz J, De Abreu F, Compos JR *et al*. Early breakdown of blood-retinal barrier in diabetics. *Br J Ophthalmol* 1975; **59**: 649–56.
53 Waltman SR, *Oestrich C, Krupin T et al*. Quantitative vitreous fluorophotometry: a sensitive technique for measuring early breakdown of blood-retinal barrier in young diabetic patients. *Diabetes* 1978; **27**: 85–7.
54 White NH, Waltman SR, Krupin T *et al*. Reversal of abnormalities in ocular fluorophotometry in insulin-dependent diabetes after five to nine months of improved metabolic control. *Diabetes* 1982; **31**: 80–5.
55 Mustard JF, Packham MA. Platelets and diabetes mellitus. *N Engl J Med* 1977; **297**: 1345–7.
56 Halushka PV, Lune D, Colwell JA. Increased synthesis of prostaglandin-E-like material by patients with diabetes mellitus. *N Engl J Med* 1977; **297**: 1306–10.
57 Silberbauer K, Schernthaner G, Sinzinger H, Piza-Katzer H, Winter M: Increased vascular prostacyclin in juvenile onset diabetes. *N Engl J Med* 1979; **300**: 367–8.
58 Barnes AJ, Locke P, Scudder PR *et al*. Is hyperviscosity a treatable component of diabetic microcirculatory disease? *Lancet* 1977; **ii**: 789–91.
59 McMillan DE, Utterback NG, La Puma J. Reduced erythrocyte deformability in diabetes. *Diabetes* 1978; **27**: 895–901.
60 Tooke JE. The microcirculation in diabetes. *Diabetic Med* 1987; **4**: 189–96.
61 Jensen T, Feldt-Rasmussen B, Bjerre-Knudsen J, Deckert T. Features of endothelial dysfunction in early diabetic nephropathy. *Lancet* 1989; **i**: 461–3.
62 Li W, Shen S, Khatami M, Rockey JH. Stimulation of retinal capillary pericyte protein and collagen synthesis in culture by high-glucose concentration. *Diabetes* 1984; **33**: 785–9.
63 King GL, Johnson S, Wu G. Possible growth modulators involved in the pathogenesis of diabetic proliferative retinopathy. In: Westermark B, Betsholtz C, Hokfelt B, eds. *Growth Factors in Health and Disease*. New York: Elsèvier, 1990, pp. 303–17.
64 Buzney SM, Frank RN, Varma SD, Tanishima T, Gabbay KH. Aldose reductase in retinal mural cells. *Invest Ophthalmol Vis Sci* 1977; **16**: 392–6.
65 Li W, Khatami M, Rockey JH. The effects of glucose and an aldose reductase inhibitor on the sorbitol content and collagen synthesis of bovine retinal capillary pericytes in culture. *Exp Eye Res* 1985; **40**: 439–44.
66 Chakravarthy U, Trimble ER. Endothelin induced pericyte contraction is altered in hyperglycaemia. *Diabetologia* 1991; **34** (suppl 2): A16.
67 Lorenzi M, Cagliero E, Toledo S. Glucose toxicity for human endothelial cells in culture: delayed replication, disturbed cell cycle, and accelerated death. *Diabetes* 1985; **34**: 621–7.
68 Porta M, La Selva M, Bertagna AS, Molinatti GM. High glucose concentrations inhibit DNA synthesis and replication without causing death or impairing injury repair in cultured human endothelial cells. *Diabetes Res* 1988; **7**: 59–63.
69 Lorenzi M, Nordberg JA, Toledo S. High glucose prolongs cell-cycle traversal of cultured human endothelial cells. *Diabetes* 1987; **36**: 1261–7.
70 Lorenzi M, Montisano DF, Toledo S, Barrieux A. High glucose induces DNA damage in cultured human endothelial cells. *J Clin Invest* 1986; **77**: 322–5.
71 Ahnstrom G, Erixon K. Measurement of strand breaks by alkaline denaturation and hydroxyapatite chromatography. In: Friedberg EC, Hanawait PC, eds. *DNA Repair. A Laboratory Manual of Research Procedures*, vol. I. New York: Marcel Dekker, 1981, pp. 403–18.
72 Mascardo RN. The effects of hyperglycaemia on the directed migration of wounded endothelial cell monolayers. *Metabolism* 1988; **37**: 378–85.
73 Cagliero E, Roth T, Roy S, Lorenzi M. Characteristics and mechanisms of high-glucose-induced overexpression of basement membrane components in cultured human endothelial cells. *Diabetes* 1991; **40**: 102–10.
74 Ono H, Umeda F, Inoguchi T, Ibayashi H. Glucose inhibits prostacyclin production by cultured aortic endothelial cells. *Throm Haemostasis* 1988; **60**: 174–7.
75 Maiello M, Boeri D, Podesta F, Cagliero E, Vichi M, Odetti P, Adezati L, Lorenzi M. Increased expression of tissue plasminogen activator and its inhibitor and reduced fibrinolytic potential of human endothelial cells cultured in elevated glucose. *Diabetes*, in press.
76 Ayo SH, Radnik RA, Glass WF II, Garoni JA, Rampt ER, Appling DR, Kreisberg JI. Increased extracellular matrix synthesis and mRNA in mesangial cells grown in high glucose medium. *Am J Physiol* 1991; **260**: F185–91.
77 Haneda M, Kikkawa R, Horide N, Togawa M, Koya D, Kajiwara N, Ooshima A, Shigeta Y. Glucose enhances type IV collagen production in cultured rat glomerular mesangial cells. *Diabetologia* 1991; **34**: 198–200.
78 Ayo SH, Radnik RA, Garoni JA, Glass WF II, Kreisberg JI. High glucose causes an increase in extracellular matrix proteins in cultured mesangial cells. *Am J Physiol* 1990; **136**: 1339–1348.
79 Ziyadeh FN, Snipes ER, Watanabe M, Alvarez RI, Goldfarb S, Haverty TP: High glucose induces cell hypertrophy and stimulates collagen gene transcription in proximal tubule. *Am J Physiol* 1990; **259**: F704–14.
80 Das A, Frank RN, Zhang NL. Sorbinil does not prevent galactose-induced glomerular capillary basement membrane thickening in the rat. *Diabetologia* 1990; **33**: 515–21.
81 Hazen-Martin DJ, Sens MA, Detrisac CJ, Blackburn JG, Sens DA. Elevated glucose alters paracellular transport of cultured human proximal tubule cells. *Kidney Int* 1989; **35**: 31–9.
82 Nahman NS, Leonhart KL, Cosio FG, Hebert CL. Effects of high glucose on cellular proliferation and fibronectin production by cultured human mesangial cells. *Kidney Int* 1992; **41**: 396–402.
83 Cagliero E, Roth T, Roy S, Maiello M, Lorenzi M. Expression of genes related to the extracellular matrix in human endothelial cells. Differential modulation by elevated glucose concentrations, phorbol esters and cAMP. *J Biol Chem* 1991; **266**: 14244–50.
84 Roy S, Lorenzi M. The memory of abnormal gene expression induced by high glucose in human endothelial cells is gene-specific. *Diabetes* 1991; **40** (suppl 1): 9A.

# 3 Biochemical Basis of Microvascular Disease

**Summary**

• Prolonged exposure to elevated glucose concentrations damages tissues by causing either acute, reversible metabolic changes (mostly related to increased polyol pathway activity, decreased myoinositol and altered diacylglycerol levels, or glycosylation of proteins), or cumulative irreversible changes in long-lived molecules (formation of advanced glycosylation end-products on matrix proteins such as collagen and on nucleic acids and nucleoproteins).
• In insulin-independent tissues such as nerve, glomerulus, lens and retina, hyperglycaemia causes elevated tissue glucose levels. The enzyme aldose reductase catalyses the reduction of glucose to its polyol, sorbitol, which is subsequently converted to fructose.
• Sorbitol does not easily cross cell membranes and its accumulation may cause damage by osmotic effects (e.g. in the lens) and by altering the redox state of pyridine nucleotides.
• In addition, increased sorbitol production is partly responsible for tissue depletion of myoinositol, a molecule structurally related to glucose. Hyperglycaemia itself also inhibits myoinositol uptake into cells.
• Animal studies indicate that tissue myoinositol depletion may cause abnormalities on peripheral nerve function. Myoinositol is a precursor of phosphatidylinositol, the turnover of which activates $Na^+-K^+-$ATPase via diacylglycerol production and the stimulation of protein kinase C activity.
• Lowered $Na^+-K^+-$ATPase activity probably causes increased intracellular $Na^+$ concentrations and slows nerve conduction velocity.
• In other tissues such as endothelial cells and aortic smooth muscle cells in culture, protein kinase C is activated by high glucose levels, because of synthesis of diacylglycerol from glucose; these changes in protein kinase C may be involved in abnormal growth and synthesis in these tissues.
• Early glycosylation products form on proteins as glucose attaches to amino groups. These Schiff base adducts then undergo 'Amadori' rearrangement to form stable products analogous to glycosylated haemoglobin. Such glycosylation may affect the function of a number of proteins and be partly responsible for free radical-mediated damage in diabetes.
• Glycosylation may be limited by oxidative cleavage of Amadori products to peptide-bound carboxymethyllysine and erythronic acid.
• In long-lived molecules, early glycosylation products slowly and irreversibly form complex cross-linkings termed 'advanced glycosylation end-products' (AGE).
• One type of AGE is probably formed from the condensation of two Amadori products and is related to furoyl-furanyl-imidazole. Another type probably derives from reaction of Amadori products with the Amadori-derived 3-deoxyglucosone, to form several types of pyrrole-based cross-links.
• Pathological consequences of AGE cross-linking include covalent binding of proteins (e.g. LDL, albumin and IgG) to vessel walls; cross-linking of matrix components in vessel walls causing resistance to enzymatic degradation; and disturbed three-dimensional structure and altered binding of anionic proteoglycans which

influence charge on the vessel wall and its interaction with blood-borne protein.
- Monocyte macrophages have a high-affinity receptor for AGE and binding of AGE may release cytokines such as tumour necrosis factor (TNF) and interleukin-1 (IL-1).
- AGE also form on nucleic acids and histones and may cause mutations and altered gene expression.
- Pharmacological modulation of AGE formation may be possible using agents such as aminoguanidine which prevent cross-linking.

### The pathogenesis of diabetic complications

Although the insulin deficiency of diabetes mellitus can be ameliorated by diet, oral hypoglycaemic agents or insulin administration, standard therapy has not been able to prevent the development of chronic complications affecting multiple organ systems. In the eye, retinal capillary damage leading to oedema, new vessel formation and haemorrhage results in visual impairment, and cataracts also develop at an accelerated rate. Chronic renal failure occurs because of capillary damage in the glomerulus associated with basement membrane and mesangial matrix accumulation. In the diabetic nerve, axonal dwindling and segmental demyelination associated with changes in the vasa nervorum produce motor, sensory and autonomic dysfunction. Large- and medium-sized vessel atheromatous disease are responsible for an increased incidence of coronary artery cerebrovascular and peripheral vascular disease.

These diverse clinical syndromes share a common pathophysiological feature: a progressive narrowing of vascular lumina in diabetes leading to inadequate perfusion of target organs. This narrowing appears to be the cumulative effect of three processes. First, an abnormal leakage of PAS-positive, carbohydrate-containing plasma proteins causes a progressive constriction of luminal area in both small and large vessels. Secondly, an increase in extracellular matrix is seen in all types of diabetic vessels. The basement membrane is thickened in many tissues, including retinal capillaries and the vasa nervorum, mesangial matrix is expanded in the renal glomerulus, and collagen is increased in developing atherosclerotic plaques. Endothelial, mesangial and arterial smooth muscle cell hypertrophy and hyperplasia comprise the third pathological process [1–3].

What causes these pathological processes? Numerous investigations (see Chapter 1) have concluded that the primary causal factor responsible for the development of most diabetic complications is probably prolonged exposure to hyperglycaemia (Fig. 3.1). Marked differences in susceptibility to glucose-mediated tissue damage observed in different diabetic patients exposed to the same degree and duration of hyperglycaemia might be accounted for by genetic polymorphism, although the identity and function of these genes have yet to be determined. Hypertension is now recognized as the most significant independent accelerating factor for diabetic microvascular disease, while both hypertension and hyperlipidaemia accelerate the development of macrovascular disease [4].

Hyperglycaemia appears to damage tissues by causing both acute, reversible changes in cellular metabolism and cumulative, irreversible alterations in stable macromolecules (Fig. 3.1). Among the reversible abnormalities are abnormal polyol metabolism and the formation of early glycosylation products on matrix, cellular and plasma proteins (Table 3.1). The cumulative, irreversible changes caused by hyperglycaemia appear to affect long-lived molecules such as extracellular matrix components and nucleic acids. In model systems,

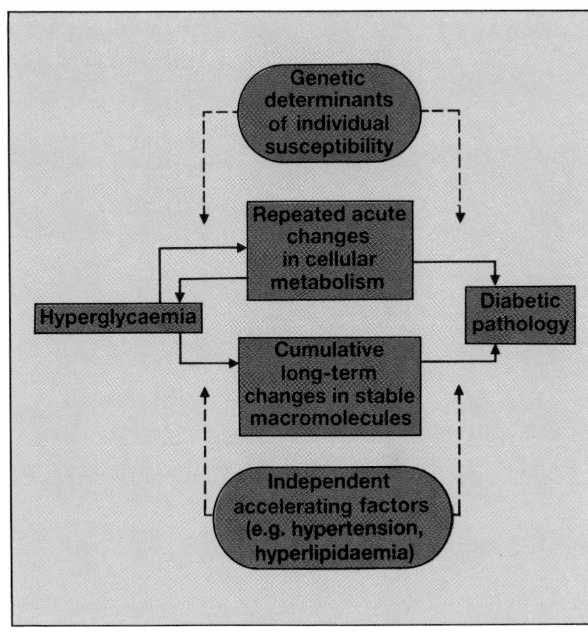


**Fig. 3.1.** Schematic representation of the mechanisms by which hyperglycaemia and independent risk factors interact to cause diabetic complications.

**Table 3.1.** Biochemical consequences of hyperglycaemia.

| |
|---|
| *Acute reversible metabolic changes* |
| Increased polyol pathway activity |
| Altered redox state of pyridine nucleotides |
| Decreased pools of myoinositol |
| Increased *de novo* synthesis of diacylglycerol |
| Increased activation of protein kinase C |
| Greater formation of early glycosylation products (EGP) and EGP-derived free radicals |
| *Cumulative changes in stable macromolecules* |
| Increased formation of advanced glycosylation end-products (AGE) on extracellular matrix components |
| Increased formation of advanced glycosylation end-products on nucleic acids and nucleoproteins |
| Disordered three-dimensional structure of basement membrane and collagen |
| Impaired matrix associative/binding properties |
| Increased rate of genetic mutations (in prokaryotes) |

these irreversible changes cause defective matrix binding of growth-inhibiting heparan sulphate proteoglycan [5], disordered three-dimensional structure of both basement membrane and collagen [6], and increased rates of genetic mutation [7]. Early in the course of diabetes, pathological changes are most likely due to the acute, reversible changes induced by hyperglycaemia. With increasing duration of diabetes, however, the cumulative, irreversible abnormalities play an increasingly prominent role.

## Acute reversible metabolic changes

The acute reversible changes in metabolism that result from hyperglycaemia include increased polyol pathway activity [8], altered redox state of pyridine nucleotides [9], decreased myoinositol in selected subcellular pools [10], increased *de novo* synthesis of diacylglycerol [11], increased activation of protein kinase C [8, 11], and greater formation of early glycosylation products [12] (Table 3.1).

### *Polyol production*

The polyol pathway includes a family of aldoketo reductase enzymes which can utilize hexoses as a substrate for reduction by NADPH to their respective sugar alcohols (polyols), e.g. glucose to sorbitol, galactose to galactitol (Fig. 3.2). Because the Km of aldose reductase is high, elevated glucose levels are needed to produce high activity of the pathway.

In insulin-independent tissues where such enzymatic activity is present, hyperglycaemia increases the intracellular concentration of glucose, and thus the net flux through the polyol pathway. In many tissues, the sorbitol produced is subsequently oxidized to fructose by a specific dehydrogenase, using NAD as a cofactor (Fig. 3.2) [8]. Sorbitol does not easily diffuse across cell membranes and osmotic damage to cells may occur where accumulated sorbitol levels are high, such as in the lens during the development of diabetic cataracts. In other tissues, such as peripheral nerve, sorbitol levels are probably too low in diabetes to cause osmotic damage and here other consequences of increased polyol pathway flux might be important. One suggestion is that the altered redox state of pyridine nucleotides is critical, since pyruvate administration, which restores $NAD^+$ levels, can prevent endothelial cell dysfunction [9]. Another suggestion, based on animal data, is that increased polyol pathway activity results in a decrease in myoinositol, perhaps limited to a specific subcellular compartment involved in phosphoinositide metabolism [8, 10].

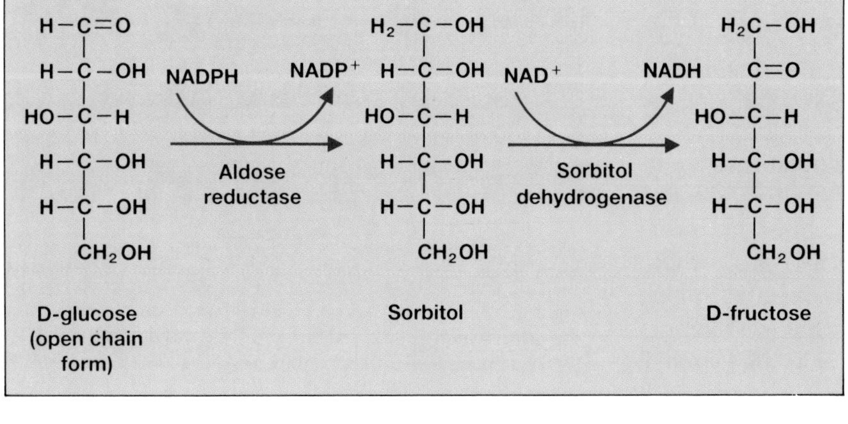

NADPH → $NADP^+$ (Aldose reductase); $NAD^+$ → NADH (Sorbitol dehydrogenase)
D-glucose (open chain form) → Sorbitol → D-fructose

**Fig. 3.2.** The polyol pathway.

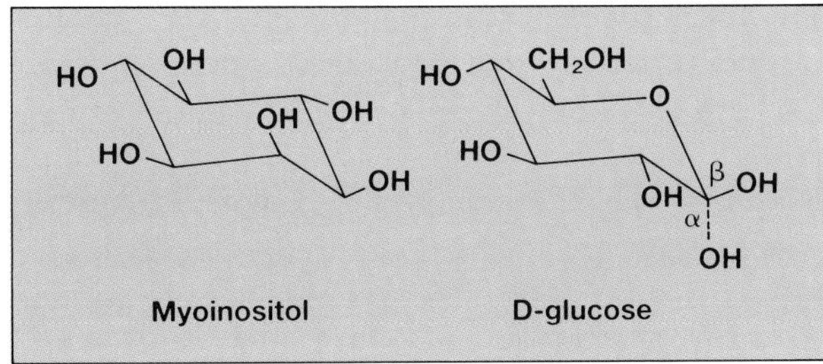


Fig. 3.3. The structures of myoinositol and glucose.

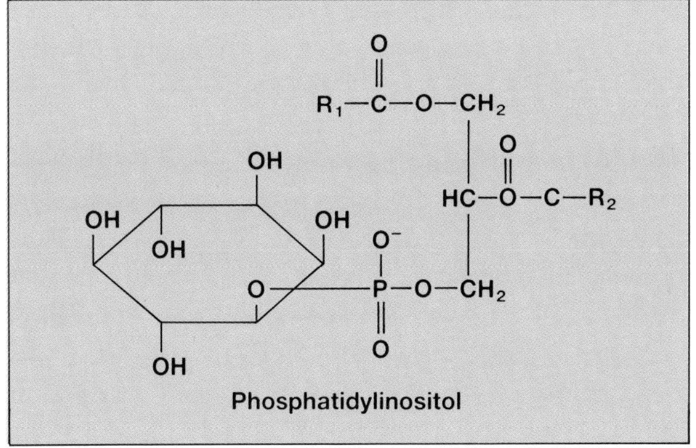


Fig. 3.4. The structure of phosphatidyl inositol. $R_1$ is usually stearate and $R_2$ arachidonate.

### *Polyols, myoinositol and protein kinase C*

Myoinositol is structurally related to glucose (Fig. 3.3) and is present in most animal and plant tissues, at higher intracellular than extracellular concentrations. It is mostly derived from the diet but is also synthesized in the cell from glucose-6-phosphate. It is actively transported inwards across cell membranes.

In rats made diabetic with streptozotocin, both motor nerve conduction velocity (NCV) and sciatic nerve myoinositol levels are decreased. Treatment with insulin to restore near-normoglycaemia increases both NCV and myoinositol content. Moreover, dietary supplements of myoinositol given to untreated diabetic rats also increase NCV and nerve myoinositol, even though nerve and blood glucose concentrations remain unaltered [8, 10].

One explanation for intracellular myoinositol depletion in diabetes is that glucose competes with myoinositol for uptake into cells. However, aldose reductase inhibitors have also been found to block the tissue depletion of myoinositol, suggesting a link between sorbitol accumulation and lowered myoinositol levels. Indeed, changes in myoinositol in diabetes are confined to those tissues susceptible to long-term complications and in which the polyol pathway is active (nerve, retina and glomerulus). The mechanism by which sorbitol affects myoinositol is unclear but may involve diminished myoinositol uptake into the cells.

Present evidence suggests that myoinositol depletion causes neuronal abnormalities by decreasing $Na^+-K^+-$ATPase activity (see Chapter 10). Myoinositol is a precursor of phosphoinositides such as phosphatidylinositol (Fig. 3.4) which activate $Na^+-K^+-$ATPase either directly or through the production of mediators (second messengers) such as inositol polyphosphates and diacylglycerol. The latter binds to and activates protein kinase C, a calcium-dependent activator of $Na^+-K^+-$ATPase. Inositol polyphosphates mobilize calcium and may thus also modulate $Na^+-K^+-$ATPase activity (see Fig. 3.5). Diminished $Na^+-K^+-$ATPase is thought to impede $Na^+$ extrusion from the nerve cell, the resultant high intracellular $Na^+$ levels blocking nodal depolarization and slowing NCV. Altered $Na^+$ levels may also affect myoinositol uptake, which is $Na^+$-dependent.

Sorbitol–myoinositol derangement has also been implicated in glomerular hyperfiltration (an early renal abnormality in diabetes), increased

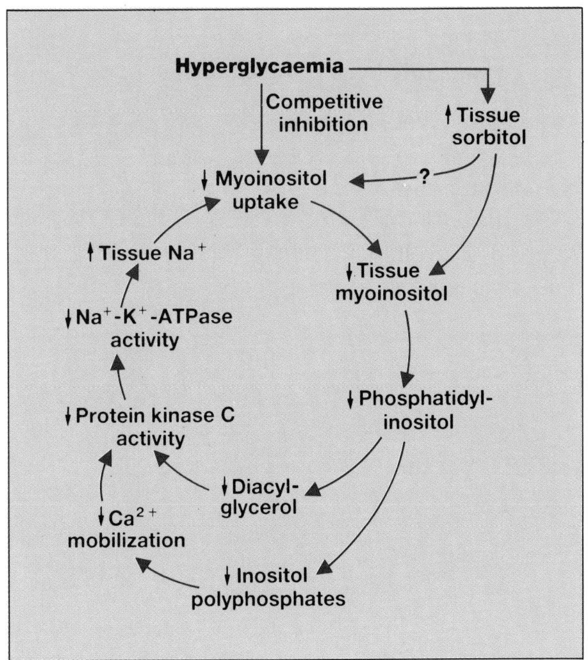


Fig. 3.5. A simplified scheme which shows some possible ways in which myoinositol depletion is involved in diabetic nerve damage. (Modified from [8] with permission from *The New England Journal of Medicine*.)

permeability of the blood/retinal barrier and possibly the association of hypertension with diabetes, as $Na^+-K^+$-ATPase in vascular smooth muscle may control the contractile response to hormones and neurotransmitters. In nerve, protein kinase C activity appears to be reduced and is associated with decreased $Na^+-K^+$-ATPase activity (see above), whereas in vascular tissues and in cell culture, hyperglycaemia is associated with an *increase* in diacylglycerol level and a corresponding increase in protein kinase C activation [8, 11]. This activation could be crucially involved in abnormal growth and synthesis in the diabetic vasculature. Increased *de novo* synthesis of diacylglycerol from glucose has been demonstrated directly in vascular tissue from diabetic animals.

### *Early glycosylation products*

Another acute reversible change induced by hyperglycaemia is the excessive formation of early glycosylation products [12], which form continuously both outside and inside cells. Glucose rapidly attaches to amino groups of proteins via the non-enzymatic process of nucleophilic addition to form Schiff base adducts (Fig. 3.6). Within hours, these adducts reach equilibrium levels which are proportional to the blood glucose concentration and subsequently undergo the Amadori rearrangement to form more stable early glycosylation products, typified by glycosylated haemoglobin, which reach equilibrium levels over a period of weeks. Excessive formation of early glycosylation products may adversely affect a variety of functions relevant to diabetic complications, including the uptake of low-density lipoprotein [13] and the regulation of free radical-mediated vascular damage [14, 15]. Glycosylated proteins can undergo auto-oxidation, generating free radicals which may contribute to protein cross-linking and degradation and other forms of molecular damage in diabetes (see below).

The two major factors determining the extent of early glycosylation product formation *in vivo* are

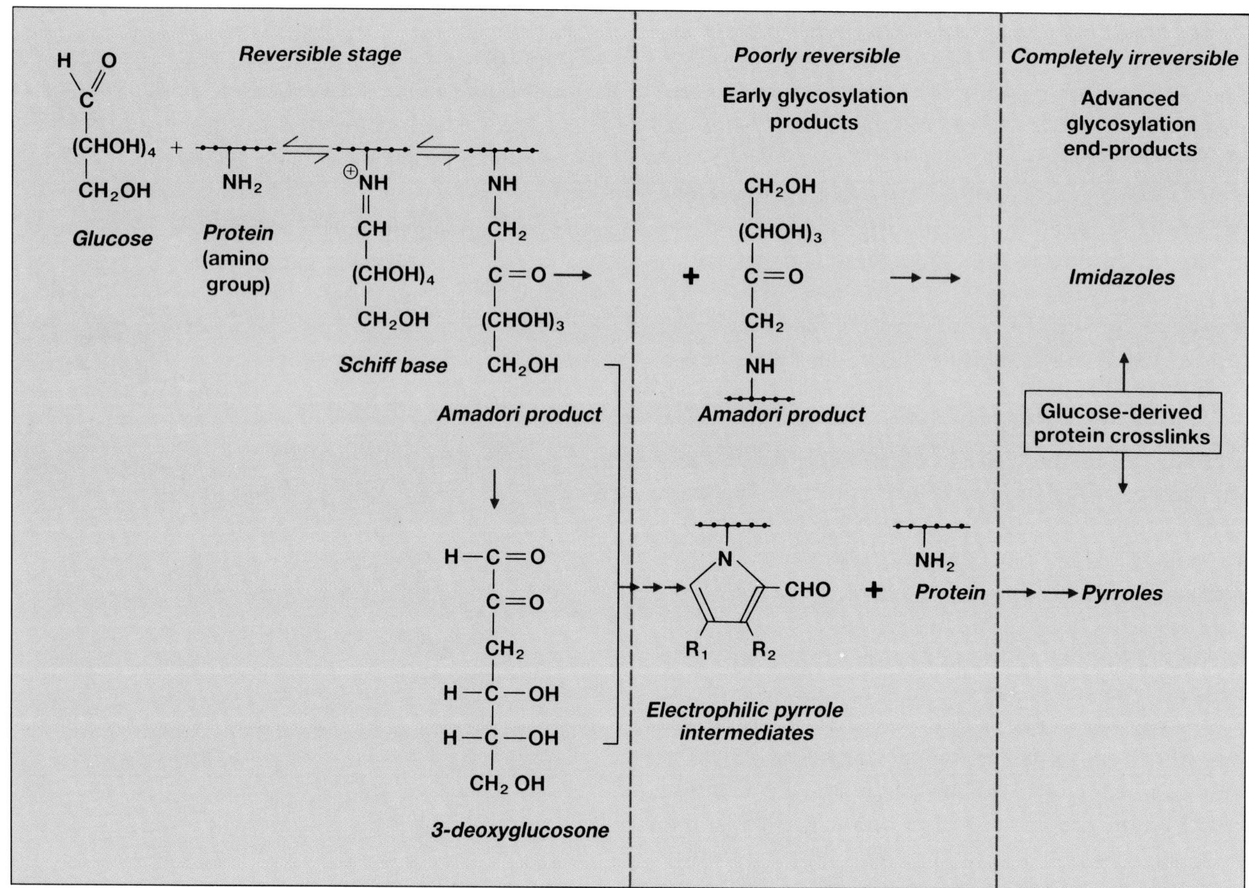


**Fig. 3.6.** Formation of reversible, early non-enzymatic glycosylation products, and of irreversible advanced glycosylation end-products (AGE). Through a complex series of chemical reactions, Amadori products can form families of imidazole-based and pyrrole-based glucose-derived cross-links.

the glucose concentration and duration of exposure to glucose. As glucose concentrations rise, the rate and equilibrium level of early glycosylation products increase proportionally through a mass action effect. One possible factor opposing this process may be a newly described pathway through which Amadori products are degraded by oxidative cleavage into peptide-bound carboxymethyllysine and erythronic acid [16]. Genetic variability in the regulation of this or analogous pathways might contribute to the wide differences in individual susceptibility to hyperglycaemia-mediated tissue damage.

### Chronic irreversible changes in stable macromolecules

Some early glycosylation products dissociate or are degraded but those formed on collagen, DNA and other long-lived macromolecules slowly undergo further complex chemical rearrangements, which are irreversible, to form advanced glycosylation end-products (AGE) [17]. Unlike the short-lived and reversible products described above, AGE are stable and therefore accumulate throughout the lifetime of the tissue or vessel wall; their levels do not return to normal if hyperglycaemia is corrected.

Glucose-derived advanced glycosylation products apparently result from covalent cross-linking of protein molecules, which apparently follows one of two patterns (Fig. 3.6) [18, 19]. One type closely resembles the heterocyclic imidazole derivative, 2-furoyl-4(5)-(2-furanyl)1-*H*-imidazole (FFI) (Fig. 3.6). This yellow-brown compound has a fluorescence spectrum characteristic of AGE proteins. This type of AGE has been found in enzymatically hydrolyzed tissue [18] and appears to form from the condensation of two Amadori products. The other pattern of AGE cross-linking apparently results from the reaction of an Amadori product with the Amadori-derived compound, 3-deoxyglucosone [19]. This highly reactive dicarbonyl compound cyclizes to form electrophilic pyrrole intermediates with reactive hydroxyl groups in benzylic positions, which then react with amino groups to form pyrrole-based cross-links. Examples of this latter type of AGE include the 1-alkyl-2-formyl-3, 4-diglycosyl pyrroles (AFGP), an arginine-ribose-lysine cross-linked compound termed 'pentosidine', a fluorescent HPLC peak designated 'peak L1', and the newly identified Maillard fluorescent product-1 (MFP-1). Formation of other AGE apparently involves generation of glycolaldehyde from Schiff bases through a reversed aldol condensation reaction; the resulting product is an even more reactive cross-linking agent than 3-deoxyglucosone.

### *Pathological consequences of advanced glycosylation product formation*

A number of these irreversible advanced glycosylation products are capable of forming covalent bonds with nearby amino groups on other proteins and nucleotides, resulting in glucose-derived cross-links. The formation of advanced glycosylation products could contribute to the development of diabetic tissue damage in several ways, including effects on extracellular matrix proteins, specific cellular receptors, or nucleic acids and nucleoproteins.

#### CROSS-LINKING OF EXTRACELLULAR MATRIX PROTEINS (see Table 3.2)

Diabetic blood vessels characteristically show early and progressive accumulation of various plasma proteins. In the arterial subintima, extracellular accumulation of extravasated low-density lipoprotein (LDL) makes up the bulk of such material, whereas PAS-positive plasma glycoprotein deposits are most prominent in the media [20]. This accumulated lipoprotein can only be released from atherosclerotic plaques by treatment with proteolytic enzymes, suggesting that it is chemically attached to vessel wall matrix components [21].

*In vitro*, human LDL binds covalently to collagen modified by advanced glycosylation in direct proportion to the content of AGE, indicating that LDL binds specifically to AGE [22]. These findings suggest that excessive cross-linking by hyperglycaemia-induced AGE may accelerate atherosclerosis in diabetic patients, even at normal levels of plasma LDL.

**Table 3.2.** Pathological consequences of advanced glycosylation product accumulation: extracellular protein cross-linking.

Extracellular protein cross-linking:
- Irreversibly traps deposited plasma proteins
- Reduces susceptibility to enzymatic degradation
- Interferes with basement membrane self-assembly
- Decreases binding affinity for growth-modulating heparan sulphate proteoglycans

In the diabetic microcirculation, PAS-positive material is deposited in retinal, glomerular and endoneurial arterioles together with plasma proteins such as IgG, albumin and IgM which accumulate in the basement membrane [23, 24]. These proteins are tightly bound to matrix components and cannot be extracted even with high-salt buffers or thiocyanate treatment. Similarly, serum albumin or IgG added *in vitro* to non-enzymatically glycosylated collagen or basement membrane become covalently bound to matrix [25, 26]. Once normally short-lived plasma proteins such as LDL and IgG become covalently attached to vascular matrix AGE, further AGE form on these incorporated proteins and in turn serve as attachment sites for additional molecules of extravasated plasma proteins.

AGE on matrix proteins can also cross-link adjacent matrix components such as collagen, forming covalent and heat-stable bonds throughout the collagen molecule [27]; aortic collagen from diabetic rats is three times more cross-linked than that from non-diabetic animals [28].

Matrix components cross-linked by glucose probably accumulate in diabetic vessel walls because they are less susceptible to normal enzymatic degradation. *In vitro*, non-enzymatically glycosylated glomerular basement membrane is considerably more resistant to digestion by pepsin, papain, trypsin and endogenous glomerular proteases than is normal basement membrane [29]. Overall, accumulation within large- and small-vessel walls of cross-linked material involving matrix, plasma proteins, collagen and other proteins would directly cause progressive luminal narrowing. Further tissue injury could result from AGE-catalysed oxygen radical formation.

As well as impeding its enzymatic removal, cross-linking by AGE has detrimental effects on other matrix protein properties. For example, self-assembly of the basement membrane structure, which normally involves precise geometrical interactions between Type IV collagen, laminin, heparan sulphate proteoglycan and entactin, is disordered [5, 6]. There is an associated increase in the effective intermolecular pore size, which together with alterations in anionic proteoglycans of the vascular matrix, may damage the integrity of the charge-selective matrix filtration barrier which prevents circulating proteins from escaping into the vessel wall.

The anionic proteoglycans, such as heparan sulphate, also appear to inhibit the proliferation of adherent cells [30], either through direct transmembrane inhibition of cellular activity via specific glycosaminoglycan (GAG) receptors, or indirectly by down-regulating receptors for growth factors such as interleukin-1 (IL-1), insulin-like growth factor-1 (IGF-1) and platelet-derived growth factor (PDGF). In long-standing diabetes, the basement membrane content of anionic proteoglycan is markedly decreased in several tissues including the renal glomerulus [31, 32] (Chapter 14), and there is evidence that loss of this inhibitory matrix signal results in a compensatory increase in basement membrane production [33].

Accumulation of AGE on collagen and basement membrane contributes to this permanent loss of proteoglycan by reducing the ability of these long-lived matrix proteins to bind heparin.

These glycosylation-induced matrix defects would both increase leakage of plasma proteins and stimulate matrix overproduction. AGE-induced conformational changes in matrix components such as fibronectin, laminin, vitronectin and collagen are likely to cause further abnormalities in diabetic blood vessels by altering the interactions between the matrix and platelets and vessel-wall cells. These abnormalities, mediated by specific transmembrane signalling receptors called integrins [34], may result in microthrombus formation, hyper-responsiveness to growth factors, and enhanced secretion of vasoconstrictor molecules.

### EFFECTS ON CELLULAR RECEPTORS (see Table 3.3)

Accumulation of vascular matrix in diabetes is due not only to reduced degradation but also to a significant increase in the synthesis of its components [35], which is frequently accompanied by proliferation of adjacent cells such as retinal endothelium, glomerular mesangial cells and arterial smooth muscle. These processes may be chronically stimulated by increased local production of growth-promoting factors such as IGF-1 [36], tumour necrosis factor (TNF), IL-1 and PDGF.

Both murine and human monocyte macrophages are now known to carry a high-affinity receptor for AGE proteins [37], which may also exist on endothelial cells [38]. As it does not recognize proteins with early glycosylation products alone, this receptor enables macrophages to identify and remove preferentially vascular matrix macromolecules which have been cross-linked through long-term exposure to glucose.

In non-diabetic individuals, AGE-protein binding to its cellular receptor appears to release TNF, IL-1 and possibly other monokines [39], which then initiate a cascade of homeostatic events within the vessel wall. The monokines act upon mesenchymal cells, which release extracellular hydrolases including collagenase [39] and a mesangial neutral protease [40], and upon endothelial cells to produce growth factors which enhance the growth-promoting effects of the monokines themselves [41, 42] (Fig. 3.7). Normally, these degradative and proliferative responses are balanced and the turnover of AGE-containing vascular elements is carefully regulated. The proliferative responses may, however, predispose to thrombus formation. The binding of TNF to its specific endothelial cell receptors induces a procoagulatory state, which in turn promotes the release of PDGF-like activity in response to stimulation of endothelial cells by thrombin and factor Xa [43]. In diabetic vessels, platelet aggregation and thrombosis might be induced by the rapid fall in thrombomodulin activity caused directly by binding of AGE proteins to endothelial cells [44]. The relative activity of the proliferative responses, and therefore the tendency to thrombosis in response to glucose-derived AGE in vessel walls, may be modulated by genetic factors. These could perhaps affect the magnitude of the monokine response elicited by AGE-protein binding to macrophages, or the sensitivity of the endothelial and mesenchymal cells to the monokines. Such

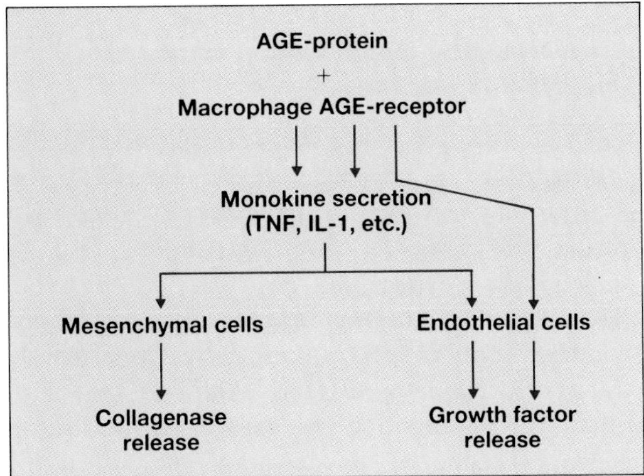


**Fig. 3.7.** Schematic representation of the proposed mechanism by which monokine production stimulated by AGE-protein binding to its macrophage receptor may regulate normal vessel wall homeostasis. (Redrawn with permission from [17].)

**Table 3.3.** Pathological consequences of advanced glycosylation product accumulation: interaction with cellular receptors.

Interaction with cellular receptors increases production of growth-promoting cytokines that:
- Augment matrix synthesis
- Stimulate hypertrophy/hyperplasia
- Induce procoagulatory changes in endothelial surface

factors could account for some of the great individual variation in susceptibility to hyperglycaemia-mediated cell damage.

INTRACELLULAR NUCLEIC ACID CROSS-LINKING (see Table 3.4)

The primary amino groups of nucleotides are chemically less reactive nucleophiles than the ε-amino groups of lysine. None the less, reducing sugars found intracellularly can react *in vitro* with amino groups on DNA nucleotides in a manner analogous to the non-enzymatic glycosylation of protein amino groups [45], forming AGE whose spectral and fluorescent properties are similar to those of AGE on proteins. AGE also form readily on all classes of histones, suggesting that hyperglycaemia may also result in cross-linking of DNA with nucleoproteins [46].

In prokaryotic cells, formation of AGE on DNA is associated with mutations (either deletions or insertions) and altered gene expression [7]. Hyperglycaemia also affects DNA from eukaryotic cells [47]. Human endothelial cells cultured in 30 mmol/l glucose display an increase in single-strand DNA breaks and in DNA repair synthesis. Increased single-strand DNA breaks also occur in lymphocytes from chronically hyperglycaemic diabetic patients, but the extent of AGE formation in these human DNA preparations is not yet known. Accumulation of AGE on nucleic acids of diabetic vascular wall cells may eventually interfere with normal physiology, perhaps resulting in the early loss of pericytes from diabetic retinal capillaries (Chapter 7) and possibly explaining the expression of transforming genes by human coronary artery plaque cells [48].

## Relationship of AGE formation to other pathogenic factors

### *Hypertension*

In recent years, hypertension has been increasingly

**Table 3.4.** Pathological consequences of advanced glycosylation product accumulation: intracellular nucleic acid cross-linking.

- Increases single-strand breaks in DNA
- Increases DNA excision/repair
- Increases mutation frequency
- Decreases transcriptional regulatory protein binding

recognized as one of the most significant secondary risk factors for both microvascular and macromuscular diabetic complications (Chapter 1) [4, 49]. Effective anti-hypertensive treatment significantly reduces the rate of renal function decline in nephropathic patients (Chapter 14); a natural corollary is that unilateral ophthalmic or renal artery stenosis greatly reduces the severity of retinopathy or nephropathy on the affected side. Increased intravascular pressure probably accelerates the development of AGE-induced pathological changes by increasing the extravasation of plasma proteins. This would both accelerate the accumulation of AGE cross-linked protein deposits in the vascular matrix and increase the concentration of AGE proteins available to stimulate growth-factor production by cells carrying AGE receptors.

### *Aldose reductase inhibitors*

Aldose reductase inhibitors (ARI) produce various biochemical effects which may retard the progression of diabetic complications [50]. For example, ARI can improve the 1.5-fold increase in vascular permeability associated with diabetes of short duration [51] and would thereby reduce the deposition of AGE proteins. Recent evidence indicates that ARI may also directly inhibit the excess formation of fructose-derived AGE in tissues with increased polyol pathway activity. Administration of ARI to rats induces both a decrease in collagen AGE content [52] and a reduction in collagen cross-linking [53]. However, such fructose-derived products appear to constitute only 10–20% of the total AGE in long-lived proteins [54].

### *Hypercoagulability and platelet aggregation*

Diabetes is associated with several thrombogenic abnormalities, including a probable increase in coagulation cascade activity, hyperaggregable platelets, and decreased fibrinolysis [55]. Together, these processes are thought to accelerate the development of both microvascular and macrovascular disease. Excessive AGE formation is now known to promote thrombogenic changes at the endothelial cell surface by stimulating TNF and IL-1 secretion by macrophages. These monokines induce endothelial cells to produce a tissue-factor-like procoagulant (which suppresses the activity of the anticoagulant protein C pathway) and to synthesize an inhibitor of plasminogen activator [43]. These changes generate thrombin and activated factor Xa, which stimulate the release of PDGF which in turn accelerates both hyperplasia and hypertrophy in the diabetic vessel wall. Other thrombogenic effects include endothelial cell binding to AGE proteins, causing a rapid reduction in thrombomodulin activity [44], and increased AGE-protein cross-linking, which encourages platelet aggregation [56].

### *Dyslipoproteinaemia*

Although diabetes is associated with greatly increased risks of developing coronary, cerebral and peripheral arteriosclerosis, plasma LDL levels are not consistently abnormal [57]. At any level of plasma LDL, however, accumulation of AGE on arterial wall collagen would enhance the extracellular deposition of lipoprotein [22], which would act as a nucleus for AGE formation and, by interaction with cellular AGE receptors, would stimulate growth-factor release (Fig. 3.7) [39]. AGE attached to LDL or collagen in the vessel wall could aggravate vascular injury by catalysing the formation of toxic free radicals [14, 15].

## Pharmacological modulation of advanced glycosylation reactions

As AGE formation has been implicated in the pathogenesis of chronic diabetic complications, pharmacological agents have been sought to inhibit this process. Aminoguanidine HCl, a nucleophilic hydrazine derivative, selectively blocks reactive carbonyl groups on early glycosylation products and on their derivatives such as 3-deoxyglucosone and glycolaldehyde (see Fig. 3.8). Aminoguanidine is essentially non-toxic ($LD_{50}$ = 1800 mg/kg in rodents) and does not interfere with the formation of normal, enzymatically derived collagen cross-links, as determined both indirectly [28] and by direct quantitation of lysyl oxidase-dependent cross-link products.

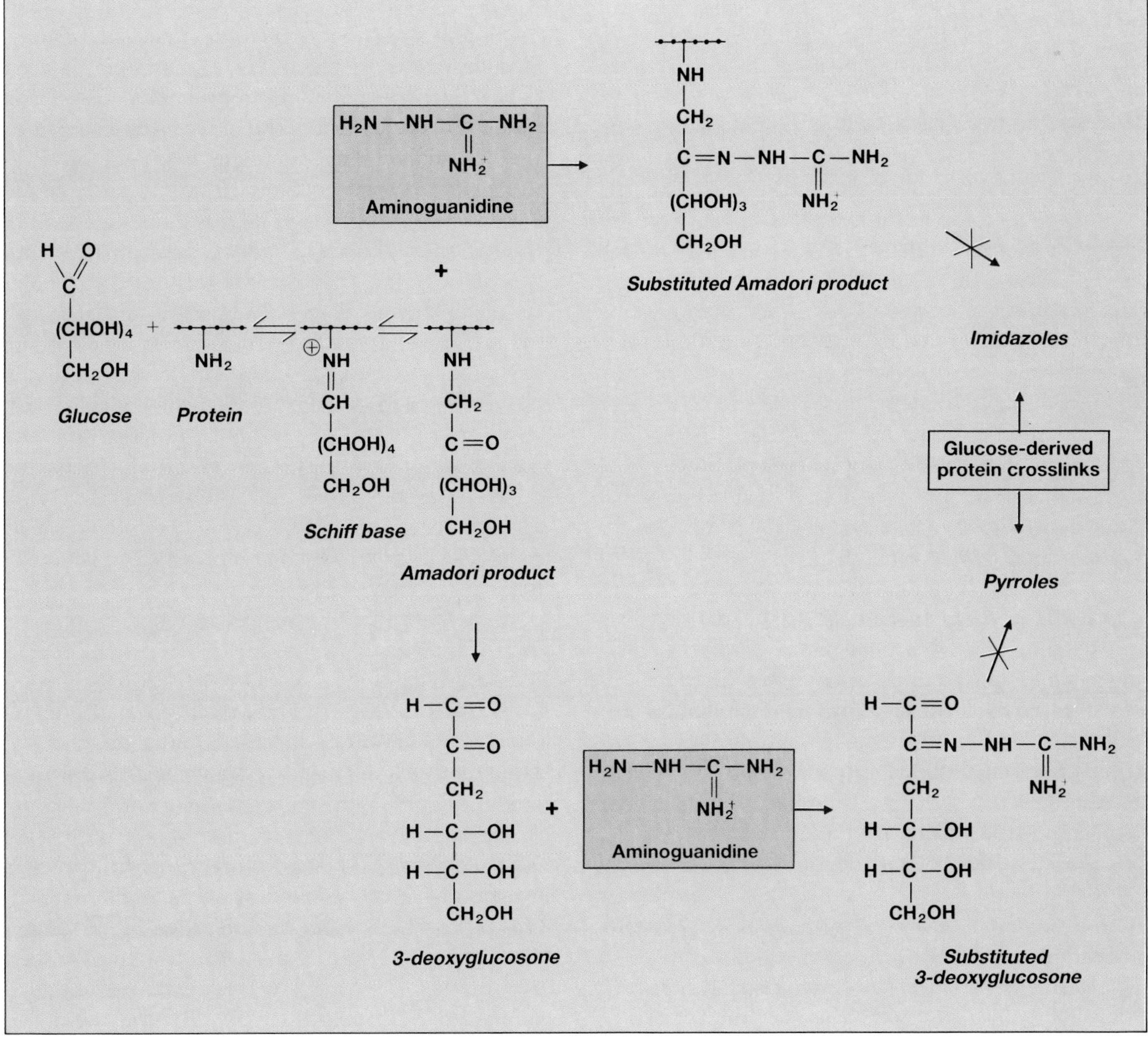


**Fig. 3.8.** Prevention of AGE-protein cross-link formation by aminoguanidine. Aminoguanidine binds preferentially to reactive AGE cross-link precursors, forming unreactive substituted products which can no longer participate in AGE cross-link formation.

*In vitro*, aminoguanidine effectively inhibits the formation of AGE, and blocks the AGE cross-linking of soluble proteins to matrix and of collagen. It also prevents defects due to cross-linking in the binding of heparin to collagen/fibronectin and of heparan sulphate proteoglycan to basement membrane [28, 58].

*In vivo*, the effect of aminoguanidine on diabetic early vascular lesions has been examined in diabetic rats. After 16 weeks of untreated diabetes, the matrix contents of AGE and of cross-linked plasma proteins in both aorta and kidney were four-fold higher than in non-diabetic controls [28, 59]. By contrast, these defects were nearly normalized in tissues from aminoguanidine-treated diabetic animals. Preliminary data from long-term studies suggest that aminoguanidine treatment also inhibits the development of experimental diabetic retinopathy. This is discussed further in the recent developments section at the end of this chapter.

The therapeutic potential of aminoguanidine and its analogues is currently being further evaluated in several animal and cell culture model systems, while the pharmacokinetics and potential toxicity of this agent are being determined in human studies.

### Recent developments

A causal relationship between chronic hyperglycaemia and diabetic microvascular disease has been inferred from a variety of animal and clinical studies [60]. This relationship has now been definitely established by data from the Diabetes Control and Complications Trial (DCCT), a multicentre randomized, prospective controlled clinical study. The relationship between hyperglycaemia and macrovascular disease is complicated by the many other factors which influence atherogenesis in non-diabetic subjects. Nevertheless, a strong independent association was found between hyperglycaemia and macrovascular disease in older women in the Framingham Heart Study [61], and hyperglycaemia was found to be the most important coronary risk factor in elderly men in Gothenberg, Sweden [62].

As discussed earlier in this chapter, hyperglycaemia appears to damage tissues by causing both acute, reversible changes in cellular metabolism, and cumulative, irreversible changes in stable macromolecules. Acute, reversible changes are associated with reversible abnormalities in blood flow and vascular permeability [63–65]. Hyperglycaemia-induced alterations in several biochemical pathways have been linked to early changes in diabetic microvessels. These include the polyol pathway (Fig. 3.2); the *de novo* synthesis of diacylglycerol (DAG) which can lead to the activation of several isoforms of protein kinase C; decreased cellular uptake of myoinositol; reduced $Na^+-K^+-$ATPase activity (p. 23); and the rapid covalent modification of intracellular proteins by glycolytic intermediates such as glyceraldehyde-3-phosphate.

Recently, it has been proposed that each of these separate acute alterations may reflect a common abnormality in the cytosolic $NADH/NAD^+$ ratio [66]. Polyol pathway-linked reactions such as the oxidation of sorbitol to fructose by sorbitol dehydrogenase lead to an increase in the cytosolic $NADH/NAD^+$ ratio [67]. This increase, in turn, favours the *de novo* synthesis of diacylglycerol by inhibiting the glycolytic oxidation of glyceraldehyde-3-phosphate and promoting the reduction of dihydroxyacetone phosphate. Myoinositol depletion may reflect increased incorporation into phosphatidylinositol. Reduced $Na^+-K^+-$ATPase activity has been linked to protein kinase C activity. An increase in the cytosolic $NADH/NAD^+$ ratio would also amplify the non-enzymatic glycation of intracellular proteins by glycolytic intermediates such as glyceraldehyde-3-phosphate, since inhibition of the $NAD^+$-dependent glyceraldehyde-3-phosphate dehydrogenase reaction would further elevate the concentration of this highly-reactive glycating sugar.

These reversible biochemical abnormalities almost certainly play a role in the pathogenesis of the early functional changes in the diabetic microvasculature, but they cannot account for a major characteristic of diabetic complications so-called 'hyperglycaemic memory'. This term refers to the persistence or progression of hyperglycaemia-induced microvascular alterations during subsequent periods of normal ambient glucose concentrations. A striking example of this is the delayed development of severe retinopathy in diabetic dogs after a 2.5-year period of near-normoglycaemia which followed 2.5 years of hyperglycaemia; at the start of the normoglycaemic period, there were no histological signs of retinal damage [68].

In chemical terms, pathogenic changes induced by antecedent hyperglycaemia imply that glucose irreversibly modifies long-lived macromolecules. The most well-characterized and best understood model of such irreversible modification by sugars is the formation and accumulation of advanced AGE. As described on p. 25, AGE accumulate as a function of glucose concentration and time [69], but their formation may be retarded by the action of reductase enzymes that reduce compounds such as 3-D-deoxyglucosone to less reactive ones such as 3-deoxy-D-fructose [70]. Recent evidence suggests that accumulated AGEs may blunt the effect of vasodilator and antiproliferative factors such as nitric oxide (EDRF) [71, 72]. The AGE receptor which mediates procoagulatory changes in endothelium [73] has been cloned, and appears to be a new 35 kD member of the immunoglobulin superfamily of proteins [74].

Inhibition of *in vivo* AGE formation by aminoguanidine has now been shown convincingly to prevent or ameliorate diabetic retinopathy [75], nephropathy [76–78], and neuropathy [79, 80] in animal models. Current clinical studies in diabetic patients have been designed to assess the effects of aminoguanidine on various endpoints in different stages of diabetic nephropathy; the results of these investigations are awaited with interest.

CATHLEEN J. MULLARKEY
MICHAEL BROWNLEE

## References


1 Keen H, Jarrett J, eds. *Complications of Diabetes* 2nd ed. London: Edward Arnold, 1982: 1–331.

2 Bloodworth JMB Jr, Greider MH. The endocrine pancreas and diabetes mellitus. Bloodworth JMB Jr ed. In: *Endocrine Pathology, General and Surgical*, 2nd ed. Baltimore: Williams and Wilkins, 1982: 556–721.

3 Dyck PJ. Hypoxic neuropathy: Does hypoxia play a role in diabetic neuropathy? *Neurology* 1989; **39**: 111–18.

4 Krolewski A, Canessa M, Warram JH *et al*. Predisposition to hypertension and susceptibility to renal disease in insulin-dependent diabetes mellitus. *N Engl J Med* 1988; **318**: 140–6.

5 Tarsio JF, Reger LA, Furcht LT. Decreased interaction of fibronectin, type IV collagen and heparin, due to non-enzymatic glycosylation. Implications for diabetes mellitus. *Biochemistry* 1987; **26**: 1014–20.

6 Tsilibary EC, Charonis AS, Reger LA, Wohlhueter RM, Furcht LT. The effect of non-enzymatic glucosylation on the binding of the main non-collagenous NC1 domain to type IV collagen. *J Biol Chem* 1988; **263** (suppl 9): 4302–8.

7 Lee AT, Cerami A. Elevated glucose 6-phosphate levels are associated with plasmid mutations *in vivo*. *Proc Natl Acad Sci USA* 1987; **84**: 8311–14.

8 Greene DA, Lattimer SA, Sima AAF. Sorbitol, phophoinositides, and sodium–potassium–ATPase in the pathogenesis of diabetic complications. *N Engl J Med* 1987; **316**: 599–606.

9 Williamson JR, Change K, Ostrow E, Allision W, Harlow J, Kilo C. Sorbitol-induced increases in vasculâr albumin clearance are prevented by pyruvate but not by myoinositol. *Diabetes* 1989; **38** (suppl 2): 94A.

10 Winegrad AI. Does a common mechanism induce the diverse complications of diabetes? *Diabetes* 1987; **36**: 396–406.

11 Lee TS, Saltsman KA, Ohashi H, King GL. Activation of protein kinase C by elevation of glucose concentration: Proposal for a mechanism in the development of diabetic vascular complications. *Proc Natl Acad Sci USA* 1989; **86**: 5141–5.

12 Brownlee M, Vlassara H, Cerami A. Non-enzymatic glycosylation and the pathogenesis of diabetic complications. *Ann Inter Med* 1984; **101**: 527–37.

13 Witztum JL, Mahoney EM, Branks MJ *et al*. Non-enzymatic glucosylation of low-density lipoprotein alters its biologic activity. *Diabetes* 1982; **3**: 283–91.

14 Gillery P, Monboisse JC, Maquart FX, Borel JP. Glycation of proteins as a source of superoxide. *Diabètes Métab* 1988; **14**: 25–30.

15 Hicks M, Delbridge L, Yue DK, Reeve TS. Catalysis of lipid peroxidation by glucose and glycosylated collagen. *Biochem Biophys Res Commun* 1988; **151**: 649–55.

16 Ahmed MU, Thorpe SR, Baynes JW. Identification of N-carboxymethyllysine as a degradation product of fructosyllysine in glycated protein. *J Biol Chem* 1986; **261**: 4889–94.

17 Brownlee MB, Cerami A, Vlassara H. Advanced glycosylation end-products in tissue and the biochemical basis of diabetic complications. *N Engl J Med* 1988; **318**: 1315–21.

18 Chang JCF, Ulrich PC, Bucala R, Cerami A. Detection of an advanced glycosylation product bound to protein *in situ*. *J Biol Chem* 1985; **260**: 7970–4.

19 Baines JW, Monnier VM, eds. *The NIH Conference on the Maillard Reaction in Ageing, Diabetes and Nutrition*. New York: Alan R Liss, 1989.

20 Dybdahl H, Ledet TS. Diabetic macroangiopathy: Quantitative histopathological studies of the extramural coronary arteries from Type 2 (non-insulin-dependent) diabetic patients. *Diabetologia* 1987; **30**: 882–6.

21 Smith EB, Massie IB, Alexander KM. The release of an immobilized lipoprotein fraction from atherosclerotic lesions by incubation with plasmin. *Atherosclerosis* 1976; **25**: 71–84.

22 Brownlee M, Vlassara H, Cerami A. Non-enzymatic glycosylation products on collagen covalently trap low-density lipoprotein. *Diabetes* 1985; **34**: 938–41.

23 Michael AF, Brown DM. Increased concentrations of albumin in kidney basement membranes in diabetes mellitus. *Diabetes* 1981; **30**: 843–6.

24 Graham AR, Johnson PC. Direct immunofluorescence findings in peripheral nerve from patients with diabetic neuropathy. *Ann Neurol* 1985; **17**: 450–4.

25 Brownlee M, Pongor S, Cerami A. Covalent attachment of soluble proteins by non-enzymatically glycosylated collagen: Role in the *in situ* formation of immune complexes. *J Exp Med* 1983; **158**: 1739–44.

26 Sensi M, Tanzi P, Bruno MR *et al*. Human glomerular basement membrane: altered binding characteristics following *in vitro* non-enzymatic glycosylation. *Ann NY Acad Sci* 1986; **488**: 549–52.

27 Kent MJC, Light ND, Bailey AJ. Evidence for glucose-mediated covalent cross-linking of collagen after glycosylation *in vitro*. *Biochem J* 1985; **225**: 745–52.

28 Brownlee M, Vlassara H, Kooney T, Ulrich P, Cerami A. Aminoguanidine prevents diabetes-induced arterial wall protein cross-linking. *Science* 1986; **232**: 1629–32.

29 Lubec G, Pollak A. Reduced susceptibility of non-enzymatically glucosylated glomerular basement membrane to proteases: is thickening of diabetic glomerular basement due to reduced proteolytic degradation? *Renal Physiol* 1980; **3**: 4–8.

30 Klahr S, Schreiner G, Ichikawa I. The progression of renal disease. *N Engl J Med* 1988; **318**: 1657–66.

31 Klein DJ, Brown DM, Oegema TR. Glomerular proteoglycans: partial structural characterization and metabolism of *de novo* synthesized heparan-$^{35}SO_4$ proteoglycan in streptozotocin-induced diabetic rats. *Diabetes* 1986; **35**: 1130–42.

32 Shimomura H, Spiro RG. Studies on macromolecular components of human glomerular basement membrane and alterations in diabetes: decreased levels of heparan sulfate proteoglycan and laminin. *Diabetes* 1987; **36**: 374–81.

33 Rohrbach DH, Hassel JR, Kleinman HK, Martin GR. Alterations in basement membrane (heparan sulfate) proteoglycan in diabetic mice. *Diabetes* 1982; **31**: 185–8.

34 Ruoslahti E, Pierschbacher MD. New perspectives in cell adhesion: RGD and integrins. *Science* 1987; **238**: 491–7.

35 Brownlee M, Spiro RG. Glomerular basement membrane metabolism in the diabetic rat. *In vivo* studies. *Diabetes* 1979; **28**: 121–5.

36 King GL, Goodman AD, Buzney S, Moses A, Kahn CR. Receptors and growth-promoting effects of insulin and insulin-like growth factors on cells from bovine retinal capillaries and aorta. *J Clin Invest* 1985; **75**: 1028–36.

37 Vlassara H, Brownlee M, Cerami A. High-affinity receptor-mediated uptake and degradation of glucose-modified proteins: A potential mechanism for the removal of senescent macromolecules. *Proc Natl Acad Sci USA* 1985; **82**: 5588–92.

38 Williams SK, Devenny JJ, Bitensky MW. Micropinocytic ingestion of glycosylated albumin by isolated microvessels: possible role in pathogenesis of diabetic microangiopathy.

*Proc Natl Acad Sci USA* 1981; **78**: 2393–7.
39 Vlassara H, Brownlee M, Monogue K *et al*. Cachectin/TNF and IL-1 induced by glucose-modified proteins: role in normal tissue remodelling. *Science* 1988; **240**: 1546–8.
40 Lovett DH, Sterzel M, Kashgarian M, Ryan JL. Neutral proteinase activity produced *in vitro* by cells of the glomerular mesangium. *Kidney Int* 1983; **23**: 342–9.
41 Lovett DH, Ryan JL, Sterzel RB. Stimulation of rat mesangial cell proliferation by macrophage interleukin 1. *J Immunol* 1983; **136**: 3700–5.
42 Libby P, Warner SJC, Freidman GB. Interleukin 1: a mitogen for human vascular smooth muscle cells that induces the release of inhibitory prostanoids. *J Clin Invest* 1988; **81**: 487–98.
43 Bevilacqua MP, Pober JS, Majeau GR, Fiers W, Cotran RS, Giambrone MA. Recombinant tumor necrosis factor induces procoagulant activity in cultured human vascular endothelium: Characterization and comparison with the actions of interleukin 1. *Proc Natl Acad Sci USA* 1986; **83**: 4533–7.
44 Vlassara H, Esposito C, Gerlach H, Stern D. Receptor-mediated binding of glycosylated albumin to endothelium induces tissue necrosis factor and acts synergistically with TNF procoagulant activity. *Diabetes* 1989; **38** (suppl 2): 32A.
45 Bucala R, Model P, Cerami A. Modification of DNA by reducing sugars: a possible mechanism for nucleic acid aging and age-related dysfunction in gene expression. *Proc Natl Acad Sci USA* 1984; **81**: 105–9.
46 De Bellis D, Horowitz MI. *In vitro* studies of histone glycation. *Biochem Biophys Acta* 1987; **926**: 365–8.
47 Lornezi M, Montisano DF, Toledo S, Barrieux A. High glucose and DNA damage in endothelial cells. *J Clin Invest* 1986; **77**: 322–5.
48 Penn A, Garte SJ, Warren L, Nesta D, Mindich B. Transforming gene in human atherosclerotic plaque DNA. *Proc Natl Acad Sci USA* 1986; **83**: 7951–5.
49 *Diabetes in America: Diabetes Data Compiled 1984*. NIH Publication No. 85–1468, 1985.
50 Kador PF, Robison WG, Kinoshita JH. The pharmacology of aldose reductase inhibitors. *Ann Rev Pharmacol Tox* 1985; **25**: 691–714.
51 Williamson JR, Chang K, Tilton RC *et al*. Increased vascular permeability in spontaneously diabetic BB/W rats and in rats with mild versus severe streptozocin-induced diabetes: prevention by aldose reductase inhibitors and castration. *Diabetes* 1987; **36**: 813–21.
52 Suarez G, Rajaram R, Bhuyan KC, Oronsky AL, Goidl JA. Administration of an aldose reductase inhibitor induces a decrease of collagen fluorescence in diabetic rats. *J Clin Invest* 1988; **82**: 624–7.
53 Tamas C, Monnier VM. Aldose reductase inhibition partly prevents the browning and cross-linking of collagen in chronic experimental hyperglycaemia. In: Baines JW, Monnier VM, eds. *Proceedings of the NIH Conference on the Maillard Reaction in Aging, Diabetes and Nutrition*, New York: Elsevier, in press.
54 McPherson JD, Shilton BH, Walton DJ. Role of fructose in glycation and cross-linking of proteins. *Biochemistry* 1988; **27**: 1901–7.
55 Brownlee M, Cerami A. The biochemistry of the complications of diabetes mellitus. *Annu Rev Biochem* 1981; **50**: 385–432.
56 Le Pape A, Gutman N, Guitton JD, Legrand Y, Muh JP. Non-enzymatic glycosylation increases platelet aggregating potency of collagen from placenta of diabetic human beings. *Biochem Biophys Res Commun* 1983; **111**: 602–10.
57 Briones ER, Mao SJT, Palumbo WM *et al*. Analysis of plasma lipids and apolipoproteins in insulin-dependent and non-insulin-dependent diabetes. *Metabolism* 1984; **33**: 42–9.
58 Brownlee M, Vlassara H, Cerami A. Aminoguanidine prevents hyperglycemia-induced defect in binding of heparin by matrix molecules. *Diabetes* 1987; **36**: 85A.
59 Nicholls K, Mandel TE. Advanced glycosylation end-products in experimental murine diabetic nephropathy: effect of islet isografting and aminoguanidine. *Lab Invest* 1989; **60**: 486–93.
60 Skyler JS. Relation of metabolic control of diabetes mellitus to chronic complications. In: Rifkin H, Porte D Jr, eds. *Diabetes Mellitus, Theory and Practice*. New York: Elsevier, 1990, pp. 856–68.
61 Singer DE, Nathan DM, Anderson KM, Wilson PWF, Evans JC. Association of $HbA_{1c}$ with prevalent cardiovascular disease in the original cohort of the Framingham Heart Study. *Diabetes* 1992; **41**: 202–9.
62 Welin L, Eriksson H, Larsson B, Ohlson L-O, Svardsudd K, Tibblin G. Hyperinsulinaemia is not a major coronary risk factor in elderly men. *Diabetologia* 1992; **35**: 766–70.
63 Williamson JR, Wolf BA, Ostrow E, Turk J. Relationship of glucose-induced vascular function changes to diacylglycerol (DAG) levels and protein kinase C (PKC) activity. *Diabetes* 1990; **39**: 157A.
64 Williamson JR, Ostrow E, Eades D *et al*. Glucose-induced microvascular functional changes in nondiabetic rats are stereospecific and are prevented by an aldose reductase inhibitor. *J Clin Invest* 1990; **85**: 1167–72.
65 Wolf BA, Williamson JR, Eason RA, Chang K, Sherman WR, Turk J. Diacylglycerol accumulation and microvascular abnormalities induced by elevated glucose levels. *J Clin Invest* 1991; **87**: 31–8.
66 Ruderman NB, Williamson JR, Brownlee M. Glucose and diabetic vascular disease. *FASEB* 1992; **6**: 2905–14.
67 Tilton RG, Baier LD, Harlow JE, Smith SR, Ostrow E, Williamson JR. Diabetes-induced glomerular dysfunction: Links to a more reduced cytosolic ratio of $NADH/NAD^+$. *Kidney Int* 1992; **41**: 778–88.
68 Engerman RL, Kerns TS. Progression of incipient diabetic retinopathy during good glycemic control. *Diabetes* 1987; **36**: 808–12.
69 Makita Z, Radoff S, Rayfield EJ *et al*. Advanced glycosylation end products in patients with diabetic neuropathy. *N Engl J Med* 1991; **325**: 836–42.
70 Knecht KJ, Feather MS, Baynes JW. Detection of 3-deoxyglucosone in human plasma: evidence for intermediate states of the Maillard reaction *in vivo* (abstract). *Diabetes* 1992; **41** (suppl 1): 23A.
71 Bucala R, Tracey KJ, Cerami A. Advanced glycosylation products quench nitric oxide and mediate defective endothelium-dependent vasodilation in experimental diabetes. *J Clin Invest* 1991; **87**: 432–8.
72 Hogan M, Cerami A, Bucala R. Advance glycosylation end products block the antiproliferative effect of nitric oxide. *J Clin Invest* 1992; **90**: 1110–15.
73 Esposito C, Gerlach H, Brett J, Stern D, Vlassara H. Endothelial receptor-mediated binding of glucose modified albumin is associated with increased mono-layer permeability and modulation of cell surfact coagulant properties. *J Exp Med* 1989; **170**: 1387–407.
74 Neeper M, Schmidt AM, Brett J, Du Yan S, Wang F, Shaw A. Cloning and expression of RAGE: a cell surface receptor for advanced glycosylation end products of proteins. *J Biol Chem* 1992; **267**: 14998–5004.
75 Hammes H-P, Martin S, Federlin K, Geisen K, Brownlee M. Aminoguanidine treatment inhibits the development of

experimental diabetic retinopathy. *Proc Natl Acad Sci USA* 1991; **88**: 11555–58.
76 Soules-Liparota T, Cooper M, Papazoglou D, Clarke B, Jerums G. Retardation by aminoguanidine of development of albuminuria, mesangial expansion, and tissue fluorescence in streptozocin-induced diabetic rat. *Diabetes* 1991; **40**: 1328–35.
77 Edelstein D, Brownlee M. Aminoguanidine ameliorates albuminuria in diabetic hypertensive rats. *Diabetologia* 1992; **35**: 96–7.
78 Ellis EN, Good BH. Prevention of glomerular basement membrane thickening by aminoguanidine in experimental diabetes mellitus. *Metabolism* 1991; **40**: 1016–19.
79 Kihara M, Schmelzer JD, Poduslo JF, Curran GL, Nickander KK, Low PA. Aminoguanidine effects on nerve blood flow, vascular permeability, electrophysiology and oxygen free radicals. *Proc Natl Acad Sci USA* 1991; **88**: 6107–11.
80 Yagihashi S, Kamijo M, Baba M, Yagihashi N, Nagai K. Effect of aminoguanidine on functional and structural abnormalities in peripheral nerve of STZ-induced diabetic rats. *Diabetes* 1992; **41**: 47–52.

# 4 The Regulation of Microvascular Function in Diabetes Mellitus


**Summary**

• Blood flow through the microcirculation is normally tightly regulated by central neural mechanisms, local reflexes, circulating mediators and locally produced vasoactive substances including nitric oxide (vasodilator) and endothelin (vasoconstrictor).
• Haemodynamic disturbances accompany and precede the natural history of diabetic microangiopathy and may contribute to its pathogenesis.
• Early haemodynamic abnormalities include increased basal blood flow in skin, retina and kidney, together with relatively impaired responses to various hyperaemic stimuli in skin. These abnormalities occur early in IDDM, before evidence of structural microvascular damage appears.
• Haemodynamic disturbances often worsen during puberty or pregnancy, paralleling the tendency of microvascular disease to deteriorate.
• Like microvascular disease, haemodynamic abnormalities are generally related to the duration of diabetes and the degree of hyperglycaemia. Early in the disease, haemodynamic changes may be reversible with tight glycaemic control but later become irreversible.
• Patients with uncomplicated diabetes of long duration often show preserved haemodynamic responses. Microvascular disease may therefore develop specifically in a susceptible subgroup of patients.
• Failure of autoregulation of capillary blood flow, together with a reduction in perfusion which tends to follow a fall in blood glucose levels, may compromise tissue nutrition when diabetic control is suddenly tightened. This may explain the acute deterioration in microvascular disease (the 'glycaemic re-entry' phenomenon) which sometimes occurs at this time.
• Haemodynamic changes, notably increased capillary pressure and flow, could stimulate capillary basement membrane thickening and cause arteriolar sclerosis. These changes could lead to failure of autoregulation, leakage of albumin and ultimately to impaired tissue nutrition.


It is generally accepted that damage to the smallest blood vessels underlies most of the late complications of diabetes but the nature of diabetic microangiopathy is far less certain. Clarification of the disease process depends upon understanding the normal physiology of the microvasculature, which in health is able to balance a series of conflicting demands. Flow must match local metabolic needs, yet pressure must be carefully regulated in order to prevent large shifts of fluid across the capillary endothelium. At the same time, general body functions which depend critically upon blood flow in various vascular beds — such as arterial blood pressure and core temperature — must be tightly controlled. These complicated specifications demand a sophisticated array of local and extrinsic mechanisms controlling flow through the microcirculation.

## Microvascular control systems

### *Extrinsic control*

Blood vessel diameter is regulated by both neural and humoral factors. The degree to which an organ is subject to central neural control is a function of both its metabolic needs and its capacity to withstand circulatory deprivation. Accordingly, the cerebral circulation is under little neurogenic control by comparison with the splanchnic bed. On the other hand, core temperature is largely regulated by the sympathetic nervous control of skin blood flow in the extremities, and arterial pressure by the sympathetic innervation supplying the various vascular beds which determine peripheral vascular resistance.

Receptors exist on the endothelium and vascular smooth muscle cells for a wide variety of peptide and non-peptide neurohumoral mediators, and the distribution of receptors may determine in part the reactivity of a particular vascular bed [1].

### *Intrinsic control mechanisms*

Local systems which affect flow through capillaries by influencing pre- and postcapillary resistance could clearly be important in supplying the tissues' needs while maintaining tissue fluid economy, especially in the face of changing arterial blood pressure. There is considerable evidence that the local accumulation of metabolites may modify local vascular tone and hence blood flow. Furthermore, vascular smooth muscle responds directly to stretch and/or tension by contracting, thereby limiting any imposed increase in pressure or flow [2]. Recent work suggests that the sensor for this process may reside in the endothelial cell [3], although isolated vascular smooth muscle cells also possess this capacity, the so-called 'myogenic response' of Bayliss [4]. It is now firmly established that the vascular endothelium produces vasoactive mediators, notably the vasodilator, endothelium-derived relaxing factor (EDRF, recently identified as nitric oxide [5]) and endothelin, an extremely powerful vasoconstrictor peptide [6], as well as a variety of prostanoids. Endothelin receptors have also recently been identified on retinal capillary pericytes [7], supporting the possibility that these enigmatic cells are involved in vasoconstriction (see Chapter 6).

Local nervous mechanisms may also exist. Stimulation of pain fibres results in the axon reflex responsible for the flare component of Lewis's triple response in the skin [8] and a sympathetic axon reflex has been proposed to explain the precapillary vasoconstriction which accompanies a rise in venular pressure. The latter, the veno-arteriolar response, can be demonstrated in both skin [9] and subcutaneous tissue [10], and probably acts in health as a mechanism preventing oedema [11].

From the above, it is clear that microvascular control depends upon the integrity of the peripheral and central autonomic nervous systems, sensory nerves, vascular smooth muscle, pericytes and endothelium, all of which may be adversely affected by diabetes. The profound haemodynamic disturbances in the microcirculation of various tissues, particularly the kidney, retina and skin, are therefore to be anticipated. Indeed, haemodynamic abnormalities accompany and often precede the natural history of microangiopathy and, although other biochemical, rheological and cellular factors are also undoubtedly involved, haemodynamic factors fulfil several key criteria for a fundamental cause of microvascular disease. These observations are outlined in Table 4.1 and are discussed in more detail below.

## Relationship of haemodynamic changes to microangiopathy

### *Early expression*

To be considered a prime mover, a putative aetiological factor must be present from the outset of diabetes. Early haemodynamic abnormalities have been demonstrated in IDDM patients, including increased basal blood flow in various organs, including the kidney [12], retina [13] and limbs [14]. In the skin, which is accessible to various measurement techniques, haemodynamic disturbances have been characterized in detail. Character-

**Table 4.1.** Evidence suggesting that haemodynamic abnormalities may cause or contribute to diabetic microvascular disease.

*Time-course of haemodynamic abnormalities*:
- Present from early in untreated IDDM (i.e. precede microvascular disease)
- Accelerated progression during puberty (similar to microvascular complications)
- Related to duration of diabetes (similar to microvascular complications)

*Relationship of haemodynamic abnormalities to glycaemic control*:
- Reversible initially with improved metabolic control; poorly reversible in established disease (similar to microvascular disease)
- Consistent with 'glycaemic re-entry' phenomenon

*Evidence for a susceptible subgroup*
(as with microvascular disease)

istically, resting flow is increased [15], particularly in areas with numerous arteriovenous shunts, and probably reflects the increased metabolic rate [16] and the need to dissipate heat in the newly diagnosed patient with uncontrolled IDDM. In addition to high resting values, impaired microvascular responses can be demonstrated within the first year of diabetic life [17]: the time taken to reach the peak of reactive hyperaemia (determined in single capillaries) is prolonged and the veno-arteriolar response is blunted. Even in children with IDDM, the maximum transcutaneous oxygen tension observed after release of ischaemia is reduced in the first few months of the disease [18].

In NIDDM, early expression of haemodynamic abnormalities is difficult to demonstrate because of the uncertain duration of the disease before presentation. NIDDM patients display a spectrum of microvascular haemodynamic defects which may represent the various stages of the evolution of microangiopathy.

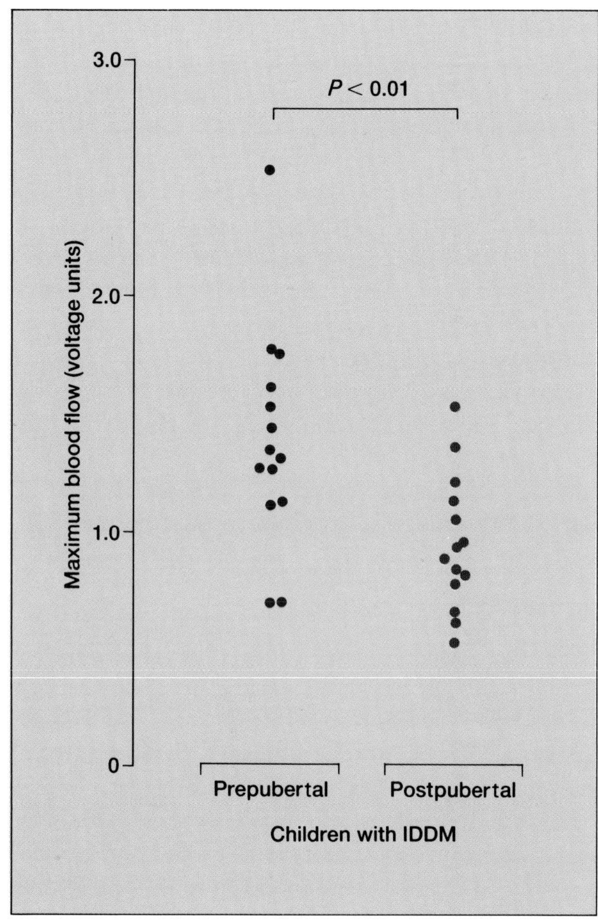


**Fig. 4.1.** Maximum microvascular blood flow values determined by laser Doppler flowmetry on the dorsum of the foot in pre- and postpubertal diabetic children matched for age and duration of IDDM.

### *Acceleration of abnormalities with passage through puberty*

Clinically significant microangiopathic complications are rarely seen before puberty, but the rate of development of retinopathy is faster in the postpubertal years even when corrections are made for the overall duration of diabetes. In animal models, sex hormones and growth factors have been shown to influence the activity of the polyol pathway and the degree of collagen cross-linking [19], which may both be implicated in the development of microangiopathy (see Chapter 3).

Functional haemodynamic abnormalities also progress with passage through puberty, in parallel with the tendency of microvascular disease to deteriorate. Figure 4.1 shows maximum skin microvascular blood flow values in pre- and postpubertal children of similar disease duration. The significant reduction in the postpubertal group cannot be attributed to age differences alone.

### *Relationship to disease duration*

The likelihood of developing microangiopathy rises with increasing disease duration, and abnormalities in microvascular reactivity demonstrate the same relationship. Maximum cutaneous microvascular blood flow falls with increasing disease duration in both children [20] and young adults [21]. Limitation of blood flow which is related to the duration of diabetes may also be demonstrated in the renal [22] and retinal circulations using indirect techniques.

### *Relationship to glycaemic control*

Although protracted hyperglycaemia is a prerequisite, the relationship between the development of microangiopathy and glycaemic control is not direct, and correcting hyperglycaemia does not necessarily reverse the damage. The pattern of microvascular functional impairment exhibits a similar relationship. Relatively early in diabetic life, effective control of diabetes will correct the impairment of maximum transcutaneous oxygen tension [18]. With increasing disease duration, however, the relationship to current diabetic control becomes more tenuous. After 10 years of diabetes, a protracted period (at least 1 year) of 'good' control improves microvascular reactivity in some tissues but not others [17]. Short-term treatment (12 weeks) with an aldose reductase inhibitor in patients of short to moderate disease duration has conferred no apparent benefit on a variety of cutaneous microvascular responses (J.E. Tooke, M. Boolell, unpublished observations).

### *Is there a susceptible subgroup?*

One possible explanation for the lack of a direct relationship between glycaemic control and the development of microangiopathy is that there may exist subsets of patients who are less vulnerable to the effects of sustained hyperglycaemia. Studies of patients who have survived IDDM for more than 40 years without developing nephropathy or significant retinopathy have revealed that microvascular responses which do not depend upon neural integrity are normal in this group, although neurally-dependent mechanisms may be impaired [23]. Maximum cutaneous perfusion capacity is also relatively preserved in patients with uncomplicated disease of long duration [24].

### *Relationship to the 'glycaemic re-entry' phenomenon*

Changes in microvascular reactivity may also provide an explanation for the acute deterioration in microvascular disease sometimes observed when glycaemic control is suddenly and markedly improved, the so-called 'glycaemic re-entry' phenomenon. A characteristic of the diabetic microcirculation after a moderate disease duration is impairment of autoregulation [25–27], i.e. the capacity to maintain constant flow in the face of a changing pressure head. A fall in blood glucose is accompanied by changes in plasma volume, sympathetic nervous activity and endothelial function, all of which may influence capillary pressure and flow if local control systems are impaired. Allied to this is the fact that improved diabetic control inevitably results in more episodes of hypoglycaemia, which not only influence the rheological properties of blood and encourage a prothrombotic tendency [28], but may also cause a transient increase in arterial blood pressure. In the presence of impaired autoregulation, increased systemic pressure may be transmitted to the microvascular bed and so cause tissue damage. Furthermore, in the retina (where nutrient supply is very closely matched to metabolic demand), a sudden reduction in glucose availability may seriously compromise tissue nutrition until adaptive changes can occur.

### *Exacerbation during pregnancy*

A transient but sometimes marked advancement of nephropathy [29] and retinopathy [30] may occur during pregnancy; the physiological changes in microvascular haemodynamics which accompany pregnancy may offer a ready explanation. In normal pregnancy, plasma volume is increased and vascular resistance in the periphery and kidney is reduced, overall causing a rise in peripheral capillary pressure [31]. Similar increases in capillary pressure are seen in women receiving the oral contraceptive pill [32], which may also be associated with an exacerbation of microangiopathy.

## The haemodynamic hypothesis

These compelling data may suggest a primary role for microvascular haemodynamic changes in the pathogenesis of diabetic microangiopathy [33] (Table 4.2). According to this 'haemodynamic' hypothesis, capillary pressure and flow are increased in the relevant tissues, early in the disease. This acts as a stimulus to the basement membrane thickening and arteriolar sclerosis which are characteristic of long-standing diabetes and which, in turn, limit maximum perfusion and the capacity to autoregulate. Several studies have now demonstrated a link between microvascular histological changes and the later functional abnormalities [34, 35].

The central tenet of the hypothesis, that capillary pressure is pathologically raised, has until recently lacked direct experimental proof in humans, although direct micropuncture measurements in diabetic rats have demonstrated elevated glomerular capillary pressures [36]. Recent human studies have shown that nailfold capillary pressure

**Table 4.2.** The 'haemodynamic hypothesis' for the development of diabetic microangiopathy.

| |
|---|
| Increased microvascular pressure and flow |
| ↓ |
| Microvascular sclerosis |
| ↓ |
| Limitation of maximum perfusion |
| ↓ |
| Loss of autoregulation |

is elevated in dependent feet [37] and that complication-prone patients may fail to prevent rises in arterial blood pressure from being transmitted to the capillary bed (Fig. 4.2). Not only is mean capillary pressure increased, but subtle changes in capillary pulse timing and wave-form are demonstrable which may have a bearing on endothelial cell function and transcapillary exchange.

### The relationship between haemodynamic disturbances and other factors involved in the pathogenesis of diabetic microangiopathy

As discussed in Chapters 2 and 3, various biochemical, rheological and other factors are also

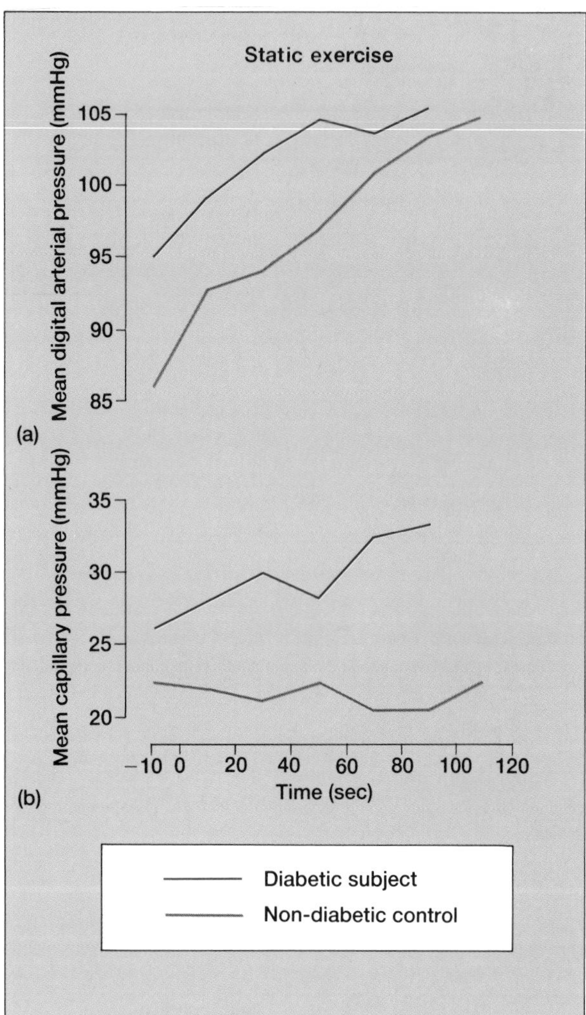


**Fig. 4.2.** Changes in digital arterial pressure (a) and capillary pressure (b) during isometric exercise in a diabetic subject and a matched control. Arterial blood pressure rises in both but only in the diabetic subject is a pressure increment transmitted to the capillary. This is evidence of loss of pressure autoregulation.

convincingly implicated in the development of diabetic microvascular disease. Figure 4.3 represents a possible sequence of events in which microangiopathy results from interactions between these various factors and haemodynamic abnormalities. Initially, precapillary resistance is reduced, increasing flow through the capillary bed. Hyperaggregable red cells are forced to disaggregate as the vessel diameter narrows, resulting in greater tangential stress on the microvascular endothelium. In functional terms, this will result in greater filtration of fluid (for which there is experimental evidence) [38] as well as increased passage, mainly through solvent drag [39], of plasma albumin across the capillary wall. Alterations in endothelial charge characteristics will also facilitate the passage of albumin. Increased tangential stress also stimulates the endothelial cell to release vasodilator compounds such as nitric oxide and prostacyclin and to synthesize basement membrane components. As well as becoming thicker, the chemical composition of the capillary basement membrane will be chemically modified by the glycaemic and humoral environment (see Chapter 3).

In established disease (Fig. 4.4), sclerosis (thickening) of the capillary wall has supervened and effectively limits maximum vasodilation. The endothelium has been denuded, exposing the subintima and allowing the activation and aggregation of platelets. The break in the endothelial barrier further increases permeability, which is not offset by basement membrane thickening as the latter is architecturally distorted and has lost its chemical and electrostatic integrity. The autoregulation of pressure and flow becomes progressively impaired, exposing the microvascular bed to the vagaries of arterial blood pressure. The local 'fine tuning' of precapillary resistance which normally regulates vasomotion and ensures a uniform distribution of blood flow breaks down, causing heterogenous flow [40] and microvascular 'steal' which compromises the capillary supply to the tissues.

### Implications for therapy

Consistent with the haemodynamic hypothesis is the fact that various agents which alter haemodynamic variables can also influence the course of microvascular disease in diabetes and certain other conditions. An important example is the lowering of arterial blood pressure, which has been shown

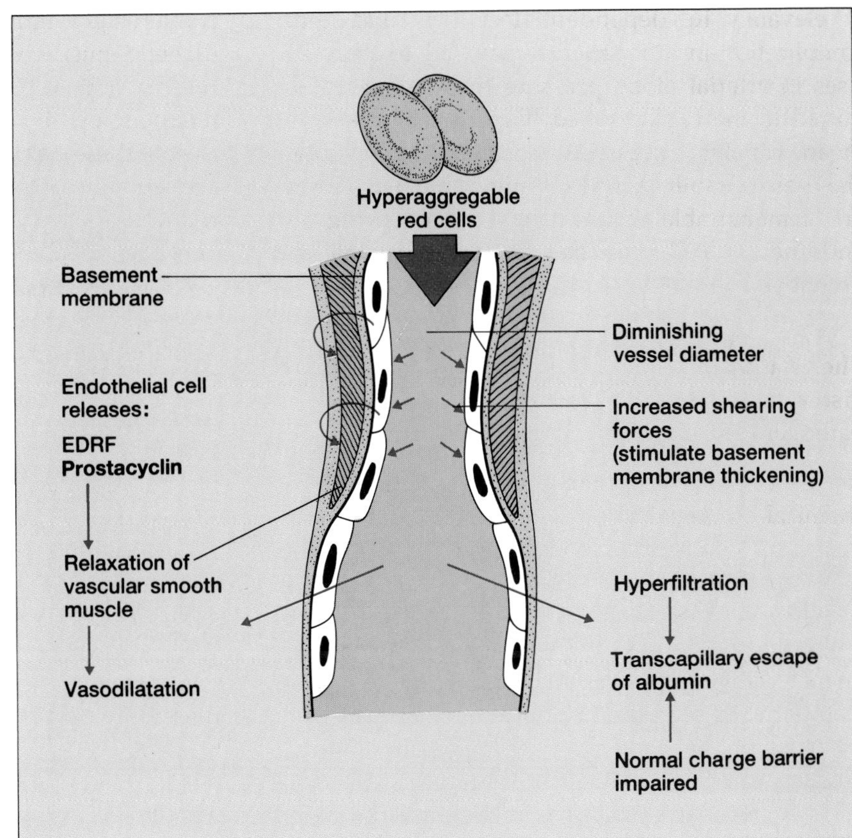


**Fig. 4.3.** Schematic diagram of pathogenic mechanisms which may operate early in diabetic microangiopathy.

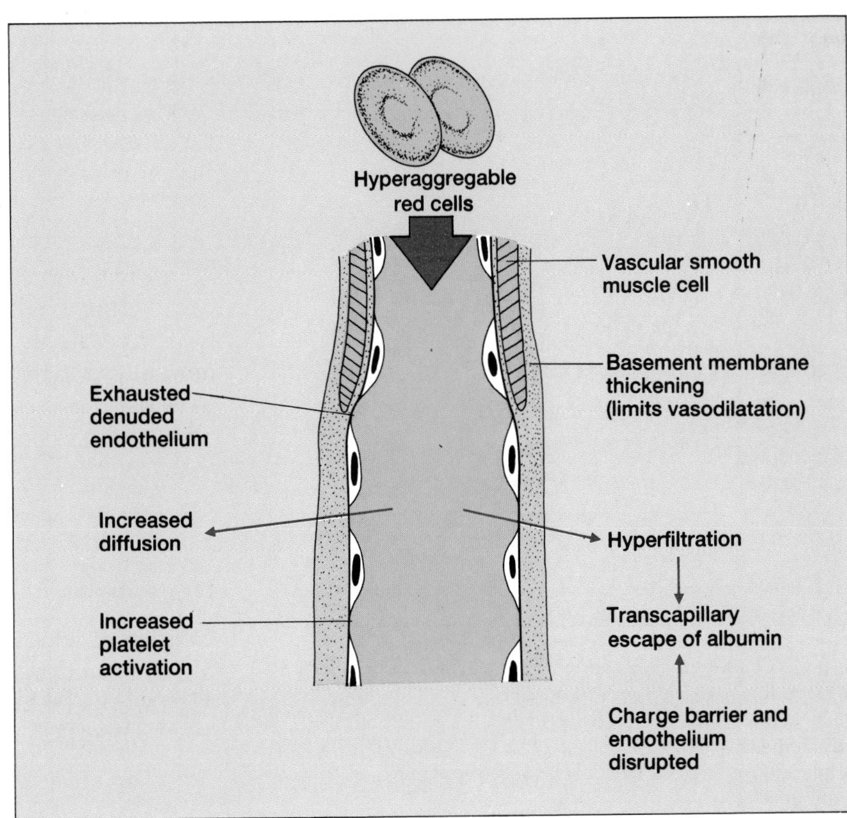


**Fig. 4.4.** Schematic diagram of possible pathogenic mechanisms operating in advanced microangiopathy.

to decrease capillary pressure in patients with essential hypertension [41] and to reduce the abnormally enhanced passage of retinal fluorescein in diabetes [42]. Furthermore, blood pressure regulation is the only strategy that has been demonstrated to slow the progression of a clinical complication of diabetes, namely nephropathy [43] (see Chapters 14 and 16). Insulin may alter the distribution of peripheral blood flow in favour of the capillary bed [44]; theoretically, this may represent a disadvantage during evolving disease but may be a positive advantage in the foot threatened by ischaemia. It may ultimately be possible to manipulate capillary pressure separately from arterial blood pressure by using low doses of certain hypotensive drugs, but at present, the early control of blood glucose — before the development of irreversible impairment of microvascular control mechanisms — is of key importance. In the future, it may become possible to detect subtle microvascular functional changes before the appearance of clinical microangiopathy, or even of the early stage of microalbuminuria. This in turn may enable us to intervene in susceptible subjects at a stage when they may be more responsive to therapy.

JOHN E. TOOKE
ANGELA C. SHORE

## References


1 Vanhoutte PM. Serotonin, adrenergic nerves, endothelial cells and vascular smooth muscle. *Prog Appl Microcirc* 1986; **10**: 1–11.

2 Johansson B. Myogenic tone and reactivity: definitions based on muscle physiology. *J Hypertens* 1989; **7** (suppl 4): 55–8.

3 Harder DR. Pressure-induced myogenic activation of cat cerebral arteries is dependent on intact endothelium. *Circ Res* 1987; **60**: 102–7.

4 Bayliss WM. On the local reactions of the arterial wall to changes of internal pressure. *J Physiol* (Lond) 1902; **28**: 230–41.

5 Furchgott RF. Role of the endothelium in responses of vascular smooth muscle. *Circ Res* 1983; **53**: 557–73.

6 Yanagisawa M, Kurihara H, Kimura S *et al.* A novel potent vasoconstrictor peptide produced by vascular endothelial cells. *Nature* 1988; **332**: 411–15.

7 Takahashi K, Brooks R, Kanse S *et al.* Production of endothelin 1 by cultured bovine retinal endothelial cells and presence of endothelin receptors on associated pericytes. *Diabetes* 1989; **38**: 1200–2.

8 Lewis T. *Blood Vessels of the Human Skin and their Responses.* London: Shaw and Sons, 1927.

9 Rayman G, Hassan AAK, Tooke JE. Blood flow in the skin of the foot related to posture in diabetes mellitus. *Br Med J* 1986; **292**: 87–90.

10 Henriksen O. Local nervous mechanism in regulation of blood flow in human subcutaneous tissue. *Acta Physiol Scand* 1976; **97**: 385–91.

11 Hassan AAK, Tooke JE. The relationship between foot swelling rate and postural vasoconstriction in man. *J Physiol* (Lond) 1987; **387**: 76P.

12 Christiansen JS, Gammelgaard J, Tronier B, Svendsen PAa, Parving H-H. Kidney function and size in diabetes, before and during initial insulin treatment. *Kidney Int* 1982; **21**: 683–8.

13 Kohner EM, Hamilton AM, Saunders SJ, Sutcliffe BA, Bulpitt CJ. The retinal blood flow in diabetes. *Diabetologia* 1975; **11**: 27–33.

14 Gundersen HJG. Peripheral blood flow and metabolic control in juvenile diabetes. *Diabetologia* 1974; **10**: 225–31.

15 Tymms DJ, Tooke JE. The effect of continuous subcutaneous insulin infusion (CSII) on microvascular blood flow in diabetes mellitus. *Int J Microcirc Clin Exp* 1988; **7**: 347–56.

16 Leslie P, Jung RT, Isles TE *et al.* Effect of optimal glycaemic control with subcutaneous insulin infusion on energy expenditure in type 1 diabetes mellitus. *Br Med J* 1986; **293**: 1121–6.

17 Tooke JE, Lins P-E, Østergren J, Fagrell B. Skin microvascular autoregulatory responses in Type I diabetes: the influence of duration and control. *Int J Microcirc Clin Exp* 1985; **4**: 249–56.

18 Kobbah AM, Ewald U, Tuvemo T. Impaired vascular reactivity during the first 2 years of diabetes mellitus after initial restoration. *Acta Universitatis Uppsaliensis*, Doctoral Thesis, 1988.

19 Williamson JR, Chang K, Tilton RG, Kilo C. Sex steroid modulation of vascular leakage and collagen metabolism in diabetic rats. *Pediatr Adolesc Endocr* 1988; **17**: 12–17.

20 Shore AC, Price KS, Tripp JH, Tooke JE. Impaired microvascular hyperaemia in children with diabetes mellitus (abstract). *Clin Sci* 1989; **76** (suppl 20): 15P.

21 Rayman G, Williams SA, Spencer PD *et al.* Impaired microvascular hyperaemic response to minor skin trauma in Type I diabetes. *Br Med J* 1986; **292**: 1295–8.

22 Mogenson CE, Christensen CK, Vittinghus E. The stages in diabetic renal disease. *Diabetes* 1983; **32** (suppl 2): 64–78.

23 Tooke JE, Østergren J, Lins P-E, Fagrell B. Skin microvascular blood flow control in long duration diabetics with and without complications. *Diabetes Res* 1987; **5**: 189–92.

24 Walmsley D, Wales JK, Wiles PG. Reduced hyperaemia following skin trauma: evidence for an impaired microvascular response to injury in the diabetic foot. *Diabetologia* 1989; **32**: 736–9.

25 Grunwald JE, Riva CE, Sinclair SH, Brucker AV. Altered retinal vascular response to 100% $O_2$ breathing in diabetes mellitus (abstract 35). *Microvasc Res* 1983; **25**: 236.

26 Parving H-H, Kastrup H, Smidt UM, Andersen AR, Feldt-Rasmussen BF, Sandahl Christiansen J. Impaired autoregulation of glomerular filtration rate in Type I (insulin dependent) diabetic patients with nephropathy. *Diabetologia* 1984; **27**: 247–552.

27 Faris I, Vagn Nielsen H, Henriksen O, Parving H-H, Lassen NA. Impaired autoregulation of blood flow in skeletal muscle and subcutaneous tissue in long-term Type 1 (insulin-dependent) diabetic patients with microangiopathy. *Diabetologia* 1983; **25**: 486–8.

28 Frier BM, Hilsted J. Does hypoglycaemia aggravate the complications of diabetes? *Lancet* 1985; **ii**: 1174–6.

29 Zitzmiller JL, Brown ER, Phillipe M *et al.* Diabetic nephropathy and perinatal outcome. *Am J Obstet Gynecol* 1981; **141**: 741–6.

30 Phelps RL, Sakol P, Metzger BE *et al*. Changes in diabetic retinopathy during pregnancy: correlations with regulation of hyperglycaemia. *Arch Ophthalmol* 1986; **104**: 1806–10.

31 Tooke JE. The study of human capillary pressure. In: Tooke JE, Smaje LH, eds. *Clinical Investigation of the Microcirculation*. Massachusetts, USA: Martinus Nijhoff, 1987.

32 Tooke JE, Tindall H, McNicol GP. The influence of a combined oral contraceptive pill and menstrual cycle phase on digital microvascular haemodynamics. *Clin Sci* 1981; **61**: 91–5.

33 Henriksen O. Effect of chronic sympathetic denervation upon local regulation of blood flow in human subcutaneous tissue. *Acta Physiol Scand* 1976; **97**: 377–84.

34 Parving H-H, Viberti GC, Keen H, Christiansen JS, Lassen NA. Haemodynamic factors in the genesis of diabetic microangiopathy. *Metabolism* 1983; **32**: 943–9.

35 Rayman G, Malik RA, Metcalfe J *et al*. Relationship between impaired skin microvascular responses to injury and abnormal capillary morphology in the feet of Type I diabetics (abstract). *Diabetic Med* 1989; **6** (suppl 1): 7.

36 Zatz R, Dunn R, Meyer TW *et al*. Prevention of diabetic glomerulopathy by pharmacological amelioration of glomerular capillary hypertension. *J Clin Invest* 1986; **77**: 1925–30.

37 Rayman G, Williams SA, Hassan AAK, Gamble J, Tooke JE. Capillary hypertension and overperfusion in the feet of young diabetics (abstract). *Diabetic Med* 1985; **2**: A30.

38 Parving H-H, Noer I, Deckert T *et al*. The effect of metabolic regulation on microvascular permeability to small and large molecules in short-term juvenile diabetics. *Diabetologia* 1976; **12**: 161–6.

39 Renkin EM. Relation of capillary morphology to transport of fluid and large molecules: a review. *Acta Physiol Scand* 1979; **463**: 81–91.

40 Junger M, Frey-Schnewlin G, Bollinger A. Microvascular flow distribution and transcapillary diffusion at the forefoot in patients with peripheral ischaemia. *Int J Microcirc Clin Exp* 1989; **8**: 3–24.

41 Tooke JE. Microvascular dynamics in diabetes mellitus. *Diabète Métab* 1988; **14**: 530–4.

42 Parving H-H, Larsen M, Hommel E, Lund-Andersen H. Effect of antihypertensive treatment on blood–retinal barrier permeability to fluorescein in hypertensive. Type I (insulin-dependent) diabetic patients with background retinopathy. *Diabetologia* 1989; **32**: 440–4.

43 Parving H-H, Andersen AR, Smidt UM, Svendsen PAa. Early aggressive antihypertensive treatment reduces rate of decline in kidney function in diabetic nephropathy. *Lancet* 1983; **i**: 1175–9.

44 Tooke JE, Lins P-E, Østergren J, Adamson U, Fagrell B. The effects of intravenous insulin infusion on skin microcirculatory flow in Type I diabetes. *Int J Microcirc Clin Exp* 1985; **4**: 69–83.

# PART 2
# DIABETIC EYE DISEASE

# 5 The Epidemiology of Diabetic Retinopathy

**Summary**

- The *prevalence* of retinopathy (of any degree) is highest in young-onset, insulin-treated diabetic patients and lowest in older-onset diabetic patients not taking insulin.
- The prevalence of retinopathy increases with duration of diabetes. In young-onset, insulin-treated diabetic patients, proliferative retinopathy is generally absent below 5 years' duration of diabetes and present in about 25% at 15 years and over 50% at 20 years of diabetes. In older-onset diabetic patients, retinopathy can be present in the first few years of diabetes (about 3–4% for proliferative retinopathy) but the prevalence is lower than in young-onset diabetic patients after 15 or more years (about 15–20%).
- Macular oedema is also associated with increasing duration of diabetes. It is commoner in older-onset diabetic patients, particularly in the first few years after diagnosis.
- The *incidence* of retinopathy is highest in younger-onset patients.
- In younger-onset patients, the incidence of proliferative retinopathy is close to zero with less than 5 years' duration of disease. The 4-year incidence of proliferative retinopathy rises to 28% after 13–14 years of diabetes and is stable at 14–16% after 15 years.
- In older-onset patients, the 4-year incidence of proliferative retinopathy is 2–3%, even in those with disease of short duration (2 years or less).
- These findings suggest that full ophthalmological examination should be carried out at the time of diagnosis and at least annually thereafter in patients diagnosed after 30 years of age. In those diagnosed diabetic before this age, examination should be performed at least annually after 5–9 years of diabetes.

Epidemiological data are essential for estimating the frequency, severity, development and progression of diabetic retinopathy in a given population. Such data are also needed in order to predict the demand for medical counselling and rehabilitative services, for developing screening programmes, for projecting costs, and for measuring temporal trends. Moreover, causal and risk factors may be identified, raising the possibility that such factors might be modified to ameliorate or prevent diabetic retinopathy.

Data on the frequency and incidence of diabetic retinopathy have come from specialized clinics for diabetes [1, 2] or eye disease [3], hospitals [4] and clinical trials [5]. Unfortunately, data from many of these studies cannot be extrapolated to a larger unselected population of diabetic patients. Other factors such as intervention, failure to use standardized protocols, inconsistent follow-up times and inadequate documentation of the retinopathy further limit the use of such data. For these reasons, the present description of prevalence and incidence of diabetic retinopathy is focused on a population-based study, the Wisconsin Epidemiologic Study of Diabetic Retinopathy (WESDR), which used grading of photographs to determine objectively the presence and severity of retinopathy [6–9].

## Incidence and progression

Few population-based data exist which describe

**Table 5.1.** Selected list of population-based studies describing the prevalence and/or incidence of diabetic retinopathy.

| Author | Reference | Site | Type of diabetes | Duration of diabetes (y) | Retinopathy detection* | Crude prevalence (%) | Crude incidence |
|---|---|---|---|---|---|---|---|
| Nilsson *et al.* | 10 | Kristianstad, Sweden | — | 0–16+ | O | 35 | — |
| Dorf *et al.* | 11 | Pima Indians Arizona, USA | II | 0–10+ | O | 18 | — |
| Leibowitz *et al.* | 12 | Framingham Massachusetts, USA | II | — | O | 20 | — |
| West *et al.* | 13 | Oklahoma Indians, USA | II | — | O | — | — |
| Houston | 14 | Poole, England | I & II | 0–30+ | O, P | Not reported | — |
| King *et al.* | 15 | Nauru, Central Pacific | II | 0–10+ | O | 24 | — |
| Dwyer *et al.* | 16 | Rochester, Minnesota USA | I | — | — | — | 45.8/1000 person-y |
| | | | II | — | O | — | 15.6/1000 person-y |
| Sjolie | 17 | County of Fynn, Denmark | I | 0–30+ | O | 47.7 | ? |
| Nielsen | 18, 19 | Falster, Denmark | I | 0–58 | P | 66.3 | 1 y = 3.7% |
| | | | II | 0–42 | P | 40.9 | 1 y = 3.7% |
| Teuscher *et al.* | 20 | Switzerland | I | 0–30+ | O | 51 | 8 y = 39% |
| | | | II | | | 9 | 8 y = 19% |

* O: ophthalmoscopy; P: photography; I: IDDM; II: NIDDM.

**Table 5.2.** Prevalence and severity of retinopathy by sex (Wisconsin Epidemiologic Study of Diabetic Retinopathy).

| | Younger-onset taking insulin | | | Older-onset taking insulin | | | Older-onset not taking insulin | | |
|---|---|---|---|---|---|---|---|---|---|
| Retinopathy status | Male (%) ($n = 512$) | Female (%) ($n = 484$) | Total (%) ($n = 996$) | Male (%) ($n = 321$) | Female (%) ($n = 352$) | Total (%) ($n = 673$) | Male (%) ($n = 313$) | Female (%) ($n = 379$) | Total (%) ($n = 692$) |
| None | 31.1 | 27.5 | 29.3 | 26.8 | 32.7 | 29.9 | 64.5 | 58.6 | 61.3 |
| Early non-proliferative | 26.4 | 34.7 | 30.4 | 34.0 | 27.6 | 30.6 | 25.9 | 28.5 | 27.3 |
| Moderate to severe non-proliferative | 18.2 | 16.9 | 17.6 | 27.7 | 23.9 | 25.7 | 6.4 | 10.3 | 8.5 |
| Proliferative — without DRS high-risk characteristics | 12.3 | 14.0 | 13.2 | 8.1 | 9.9 | 9.1 | 1.9 | 1.1 | 1.4 |
| Proliferative — with DRS high-risk characteristics or worse | 12.1 | 6.8 | 9.5 | 3.4 | 6.0 | 4.8 | 1.3 | 1.6 | 1.4 |

DRS: Diabetic Retinopathy Study [23].

the prevalence and/or incidence of diabetic retinopathy [6–20]. Some recent and continuing studies of retinopathy are listed in Table 5.1, together with their method of detecting retinopathy, and their reported crude rates of prevalence and incidence of diabetic retinopathy. Caution must be observed in attempting to compare studies, because of the differences in the populations and the methods used to detect retinopathy (for example, direct ophthalmoscopy versus grading of stereoscopic colour photographs of standard retinal fields).

In the WESDR, a large population of diabetic persons living and receiving their primary medical care in an 11-county area of south-western Wisconsin was identified in 1979–1980. The population, consisting of all younger-onset, insulin-taking diabetic persons diagnosed before 30 years of age ($n = 996$) and a probability sample of older-onset diabetic persons taking insulin ($n = 673$) and not taking insulin ($n = 692$), diagnosed at or after 30 years of age, was first examined in 1980–1982 and again 4 years later. At both examinations, the presence and severity of diabetic retinopathy was identified by masked grading of stereoscopic colour fundus photographs using modifications of the Wisconsin '191' system and the Airlie House classification system [3].

### *Prevalence*

Prevalence rates of retinopathy in different populations are shown in Table 5.1. In the WESDR baseline examination, the highest rates of prevalence of any degree or of severe retinopathy were found in the younger-onset, insulin-taking group; the lowest rates were found in the older-onset group not taking insulin (Table 5.2) [6, 7]. The relationship of the prevalence of any or proliferative retinopathy to the duration of diabetes is shown in Figs 5.1 and 5.2.

For the younger-onset group, the prevalence of any retinopathy varied from 2% in persons with fewer than 2 years of diabetes to 98% in persons with 15 or more years of disease. The prevalence of proliferative retinopathy varied from 0 in persons with fewer than 5 years of disease to 26% in patients with 15–16 years, and to 56% in those with 20 or more years of disease. The lower prevalence of proliferative retinopathy after 35 years of diabetes (Fig. 5.1) was most likely due to the higher mortality in this group as well as to a decreased progression to proliferative retinopathy after 19 years of disease.

In the older-onset groups, the prevalence of diabetic retinopathy was also positively associated with duration of diabetes [7]. During the first 2 years of diabetes, higher rates of retinopathy (23% in those taking insulin and 20% in those not taking insulin) were found in the older-onset groups compared with the younger-onset group (2%). The higher rates in the older-onset group probably reflect the difficulty of accurately determining the actual onset of disease in these persons; they might also be due to increased sensitivity of retinal tissue to the diabetic process in older people. Four per cent of older-onset persons taking insulin and 3% of those not taking insulin, who had a history of diabetes of 4 years or less, had proliferative retinopathy. The prevalence of any retinopathy or of proliferative retinopathy was significantly lower in older-onset people compared

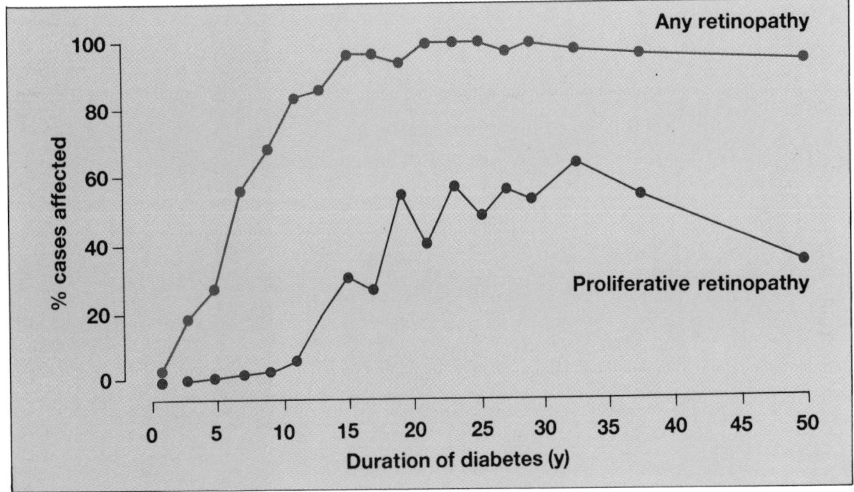


**Fig. 5.1.** Frequency of retinopathy (any degree) or proliferative retinopathy by duration of diabetes (in years) in persons taking insulin who were diagnosed as diabetic before 30 years of age and who participated in the Wisconsin Epidemiologic Study of Diabetic Retinopathy, 1980–1982. (Redrawn from [6]. Reproduced by permission of the American Medical Association.)

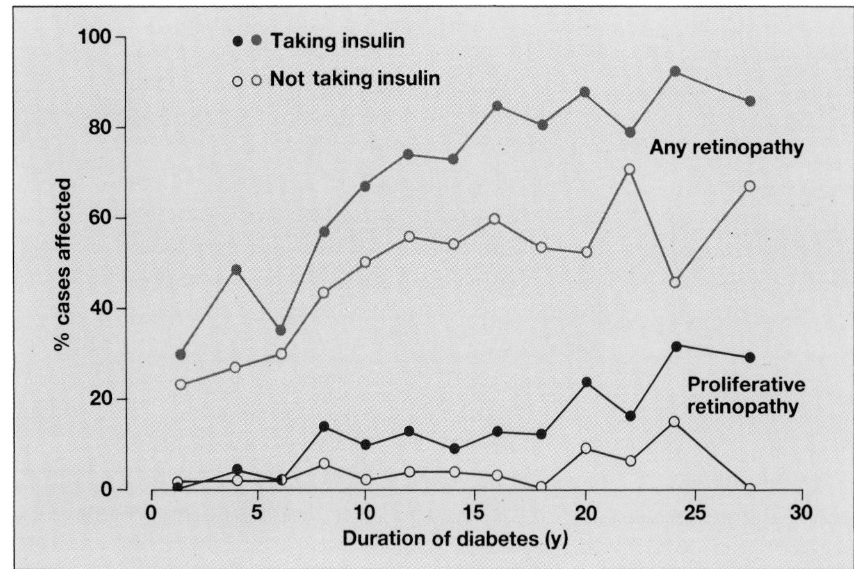


**Fig. 5.2.** Frequency of retinopathy (any degree) or proliferative retinopathy by duration of diabetes (in years) in persons receiving or not receiving insulin who were diagnosed to have diabetes at or after 30 years of age. (Redrawn from [7]. Reproduced by permission of the American Medical Association.)

with younger-onset patients with 15 or more years of diabetes (Figs 5.1 and 5.2).

Clinically significant macular oedema (defined as the presence of any one of the following: thickening of the retina located 500 µm or less from the centre of the macula; hard exudates with thickening of the adjacent retina, 500 µm or less from the centre of the macula; or a zone of retinal thickening one disc area or larger in size, located one disc diameter or less from the centre of the macula) [21] was also found to be significantly associated with increasing duration of diabetes in all three groups in the WESDR (Fig. 5.3). The prevalence of clinically significant macular oedema was consistently higher in older-onset patients taking insulin. In comparison with younger-onset diabetic patients, macular oedema was found to be present more frequently in older-onset people during the first few years after diagnosis of the disease. In addition, visual acuity was worse in older-onset persons as compared with younger-onset subjects when macular oedema was present [22].

## Incidence and practical guidelines for ophthalmological care

The 4-year incidence rates and rates of progression of retinopathy for the three groups are reported in Table 5.3. Incidence rates were highest for the younger-onset group taking insulin (59%) and lowest for the older-onset group not taking insulin (34%). There was no significant difference between the males and females.

Information on the relationship of incidence to the duration of diabetes is of importance in determining guidelines for ophthalmological care. Because proliferative diabetic retinopathy is often

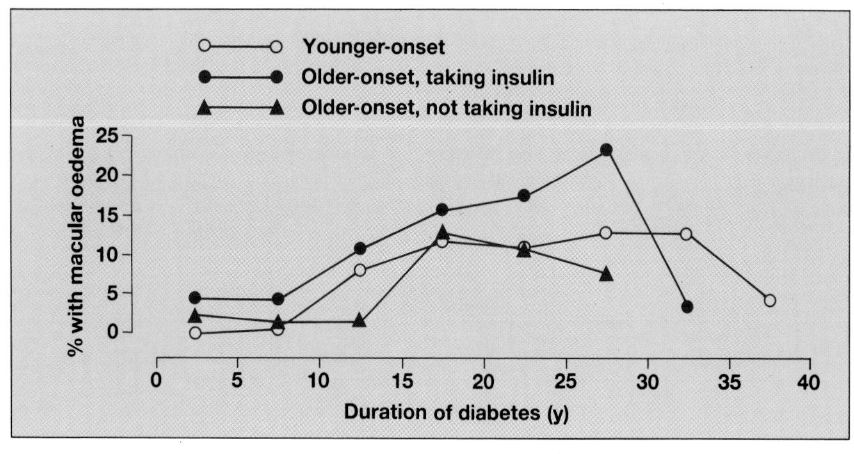


**Fig. 5.3.** Frequency of clinically significant macular oedema (CSME, as defined in the Early Treatment Diabetic Retinopathy Study) by duration of diabetes in younger-onset persons taking insulin ($n$ = 996) and older-onset persons taking insulin ($n$ = 674) or not taking insulin ($n$ = 696) who participated in the Wisconsin Epidemiologic Study of Diabetic Retinopathy (WESDR), 1980–1982 [21].

**Table 5.3.** Four-year incidence of retinopathy or progression to proliferative retinopathy by sex (from the WESDR).

| Diabetic group | No. at risk | Incidence (%) | No. at risk | Progression to proliferative retinopathy (%) |
|---|---|---|---|---|
| Younger-onset, taking insulin | | | | |
| Male | 143 | 56 | 354 | 11 |
| Female | 128 | 63 | 359 | 10 |
| Total | 271 | 59 | 713 | 11 |
| Older-onset, taking insulin | | | | |
| Male | 62 | 47 | 193 | 7 |
| Female | 92 | 48 | 225 | 8 |
| Total | 154 | 47 | 418 | 7 |
| Older-onset, not taking insulin | | | | |
| Male | 151 | 32 | 216 | 3 |
| Female | 169 | 36 | 270 | 2 |
| Total | 320 | 34 | 486 | 2 |

asymptomatic and difficult to detect accurately by non-specialists, and because pan-retinal photocoagulation treatment has been proven to be effective in preventing visual loss, it is important to be aware of the best time to refer diabetic patients to ophthalmologists [23]. The relationship of incidence of any retinopathy and progression to proliferative retinopathy to the duration of diabetes in the WESDR population is presented in Figs 5.4 and 5.5. None of the younger-onset, insulin-taking participants in the study who had less than 5 years duration at the baseline examination developed proliferative diabetic retinopathy over the 4-year follow-up period. Thereafter, the incidence of proliferative retinopathy rose from 0.6% in younger-onset persons with 5–6 years of diabetes at the baseline examination to 27.9% in persons with 13–14 years of diabetes; after 15 or more years of diabetes, the incidence of proliferative retinopathy remained stable at 14–16%. For older-onset patients not taking insulin, some cases of proliferative retinopathy were found even in those with fewer than 2 years of diabetes at the baseline examination. Because of the possibility of developing proliferative retinopathy shortly after diagnosis of diabetes in this group, current guidelines for ophthalmological care for diabetic retino-

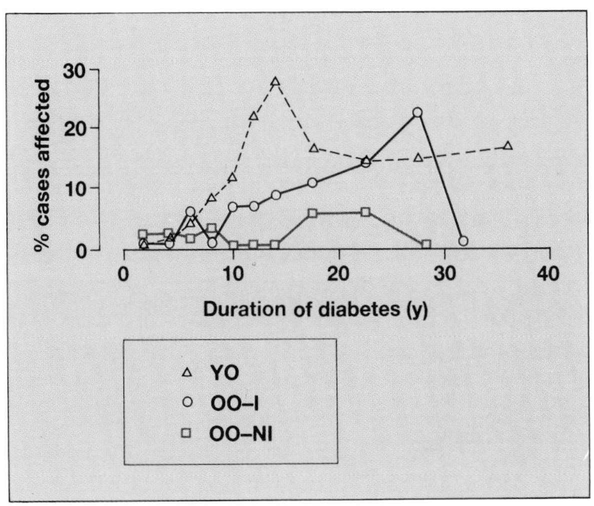


**Fig. 5.5.** Four-year incidence of proliferative retinopathy by duration of diabetes (in years) in younger-onset persons (YO, $n = 713$), and older-onset persons taking insulin (OO–I, $n = 418$) or not taking insulin (OO–NI, $n = 486$) who participated in both baseline and follow-up examinations of the WESDR.

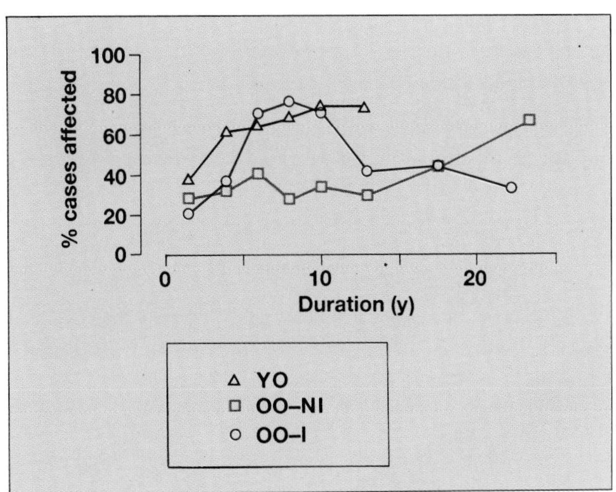


**Fig. 5.4.** Four-year incidence of any retinopathy by duration of diabetes in persons taking insulin who were diagnosed as diabetic before 30 years of age (YO, $n = 271$) and older-onset persons taking insulin (OO–I, $n = 154$) or not taking insulin (OO–NI, $n = 320$) who participated in both baseline and follow-up examinations of the WESDR.

pathy should include careful ophthalmological examination at the time of diagnosis for *all* older-onset diabetic persons (i.e. those diagnosed after 30 years of age) followed by regular yearly (or more frequent) review, as determined by the findings on examination. The WESDR data suggest the need for careful ophthalmological examinations for younger-onset persons 5–9 years after the diagnosis of diabetes. After 10 years of diabetes, because of the increased incidence of proliferative diabetic retinopathy and clinically significant macular oedema, younger-onset patients should be examined on a yearly basis or more often, depending on the severity of the retinopathy present [24].

While incidence rates are significantly higher in the younger than the older-onset diabetic groups in the WESDR, the estimated number of incident cases of proliferative retinopathy (and of severe proliferative retinopathy with high risk for visual loss to 5/200 or worse) over a 4-year period is higher in the older compared with the younger-onset diabetic group (120 versus 83, estimated or a total population of persons living in the 11-county area of 839 000 in south-western Wisconsin). These data suggest that a greater burden will be imposed on the health care delivery system by the treatment of ocular complications developing in older-onset diabetic persons.

## Ophthalmological care in the WESDR

The WESDR also provided an opportunity to evaluate ophthalmological care in the population [23]. In the WESDR, 22% of younger-onset diabetic people and 40% of older-onset diabetic patients had not seen an ophthalmologist. In addition, 11% of younger and 7% of older-onset people with high-risk characteristics for severe visual loss (as defined by the Diabetic Retinopathy Study) had never been seen by an ophthalmologist or were seen more than 2 years before the time of the study. These data suggest the need for further education of diabetic patients about the importance of periodic examinations by those experienced in evaluating the retina, and referral to retinal specialists or ophthalmologists interested in retinal disease, of all those individuals found to have either severe non-proliferative retinopathy, proliferative retinopathy and/or macular oedema, or decreased vision not correctable by refraction. This is important because patients with severe retinopathy are often asymptomatic and timely treatment with pan-retinal photocoagulation and/or focal photocoagulation may prevent visual loss.

RONALD R. KLEIN

## References


1 Pirart J. Diabetes mellitus and its degenerative complications: A prospective study of 4400 patients observed between 1947 and 1973. *Diabetes Care* 1978; **1**: 168–88.

2 Krolewski AS, Warram JH, Rand LI *et al*. Risk of proliferative diabetic retinopathy in juvenile-onset Type I diabetes: A 40-year follow-up study. *Diabetes Care* 1986; **9**: 443–52.

3 Klein BEK, Davis MD, Segal P *et al*. Diabetic retinopathy: Assessment of severity and progression. *Ophthalmology* 1984; **91**: 10–17.

4 Miki E, Fukuda M, Kuzuya T *et al*. Relation of the course of retinopathy to control of diabetes, age, and therapeutic agents in diabetic Japanese patients. *Diabetes* 1969; **18**: 773–80.

5 University Group Diabetes Program. A study of the effects of hypoglycemic agents on vascular complications in patients with adult-onset diabetes. *Diabetes* 1982; **5** (suppl 31): 1–81.

6 Klein R, Klein BEK, Moss SE *et al*. The Wisconsin Epidemiologic Study of Diabetic Retinopathy: II. Prevalence and risk of diabetic retinopathy when age at diagnosis is less than 30 years. *Arch Ophthalmol* 1984; **102**: 520–6.

7 Klein R, Klein BEK, Moss SE *et al*. Wisconsin Epidemiologic Study of Diabetic Retinopathy: III. Prevalence and risk of diabetic retinopathy when age at diagnosis is 30 or more years. *Arch Ophthalmol* 1984; **102**: 527–32.

8 Klein R, Klein BEK, Moss SE *et al*. The Wisconsin Epidemiologic Study of Diabetic Retinopathy: IX. Four-year incidence and progression of diabetic retinopathy when age at diagnosis is less than 30 years. *Arch Ophthalmol* 1989; **107**: 237–43.

9 Klein R, Klein BEK *et al*. The Wisconsin Epidemiologic Study of Diabetic Retinopathy: X. Four-year incidence and progression of diabetic retinopathy when age at diagnosis is 30 or more years. *Arch Ophthalmol* 1989; **107**: 244–9.

10 Nilsson SE, Nilsson JE, Frostberg N *et al*. The Kristianstad Survey II. *Acta Med Scand* 1967; **469** (suppl): 1–42.

11 Dorf A, Ballintine EJ, Bennett PH *et al*. Retinopathy in Pima Indians. Relationships to glucose level, duration of diabetes, age at diagnosis of diabetes, and age of examination in a population with a high prevalence of diabetes mellitus. *Diabetes* 1976; **25**: 554–60.

12 Leibowitz HM, Krueger DE, Maunder LR *et al*. The Framingham Eye Study monograph. *Survey Ophthalmol* 1980; **24**: 335–610.

13 West KM, Erdreich LJ, Stober JA *et al*. A detailed study of risk factors for retinopathy and nephropathy in diabetes. *Diabetes* 1980; **19**: 501–8.

14 Houston A. Retinopathy in the Poole area: An epidemiological inquiry. In: Eschwege E, ed. *Advances in Diabetes Epidemiology. INSERM Symposium No 22*. Amsterdam: Elsevier Biomedical Press, 1982: 199–206.

15 King H, Balkau B, Zimmet P *et al*. Diabetic retinopathy in Nauruans. *Am J Epidemiol* 1983; **117**: 659–67.

16 Dwyer MS, Melton LJ, Ballard DJ *et al*. Incidence of diabetic retinopathy and blindness: A population-based study in Rochester, Minnesota. *Diabetes Care* 1985; **8**: 316–22.

17 Sjolie AK. Ocular complications in insulin treated diabetes mellitus. An epidemiological study. *Acta Ophthalmol* 1985;

**172** (suppl): 1–72.

18 Nielsen NV. Diabetic retinopathy. I. The course of retinopathy in insulin-treated diabetics. A one-year epidemiological cohort study of diabetes mellitus. The Island of Falster, Denmark. *Acta Ophthalmol* 1984; **62**: 256–65.

19 Nielsen NV. Diabetic retinopathy. II. The course of retinopathy in diabetics treated with oral hypoglycaemic agents and diet regime alone. A one-year epidemiological cohort study of diabetes mellitus. The Island of Falster, Denmark. *Acta Ophthalmol* 1984; **62**: 266–73.

20 Teuscher A, Schnell H, Wilson PWF *et al*. Incidence of diabetic retinopathy and relationship to baseline plasma glucose and blood pressure. *Diabetes Care* 1988; **11**: 246–51.

21 Early Treatment Diabetic Retinopathy Study Research Group. Photocoagulation of diabetic macular edema. *Arch Ophthalmol* 1985; **103**: 1796–1806.

22 Klein R, Klein BEK, Moss SE *et al*. The Wisconsin Epidemiologic Study of Diabetic Retinopathy. IV. Diabetic macular edema. *Ophthalmology* 1984; **91**: 1464–74.

23 Diabetic Retinopathy Study Group. Photocoagulation treatment of proliferative diabetic retinopathy: clinical application of Diabetic Retinopathy Study (DRS) findings (DRS Report No 8). *Ophthalmology* 1981; **88**: 583–600.

24 Klein R, Moss SE, Klein BEK. New management concepts for timely diagnosis of diabetic retinopathy treatable by photocoagulation. *Diabetes Care* 1987; **10**: 633–8.

25 Witkin SR, Klein R. Ophthalmologic care for persons with diabetes. *J Am Med Ass* 1984; **251**: 2534–7.

# 6 The Pathogenesis of Diabetic Retinopathy and Cataract


**Summary**

• The earliest lesions of diabetic retinopathy, detectable histologically, are thickening of the capillary basement membrane and loss of pericytes which may have a contractile function.
• Capillary dilatation is the first abnormality recognizable on fluorescein angiography and is probably partly functional (secondary to increased retinal blood flow) and partly due to true anatomical widening of the vessel; dilatation is most marked in areas of pericyte fallout. Microaneurysms are localized capillary dilatations; they may give rise to haemorrhages or exudates.
• Capillary leakage of plasma lipids and proteins is probably due to a functional increase in permeability across the cells in early stages. Interruption of the tight junctions may occur later.
• Increased polyol pathway activity in pericytes (which contain aldose reductase, the pathway's rate-limiting enzyme) generates sorbitol under hyperglycaemic conditions. Accumulation of sorbitol, or of other polyols in galactosaemic animals, is associated with basement membrane thickening and pericyte loss; associated abnormalities such as myoinositol depletion and reduced $Na^+-K^+-$ATPase activity may also contribute.
• Aldose reductase inhibitors can prevent certain early features of galactosaemic retinopathy in animals but so far have no proven benefit in man, possibly because treatment is not started early enough in the course of retinopathy.
• Vascular occlusion, initially of capillaries and later of arteries and veins, leads to nonperfusion of areas of retina. Large ischaemic areas are the stimulus to new vessel formation. Vascular occlusion may be due to microthrombi; the possible contributions of increased platelet aggregability, coagulation factor activity and endothelial damage are uncertain. Treatment with drugs which prevent platelet aggregation has only a small beneficial effect in reducing microaneurysm formation.
• Neovascularization begins with dissolution of extracellular matrix and proliferation of vascular cells into a solid cord which later canalizes. New vessel growth may be stimulated by factors such as retina-derived growth factor (fibroblast growth factor) which is produced locally, and insulin-like growth factor-1 (IGF-1) which is produced in the liver under the influence of growth hormone. Various factors which inhibit neovascularization are also released by the retina.
• Retinal blood flow is increased in untreated or poorly controlled diabetes and may damage endothelial cells. Retinal blood flow is reduced by correcting hyperglycaemia; an acute and profound glycaemic fall may cause retinal ischaemia and a deterioration in retinopathy.
• The presence of diabetes accelerates the development of senile cataracts, by two- to three-fold in patients in their 50s and 60s. 'Juvenile' cataracts with a snowflake appearance may be precipitated acutely by a period of poor metabolic control.
• The maintenance of lens shape and transparency depends on active metabolism by the lens epithelium, which contains aldose reductase and therefore accumulates sorbitol

under high glucose concentrations. Sorbitol accumulation, myoinositol depletion or other associated factors may contribute to cataract formation.

• Non-enzymatic glycation of the lens protein, crystallin, could also interfere with light transmission by forming disulphide-linked aggregates.

Diabetic retinopathy is a long-term sequel or complication of diabetes. While the exact cause of the abnormalities seen is not known, in recent years a considerable amount of work has been done to unravel the sequence of events which finally lead to sight-threatening forms of the disease. The three principal abnormalities are capillary occlusion, leakage (usually associated with vascular dilatation), and finally new vessel formation. This last event only occurs when, in addition to the capillaries, larger vessels, both arteries and veins, are also occluded. When considering pathogenic mechanisms in the evolution of diabetic retinopathy, these three steps, which are not independent from one another, have to be explained.

**Structure of the capillary wall**

Throughout the vascular network, the capillaries have two types of cells in their wall, endothelial cells and pericytes. In most tissues the number of endothelial cells is far larger than that of the pericytes, and only in the retina is there a one-to-one relationship between the two. This is important because it has been shown that, the higher the number of pericytes in relation to the number of endothelial cells, the slower is the turnover of the cells under normal conditions [1]. The endothelial cells in the retina are also different from other vascular cells in the body (with the exception of the brain endothelial cells) in that they have tight junctions between adjacent cells, *zonae occludentes*, which under normal circumstances prevent leakage of certain substances such as sodium fluorescein and horseradish peroxidase from the intravascular to the extravascular space.

The endothelial cells have many functions, and these have recently been surveyed by Petty and Pearson [2]. They include both thrombotic and anticoagulant, fibrinolytic, antiplatelet and immunological properties, secretion of basement membrane, production of growth factors and vasoactive properties. In addition, the cells, together with the basement membrane, are responsible for the permeability of the capillaries.

The function of the pericytes is less clear. In the 1960s, Cogan and Kuwabara developed the technique of the retinal digest preparation [3]. This enabled the study of the vasculature of the retina without interference from neuronal elements. These authors noted the selective loss of pericytes in the diabetic retina [4], and observed a number of other changes, such as dilatation of some capillaries, while others lost their endothelial cells and became simple basement membrane tubes. Earlier work by Ashton [5] using Indian ink injection, showed that there were large areas of non-perfused retina in diabetes, these areas being the acellular capillaries demonstrated by Cogan and Kuwabara. Because of the changes noted, in particular the dilatation of some capillaries without pericytes in their wall, Cogan and Kuwabara suggested that the pericytes may have a muscle cell-like action on the capillaries, controlling their diameter. They also suggested that some capillaries may become occluded because these dilated vessels act as shunt vessels, diverting blood away from the capillaries. Kohner *et al.* [6] demonstrated that only rarely did dilated vessels act as true shunts, in the sense of high-flow, low-resistance channels. However, recent work supports the muscle cell-like activity of pericytes. In most vascular systems, smooth muscles control vascular tone. In the retinal vessels, there are relatively few muscle cells. Endothelin, a recently isolated vasoactive peptide [7], is secreted by endothelial cells and acts on smooth muscle cells causing vascular constriction. Though initially thought to be absent in brain, and by inference in retinal vessels [8], this has not subsequently proved to be the case. The Hammersmith Hospital group found that bovine retinal endothelial cells, but not pericytes, secreted endothelin *in vitro* and that the receptors normally found on smooth muscle cells were on pericytes [9]. Thus, pericytes may well control small vessel tone in the retina.

The controlling role of the pericytes on endothelial cells was demonstrated in elegant co-culture studies by Orlidge and D'Amore [10]. These workers were able to demonstrate that pericytes and smooth muscle cells grown in co-cultures allowing cell-to-cell contact with endothelial cells inhibited endothelial cell growth and multiplication. In the absence of contact, but with free access of diffusible factors, this inhibition was absent. Other cells such as epithelial cells, fibroblasts and 3T3 cells did not have this effect. Further work by the same group identified the inhibiting factor as activated transforming growth factor β (TGF-β). Purified antibodies to TGF-β added to the co-culture abolished the inhibitory effect on cell growth [11]. We still do not know whether the TGF-β is produced by the endothelial cells and then activated by the pericytes, or whether pericytes produce TGF-β.

This recent work indicates why the capillaries could become abnormal when pericytes are lost. The exact cause of the pericyte damage, and indeed of the damage to endothelial cells, has not been fully established.

### Metabolic causes of damage to endothelial cells and pericytes

Since pericyte loss is the earliest abnormality seen in histological preparations of the diabetic retina (with perhaps the exception of basement membrane thickening), it is important to explain this abnormality. Until recently, there were no good explanations, but in 1977 Buzney *et al.* demonstrated in cell culture work the presence of the polyol pathway in pericytes [12]. In 1984, Engerman and Kern [13] reported that dogs fed a high galactose diet developed a diabetic-like retinopathy, consisting of pericyte loss, microaneurysms and acellular capillaries. In galactosaemia, the galactose is converted by aldose reductase to dulcitol. This substance then accumulates in cells which contain aldose reductase. This finding led to a large amount of work by many investigators, mainly those of the National Eye Institute and the St Louis group. Williamson's group, in elegant studies, showed that thickening of basement membrane in both BB and streptozotocin-induced diabetic rats could be inhibited by aldose reductase inhibitors [14]. Increased basement membrane production is probably more related to an endothelial cell abnormality than abnormal pericyte function, but Li *et al.* [15] showed in cell culture work of bovine retinal pericytes, that in high glucose medium more basement membrane collagen was produced. Williamson's group [16] also showed decreased degradation of Type IV collagen in basement membrane in renal glomeruli of diabetic rats. The fact that rats fed a galactose-rich diet develop increased basement membrane thickening and that this can be prevented by aldose reductase inhibitors has been shown by various observers [17–19]. It again suggests that the basement membrane excess comes from pericytes rather than endothelial cells, as there is no evidence that the polyol pathway plays an important role in the endothelial cells. Although most workers have not found aldose reductase in endothelial cells of the retina, a notable exception is the work of Chakrabati *et al.* [20] who found aldose reductase in the retinal endothelial cells of BB rats.

Kinoshita's group has shown recently that there is not only basement membrane thickening in galactosaemic rats, but also formation of microaneurysms, and this too is prevented by aldose reductase inhibitors [21]. Kador *et al.* have performed most interesting experiments; they used galactosaemic dogs, and randomly allocated them to galactose only or to galactose and an aldose reductase inhibitor. They found that microaneurysms were seen after 3–6 months in those on the high galactose diet, but this was prevented by aldose reductase inhibitors. In particular, they noted that pericyte loss did not occur in the first several months in animals fed with the inhibitors as well as the high galactose. However, at 32 months high galactose feeding resulted in at least some microaneurysms, even in those on aldose reductase inhibitors [22]. Unfortunately, the experiments were not continued after 36 months, and therefore the long-term effect of aldose reductase inhibitors cannot be certain, even in the galactosaemic animals. Engerman, whose experiments were of longer duration, and who also studied diabetic animals receiving aldose reductase inhibitors, did not find the dramatic effects seen by Kador [23]. It appears that most of the lesions only appear after about 42 months. In addition, human studies with the aldose reductase inhibitor sorbinils in some 600 diabetic patients with minimal or no retinopathy have not yet produced any striking results. The work of Kador suggests that studies in humans with diabetes of some years duration may be non-productive because by then many of the pericytes are lost, and thus the disease is probably self-perpetuating. Indeed, a study to show the effectiveness of aldose reductase inhibitors would have to start when diabetes was diagnosed.

How the polyol pathway is involved in pericyte damage is not completely clear. It is unlikely to be the accumulation of sorbitol itself (although in galactosaemic animals dulcitol accumulation may be harmful); it could be a consequence of the associated reduction in myoinositol or the reduced

$Na^+-K^+-ATPase$ activity which damages cells [24, 25].

Retinal endothelial cells are probably not directly affected by the polyol pathway, as aldose reductase has not been found in these cells by most observers. Endothelial cells of larger vessels may contain this enzyme, as the Newcastle group [26] found it in umbilical vein endothelial cells. Even in the absence of aldose reductase, high glucose concentrations may nevertheless affect endothelial cell function, as suggested by the work of Lorenzi *et al.* [27], who found reduced cell replication and increased cell death of cultured umbilical vein endothelial cells in a high glucose medium. Prolonged exposure of these cultured cells also resulted in changes in the DNA which manifested an accelerated rate of unwinding in alkali, suggestive of an increased number of single-strand breaks [28]. Such changes have not yet been demonstrated in retinal endothelial cells. Damage may also occur if there is interference with the controlling influence of pericytes. This could of course occur simply by increased basement membrane thickening, which interrupts cell-to-cell interaction between endothelial cells and pericytes.

Although these metabolic abnormalities can explain many of the features of endothelial cell damage in diabetes, changes in blood flow may also be involved.

### Haemodynamic changes in diabetic retinopathy

In early and uncontrolled diabetes, blood flow in the retina is probably increased [27–29]. Experimental work by Atherton *et al.* [30] suggested that high blood glucose levels (approximately 26 mmol/l), achieved by bolus injection in experimental animals, increased blood flow significantly. Recent studies by Sullivan *et al.* (unpublished observations), using laser Doppler velocimetry (LDV) for blood flow measurement in miniature swine, demonstrated that a gradual rise in blood glucose concentrations caused an even bigger rise in blood flow already noticeable at 17 mmol/l. Reducing the glucose to hypoglycaemic levels also caused an increase in blood flow [31]. This latter finding was somewhat unexpected. Though, on the one hand nerve tissue needs glucose for metabolism (and if this is reduced, autoregulation would be expected to cause a compensatory increase in blood flow) on the other hand Grunwald and co-workers [32] noted that in NIDDM patients with poor control normalization of glucose over a 2-h period reduced blood flow, and at the same time improved vessel reactivity to oxygen. Using the blue light entopic technique, Fallon *et al.* found that in diabetic patients with early retinopathy blood flow was increased compared with normal controls [33], and this has recently been confirmed by work from the Joslin Clinic [34]. Thus, increases in blood flow occur in diabetes at high and at very low glucose levels, and at these levels the flow may be associated with reduced vascular reactivity. The blood flow changes noted by Kohner *et al.* [29], and those seen in experimental animals are of sufficient magnitude to damage the vascular endothelium [35]. It is not only the increased blood flow, but also the frequent changes in flow which may cause much of the damage. Once retinopathy is present, flow in the peripheral retina is probably reduced [35] as a result of the reduced capillary bed, and this serves to maintain blood flow in the functionally more important central, perifoveal retina. Only when there are large areas of capillary non-perfusion, as seen in preproliferative and proliferative diabetic retinopathy, is there significant reduction in the perifoveal blood flow [33]. Diabetic control is often improved in patients when they become aware of the presence of retinopathy, and in studies with continuous subcutaneous insulin infusion (CSII) this was also achieved [36–38]. By this time there is already significant vascular damage, and reduction of blood flow may actually worsen retinopathy, as was seen in these studies. The lesions noted to deteriorate were microaneurysms, haemorrhages and cotton-wool spots, all indicative of increasing ischaemia. Indeed, the work of Sleightholm *et al.* (unpublished observations), also using the blue light entoptic technique, showed that retinopathy did not deteriorate in those patients in whom blood flow increased during the first week following CSII.

Thus, endothelial cells could be damaged by the increased blood flow through them, which could be due to abnormal glucose levels initially, but also to reduced peripheral resistance in dilated capillaries when pericytes are lost. Damage to the endothelial cells is always present when there is capillary occlusion.

### Capillary dilatation and leakage

Capillary dilatation is an early manifestation of diabetic retinopathy. Vink found this to be the earliest feature recognizable on fluorescein angiograms [39]. Work by Sosula in diabetic rats [40] confirmed that dilatation did indeed occur early, that the endothelial cells were not flattened, while the vessel diameter was increased, suggesting true dilatation with anatomical changes. Even before there are anatomical alterations, the increased blood flow associated with high glucose could cause capillary dilatation of a functional nature in patients. As noted by Kuwabara and Cogan [3, 4], capillary dilatation occurs when there is loss of pericytes, but it could occur before if the pericyte control over the endothelial cells is lost. Thickening of the basement membrane, another early manifestation of retinopathy, could interfere with cell-to-cell contact between pericytes and endothelial cells, and thus endothelial cells may lose the controlling influence of the pericytes. Transient leakage can occasionally be seen at this early stage in diabetic patients investigated with fluorescein angiograms. This leakage is probably also functional, and indicates transfer of fluorescein through endothelial cells into the extracellular space.

That leakage is initially functional is suggested by the work of Parving *et al.* [41], who showed that in diabetic patients with mild hypertension, the normal or only slightly increased leakage, as measured by vitreous fluorophotometry, could be reduced by an angiotensin-converting enzyme (ACE) inhibitor. Parving proposed that this was due to the reduced intravascular pressure, but it could also be due to an effect of the drug on the endothelial cells, since these produce ACE. A direct effect on the endothelial cells is suggested by the fact that ACE inhibitors are therapeutically useful in idiopathic peripheral oedema.

Later, after long-standing disease, there is damage to the tight junctions between endothelial cells, at least in diabetic dogs [42], and this will allow free escape of fluorescein. New vessels invariably leak fluorescein, and this may indicate that tight junctions are missing at the time of active growth of vessels, though fenestrated junctions were only rarely seen in new vessels of fibrovascular membranes removed at vitrectomy [43].

The leakage seen in diabetic maculopathy is almost invariably associated with dilated vessels, and this dilatation is also associated with loss of some capillaries. It has not been established whether the leakage is across the cells or between them.

**Vascular occlusion**

The causes of capillary occlusion have not yet been established. The most plausible explanation remains the more active haemostasis and platelet coagulation of the blood of patients with retinopathy. The formation of microthrombi could be facilitated by the reduced fibrinolytic and antithrombin activities of the vessel wall, a direct result of the endothelial cell damage, consequent on increased blood flow and altered physical properties of the blood, such as increased viscosity and reduced red cell deformability.

Recent work, however, has questioned whether platelets are hyperactive in patients with diabetic complications. Alessandrini *et al.* [44] measured the levels of urinary 2,3-dinor metabolites of thromboxane A2, the major promoter, and prostacyclin, the major inhibitor, of platelet aggregation. No differences were found between normal controls and diabetic patients with or without retinopathy. Other widely used *in vitro* and *in vivo* indicators of platelet function also failed to discriminate between these groups. The measurement of 2,3-dinor metabolites appears to be more reliable than previous methods, overcoming the problems of cross-reactivity with other prostaglandins present in higher quantities in the plasma. By suggesting that the thromboxane/prostacyclin balance is not altered in diabetic retinopathy, these results fail to support the hypothesis that platelets are involved in capillary plugging in the retina, or elsewhere. Further negative evidence derives from the observed normal survival of $^{111}$In-labelled platelets in patients with retinopathy [45], confirming earlier reports from the Hammersmith Hospital [46].

There is no uniform agreement about the role of platelets in diabetic retinopathy, but there are several reports of abnormal *in vitro* behaviour of platelets. In trying to identify the abnormality Watanabe *et al.* [47] reported that LDL isolated from patients with IDDM significantly potentiates platelet aggregation induced by thrombin, and that this activity correlates directly with the degree of LDL glycosylation *in vivo*. LDL glycosylated *in vitro* enhances thrombin-, collagen- and ADP-induced platelet aggregation. Platelets exhibit higher uptake for glycosylated rather than native LDL and this may lead to alteration of their membrane lipid composition in poorly controlled diabetes. Insulin, on the other hand, may modify platelet membranes so as to decrease aggregability, as observed in the course of clamp studies at steady-state levels as low as 40 mU/l [48]. Other mechanisms suggested to account for *in vitro* platelet hyperactivity include an increased content of histamine [49], increased $Ca^{++}$ influx [50], potentiation by catecholamines released during hypoglycaemia [51], and reduced vitamin E content. This last observation was originally reported by Karpen *et al.* [52], and led to trials of vitamin E supplements. Normalization of thromboxane A2 production by platelets in response to ADP and collagen *in vitro* was reported by Gisinger *et al.* [53], after 4 weeks of treatment with 400 mg/day tocopherol acetate and by Colette *et al.* [54] after 5 weeks on the rather large dose of 1 g daily.

Thus, platelet abnormalities in diabetic retinopathy are more evident *in vitro* than *in vivo*. One way of ascertaining whether such changes are indeed relevant to the pathogenesis of diabetic retinopathy is by randomized controlled clinical trials where antiaggregating agents and placebo are administered and the effects on disease progression studied. The result of one major trial of aspirin alone, aspirin together with dipyridamole and placebo was reported recently by the DAMAD study group [55]. This study showed that aspirin alone or in conjunction with dipyridamole significantly (though marginally) reduced the formation of new microaneurysms in early background retinopathy.

The main problem remains the relevance of phenomena observed *in vitro* to the situation in life. Most tests look at platelet function either indirectly or under highly artificial experimental conditions, such as during anti-coagulation and after separation of platelets from red and white cells. This alone makes it difficult to translate observations into general pathogenic terms. In addition, patient selection and laboratory techniques are not standardized, contributing to the heterogeneity of reports in the literature. Major doubts still remain as to whether platelets play a significant role in the vascular occlusion of diabetic retinopathy.

### New vessel formation

New vessel formation is not unique to diabetic retinopathy; it occurs in several conditions where there is widespread vascular occlusion which is not sufficient to cause total death of the retina. Thus, it is seen in sickle cell disease, retinal vasculitis and retinal vein occlusion. In all these conditions, as in diabetes, occlusion of arterioles and venules, as well as capillaries occurs before the new vessels develop.

The steps in the development of new vessels are: first, dissolution of extracellular matrix, followed by cellular migration and proliferation, and finally the formation of a vascular lumen. Proteoglycans secreted by endothelial cells cause dissolution of the basement membrane, which allows migration of endothelial cells. The first suggestion that a retina-derived angiogenic factor was produced to initiate and promote these changes came from Michaelson [56] as long ago as 1948. But only in the last few years have real advances been made in the isolation of several growth-promoting and growth-inhibiting substances. Retina-derived angiogenic factor [57] and retina-derived growth factor [58] have been found to be homologous to fibroblast growth factor (FGF), which exists in two closely related forms, acidic and basic FGF [59]. Basic FGF (bFGF) is widely distributed and endothelial cells from brain and adrenal cortex have been shown to express the bFGF gene. bFGF is produced by the endothelial cells and is stored in the extracellular matrix, from where it is released at the time of cell death [59].

Herman and D'Amore have shown that retina-derived growth factor, by implication FGF, has the ability of transforming endothelial cells from a stationary to a motile spindle shape [60]. FGF also stimulates cell proliferation [61]. There are other angiogenic substances, insulin-like growth factor-1 (IGF-1) being a prime candidate, especially, as this substance has been found in the vitreous of patients with proliferative retinopathy [62]. The pigment epithelium also induces growth promotion under certain circumstances [63]. In health, there is a balance between the growth-promoting and growth-inhibiting substances produced by endothelial cells and pigment epithelium [62, 63], and it is this balance which is upset at the time of new vessel growth.

Among the many regulatory peptides, growth hormone (GH) is the one which has been most implicated in retinal neovascularization. Following a case report by Poulsen in 1953 [64] reporting regression of retinopathy following postpartum pituitary haemorrhage, hypophysectomy came to be used for the treatment of proliferative diabetic retinopathy. Long-term follow-up of patients treated with yttrium-90 implantation was reported by Sharp *et al.* [65]. This showed a dramatic regression and cessation of new vessel growth of the optic disc, and by 10 years there was no disc neovascularization in any eye. Since the benefits of pituitary destruction were related to the degree of GH deficiency [66, 67] it was reasonable to suggest that GH had some influence on the neovascular process. As GH acts through IGF-1 this latter peptide has become of paramount interest. It was, therefore, surprising that patients with diabetes had no higher IGF-1 levels than normals, and even patients with proliferative retinopathy had levels in the normal range [68]. This could be due in part to the fact that lower levels of IGF-1 are produced in poorly controlled diabetic children in response to a standard dose of GH than in those with better control [69]. Since insulin regulates the expression of hepatic GH receptors in more severe diabetes, there may be reduction in these receptors [70]. That IGF-1 could be of importance, at least in the proliferative stage of diabetic retinopathy, has been suggested by Merimee *et al.* [71], who found increased levels of IGF-1 in those patients with rapidly advancing 'florid' retinopathy. Recently, Hyer *et al.* [72] reported on a longitudinal study of patients with preproliferative diabetic retinopathy, and found that these patients had IGF-1 levels in the normal range. During the period of follow-up, eight of the patients developed active vascular proliferation. At the time of active neovascularization, IGF-1 levels rose in these patients, though they still remained in the normal range. The elevation of IGF-1 was restricted to these eight patients, and it returned to normal soon after effective photocoagulation. This fact, together with the finding that following photocoagulation patients with retinopathy have lower than normal IGF-1 levels [72], suggests the possibility that IGF-1 is produced in the retina. Indeed, IGF-1 receptors have been found by King *et al.* [73] in both cultured retinal endothelial cells and pericytes.

In summary, it appears that the neovascular process starts with loss of the pericyte–endothelial cell interaction, allowing proliferation of the endothelial cells. This leads to vascular dilatation and increased retinal blood flow which is also stimulated by the high glucose levels. Metabolic changes and sheer stress damage endothelial cells, and endothelial–platelet interaction, together with decreased fibrinolytic activity, leads to vascular occlusion. Cell death releases FGF and imbalance between inhibitory and stimulatory factors results in neovascularization.

Although many details in the neovascular process are still not known, and the interrelationships between the factors produced by retinal endothelial and other cells are uncertain, the picture is gradually becoming clearer, and it is hoped that a full understanding of all the processes is not too far away.

## Pathogenesis of cataract in diabetes

Diabetes is undoubtedly a significant risk factor for the development of cataracts [74–78]. In the Framingham Eye Study [74–76], senile lens change was consistently commoner in diabetic than in non-diabetic subjects up to the age of 69 years and other reports have shown an increased frequency of senile cataract in diabetic patients in their 40s and a two- to three-fold increase in patients in their 50s and 60s. Beyond the age of 69 years, however, there is little increased risk [74–78]. Overall, the available epidemiological data strongly suggest that the presence of diabetes accelerates the development of senile cataracts in man.

In addition, typical diabetic cataracts with a characteristic 'snowflake' appearance have long been recognized, particularly in adolescents with poor diabetic control. They are rarely seen today.

### *Lens metabolism*

The lens retains its shape and transparency by virtue of active metabolic processes. Nutrients and oxygen required for metabolism are taken up from the aqueous humour across a single-cell layer of cuboidal epithelial cells which maintain the ionic equilibrium within the lens [79]. These cells derive energy from glucose metabolism, mainly through anaerobic glycolysis. Control of lens glycolysis, which must be precisely regulated to avoid excessive lactate production, apparently depends on two enzymes, phosphofructokinase and hexokinase. Phosphofructokinase activity is regulated by ATP availability and hexokinase by the level of its product, glucose-6-phosphate [80]. At physiological glucose levels, both enzymes are saturated. Raising the glucose concentration in blood or aqueous humour does not, therefore, lead to increased glycolytic activity [81] and intracellular glucose levels will tend to rise. Excess glucose within the lens is metabolized by the hexose monophosphate shunt or, more importantly, by the polyol pathway which is made possible by the presence of aldose reductase in the lens epithelium.

The low activities of glycolytic enzymes and polyol (sorbitol) dehydrogenase in lens epithelium also favour sorbitol accumulation during exposure to high glucose levels [82] (see Chapter 3).

#### THE POLYOL PATHWAY AND CATARACT FORMATION IN EXPERIMENTAL DIABETES

Polyol pathway activity has been implicated in cataract formation in animals. Those species with high lenticular aldose reductase activity (such as the Mongolian gerbil, the degu and the rat) develop cataracts when diabetes is induced using streptozotocin or alloxan; the cataracts develop faster if the hyperglycaemia is more severe and the animals are young [83–85]. Sorbitol accumulation in the lens can be demonstrated in these models [86]. Similar cataracts can also be induced in these species by feeding diets with high contents (35%) of galactose or xylose which are converted by aldose reductase into their respective polyols, dulcitol and xylitol [86]. This suggests a common mechanism, namely accumulation of polyol within the lens. By contrast, in animals with absent or very low aldose reductase activity in the lens (e.g. CFW, *db/db* and *ob/ob* mice), cataract formation cannot be induced by either prolonged hyperglycaemia for up to six months or diets containing as much as 50% galactose [87, 88]. Polyol levels remain very low in the lenses of these animals.

Cell membranes are relatively impermeable to polyols and, once formed, these substances will accumulate, creating a hypertonic environment within the lens epithelium and lens fibres, which will attract water by osmosis. Opacification of the lens and cataract formation could result from secondary changes, such as loss of amino acids, myoinositol, and potassium ions due, in turn, to membrane damage associated with cellular swelling. Kinoshita's postulate that aldose reductase is pivotal in the pathogenesis of 'sugar cataract' [89] stimulated a search for inhibitors of the enzyme which might prevent this complication. Aldose reductase inhibitors have been reported to delay or prevent the onset of cataracts in diabetic and galactosaemic rats [90]. The effectiveness of these agents is critically dependent on the timing of their administration relative to the onset of galactose-feeding or induction of diabetes, suggesting an effect on an early, reversible phase before membrane damage has occurred [91].

#### THE POLYOL PATHWAY AND THE HUMAN DIABETIC LENS

A direct correlation between plasma glucose concentration and the levels of sorbitol and fructose in the lenses of diabetic patients has been reported [92]. A further study has demonstrated a strong correlation between sorbitol levels in human cataracts and both fasting blood glucose and $HbA_1$ levels [93]. The reduction in phosphofructokinase activity which occurs in the human diabetic cataract [94] will result in less efficient clearing of accumulated sorbitol. As in animals, sorbitol accumulation is therefore apparently related to cataract formation, but its pathogenic role is uncertain. It also remains to be shown whether aldose reductase inhibitors will delay or prevent cataract formation in human diabetes. It is possible that such agents will need to be administered soon after the diagnosis of diabetes if they are to be effective, a stratagem which is difficult to justify in current clinical trials.

### *Non-enzymatic glycation of lens proteins*

The soluble protein of the lens, crystallin, contained within the fibre cells, has a much slower turnover than other proteins in the body. As it ages, human lens crystallin undergoes various post-translational modifications including non-enzymatic glycation [95] (see Chapter 3). The extent of crystallin glycation in human diabetic lenses is reported to be 2–3%, about twice as high as in non-diabetic lenses [95]. In another study [96] glycation of lens cortical proteins but not of nuclear proteins was significantly higher in diabetic patients than in control subjects with senile cataracts. This implies that the lens nucleus is exposed to less metabolic variation than the lens cortex. Glycation has also been demonstrated in the human lens capsule and again was significantly greater in diabetic patients [97].

Glycation offers another possible mechanism for cataract formation. Changes in the tertiary structure of crystallin after glycation expose sulphydryl groups to oxidation, thus favouring the formation of disulphide-linked aggregates within the lens [98]. Such cross-linkages could form the basis of lens opacities and eventually cataract, although the available evidence is not sufficient to establish a definite link between the extent of lens protein glycation and the initiation of cataract formation. There is no evidence that non-enzymatic glycation is involved in the development of cataract in experimental animals fed on a high galactose diet [99].

## Conclusions

These two postulated biochemical mechanisms of cataract formation — polyol pathway activity and non-enzymatic glycation of lens proteins — are not mutually exclusive. Prevention of this complication will probably require therapeutic intervention early in the natural history of the disease before irreversible damage has taken place.

EVA M. KOHNER
MASSIMO PORTA
STEPHEN L. HYER

## References

1 Tilton RG, Miller EJ, Kilo C, Williamson JK. Pericyte form and distribution in rat retinal and uveal capillaries. *Invest Ophthalmol Vis Sci* 1985; **26**: 60–73.

2 Petty RG, Pearson JD. Endothelium — the axis of vascular health and disease. *J Roy Coll Phys London* 1989; **23**: 92–102.

3 Cogan DG, Toussaint D, Kuwabara T. Retinal vascular patterns IV: diabetic retinopathy *Arch Ophthalmol* 1961; **60**: 100–12.

4 Kuwabara T, Cogan DG. Retinal vascular patterns VI. Mural cells of the retinal capillaries. *Arch Ophthalmol* 1963; **69**: 492–502a.

5 Ashton N. Injection of the retinal vascular system in enucleated eyes in diabetic retinopathy. *Br J Ophthalmol* 1950; **54**: 38–44.

6 Kohner EM, Dollery CT, Patterson JW, Oakley WN. Arterial fluorescein studies in diabetic retinopathy. *Diabetes* 1967; **16**: 1–10.

7 Yanagisawa M, Kurihara H, Kimura S *et al*. A novel potent vasoconstrictor peptide produced by vascular endothelial cells. *Nature* 1988; **332**: 411–15.

8 Yanagisawa M, Inoue A, Ishikawa T *et al*. Primary structure synthesis and biological activity of rat endothelin as endothelium derived vasoconstrictor peptide. *Proc Natl Acad Sci USA* 1988; **85**: 6964–7.

9 Takahashi K, Brooks RA, Kanse SM, Ghatei MA, Kohner EM, Bloom SR. Endothelin I is produced by cultured bovine retinal endothelial cells and endothelin receptors are present on the associated pericytes. *Diabetes* 1989; **38**: 1200–2.

10 Orlidge A, D'Amore PA. Inhibition of capillary endothelial cell growth by pericytes and smooth muscle cells. *J Cell Biol* 1987; **105**: 1455–62.

11 Antonelli-Orlidge A, Saunders KB, Smith SR, D'Amore P. An activated form of transforming growth factor β is produced by cocultures of endothelial cells and pericytes. *Proc Natl Acad Sci USA* 1989; **86**: 4544–8.

12 Buzney SM, Frank RN, Varma SD. Aldose reductase in retinal mural cells. *Invest Ophthalmol* 1977; **16**: 392–6.

13 Engerman RL, Kern TS. Experimental galactosemia produces a diabetic like retinopathy. *Diabetes* 1984; **33**: 97–100.

14 Williamson JR, Chang K, Tilton RG *et al*. Increased vascular permeability in spontaneously diabetic *BB/W* rats with mild versus severe streptozotocin induced diabetes: prevention by aldose reductase inhibitors and castration. *Diabetes* 1987; **36**: 813–21.

15 Li W, Shen S, Khatami M, Rochley JH. Stimulation of retinal capillary pericyte protein and collagen synthesis in culture by high glucose concentration. *Diabetes* 1984; **33**: 785–9.

16 Williamson JR, Kilo C. Extracellular matrix changes in diabetes mellitus. In: Scarpelli DG, Migaki G, eds, *Comparative Pathobiology of Major Age-related Disease*. New York: Alan R Liss, 1984: 269.

17 Robinson WG Jr, Kador PF, Kinoshita JH. Retinal capillaries: Basement membrane thickening by galactosemia prevented with aldose reductase inhibitors. *Science* 1983; **221**: 1177–9.

18 Lightman S, Rechthand E, Teruyabshi H, Palestine A, Rapaport S. Permeability changes in blood retinal barrier of galactosemic rats are prevented by aldose reductase inhibitors. *Diabetes* 1986; **36**: 1271–5.

19 Akagi Y, Yajima Y, Kador PF, Kuwabara T, Kinoshita JH. Localisation of aldose reductase in the human eye. *Diabetes* 1984; **33**: 562–6.

20 Chakrabati S, Sima AAF, Nakajima T, Yagihashi S, Green DA. Aldose reductase in the BB rat — isolation, immunological identification and localisation in the retina and peripheral nerve. *Diabetologia* 1987; **30**: 244–57.

21 Kador PF, Akagi Y, Terubayashi H, Nyman M, Kinoshita JH. Prevention of pericyte ghost formation in retinal capillaries of galactose fed dogs by aldose reductase inhibitors. *Invest Ophthalmol Vis Sci* 1988; **29** (suppl 1): 180.

22 Kador PF, Akagi Y, Ikebe H, Takahasi Y, Ymar M, Kinoshita SH. Prevention of retinal vessel changes associated with diabetic retinopathy in galactose fed dogs by aldose reductase inhibitor. *Invest Ophthalmol Vis Sci* 1989; **30** (suppl 1): 139.

23 Engerman RL, Kern TS. Retinal vasculature in sorbinil treated galactosaemic dogs. *Invest Ophthalmol Vis Sci* 1989; **30** (suppl 1): 139.

24 Greene DA, Lattimer SA, Sima AAF. Sorbitol, phosphoinositides, and sodium-potassium ATP-ase in the pathogenesis of diabetic complications. *N Engl J Med* 1987; **316**: 559–606.

25 MacGregor LC, Matschinsky FM. Treatment with aldose reductase inhibitor of myoinositol arrests deterioration of the electroretinogram of diabetic rats. *J Clin Invest* 1985; **24**: 1250–8.

26 Hawthorne GC, Bartlett K, Hetherington CS, Alberti KGMM. The effect of high glucose on polyol pathway activity and myoinositol mechanism in cultured human endothelial cells. *Diabetologia* 1989; **32**: 163–6.

27 Lorenzi M, Cagliero E, Toledo S. Glucose toxicity for human endothelial cells in culture. *Diabetes* 1985; **34**: 621–3.

28 Lorenzi M, Montisano DF, Toledo S, Barrieux A. High glucose induces DNA damage in cultured human endothelial cells. *J Clin Invest* 1986; **77**: 322–5.

29 Kohner EM. The problems of retinal blood flow in diabetes. *Diabetes* 1976; **25** (suppl 2): 839–44.

30 Atherton A, Hill DW, Keen H, Young S, Edwards EJ. The effect of acute hyperglycaemia on the retinal circulation of the normal cat. *Diabetologia* 1980; **18**: 233–7.

31 Caldwell G, Davies EG, Sullivan P, Morris A, Kohner EM. The effect of hypoglycaemia on retinal blood flow measured by the laser doppler velocimeter. (Submitted for publication).

32 Grunwald JE, Riva CE, Martin DB, Quint AR, Epstein PA. Effect of an insulin induced decrease in blood glucose on the human diabetic retinal circulation. *Ophthalmology* 1987; **94**: 1614–20.

33 Fallon TJ, Chowiencyzk P, Kohner EM. Measurement of

retinal blood flow in diabetes by the blue light entoptic phenomenon. *Br J Ophthalmol* 1986; **70**: 43–6.

34 McMillan DE. Rheological and related factors in diabetic retinopathy. In: Kohner EM, ed. *International Ophthalmology Clinics*. Boston: Little, Brown and Co, 1978, 35.

35 Grunwald JE, Riva CE, Sinclair SH, Bruckner SJ, Petrig BL. Laser doppler velocimetry study of retinal circulation in diabetes mellitus. *Arch Ophthalmol* 1986; **104**: 991–6.

36 Lauritzen T, Frost Larson K, Larson HW, Deckert T, the Steno Study Group. Effect of 1 year of near normal blood glucose levels on retinopathy in insulin dependent diabetics. *Lancet* 1983; **i**: 200–4.

37 The KROC Collaborative Study Group. Blood glucose control and the evolution of diabetic retinopathy and albuminuria. *N Engl J Med* 1984; **311**: 365–72.

38 Ballegooie van E, Hooymans J, Timmerman Z, Reitsma W, Sluiter WJ, Schweitzer NMJ, Doorenbas H. Rapid deterioration of diabetic retinopathy during treatment with continuous subcutaneous insulin infusion. *Diabetes Care* 1984; **7**: 236–43.

39 Oosterhuis JA, Vink R. Fluorescein photography in diabetic retinopathy. *Perspectives Ophthalmol Excerpta Med Fed* 1967; **186**: 115–32.

40 Sosula L, Beaumont P, Hollows FC, Jonson KM. Dilatation and endothelial proliferation of retinal capillaries in streptozotocin-diabetic rats: quantitative electron microscopy. *Invest Ophthalmol* 1972; **11**: 926–35.

41 Parving HH, Larson M, Hommel E, Lund-Anderson H. Effect of antihypertensive treatment on blood retinal permeability to fluorescein in hypertensive type I diabetic patients with background retinopathy, in press.

42 Wallow IHL, Engerman RL. Permeability and patency of retinal blood vessels in experimental diabetes. *Invest Ophthalmol Vis Sci* 1977; **16**: 447–54.

43 Williams JM, de Juan E, Machemer R. Intrastructural characteristics of new vessels in proliferative diabetic retinopathy. *Am J Ophthalmol* 1988; **105**: 491–9.

44 Alessandrini P, McRae J, Feman S, Fitzgerald GA. Thromboxane biosynthesis and platelet function in diabetes mellitus. *N Engl J Med* 1988; **319**: 208–12.

45 Luikens B, Forstrom LA, Johnson T, Johnson G. Indium 111 platelet kinetics in patients with diabetes mellitus. *Nucl Med Comm* 1988; **9**: 223–34.

46 Porta M, Peters AM, Cousins SA, Cagliero E, Fitzpatrick ML, Kohner EM. A study of platelet-relevant parameters in patients with diabetic microangiopathy. *Diabetologia* 1983; **25**: 21–5.

47 Watanabe J, Wohltmann HJ, Klein RL, Colwell JA, Lopes-Virella MF. Enhancement of platelet aggregation by low density lipoprotein from IDDM patients. *Diabetes* 1988; **37**: 1652–7.

48 Trovati M, Anfossi G, Cavalot F, Massucco P, Mularoni E, Emanuelli G. Insulin directly reduces platelet sensitivity to aggregating agents. Studies *in vitro* and *in vivo*. *Diabetes* 1988; **89**: 780–6.

49 Gill DR, Barradas MA, Fonseca VA, Gracey L, Dandona P. Increased histamine content in leukocytes and platelets of patients with peripheral vascular disease. *Am J Clin Pathol* 1988; **89**: 622–6.

50 Bergh CH, Hjalmoarson A, Holm G, Angwald E, Jacobsson B. Studies on calcium exchange in platelets in human diabetes. *Eur J Clin Invest* 1988; **18**: 92–7.

51 Trovati M, Anfossi G, Cavelot F *et al*. Studies on mechanisms involved in hypoglycemia induced platelet activation. *Diabetes* 1986; **35**: 818–25.

52 Karpen CW, Pritchard KA, Arnold JH, Cornwell DG, Panganamala RV. Restoration of prostacyclin/thromboxane A2 balance in the diabetic rat: influence of dietary vitamin E. *Diabetes* 1982; **31**: 947–51.

53 Gisinger C, Jeremy J, Speiser P, Mikhailidis D, Dandona P, Schernthaner G. Effect of vitamin E supplementation on platelet thromboxane A2 production in type I diabetic patients. Double-blind cross-over trial. *Diabetes* 1988; **37**: 1260–4.

54 Colette C, Pares-Herbute N, Monnier LH, Cartry E. Platelet function in type 1 diabetes: effect of supplementation with large doses of vitamin E. *Am J Clin Nutr* 1988; **47**: 256–61.

55 DAMAD Study Group. Effect of aspirin alone and aspirin plus dipyridamole in early diabetic retinopathy. A multicentre randomised controlled clinical trial. *Diabetes* 1989; **38**: 491–8.

56 Michaelson IC. The mode of development of the vascular system of the retina. *Trans Ophthalmol Soc UK* 1948; **68**: 137–80.

57 D'Amore PA, Klagsbrun M. Endothelial cell mitogens derived from retina and hypothalamus, biochemical and biological stimulants. *J Cell Biol* 1984; **99**: 545–9.

58 Baird A, Esch F. Gospodarowicz D, Guillemin R. Retina and eye derived endothelial cell growth factors: partial molecular characterisation and identity with acidic and basic fibroblast growth factor. *Biochemistry* 1985; **24**: 7855–60.

59 Gospodarowicz D, Massoglia S, Cheng J, Fuji DK. Effect of retina-derived basic and acidic fibroblast growth factor and lipoproteins on the proliferation of retina-derived capillary endothelial cells. *Exp Eye Res* 1986; **43**: 459–76.

60 Herman IM, D'Amore PA. Capillary endothelial cell migration: loss of fibres in response to retina derived growth factor. *J Muscle Res Cell Motil* 1989; **5**: 697–709.

61 Schweigerer I, Neufeld G, Friedman J, Abraham JA, Fiddes JC, Gospodarowicz D. Capillary endothelial cells express basic fibroblast growth factor, a mitogen that promotes their growth. *Nature* 1987; **325**: 257–9.

62 Grant M, Russel B, Fitzgerald C, Merimee TJ. Insulin-like growth factors in vitreous. *Diabetes* 1986; **35**: 416–20.

63 Glaser BM, Campochiaro PA, Davis JL, Sato M. Retinal pigment epithelial cells release an inhibitor of neovascularization. *Arch Ophthalmol* 1985; **103**: 1870–5.

64 Poulsen JE. Recovery from retinopathy in the case of diabetes with Simmonds' disease. *Diabetes* 1953; **2**: 7–12.

65 Sharp PS, Fallon TJ, Brazier OJ, Sandler L, Joplin GF, Kohner EM. Long term follow up of patients who underwent yttrium-90 pituitary implantation for treatment of proliferative retinopathy. *Diabetologia* 1987; **33**: 199–207.

66 Wright AD, Kohner EM, Oakley NW, Hartog M. Joplin GF, Fraser TR. Serum growth hormone levels and the response of diabetic retinopathy to pituitary ablation. *Br Med J* 1969; **2**: 364–8.

67 Adams DA, Rand RW, Roth NH, Dashe AM, Gipstein RM, Heuser G. Hypophysectomy in diabetic retinopathy — the relationship between the degree of pituitary ablation and ocular response. *Diabetes* 1974; **23**: 698–707.

68 Hyer SL, Sharp PS, Brooks RA, Burrin JM, Kohner EM. Serum IGF-I concentration in diabetic retinopathy. *Diabetic Med* 1988; **5**: 356–60.

69 Lanes R, Recher B, Fort B, Liftschitz F. Impaired somatomedin generation test in children with insulin dependent diabetes mellitus. *Diabetes* 1985; **34**: 156–60.

70 Baxter RC, Brown AJ, Turtle JR. Association between serum insulin, serum somatomedin and liver receptors for human growth hormone in streptozotocin diabetes. *Horm Metab Res* 1980; **12**: 371–81.

71 Merimee TJ, Zapf F, Froesch ER. Insulin like growth factors:

studies in diabetics with and without retinopathy. *N Engl J Med* 1983; **309**: 527–30.
72 Hyer SL, Sharp PS, Brooks RA, Burrin JM, Kohner EM. A two year follow up study of serum insulin like growth factors in diabetics with retinopathy. *Metabolism* 1989; **38**: 586–9.
73 King GL, Goldman AD, Buzney S, Moses A, Kahn CR. Receptors and growth promoting effects of insulin and insulin like growth factors on cells from bovine retinal capillaries and aorta. *J Clin Invest* 1985; **75**: 108–1036.
74 Kahn HA, Leibowitz HM, Ganley JP *et al.* The Framingham Eye Study I. Outline and major prevalence findings. *Am J Epidemiol* 1977; **106**: 17–32.
75 Kahn HA, Leibowitz HM, Ganley JP *et al.* The Framingham Eye Study II. Association of ophthalmic pathology with single variables previously measured in the Framingham Heart Study. *Am J Epidemiol* 1977; **106**: 33–41.
76 Leibowitz HM, Krueger DE, Maunder LR *et al.* The Framingham Eye Study monograph. *Surv Ophthalmol* 1980; **24** (suppl): 335–610.
77 Hiller R, Kahn HA. Senile cataract extraction and diabetes. *Br J Ophthalmol* 1976; **60**: 283–6.
78 Ederer F, Hiller R, Taylor HR. Senile lens changes and diabetes: two population studies. *Am J Ophthalmol* 1981; **91**: 381–95.
79 Cheng HM, Chylack LT Jr. Lens metabolism. In: Maisel H, ed. *The Ocular Lens*. New York: M. Dekker Inc, 1985: 223–64.
80 Lou MF, Kinoshita JH. Control of lens glycolysis. *Biochem Biophys Acta* 1967; **141**: 545–59.
81 Levari R, Wertheimer E, Kornblueth W. Interrelation between the various pathways of glucose metabolism in the rat lens. *Exp Eye Res* 1964; **3**: 99–104.
82 Ahmad SS, Tsou KC, Ahmad SI *et al.* Studies on cataractogenesis in humans and rats with alloxan-induced diabetes. II. Histochemical evaluation of lenticular enzymes. *Ophthalmic Res* 1985; **17**: 12–20.
83 Patterson JW. Cataractogenic sugars. *Arch Biochem Biophys* 1955; **58**: 24–30.
84 Varma SD, Mizuno A, Kinoshita JH. Diabetic cataracts and flavonoids. *Science* 1977; **195**: 205–6.
85 El-Aguizy HK, Richards RD, Varma SD. Sugar cataracts in Mongolian gerbils. *Exp Eye Res* 1983; **36**: 839–44.
86 Van Heyningen R. Formation of polyols by the lens of the rat with sugar cataract. *Nature* 1959; **184**: 194–5.
87 Kuck JFR. Response of the mouse lens to high concentrations of glucose or galactose. *Ophthalmol Res* 1970; **1**: 166–74.
88 Varma SD, Kinoshita JH. The absence of cataracts in mice with congenital hyperglycaemia. *Exp Eye Res* 1974; **19**: 577–82.
89 Kinoshita JH. Mechanisms initiating cataract formation. *Invest Ophthalmol* 1974; **13**: 713–24.
90 Kador PF, Kinoshita JH. Diabetic galactosaemic cataracts. *Human Cataract Formation* (Ciba Foundation Symposium 106). London: Pitman, 1984: 110–31.
91 Simard-Duquesne N, Greselin E, Dubuc J *et al.* The effect of a new aldose reductase inhibitor (Tolrestat) in galactosemic and diabetic rats. *Metabolism* 1985; **34**: 885–92.
92 Varma SD, Schocket SS, Richards RD. Implications of aldose reductase in cataracts in human diabetes. *Invest Ophthalmol Vis Sci* 1979; **18**: 237–41.
93 Lerner BC, Varma SD, Richards RD. Polyol pathway metabolites in human cataracts. Correlation of circulating glycosylated hemoglobin content and fasting blood glucose levels. *Arch Ophthalmol* 1984; **102**: 917–20.
94 Jedziniak J, Arredondo LM, Meys M. Polyol dehydrogenase in the human lens. *Invest Ophthalmol Vis Sci* 1986; **27** (suppl 1): 137.
95 Garlick RL, Mazer JS, Chylack LT Jr *et al.* Non-enzymatic glycation of human lens crystallin. *J Clin Invest* 1984; **74**: 1742–9.
96 Liang JN, Hershorin LL, Chylack LT Jr. Nonenzymatic glycosylation in human diabetic lens crystallins. *Diabetologia* 1986; **29**: 225–8.
97 Mandel SS, Shiu DH, Newman BL *et al.* Glycosylation *in vivo* of human lens capsule (basement membrane) and diabetes mellitus. *Biochem Biophys Res Comm* 1983; **117**: 51–6.
98 Liang JN, Chylack LT Jr. Change in the protein tertiary structure with nonenzymatic glycosylation of calf crystallin. *Biochem Biophys Res Comm* 1984; **123**: 899–906.
99 Chou S, Chylack LT Jr, Bunn HF *et al.* Role of nonenzymatic glycosylation in experimental cataract formation. *Biochem Biophys Res Comm* 1980; **95**: 894–901.

# 7 The Lesions and Natural History of Diabetic Retinopathy


**Summary**

- The lesions of diabetic retinopathy can be grouped into those associated with background, preproliferative and proliferative retinopathy.
- Background retinopathy is characterized by: capillary dilatation (later with leakage), capillary occlusion, microaneurysms, 'blot' haemorrhages and lipid-rich hard exudates (commonly in the macular area and associated with oedema).
- In preproliferative retinopathy, there are cotton-wool spots (interruption of axoplasmic transport indicating retinal ischaemia), venous abnormalities (loops, beading and reduplication), arterial abnormalities (variation of calibre, narrowing of segments and occlusion) and intraretinal microvascular abnormalities (IRMA — clusters of dilated abnormal capillaries lying within the retina).
- In proliferative retinopathy, new vessels arise in the periphery and/or on the optic disc, eventually with a fibrous tissue covering. The visual complications are caused by vitreous retraction which leads to haemorrhage and to traction and detachment of the retina.
- New vessels on the optic disc are a 'high-risk' feature as they are particularly prone to cause complications of haemorrhage and retinal detachment.
- Uncomplicated background retinopathy is common and in most patients remains mild for many years. Turnover of microaneurysms, haemorrhages and hard exudates is relatively rapid.
- Maculopathy is heralded by rings of hard exudates approaching the fovea.
- Maculopathy occurs mostly in NIDDM and can cause severe visual loss which is often central, with preserved peripheral navigational vision. It can be exudative, oedematous (at times cystoid) or ischaemic.
- Proliferative retinopathy is the commonest sight-threatening lesion in IDDM. Advanced diabetic eye disease is its end stage, defined by long-standing vitreous haemorrhage, macular traction or detachment, or thrombotic glaucoma.
- Thrombotic glaucoma is due to new vessels and fibrous tissue proliferating in the angle of the anterior chamber, preventing drainage of the aqueous. It is associated with rubeosis iridis (neovascularization of the iris) and causes severe pain and irreversible blindness.


There are few conditions which have been studied as intensely as diabetic retinopathy. There is hardly a week in which there are not several papers on the subject in the medical literature. The tremendous effort expended on this subject has not been in vain. During the last 20 years the lesions of diabetic retinopathy have been well recognized, and the natural history described in detail. Though the condition still surprises us from time to time in its manifestations or progression, by and large there is little that we do not know about the clinical features. In addition, the last 15 years have seen the development of treatment, in the form of photocoagulation, for the sight-threatening forms of diabetic retinopathy. Microsurgery, in particular vitrectomy and membrane stripping, has also allowed eyes that are already blind to regain some vision. In spite of these advances, there is still very little that we know about the pathogenic mechanisms leading to the lesions, particularly the sight-threatening ones, and we have as yet no ideas about how to avoid the development of these events.

In this chapter, the lesions themselves and their natural history will be described. Their treatment is discussed in Chapter 8.

## The lesions of diabetic retinopathy

The lesions of diabetic retinopathy can be divided into two major groups: those associated with background or non-proliferative retinopathy, and those with proliferative retinopathy (Table 7.1). *Background* changes include capillary dilatation, capillary occlusion, microaneurysms, haemorrhages, hard exudates and retinal (especially macular) oedema. *Proliferative* retinopathy includes the formation of new vessels, arising from the disc or the retinal periphery, and fibrous tissue which accompanies and eventually replaces the new vessels. There is an additional sub-group of lesions which although considered as background changes indicate that proliferative retinopathy is likely to develop within the next 6–12 months. These *preproliferative* changes include cotton-wool spots, intraretinal microvascular abnormalities (IRMA), and venous and arterial abnormalities.

### *Non-proliferative lesions*

#### CAPILLARY DILATATION

Capillary dilatation is probably the earliest manifestation of diabetic retinopathy. True dilatation of the capillaries is suggested by the findings in diabetic rats that the number of cells forming the capillary wall was increased, and that the wall was thinned, compared with non-diabetic controls [1]. Fluorescein angiograms in diabetic patients demonstrate retinal capillaries more clearly than in non-diabetic subjects, suggesting either true dilatation or leakage of fluorescein into the capillary wall [2].

The significance of capillary dilatation early in diabetes, before any other signs of retinopathy, is not clear. It may reflect increased retinal blood flow, which has been observed by some workers [3] but not by others [4]. Other causes of the dilatation could include metabolic factors such as increased lactic acid production or reduced oxygen utilization.

At this early stage, when dilatation is uniform, it carries no prognostic significance. Later, however, when dilatation of some capillaries is secondary to occlusion of others, the dilated capillaries become leaky and are responsible for retinal and macular oedema and the formation of lipid-rich 'hard' exudates.

Capillary dilatation is not visible on fundoscopy and must be demonstrated by fluorescein angiography. Dilatation of the retinal *veins* is an early fundoscopic feature of diabetic retinopathy.

#### CAPILLARY OCCLUSION

Capillary occlusion is probably the most important of the early and even the late lesions. It precedes the development of microaneurysms, and when the area occluded is large enough, the non-perfused area is responsible for the development of new vessels. In the early stages, however, capillary non-perfusion can only be detected on high-quality fluorescein angiograms (Fig. 7.1). When extensive, especially in the retinal periphery, featureless appearance of the retina, bereft of the normal striations, can be recognized easily on retinal photographs, and with experience on fundoscopic examination.

#### MICROANEURYSMS

Microaneurysms, the hallmark of diabetic retinopathy [5] (Fig. 7.2), are localized dilatations of the capillaries which were first described in detail in 1948 by Ballantyne and Lowenstein [6]. It is important to realize that, although the appearance of the first microaneurysm indicates the appearance of diabetic retinopathy, microaneurysms are not themselves of sinister prognostic importance: as long as there are only microaneurysms, with some capillary closure and dilatation, there is no danger of loss of sight.

More severe retinopathy follows as the number of microaneurysms increases. Large numbers almost never occur as the only manifestation of diabetic retinopathy. Later, when there are increasing areas of capillary non-perfusion, the number of microaneurysms may actually fall, but this is a relatively late, preproliferative stage of diabetic retinopathy.

The pathogenesis of microaneurysms is not clearly established. The most plausible current theory is that microaneurysms only arise when pericytes are lost from the capillary wall. Normal retinal capillaries have two different cell types in their walls, endothelial cells and pericytes. In diabetes, there appears to be an early loss of peri-

**Table 7.1** Appearances of diabetic retinopathy fundoscopy and corresponding features on fluorescein angiography.

| Stage | Features on fundoscopy | Angiographic appearances |
|---|---|---|
| Non-proliferative (background) | Featureless retina | Capillary dilatation<br>Capillary occlusion (with areas of non-perfusion) |
| | Venous dilatation (generalized) | Confirmed |
| | Microaneurysms | Greater number visualized than by fundoscopy |
| | Haemorrhages*:<br>• flame (superficial)<br>• blot (deep in retina) | Haemorrhages appear as dark areas (fluorescence absorbed by haemorrhage) |
| | Exudates ('hard') | |
| Preproliferative | Cotton-wool spots** | Non-perfused areas, usually larger than cotton-wool spots and surrounded by dilated, leaky vessels |
| | Specific venous abnormalities:<br>• loops<br>• beading<br>• reduplication | Appearances confirmed |
| | Arterial abnormalities:<br>• segmental narrowing<br>• 'sheathing'<br>• occlusion | Reduced luminal size, irregularity |
| Proliferative | New vessels (neovascularization):<br>• on disc<br>• elsewhere | Abnormal configuration of leaky vessels |
| | Fibrous tissue | |
| | Advanced complications:<br>Haemorrhage<br>• preretinal<br>• vitreous | |
| | Retinal detachment | Diffuse leakage |

* A single retinal haemorrhage, in the absence of other features, is not diagnostic of diabetic retinopathy.
** A single cotton-wool spot, in the absence of other features, is not diagnostic of preproliferative retinopathy.

cytes, at a time when endothelial cell numbers are normal. The role of the pericytes is not clearly established, but recent work suggests they have a controlling influence over endothelial cell growth. In elegant co-culture studies, Orlidge and D'Amore [7] demonstrated that when pericytes and endothelial cells were in direct contact, endothelial cell proliferation was inhibited. When the cells were separated, even though diffusion of materials was still possible, the inhibition was lost. Inhibition of cell proliferation was specific to smooth muscle cells and pericytes; loss of pericytes, for whatever reason, may therefore be responsible for the formation of microaneurysms.

### HAEMORRHAGES

Haemorrhages in diabetic retinopathy occur early. A single haemorrhage in the deep or superficial retinal layer, in the absence of microaneurysms, can occur in the absence of diabetes, and accordingly is given a score on the Wisconsin grading system which is lower than that of the earliest retinopathy [8]. Once microaneurysms are present, multiple haemorrhages indicate increasing severity of diabetic retinopathy. Superficial flame-shaped haemorrhages were previously thought to indicate hypertension, but this is not necessarily the case. Deep, blot-shaped haemorrhages are more common in diabetes, and almost invariably indicate retinal ischaemia. In the early phases they are usually most numerous lateral to the macula but the later are present throughout the posterior pole, very often lying on the demarcation line between perfused and non-perfused areas (Fig. 7.3). In NIDDM, multiple blot-shaped haemorrhages are common early in the disease, when they usually carry a poor prognosis. In general,

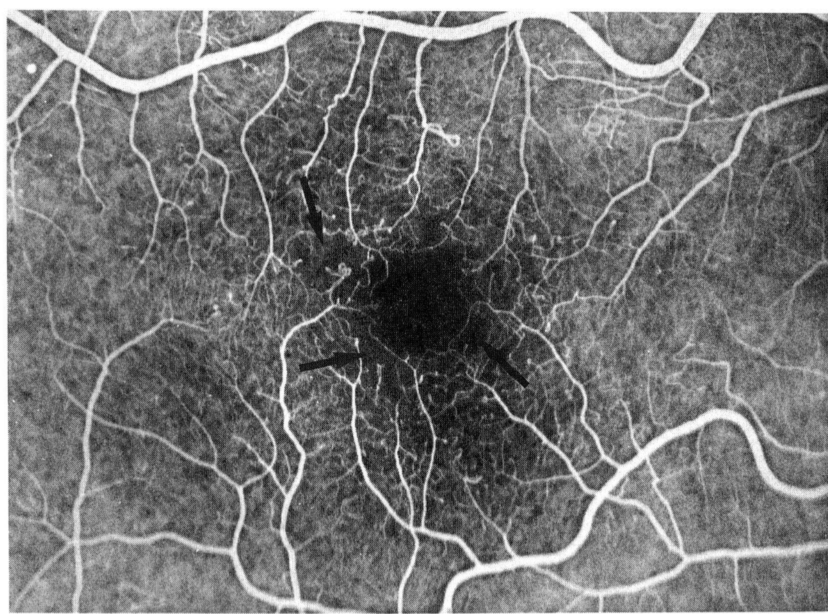

**Fig. 7.1.** Fluorescein angiogram of the perifoveal area of a patient with early diabetic retinopathy, showing small areas of non-perfusion (arrows).

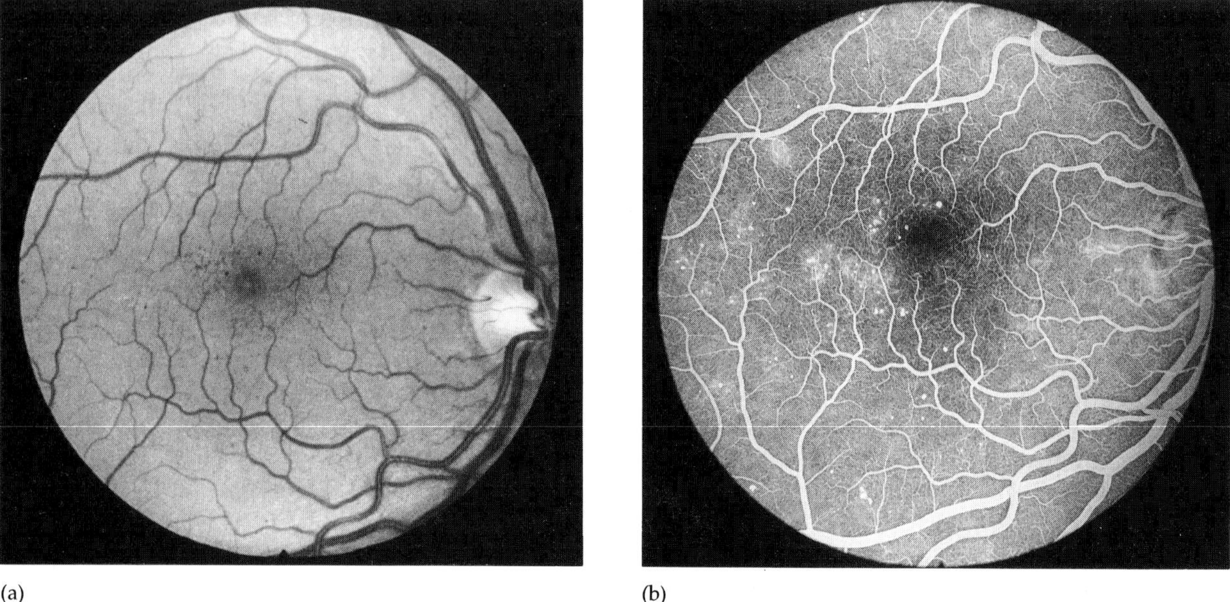

(a) (b)

**Fig. 7.2.** (a) From a colour photograph of the right macular area of a diabetic patient with mild retinopathy, showing only a few microaneurysms and early hard exudates. (b) Fluorescein photograph of area shown in (a). Note many more microaneurysms showing up as white dots.

haemorrhages have a short life, usually resolving within 6–8 weeks, but large blot haemorrhages at the margin of the perfused area may persist for much longer, especially in elderly patients.

Preretinal haemorrhages may be associated with hypertension and arise from small vessels. More commonly, they are associated with new vessels, and result from the retracting vitreous pulling on the vessels, which grow on the posterior vitreous surface. The haemorrhages may be quite large, obscuring the vessels from which they arise; they may track down to the lower half of the retina, but usually remain attached to the vessels from which they arise. If the new vessels are treated by photocoagulation, they clear up rapidly. Occasionally, the preretinal haemorrhage is partially encapsulated in fibrous tissue, in which case it may persist for a long time. Preretinal haemorrhages are only associated with visual loss if the haemorrhage covers the foveal area. Haemorrhages arising from

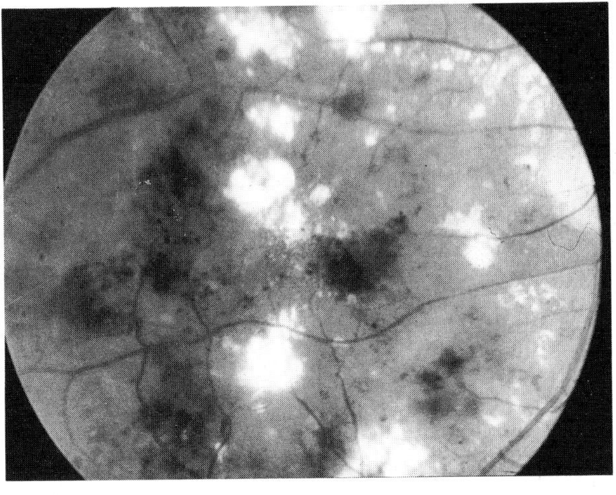

(a)

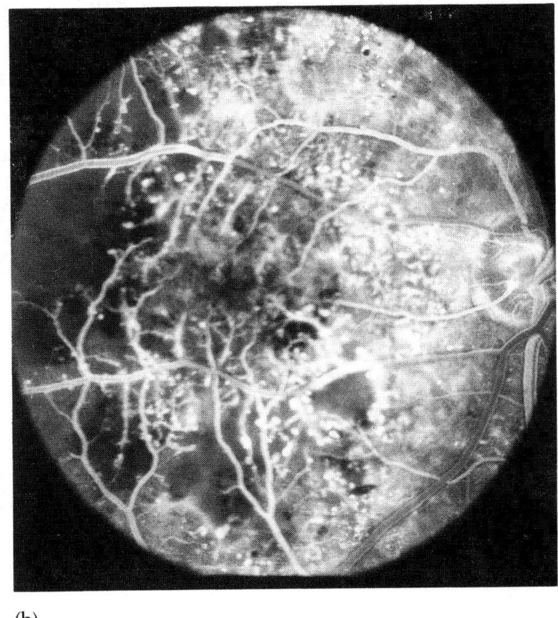

(b)

**Fig. 7.3.** (a) Right macular area of a patient with large blot haemorrhages and hard exudates. (b) Fluorescein angiogram of area shown in (a). Note large areas of non-perfusion and the darker areas indicating ischaemic haemorrhages between perfused and non-perfused retina.

new vessels, if large enough may fill the entire retrovitreal space or may break into the vitreous. Such haemorrhages are usually associated with severe visual loss.

#### HARD EXUDATES

Hard exudates are also early lesions in diabetic retinopathy and are true exudates due to leakage from abnormal vessels. Such leakage is clearly demonstrated by fluorescein angiography but the hard exudates themselves are not visualized (Fig. 7.4). In the earliest cases, hard exudates are small and scattered, but soon tend to coalesce and form plaques and ring patterns. Hard exudates can develop in any part of the retina but are most common in the macular area between the superior and inferior temporal vessels. They usually appear some distance from the fovea and gradually advance towards it, the vessels behind being leaky. Because hard exudates are true exudates, they are always associated with leakage of plasma constituents and therefore with some degree of retinal oedema, which may be focal or in later cases, more generalized and usually affects the macular area. On stereo retinal photographs, these areas appear as retinal thickening. Indeed, the Early Treatment of Diabetic Retinopathy Study defined macular oedema as macular thickening and advised focal treatment if any part of the macula was so affected [9].

The lesions described so far are all lesions of non-proliferative diabetic retinopathy. With the exception of extensive hard exudates, they do not cause visual loss unless they involve the fovea, which is rare. The remaining lesions are associated with impending or actual proliferative retinopathy (see Table 7.2).

### *Preproliferative lesions*

These lesions warn of, and may already be accompanied by, new vessel formation. They only rarely cause visual loss themselves but indicate the urgent need for treatment to prevent the develment of proliferative changes (see Table 7.2).

Preproliferative lesions are listed in Table 7.1 and illustrated in Fig. 7.5.

#### COTTON-WOOL SPOTS

Cotton-wool spots represent areas of interrupted axoplasmic transport, in which material from both orthograde and retrograde transport accumulates within an area of retinal ischaemia [10]. They are not unique to diabetes, occurring in many other conditions such as embolism, hypertension, collagen–vascular diseases and retinal vein

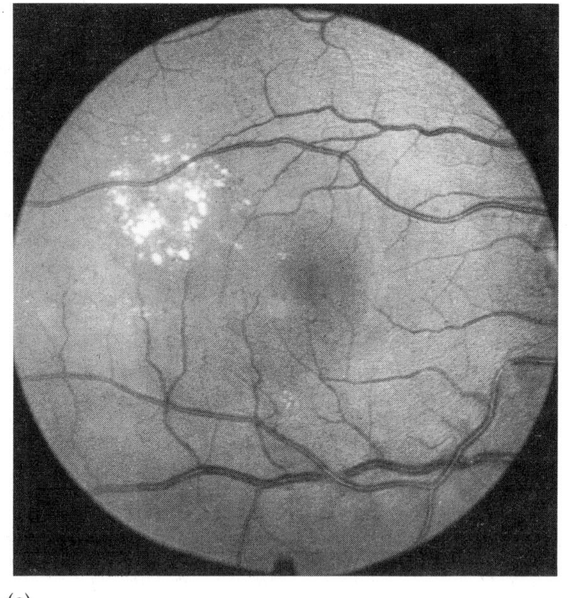

(a)

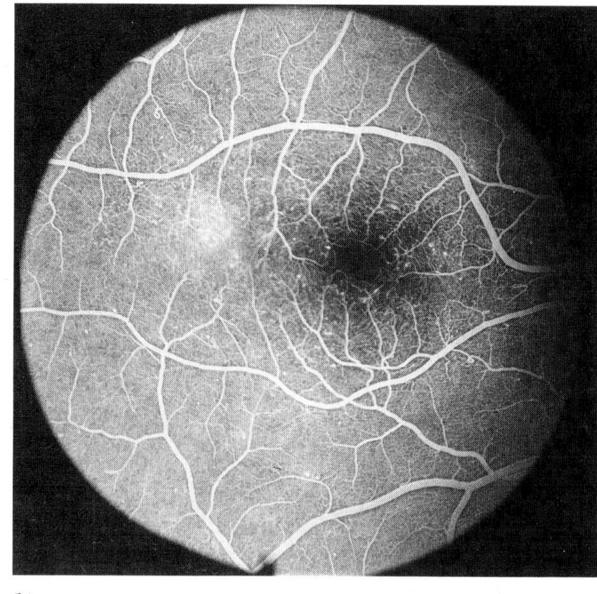

(b)

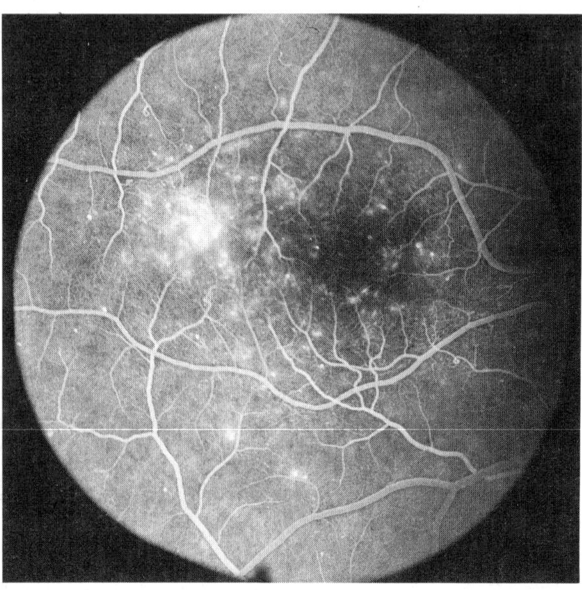

(c)

**Fig. 7.4.** (a) Vascular tree lateral to right macular area, showing an isolated hard exudate ring. (b) Fluorescein angiogram of a similarly affected area in a different patient. The capillary phase shows focal capillary dilatation, leakage and loss associated with the hard exudate rings. (c) Later phase of angiogram from same area as in (b) showing focal leakage.

occlusion. A single cotton-wool spot in a diabetic eye in the absence of microaneurysms or any other lesions is not of prognostic importance and does not necessarily herald impending diabetic retinopathy; as with a single haemorrhage, an isolated cotton-wool spot therefore has a low score according to the Wisconsin grading system. On the other hand, multiple cotton-wool spots (more than five) in an eye indicate rapidly advancing retinopathy. In a prospective study at the Hammersmith Hospital, visual prognosis at 5 years was worse in those with five or more cotton-wool spots in an eye than in those with fewer. Because of the small number of patients with over ten cotton-wool spots, it was not possible to determine whether prognosis worsened with increasing numbers of cotton-wool spots.

When fully developed, cotton-wool spots appear as shiny white areas with ragged edges, sometimes with a greyish area between the white edges where axoplasmic transport is disrupted. On fluorescein angiography cotton-wool spots always appear as non-perfused areas (Fig. 7.5), which may be considerably larger than the visible white spots. Long-standing cotton-wool spots are surrounded by microaneurysms which, on late-phase angiograms,

**Table 7.2.** Warning signs in diabetic retinopathy.

*Maculopathy*
- Hard exudates in rings approaching fovea
- Retinal thickening at macula
- Falling visual acuity without other obvious cause

*Imminent new vessel formation*
- Five or more cotton-wool spots
- Multiple IRMA
- Venous reduplication and beading

are seen to leak fluorescein into the non-perfused area.

Cotton-wool spots persist for longer in diabetes than in hypertension and other diseases, but eventually disappear as the accumulated axoplasmic debris is cleared by macrophages. In diabetes, the circulation in areas of cotton-wool spots is often markedly reduced; this probably accounts for their prolonged half-life, which may be as much as 15 months in young IDDM patients and over 40 months in older patients [11].

Multiple cotton-wool spots in an eye are of prognostic importance (see Table 7.2). However, it should be emphasized that, in the absence of venous abnormalities or IRMA (see below), the prognosis is not uniformly serious and new vessels may take over a year to appear.

### VENOUS ABNORMALITIES

Dilated veins, like capillaries, appear early in diabetes before there is any other evidence of retinopathy. Whether this indicates increased blood flow, increased viscosity, or perhaps an autoregulatory adaptation to hyperglycaemia, has not been established. Simple dilatation of retinal veins does not carry any prognostic significance in the evolution of diabetic retinopathy.

In contrast to simple venous dilatation, more severe lesions include venous loops, reduplication and beading (Fig. 7.5). These lesions are invariably associated with more severe forms of retinopathy and are always associated with occlusion of some of the veins, often only in the periphery. Of these lesions, reduplication is the least common and the most important prognostically, while loops alone are of less importance. Reduplication suggests that new vessels are not long delayed. The significance of venous beading falls between the two. It is an important preproliferative lesion and, together with clusters of blot haemorrhages and cotton-wool spots, heralds the imminent development of proliferative lesions.

### ARTERIAL ABNORMALITIES

Arterial abnormalities usually start in the retinal

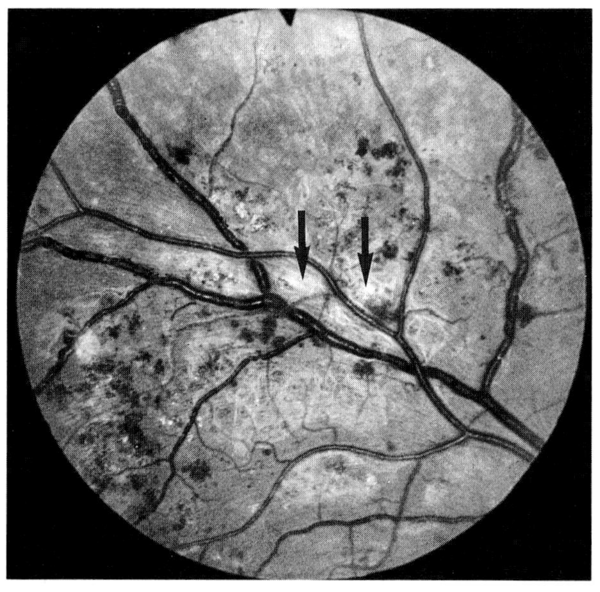

(a)

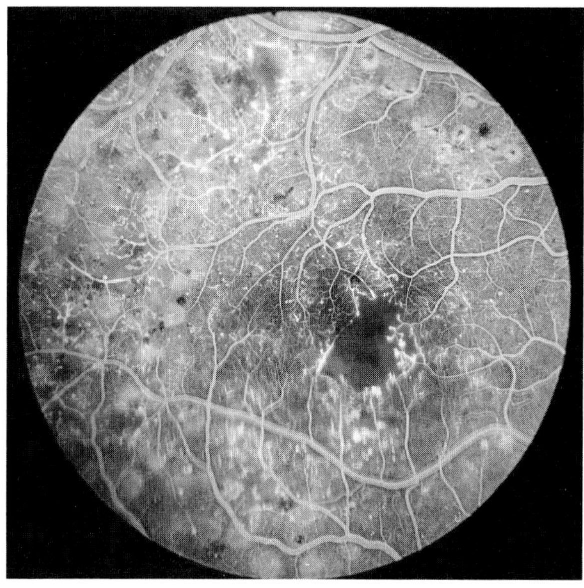

(b)

**Fig. 7.5.** (a) Right superior temporal area of patient with marked preproliferative changes, showing venous beading, haemorrhages, IRMA and a few early cotton-wool spots. The peripheral retina also appears atrophic. (b) Late phase of fluorescein angiogram of a macular area. Note blind ends of occluded small vessels, IRMA leakage and large areas of non-perfusion, some corresponding to cotton-wool spots.

periphery and extend gradually towards the posterior pole. The first notable change is marked calibre variation of the arteries, with increasing numbers of narrowed segments. Side-branches become narrowed at their origin, a feature which pre-dates eventual occlusion of the vessel. Before they become occluded, vessels are often 'sheathed' as well as irregular. The sheathing indicates that the blood flow in the vessel is reduced and there is a relative thickening of the vessel wall in comparison to the blood column. It does not necessarily mean true thickening.

Eventually, the vessels become occluded. When there is arterial occlusion, capillary perfusion in that area ceases. When the occlusion is rapid there are usually cotton-wool spots. Sudden occlusion leads to retinal infarction, and no cotton-wool spots develop. If occlusion is gradual or occurs in the retinal periphery where the retinal nerve fibre layer is thin, the disappearance of the normal striated appearance of the retina is the most marked feature, the retina looking featureless and dull. A paucity of vessels may be noted, and haemorrhages tend to occur at the junction of the perfused and non-perfused areas (see Fig. 7.3).

The crucial importance of arterial occlusion is that new vessels will not form in its absence.

#### INTRARETINAL MICROVASCULAR ABNORMALITIES

These are perhaps the most sinister of the preproliferative lesions. They occur in areas of widespread capillary occlusion, often associated with occlusion of larger vessels, and consist of dilated, abnormal capillaries which are often leaky and lie in the plane of the retina.

When widespread, their prognosis is similar to that of new vessels. Indeed, widespread IRMA are usually associated with cotton-wool spots and venous beading, often with extensive blot haemorrhages, when the prognosis is very severe indeed (Fig. 7.5). This condition is known as 'florid' diabetic retinopathy, and usually affects young patients with poorly controlled diabetes. Untreated, it leads to blindness in some 90% of cases within 1 year, and if treated with photocoagulation, requires very heavy burns and extensive treatment. This fact was not initially appreciated at the introduction of photocoagulation and explains why pituitary ablation was for a long time considered the treatment of choice for this condition [12].

### *Proliferative lesions*

#### NEW VESSELS AND FIBROUS RETINITIS PROLIFERANS

New vessels appear in the retinal periphery (Fig. 7.6) or on the optic disc (Fig. 7.7). Their origin is usually a major vein but occasionally they arise from arteries and those on the disc may grow from the choroidal circulation. Proliferative retinopathy is the commonest sight-threatening complication of retinopathy in IDDM. In the Wisconsin epi-

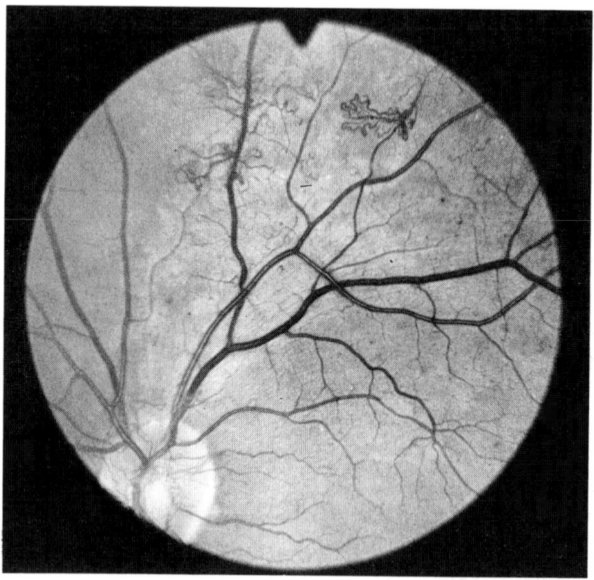

**Fig. 7.6.** New vessels arising from superior temporal vein.

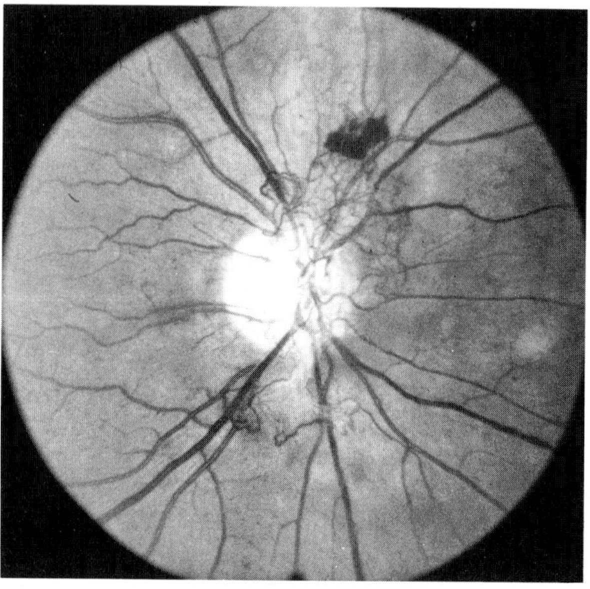

**Fig. 7.7.** New vessels arising from the optic disc.

demiogical study, up to 60% of patients diagnosed before the age of 30 years developed such lesions after about 20 years of diabetes [13]. The prevalence decreased after 30 years, probably because the patients with the worst lesions also had severe nephropathy or other fatal complications (see Chapter 5). Proliferative changes are less common in NIDDM, affecting about 40% of those treated with insulin and less than 20% of those treated by diet with or without oral agents [14].

When peripheral new vessels first form, they lie in the plane of the retina but, with accompanying mesenchyme, soon pierce the internal limiting membrane to lie in front of the retina and become attached to the posterior face of the vitreous. They may then enter the cortex of the vitreous, forming firm adhesions. The outcome of new-vessel growth depends on what happens to the vitreous. While the vitreous remains attached to the retina, the vessels are asymptomatic. Usually, however, the presence of the vessels leads to retraction of the vitreous, pulling the vascular mesenchyme forward from the site of its firm fibrovascular adhesion to the retina, forming epiretinal membranes. This event leads to the complications of new vessels which cause visual symptoms. In their early stages, vessels may break as the vitreous retracts, producing preretinal or vitreous (intragel) haemorrhage. The vessels and their fibrous tissue covering may be pulled forward, causing traction on the internal limiting membrane and retina and resulting in distortion of vision. Fibroglial tissue proliferates on the posterior vitreous face and tends to contract, applying antero-posterior traction to its attachment to vascularized fronds at the base of the vitreous. If severe, traction may result in retinal detachment, which always causes some degree of visual loss and is profound if the macula is involved. Disc vessels undergo the same process, but much faster. One reason for this may be that the vitreous is attached to the disc margin but not the surface of the disc, perhaps allowing the new vessels to grow forward at an early stage. New vessels on the disc (unless of minimal severity) are the most important 'high-risk characteristic' identified by the Diabetic Retinopathy Study [15], as they rapidly lead to visual loss if untreated. If haemorrhage is associated with new vessels, visual loss is imminent even if the initial bleed is small and retained within the new vessel fibrovascular tissue.

Clinically, new vessels are recognized by their haphazard configuration, often with microaneurysm-like dilatations at their growing ends. Later, when well established, they may form branching arborizing patterns. It must be remembered that new vessels *never* arise in an otherwise healthy retina; there are always other lesions, such as microaneurysms, haemorrhages and signs of retinal ischaemia, such as an atrophic-looking peripheral retina, cotton-wool spots, occluded arteries and veins (showing up as white lines), other venous abnormalities, and IRMA. While untreated, new vessels carry a poor prognosis for vision, but they are also the lesions most responsive to photocoagulation, when this is carried out early and adequately.

Fibrous tissue is easily recognized by its white colour. It tends to be vascular in its early stages and dry and featureless after the vessels have closed. Attached fibrous tissue puckers the retina, and traction lines can be followed to a fibrous tissue base (Fig. 7.8).

Once fibrous tissue is extensive, photocoagulation is potentially dangerous as it may cause further traction and retinal detachment. Fibrous tissue and the accompanying traction can be removed by vitrectomy, membrane splitting and peeling (see Chapter 8).

### The natural history of diabetic retinopathy

The lesions of diabetic retinopathy as indicated above can be broadly grouped into background

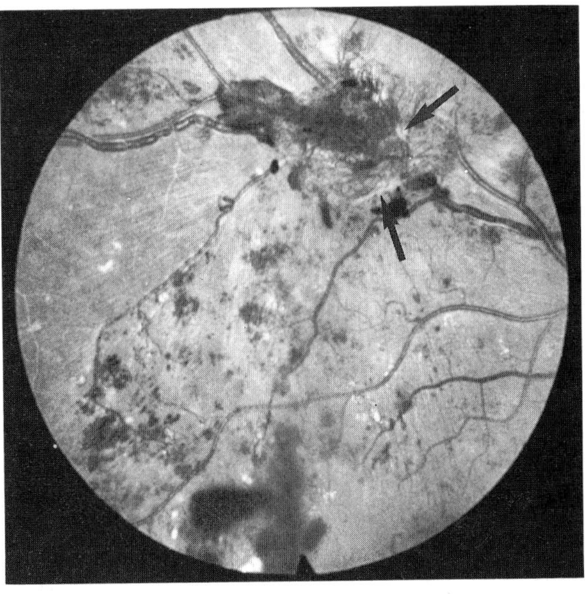

**Fig. 7.8.** Fibrous tissue (arrows) with new vessels forming the origin of traction lines distorting the internal limiting membrane.

and proliferative lesions. On a clinical basis, it is useful to subdivide retinopathy into uncomplicated background retinopathy, background retinopathy with macular oedema, proliferative retinopathy and advanced diabetic eye disease. These subdivisions also help to illustrate the natural history of the condition.

### *Uncomplicated background retinopathy*

This is the commonest form of retinopathy. It is present in up to 97% of young-onset patients after about 20 years of diabetes [13] and has been found within the first years of the disease in those diagnosed at over 30 years of age [14]. In the ongoing United Kingdom Prospective Diabetes Study, up to 30% of newly diagnosed NIDDM patients had some degree of retinopathy. Some reports suggest genetic predisposition to retinopathy, but it is difficult to believe that a condition which occurs in up to 97% of patients and is similar in appearance in IDDM, NIDDM and secondary diabetes has a genetic rather than a metabolic pathogenesis.

Although retinopathy is common, its development in patients not previously affected is more difficult to characterize and to date, has been addressed by only two good prospective studies. In Denmark, Sjolle [16], using stepwise logistic analysis, concluded that the probability of developing retinopathy depended on the duration of diabetes and insulin dosage and was greater in smokers. In a Swiss population of patients without retinopathy at an initial examination, Teuscher *et al.* [17] reported that, after 8 years of follow-up, background retinopathy had developed in 39% of 53 IDDM patients, 40% of late-onset patients treated with insulin and in only 15% of subjects treated by diet with or without oral agents.

In most patients, background retinopathy remains mild for many years. The turnover of all background lesions — microaneurysms, haemorrhages and hard exudates — is relatively high. The total number of microaneurysms tends to increase, although there is great variation between patients. Haemorrhages have a much shorter half-life, as mentioned above. Hard exudates develop gradually and tend to extend towards the fovea. It is often difficult to predict who will deteriorate within a short period of time. In general, maculopathy is imminent when hard exudates start to form rings and approach the fovea. Increasing numbers of haemorrhages suggest increasing ischaemia. In IDDM patients, preproliferative or at least more active retinopathy is heralded by increasing numbers of haemorrhages and new microaneurysms and the first appearance of IRMAs.

### *Diabetic maculopathy*

Diabetic maculopathy is background retinopathy with macular oedema. Mild degrees of macular oedema are not uncommon in IDDM, but the great majority of patients suffering from visual loss from this condition are those with NIDDM. The British Multicentre Study on Photocoagulation [18] illustrated this clearly, in that 56 of the 99 patients with maculopathy were aged 30–59 years and only nine patients were under the age of 30 years when diabetes was diagnosed.

Visual loss with maculopathy can be severe, and legal blindness is not uncommon. In the British study [18], even of those with initially good vision, 50% became blind within 5 years. The Early Treatment of Diabetic Retinopathy Study found that over 20% of patients lost two or more lines of visual acuity in eyes in which treatment was deferred [9]. It should, however, be remembered that the blindness of macular oedema is not total, as, for example, with a large vitreous haemorrhage, but is confined to central visual loss, with preservation of peripheral, navigational vision. Many of these patients can therefore be greatly helped by low-vision aids and remain able to cope with much of their everyday life (see Chapter 9).

Diabetic maculopathy can be subdivided into three groups. The commonest, and the most amenable to treatment, is *exudative maculopathy* (Fig. 7.9), in which hard exudate rings form usually lateral to the foveal area and gradually approach it. In the centre of the rings are leaky microvascular lesions which are responsible for the deposition of the exudates. The centres of the rings, and often their advancing edge are oedematous and therefore seen as retinal thickening on stereo photographs or biomicroscopy. The lesions usually progress gradually but, unless treated, will eventually affect the fovea either by forming a hard exudate plaque in its centre, or through leakage from microvascular lesions at its edge. The natural history of these rings, with new exudates forming while others disappear, was first described by Dobree [19]. Once the fovea has been involved, treatment becomes more difficult and is often impossible. Hard exudate plaques, even when in the centre of

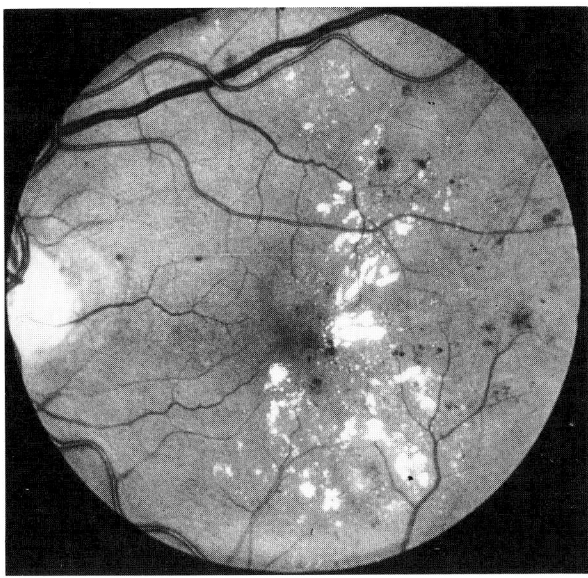
(a)

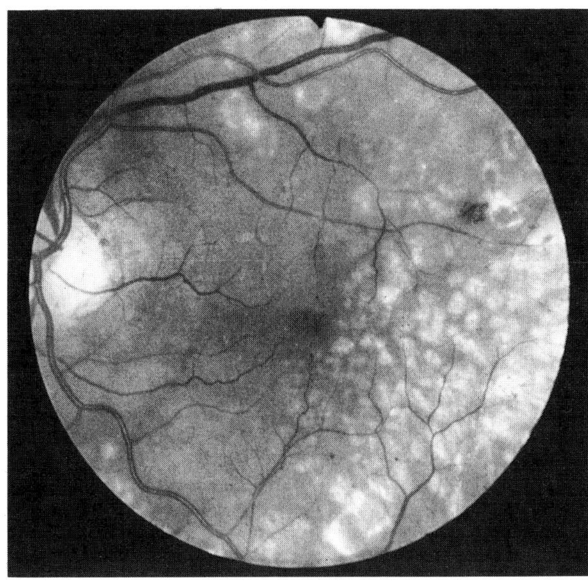
(b)

**Fig. 7.9.** (a) Hard exudate ring near the left macula, before treatment. Visual acuity 6/18. (b) Hard exudate ring has disappeared after treatment by pan-retinal photocoagulation. Visual acuity 6/9.

the fovea, eventually disappear but any resulting visual loss will remain. Similarly, long-standing oedema usually causes permanent visual loss, often with pigment epithelial changes.

*Oedematous maculopathy*, consisting of widespread and often cystoid oedema, is the other common form of maculopathy. Little is known about the natural history of this condition. In young patients, cystoid oedema can coexist with reasonable vision for long periods of time, before vision is eventually lost. In older patients, however, visual loss is more rapid and profound. In many instances of oedematous maculopathy, there is a decrease of capillaries in the perifoveal area and the remaining capillaries become dilated and leaky (Fig. 7.10).

*Ischaemic maculopathy*, carries the worse prognosis for vision (Fig. 7.11). In this condition, perifoveal capillaries are destroyed, so that the non-perfused area at the fovea is enlarged. This is compatible with normal or near-normal vision in young patients but in older patients, visual loss occurs after a relatively short period of time. In ischaemic maculopathy, peripheral as well as perifoveal capillaries are often lost. Such eyes are in danger of developing new vessels, and present a particularly difficult treatment problem, since the use of pan-retinal photocoagulation will cause loss of peripheral vision. Ischaemia is almost invariably progressive, which explains the poor prognosis.

The probability of developing maculopathy when there is no retinopathy or only mild background retinopathy has not been established, largely because the importance of maculopathy as a cause of visual loss has only recently been recognized and long-term follow-up has not been reported. Moreover, many affected patients are treated, because several studies indicate that photocoagulation is better than no treatment.

### *Proliferative diabetic retinopathy*

Proliferative diabetic retinopathy, as indicated above, is the commonest sight-threatening lesion in IDDM. The chances of developing new vessels in patients not previously affected was 3% per year in the Joslin Clinic study of IDDM patients [20]. In the 8-year follow-up study by Teuscher *et al.* [17], 9% of IDDM patients initially without retinopathy developed new vessels, which also appeared in 8% of insulin-treated NIDDM and 3% of non-insulin treated NIDDM patients. For those patients with background retinopathy at the initial examination, the chances of developing proliferative retinopathy increased to 25% of IDDM, 22% of insulin-treated NIDDM and 13% of non-insulin-treated NIDDM patients.

Proliferative retinopathy carries a poor prognosis for vision, especially if the new vessels arise from the disc. Thus, in the British Multicentre Study, no eyes with disc vessels showed

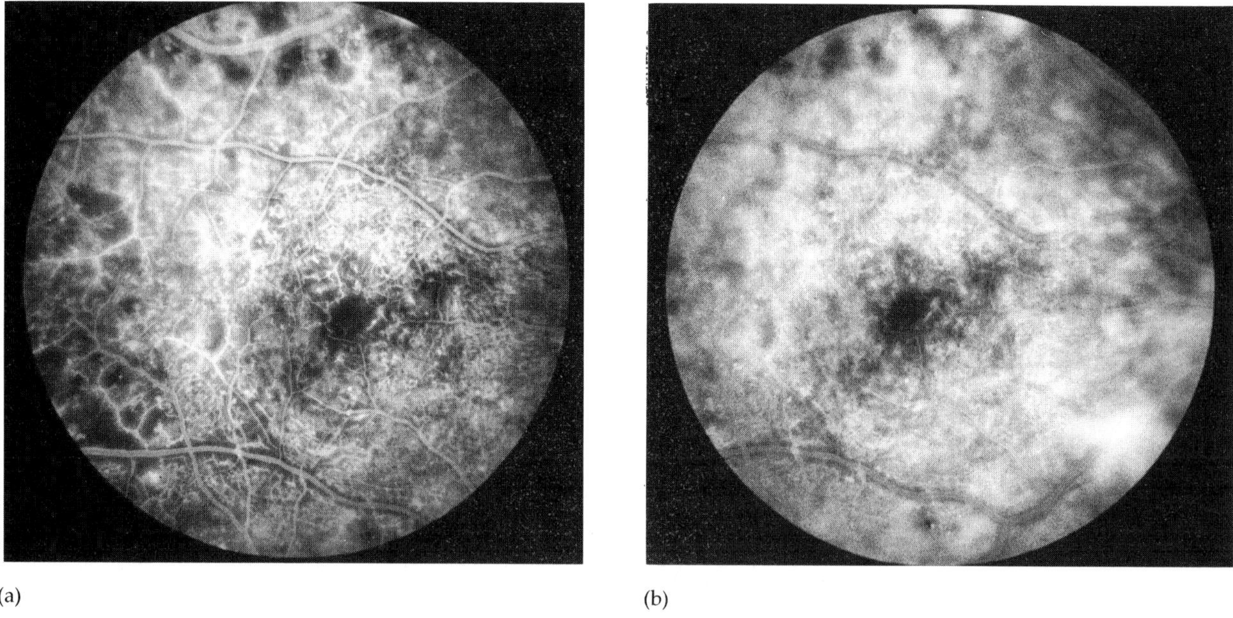

(a) (b)

**Fig. 7.10.** (a) Fluorescein angiogram from a patient with oedematous maculopathy, showing dilated leaky capillaries. (b) Late phase of fluorescein angiogram shown in (a) with widespread leakage in perifoveal area.

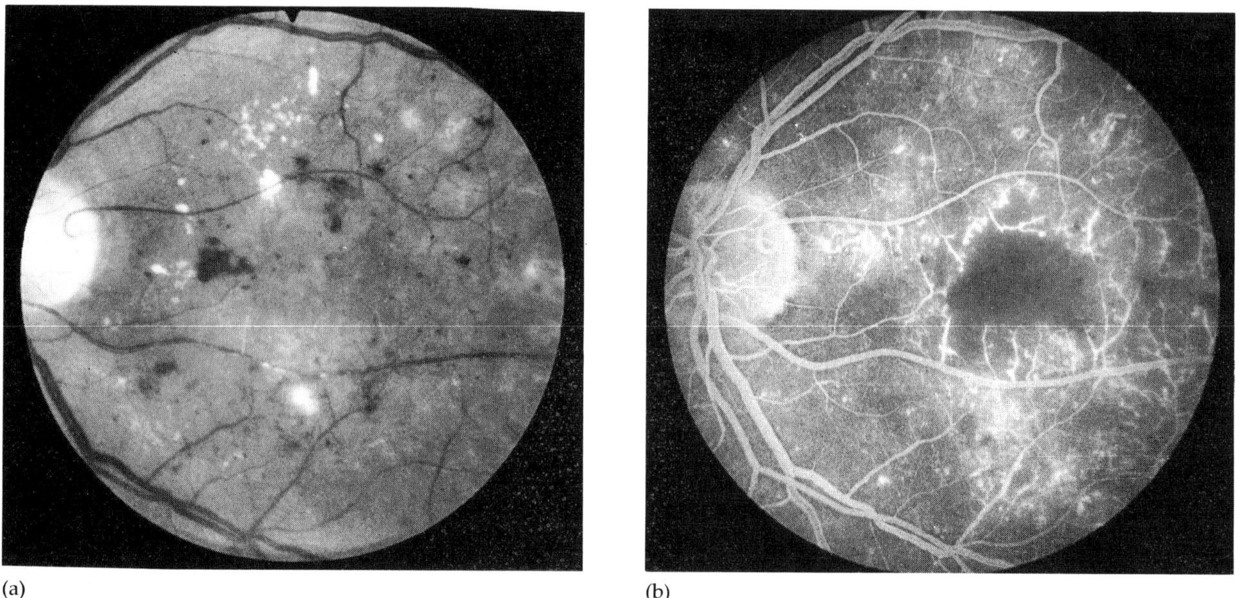

(a) (b)

**Fig. 7.11.** (a) Right macular region of patient with ischaemic maculopathy. Note large blot haemorrhages suggesting ischaemia. (b) Fluorescein angiogram of area shown in (a). Note large perifoveal and peripheral ischaemic areas.

improved vision during follow-up and 33 out of 38 eyes deteriorated, 20 of these becoming blind when untreated [21]. In a study performed at the Hammersmith Hospital before photocoagulation became available, less than one-third of eyes became blind over 5 years when new vessels arose from the retinal periphery only, and most maintained normal vision. When new vessels arose from the disc, however, 13 out of 21 eyes became blind over this period of time. The Diabetic Retinopathy Study [15] of over 1700 patients associated the worst prognosis with 'high-risk' characteristics, including more than minimal disc vessels, disc vessels with present or previous vitreous haemorrhage and peripheral new vessels with haemorrhage.

In the natural history of new vessels, vitreous haemorrhage is usually the first complication to cause visual loss. Caird *et al*. [22] found that within 1 year of the first vitreous haemorrhage, one-third of the affected eyes were blind and that within 3 years, one-third of the patients were blind in both eyes. The large follow-up study reported by Beetham in 1963 [23] found that 10% of patients with proliferative retinopathy maintained useful vision after over 10 years of follow-up.

The most important feature to note in the management of proliferative retinopathy is that new vessels by themselves do not cause significant visual loss, although leakage from them may cause macular oedema with reduction of vision. In most cases, however, vision remains normal until haemorrhage or tractional complications supervene. By then, treatment may be difficult and sometimes ineffective. Regular screening of patients at risk is therefore crucial.

### *Advanced diabetic eye disease*

Advanced diabetic eye disease is the end stage of proliferative retinopathy. Until recently, it was invariably associated with profound visual loss, leading to complete irreversible blindness. In recent years, the development of improved intraocular microsurgical techniques such as vitrectomy and membranectomy have made it possible to improve vision in most patients, as long as the diagnosis is made and treatment undertaken early. The complications of proliferative retinopathy which constitute this group of complications are long-standing vitreous haemorrhage, traction on the macula and retinal detachment, especially that involving the macula (see Chapter 8).

The other form of advanced diabetic eye disease which leads to blindness is thrombotic (neovascuar) glaucoma. This condition tends to occur in the most profoundly ischaemic eyes, and is associated with rubeosis iridis (new vessel growth in the iris). New vessels and contracting fibrous tissue proliferate in the angle of the anterior chamber and interfere with normal drainage of aqueous from the anterior chamber. The raised intra-ocular pressure causes pain, often intractable, and blindness, which is permanent.

The natural history of diabetic retinopathy is therefore unfavourable. Fortunately, however, many patients now maintain their vision due to photocoagulation. Nonetheless, as the pathogenic mechanisms are not fully known, prevention of the usual progression of retinopathy is not yet possible.

EVA M. KOHNER

## References


1 Sosula L. Capillary radius and wall thickness in normal and diabetic rat retinae. *Microvasc Res* 1974; **7**: 274–7.

2 Oosterhuis JA, Lammens AJJ. Fluorescein photography of the ocular fundus. *Ophthalmologica* 1965; **179**: 210–18.

3 Kohner EM, Hamilton AM, Saunders SJ, Sutcliffe BA, Bulpitt CJ. The retinal blood flow in diabetes. *Diabetologia* 1975; **11**: 27–33.

4 Grunwald JE, Riva CE, Sinclair SH, Bruckner SJ, Petrig BL. Laser doppler velocimetry study of retinal circulation in diabetes mellitus. *Arch Ophthalmol* 1986; **104**: 991–6.

5 Bowman W. Capillary microaneurysms in diabetic retinopathy. *Trans Ophthalmol Soc UK* 1965; **85**: 199–205.

6 Ballantyne AJ, Lowenstein A. The pathology of diabetic retinopathy. *Trans Ophthalmol Soc UK* 1943; **63**: 95–115.

7 Orlidge A, D'Amore PA. Inhibition of capillary endothelial cell growth by pericytes and smooth muscle cells. *J Cell Biol* 1987; **105**: 1455–62.

8 Early Treatment of Diabetic Retinopathy Study, *Manual of Operations*, Virginia, USA: Department of Commerce National Technical Information Service, 1985.

9 Early Treatment of Diabetic Retinopathy Study Research Group. Photocoagulation for diabetic macular edema. *Arch Ophthalmol* 1985; **103**: 1796–1806.

10 McLeod D. Clinical signs of obstructed axoplasmic transport. *Lancet* 1975; **ii**: 954–6.

11 Kohner EM, Dollery CT, Bulpitt CJ. Cotton wool spots in diabetic retinopathy. *Diabetes* 1969; **18**: 691–704.

12 Kohner EM, Hamilton AM, Joplin GF, Fraser TR. Florid diabetic retinopathy and its response to treatment by photocoagulation or pituitary ablation. *Diabetes* 1976; **25**: 104–10.

13 Klein R, Klein BEK, Moss SE, Davis MD, deMets DL. The Wisconsin Epidemiologic Study of Diabetic Retinopathy. II. Prevalence and risk of diabetic retinopathy when age of diagnosis is less than 30 years. *Arch Ophthalmol* 1984; **102**: 520–6.

14 Klein R, Klein BEK, Moss SE, Davies MD, deMets DL. The Wisconsin Epidemiologic Study of Diabetic Retinopathy. III. Prevalence and risk of diabetic retinopathy when age of diagnosis is 30 or more years. *Arch Ophthalmol* 1984; **102**: 527–32.

15 The Diabetic Retinopathy Study Grup. Preliminary report on effects of photocoagulation therapy. *Am J Ophthalmol* 1976; **81**: 383–97.

16 Sjolle AK. Ocular complications in insulin-treated diabetes mellitus. *Acta Ophthalmol* 1985; **172**: (suppl)1–77.

17 Teuscher A, Schnelle H, Wilson PWT. Incidence of diabetic retinopathy and relationship to baseline plasma glucose and blood pressure. *Diabetes Care* 1988; **11**: 246–51.

18 British Multicentre Study Group. Photocoagulation for diabetic maculopathy: A randomised controlled clinical trial using the xenon arc. *Diabetes* 1983; **32**: 1010–16.

19 Dobree JH. Simple diabetic retinopathy — evolution of lesions and therapeutic considerations. *Br J Ophthalmol* 1970; **54**: 1–10.

20 Rand LI, Krolewski AS, Aiello LM, Warram JH, Baker RS, Maki T. Multiple factors in the prediction of risk of proliferative retinopathy. *N Engl J Med* 1985; **313**: 1433–8.
21 British Multicentre Study Group. Photocoagulation for proliferative diabetic retinopathy: a randomised controlled clinical trial using the xenon arc. *Diabetologia* 1984; **26**: 109–15.
22 Caird FI, Burditt AF, Draper GJ. Diabetic retinopathy: a further study of prognosis of vision. *Diabetes* 1968; **17**: 121–3.
23 Beetham WP. Visual prognosis of proliferating diabetic retinopathy *Br J Ophthalmol* 1963; **47**: 611–19.

# 8 Laser Photocoagulation and Surgery in the Management of Diabetic Eye Disease

**Summary**

- It is now possible to treat the major sight-threatening complications of diabetic retinopathy (proliferative changes and macular oedema) using laser photocoagulation.
- Photocoagulation employs either the xenon arc lamp, which produces a relatively large, painful retinal burn, or the argon laser, which has a smaller spot size.
- Photocoagulation can be used either to destroy specific targets (e.g. new vessels) or to treat the whole retina except for the central macula and the papillomacular bundle essential for central vision; this 'pan-retinal' photocoagulation reduces overall retinal ischaemia and thus the stimulus to new vessel formation.
- Pan-retinal photocoagulation reduces by over 50% the likelihood of severe visual loss (acuity 1/60 or worse) developing in eyes with high-risk proliferative retinopathy. The place of photocoagulation in *pre*proliferative changes is not yet established.
- Photocoagulation to the peripheral macula can also seal points of capillary leakage and so reduce macular oedema; photocoagulation treatment of clinically significant macular oedema (i.e. involving or threatening the fovea) reduces the risk of visual loss by over 50%.
- 'Closed' vitreo-retinal surgery is performed using instruments and a light source inserted into the vitreous cavity through the pars plana to avoid damaging the lens or retina. The eye is kept distended by a saline infusion. Fibrous membranes, haemorrhages and vitreous can be removed and detached areas of retina can be re-attached.
- Detached retina only remains viable for some weeks; detachment must therefore be diagnosed immediately if surgical re-attachment is to restore vision. B-scan ultrasonography can identify retinal detachments behind dense vitreous haemorrhages.
- Vitreo-retinal surgery can restore and maintain useful vision in up to 70% of eyes with advanced diabetic disease.
- Diabetic patients' eyes must be examined at least annually, with formal measurements of distant and near acuity; checking for an afferent pupillary defect (a sign of serious retinal or optic nerve disease); and inspection of the lens, vitreous and retina through fully dilated pupils.
- Ophthalmological referral is indicated soon for preproliferative changes; urgently for maculopathy, new vessel formation or retinal detachment; and immediately for vitreous haemorrhage or neovascular glaucoma.

**'Next to life itself, the loss of sight is most harrowing' (Von Helmholtz)**

The principal objectives in the surgical management of diabetic eye disease are: the preservation of vision in eyes threatened by proliferative retinopathy or macular oedema; the lasting restoration of sight to eyes blinded by vitreous haemorrhage or retinal detachment; and the prevention of the ultimate horror of an eye not only blind but painful from the ravages of neovascular glaucoma. The advent and development of laser photocoagulation and closed intra-ocular microsurgery, particularly within the last decade, have made it possible to achieve these objectives in many cases.

The purpose of this chapter is to put laser treatment and vitreous surgery into clinical perspective for the physician and to discuss the nature, timing and outcome of these treatments against the background of the natural history of diabetic retinopathy. Above all, it is hoped to enable the clinician to identify the imminence of visual loss and the indications for referring specific patients for surgical management.

## Clinical classification of diabetic retinopathy

The classification of diabetic retinopathy outlined in Chapter 7 can be modified (Table 8.1) to provide a rational basis for determining treatment and for interpreting the results of recent treatment trials.

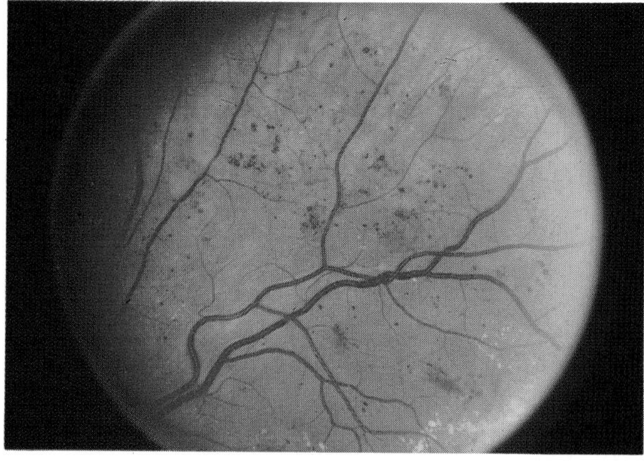

**Fig. 8.1.** Background diabetic retinopathy, showing scattered red 'dots and blots' (microaneurysms and haemorrhages) and exudates.

### *Background diabetic retinopathy without macular oedema*

This is simply the presence of scattered microaneurysms and intra-retinal haemorrhages ('dots and blots') with hard exudates which do not involve the macula (Fig. 8.1). Attempts to distinguish microaneurysms from small haemorrhages are unnecessary and unrewarding. At this stage, there is no threat to vision *per se* and monitoring is required solely to detect the possible complications of macular oedema or preproliferative changes.

### *Diabetic macular oedema*

This is defined as the presence of retinal thickening and/or hard exudate within one disc diameter (approximately 1500 μm) of the centre of the macula [1]. Macular oedema may be classified as *focal* (Fig. 8.2), where the leaking capillaries and microaneurysms are relatively discrete; *diffuse* (Fig. 8.3) where the leakage is extensive, ill-defined and accompanied by cystoid change; and *ischaemic*, in which oedema is associated with extensive areas of capillary non-perfusion, best identified by fluorescein angiography (Fig. 8.4).

This definition is independent of visual acuity, although this is generally predictable within each subgroup [2]. Visual acuity tends to be good (6/6 to 6/12) if the leakage is focal and the hard exudate is not deposited in the fovea. Acuity is moderately reduced (6/12 to 6/24) if the leakage is diffuse and the fovea oedematous, and poor (6/24 to 6/60) if the macula is ischaemic with enlargement of the normal avascular zone at the fovea (Fig. 8.4).

### *Clinically significant macular oedema*

Clinically significant macular oedema is that which threatens the fovea and central vision [3, 4] and is precisely (but lengthily) defined [3] as any one of the following:

**Table 8.1** Clinical classification of diabetic retinopathy.

| |
|---|
| Background retinopathy without macular oedema |
| Macular oedema — focal, diffuse, ischaemic |
| Clinically significant macular oedema |
| Proliferative retinopathy |
| Preproliferative retinopathy |
| Advanced diabetic eye disease:<br>• vitreous haemorrhage<br>• macular distortion<br>• tractional retinal detachment<br>• combined rhegmatogenous/tractional retinal detachment<br>• neovascular glaucoma |

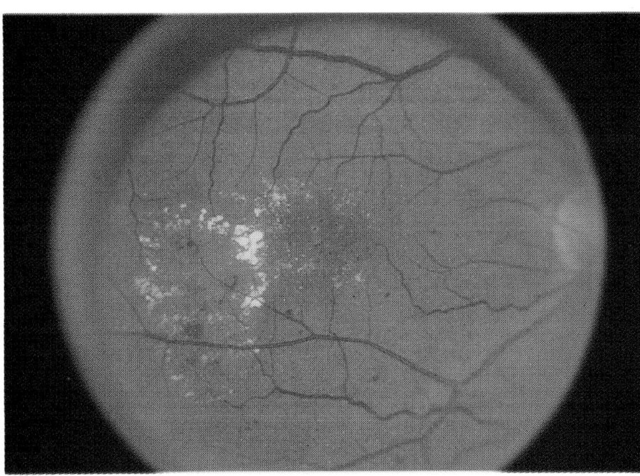

**Fig. 8.2.** Focal macular oedema, showing thickening and a greyish appearance of the retina (more easily appreciated by binocular indirect fundoscopy) restricted to the macular area adjacent to a ring of hard exudates.

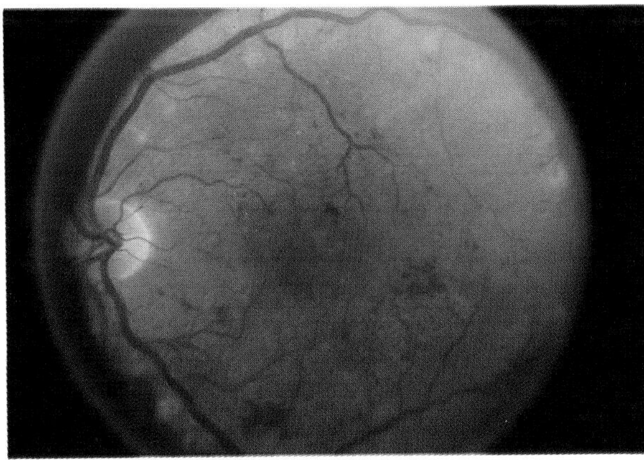

**Fig. 8.3.** Diffuse macular oedema, with widespread changes surrounding the macula. Scars from previous photocoagulation are visible peripherally.

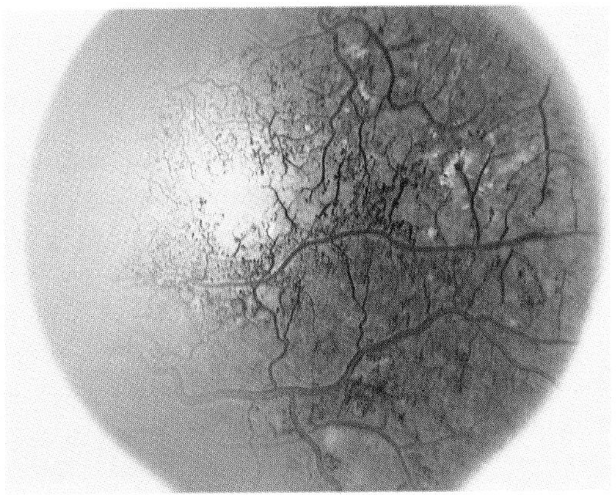

**Fig. 8.4.** Ischaemic macular oedema. The fluorescein angiogram demonstrates capillary non-perfusion and enlargement of the foveal avascular zone.

**1** Thickening of the retina at or within 500 μm of the centre of the macula (Fig. 8.5).
**2** Hard exudate at or within 500 μm of the centre of the macula, only if associated with thickening of adjacent retina (Fig. 8.6). This excludes any hard exudate remaining after retinal thickening has disappeared (Fig. 8.7).
**3** A zone or zones of retinal thickening one disc area or larger in size, any part of which falls within one disc diameter of the centre of the macula (Figs 8.8 and 8.9).

Again, this definition is purely anatomical and takes no account of visual acuity, which in patients entering the Early Treatment Diabetic Retinopathy Study (ETDRS), ranged from 6/4 to 6/60; the severity of macular oedema also varied considerably [3, 5]. The concept of *clinically significant macular oedema* is crucial to the understanding and application of the ETDRS results (see below) [3, 5–7].

### *Proliferative diabetic retinopathy*

This stage is defined as the presence of new blood vessels within the eye, which may form on the optic disc ('NVD'; Fig. 8.10), elsewhere on the retina ('NVE'; Fig. 8.11) or on the iris and drainage angle (rubeosis iridis; Fig. 8.12).

### *Preproliferative diabetic retinopathy*

Preproliferative changes comprise one or more of the following, in the absence of new vessels (Figs 8.13 and 8.14):

- Deep round haemorrhages.
- Cotton-wool spots (two or more).
- Intra-retinal microvascular abnormalities (IRMA).
- Changes in the calibre of the major vessels: venous beading, reduplication or looping and attenuation or obliteration of the smaller branch arterioles, which then appear as white lines (see Fig. 8.11).
- 'Empty' retina: the featureless appearance of ischaemic retina, devoid of its normal striations, adjacent to the above lesions.

The concept of preproliferative retinopathy is important in designing and interpreting trials of treatment to prevent or delay the onset of proliferative changes [1, 6].

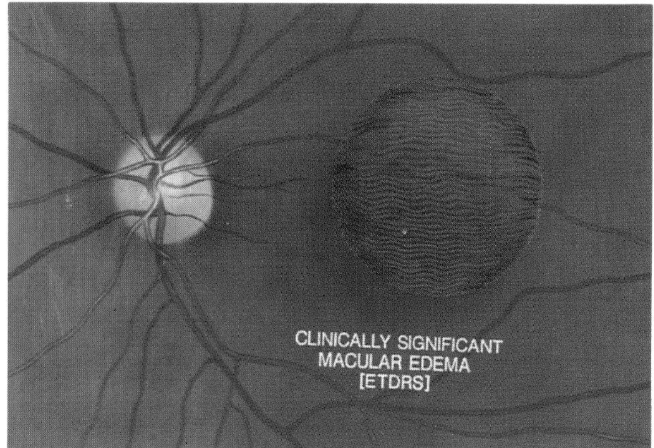


Fig. 8.5

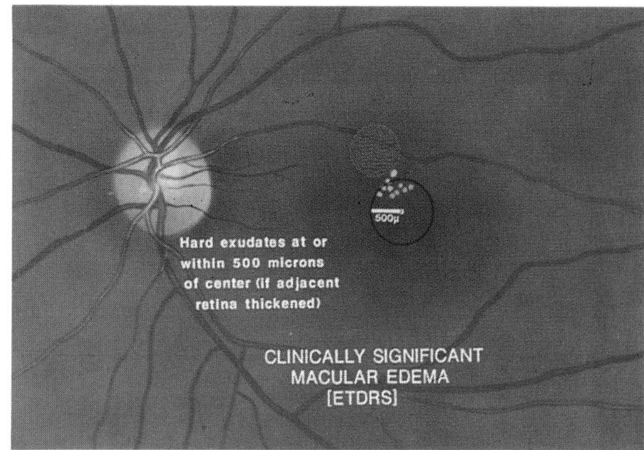


Fig. 8.6

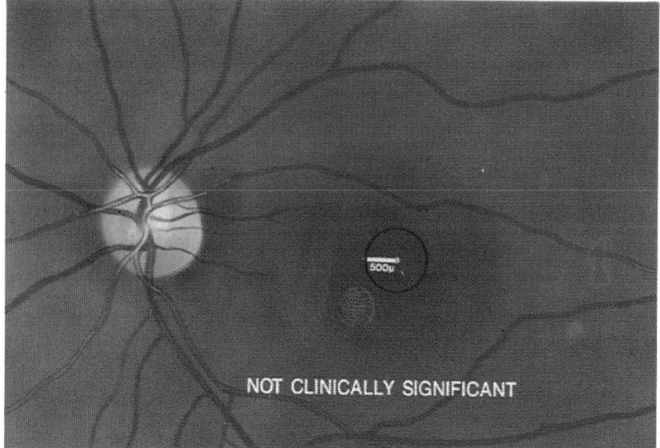


Fig. 8.7

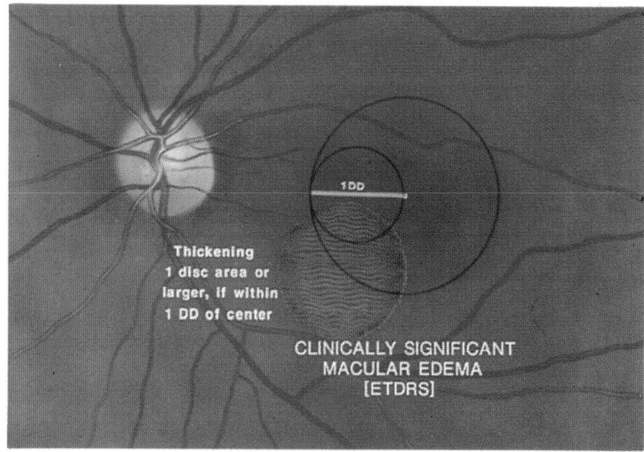


Fig. 8.8

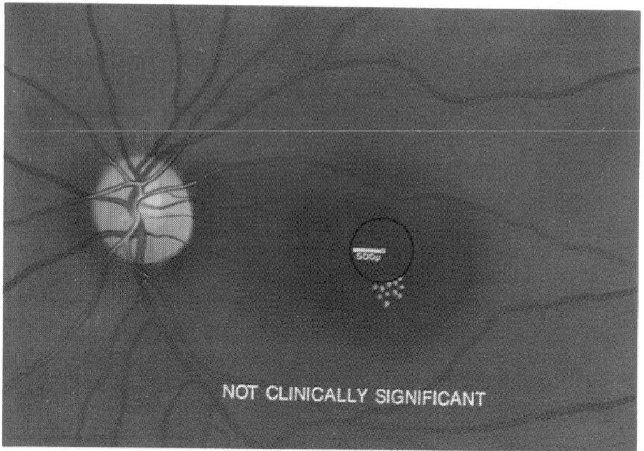


Fig. 8.9

**Fig. 8.5–8.9.** Clinically significant macular oedema, showing the variety of lesions which may threaten central vision. Retinal thickening (oedema) is shown in grey. See text for explanations. (Courtesy of Dr R. Murphy, Wilmer Institute, Baltimore, Maryland, USA.)

### *Advanced diabetic eye disease*

This is end-stage disease, defined by the presence of any of the potentially blinding complications of proliferative diabetic retinopathy:

- Severe vitreous haemorrhage (Fig. 8.15).
- Macular distortion (Fig. 8.16), due to traction by contracting fibrous tissue, which may progress to macular detachment.
- Tractional retinal detachment (TRD). This may be extramacular (Fig. 8.17), which is compatible with good vision, or involve the macula (Fig. 8.18), when vision is severely impaired.
- Combined rhegmatogenous and tractional retinal detachment. The formation of a tear or hole (Greek, *rhegma*, meaning a rent) in the retina (Fig. 8.19) permits the rapid exchange of fluid between the vitreous cavity and the subretinal space,

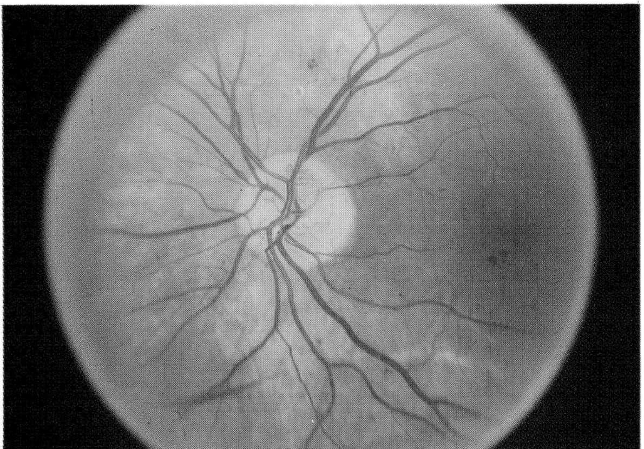

**Fig. 8.10.** Diabetic Retinopathy Study (DRS) standard photograph indicating new vessels on the disc (NVD — at 12 o'clock), and showing a preretinal haemorrhage (at 7 o'clock).

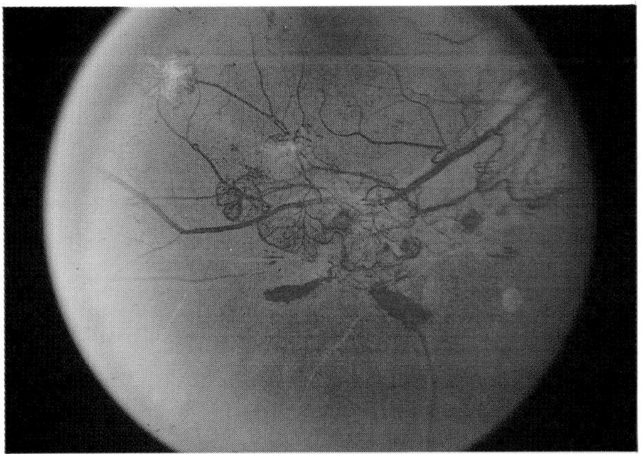

**Fig. 8.11.** New vessels elsewhere (NVE) in the retina, in this case inferior to the macula. The picture also shows arteriolar obliteration and retinal ischaemia; the columns of blood are attenuated and some occluded arterioles are reduced to whitish lines (e.g. between the two haemorrhages lying below the new vessels).

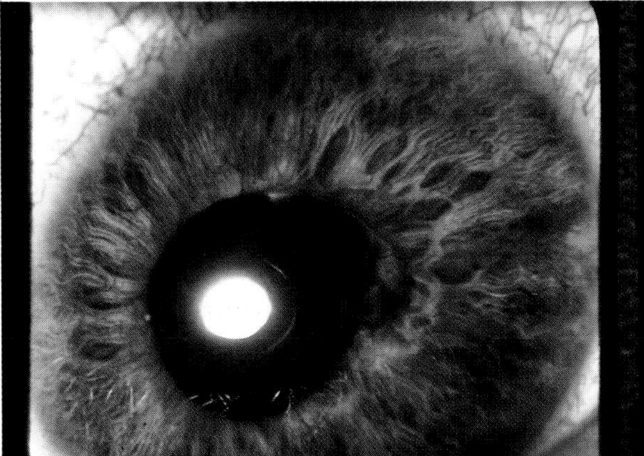

**Fig. 8.12.** Rubeosis iridis, most easily seen at 12 o'clock on the pupil margin. There is also circumcorneal injection of the sclera.

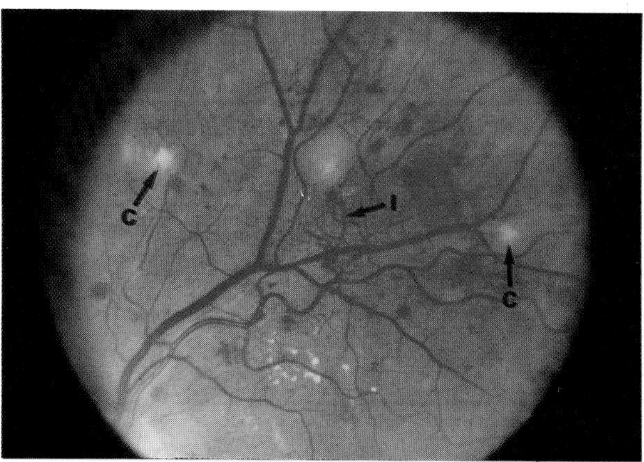


**Fig. 8.13.** Shows cotton-wool spots (C), IRMA (I), deep round haemorrhages and the 'empty retina' of preproliferative retinopathy.

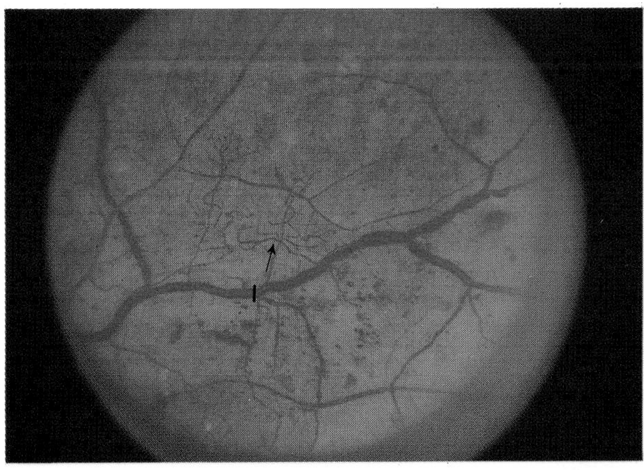


**Fig. 8.14.** Shows venous beading and IRMA (I) of preproliferative retinopathy.

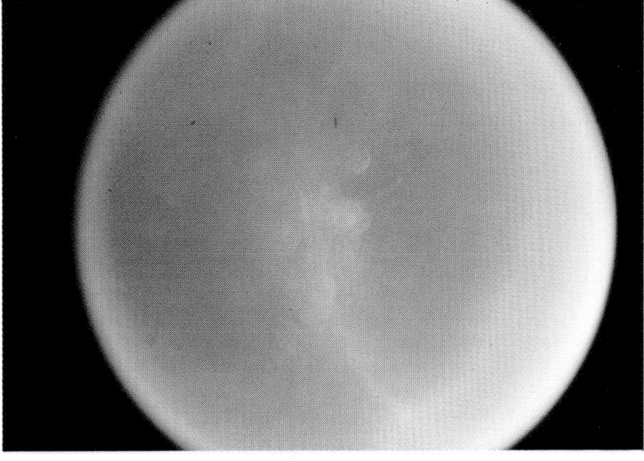

**Fig. 8.15.** Shows severe vitreous haemorrhage. The fundus is virtually invisible.

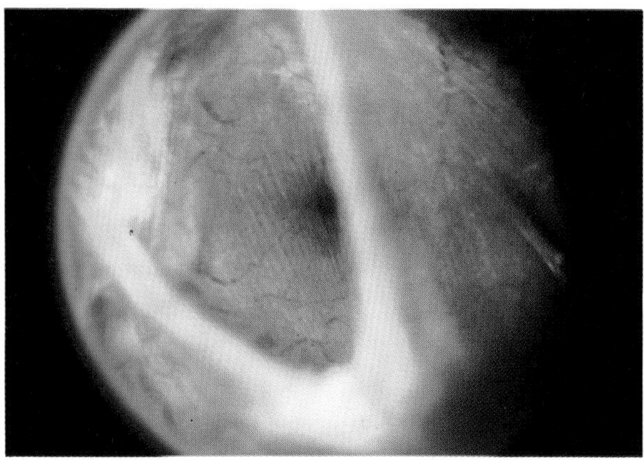

**Fig. 8.16.** Tractional macular distortion. Traction lines running obliquely are clearly visible in the retina lateral to the disc.

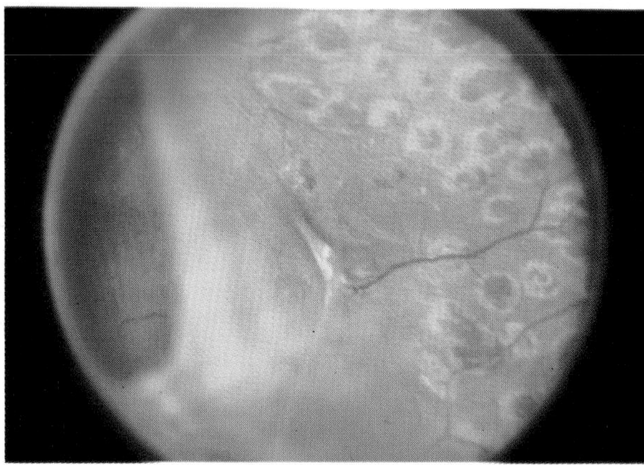

**Fig. 8.17.** Focal vitreo-retinal adhesion, with a small area of localized extramacular tractional retinal detachment, lateral to the macula. Photocoagulation scars are clearly visible.

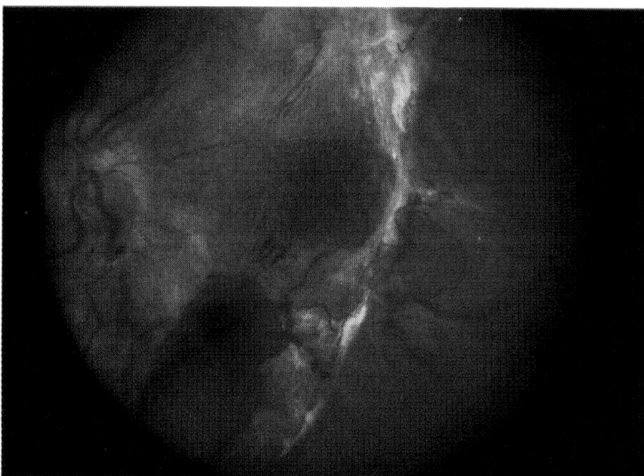

**Fig. 8.18.** Confluent epiretinal membrane with several foci of vitreo-retinal adhesion and tractional detachment involving the macula.

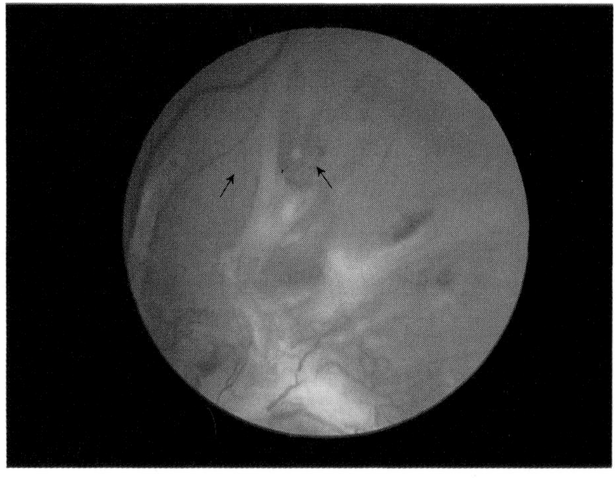

**Fig. 8.19.** Combined rhegmatogenous/tractional detachment with horseshoe-shaped retinal tear (indicated by arrowheads).

causing sudden and extensive retinal detachment accompanied by catastrophic visual loss.

• Neovascular glaucoma. This results from obstruction of the drainage angle by new vessels and accompanying fibrous tissue (Fig. 8.20). It is the final common result of untreated retinal ischaemia, progressive retinal detachment, rubeosis iridis or failed surgery and ultimately results in an eye which is often both irretrievably blind and intractably painful.

## Clinical examination

### *Visual symptoms*

Visual symptoms are extremely variable and must be elicited by careful questioning. The osmotic

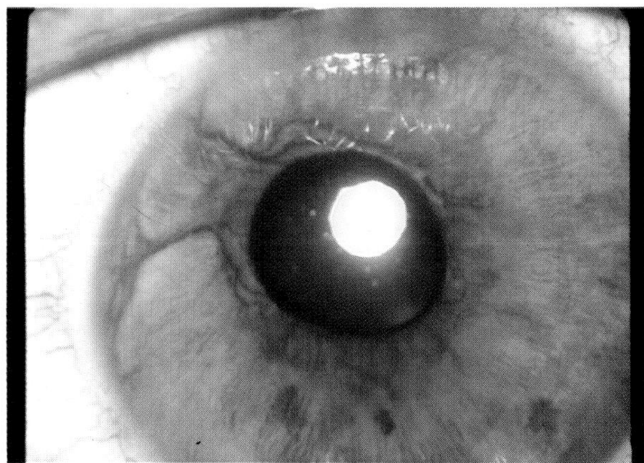

**Fig. 8.20.** Neovascular glaucoma, showing growth of new vessels and associated fibrous tissue into the drainage angle (best seen on the left of the picture). The pupil is oval and the cornea slightly hazy, suggesting corneal oedema.

effects of hyperglycaemia cause transient blurring of vision, often with hyperopia ('I cannot see the television without my *reading* glasses'). This is a common presenting symptom of diabetes but will improve with stabilization of treatment and has no long-term ill-effects.

A gradual decline in central vision ('I cannot read at all now; my new glasses are not strong enough') is often due to associated presenile cataract but demands the exclusion of diabetic macular oedema. Mild macular oedema often has no symptoms.

Sudden loss of vision — usually terrifying, especially in previously asymptomatic patients — generally denotes an extensive vitreous haemorrhage or retinal detachment; when the retina detaches behind a vitreous haemorrhage (which happens quite frequently), the patient may report a sensation 'like the light going out behind the thundercloud'. This is a crucial symptom which must not be neglected, as the duration of retinal detachment directly determines the viability of the photoreceptors and therefore the likelihood of eventual surgery failing to restore vision; long-standing, unsuspected retinal detachment is one of the greatest disappointments to the vitreoretinal surgeon and the patient.

Symptoms may be entirely absent even in patients with extensive proliferative changes, until haemorrhage or detachment occur. A lack of symptoms is therefore not necessarily reassuring and the possibility of occult retinopathy with the potential for acute severe visual loss emphasizes the importance of routine screening.

### *Physical signs*

The purpose of clinical examination (Table 8.2) is to allocate each eye to one of the above classes of retinopathy and to detect risk factors for visual loss before complications occur. It is imperative, for example, to seek retinal detachment behind a vitreous haemorrhage, proliferative changes before vitreous haemorrhage occurs, preproliferative features before neovascularization supervenes, and macular oedema before visual acuity declines.

Measurement of visual acuity is mandatory, as it is not only the end-point of clinical trials [3, 7–20] but also the property of vision most important to the patient. Acuity for distance is measured with a Snellen chart and for near vision with a standard reading chart. Distance acuity should be checked with the patient wearing spectacles for distant vision, or with a pinhole to counteract any reduction in acuity due to purely refractive problems. Poor acuity which is not improved in this way is likely to be due to serious retinal or macular disease or to dense opacities in the lens or vitreous.

Having measured the visual acuity, the presence of a relative afferent pupillary defect should be sought. If present, this sign indicates severe underlying retinal or optic nerve damage, such as retinal detachment. This applies even in the presence of vitreous haemorrhage, as opacities in the media (such as cataract or vitreous haemorrhage) do not produce such a defect.

Formal measurement of the intra-ocular pressure is the next step. Elevated intra-ocular pressure may be caused by vitreous haemorrhage or neo-

**Table 8.2.** Examination of the eyes in diabetic patients. Specialized ophthalmological examination will also include slit-lamp microscopic examination of the iris, anterior chamber and retina, indirect binocular fundoscopy and measurement of intra-ocular pressure.

*When to examine*:
- On diagnosis
- Annually after 3 years of diabetes
- Annually if background retinopathy alone is present
- Three- to 6-monthly if retinopathy is more severe than background
- Immediately if any change in vision or visual symptoms occur

*Examination should include*:
- Visual acuity:
  distant vision (Snellen chart + spectacles or pinhole)
  near vision (reading chart)
- Afferent pupillary defect
- Ophthalmoscopy through dilated pupils (1% tropicamide), unless glaucoma or previous eye surgery are present: examine lens, vitreous and retina

vascular glaucoma. A slit lamp is then used to detect rubeosis iridis and, if present, a contact lens is used to examine the drainage angle for possible occlusion by new vessels or fibrous tissue. Both pupils are then dilated with 1% tropicamide eye drops (with or without 10% phenylephrine). Patients should be warned to return should they develop symptoms of acute glaucoma; the chances of this happening are generally remote, but mydriatics should only be used by experts in patients with a known history of glaucoma or of eye surgery. Following full pupillary dilatation, the binocular indirect ophthalmoscope is used to scan the retina for the presence of background retinopathy. This is also the best instrument to detect vitreous haemorrhage or retinal detachment and, with practice, can even visualize the retina through relatively dense cataract or vitreous haemorrhage.

The traditional hand-held monocular direct ophthalmoscope can identify cataract and vitreous opacities and is particularly useful for identifying small clusters of new vessels, which are best seen by focusing slightly anterior of the retina. NVD are sought by carefully examining the disc, and NVE by following the retinal veins and their major branches out from the optic disc in each quadrant; NVE invariably arise from retinal veins, most commonly at their bifurcations (Fig. 8.11).

Detailed stereoscopic biomicroscopy of the posterior pole of the eye is performed with the slit-lamp microscope and a corneal contact lens or a 90-dioptre hand-held lens. The detection of hard exudate at the macula is easy (Fig. 8.2) but identification of retinal oedema (seen as retinal thickening) *without* hard exudate is more difficult (Fig. 8.8).

Clinical testing of colour vision and visual fields is unnecessary in routine practice, although colour vision is subtly impaired in diabetic retinopathy and could theoretically interfere with the ability to read blood glucose testing strips.

The important physical signs are illustrated in Figs 8.1–8.20.

### *Ancillary investigations*

If the retina cannot be seen through vitreous haemorrhage or dense cataract, B-scan ultrasonography can be used to determine the presence or absence of underlying retinal detachment. This technique is of great value but is expensive and requires an experienced examiner.

Fundus photography, especially stereoscopic photography, of standard retinal fields is also expensive but provides clear and permanent records and permits more detailed study of the retina than clinical examination [1]. 'Non-mydriatic' cameras can photograph the central and part of the peripheral retina through undilated pupils. The quality is not as high as with formal photography through fully dilated pupils and the photographs require skilled interpretation. However, the examination is quick and easy to perform and non-mydriatic cameras are currently being evaluated in screening for diabetic retinopathy.

Adjunctive fluorescein angiography confirms early proliferative disease and helps to confirm and classify macular oedema. The angiogram is a useful guide to the treatment of macular oedema (Figs 8.22, 8.24 and 8.25) and is essential for follow-up treatment (see below).

Electrophysiological tests such as the electroretinogram and visual evoked responses are essentially research tools and contribute little to routine clinical evaluation.

## Treatment of diabetic retinopathy

### *Laser photocoagulation*

The rationale for using photocoagulation in proliferative retinopathy is that it destroys ischaemic areas of retina which are thought to produce vasoproliferative factors which act locally to stimulate new vessel growth [21–25]. A high-energy light beam is focused through a corneal contact lens on to the target area of retina. The first device to be used was the xenon arc lamp, which produces a relatively large (1000 μm diameter) burn suitable for ablating large areas but too imprecise for small targets. Xenon arc photocoagulation is also painful and usually needs retrobulbar (or general) anaesthesia. The instrument in widest current use is the argon laser, which produces very short flashes (20 ms) of monochromatic blue-green light with a spot size of one-third of a disc diameter which allows very precise targetting. The colour is complementary to that of haemoglobin, so that vascular structures (e.g. new vessels or normal retina) will maximally absorb the radiation.

Laser photocoagulation can be used to destroy specific targets (e.g. clusters of new vessels at risk of haemorrhage) but is now generally used to perform *pan-retinal photocoagulation*, in which the the entire retina is treated, with the exception of the macula and papillomacular bundle which are essential to central vision (Figs 8.21 and 8.26). Pan-retinal photocoagulation may require 1500–2000 burns and is divided into several treatment sessions to minimize possible adverse effects [20]. By partly destroying the retina, the remaining retina can survive and function on its limited blood supply; the stimulus to neovascularization is removed, existing new blood vessels regress and further neovascularization is aborted. As the new vessels shrink or disappear, the incidence and severity of vitreous haemorrhage are reduced. The benefits of this treatment are evident from the results discussed below.

Apart from pain with the xenon arc, the most disturbing adverse effect of photocoagulation is exacerbation of pre-existing macular oedema, leading to a fall in central visual acuity [26]. This can destroy the patient's faith in photocoagulation, especially when he has asymptomatic new vessels, but can largely be avoided by careful staging of treatment. There must also be detailed discussion with the patient about the natural history of the condition and the potential benefits and limitations of photocoagulation. Patients generally welcome laser photocoagulation after their first vitreous haemorrhage, when it is often too little and too late; asymptomatic subjects must be treated carefully and considerately, or many will be lost to follow-up.

As well as its use in proliferative retinopathy, photocoagulation has also been found to improve macular oedema. Leaking capillaries and microaneurysms are directly treated and sealed. Indirect effects on the retinal pigment epithelial pump and secondary alterations in capillary integrity result in the clearing of macular oedema and hard exudate [21, 22]. Again, technical skill is crucial, particularly in patients with normal or nearly normal vision.

Recent trials of photocoagulation have suggested guidelines for the routine clinical management of these two indications.

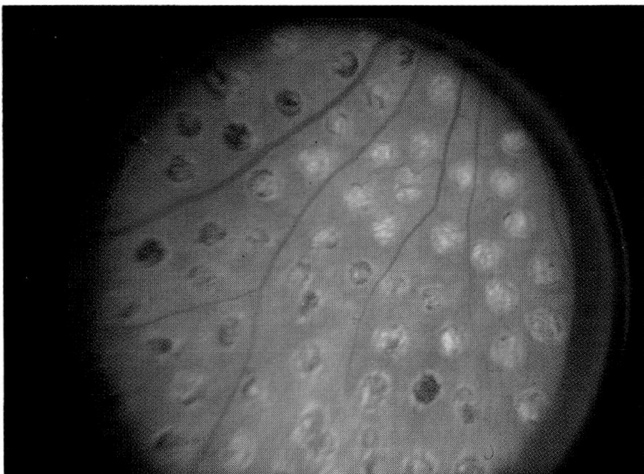

**Fig. 8.21.** Standard pan-retinal photocoagulation. The papillomacular bundle is not treated, in order to preserve central vision (see Fig. 8.26).

### *Photocoagulation treatment of proliferative retinopathy*

Several studies have now demonstrated beyond all doubt that laser photocoagulation improves the outcome of proliferative diabetic retinopathy. The Diabetic Retinopathy Study (DRS), which withstands any criticism [27], showed that pan-retinal photocoagulation reduces by more than 50% the risk of severe visual loss in proliferative retinopathy, as compared with untreated control eyes [8, 9].

The DRS identified three high-risk characteristics for severe visual loss (Table 8.3) [8, 9], defined as a visual acuity of 1/60 at two consecutive visits 4 months apart. The high-risk characteristics, which serve as indications for photocoagulation to be performed soon, are:

**1** New vessels on the optic disc (NVD) which are more extensive than in a standard photograph (Fig. 8.10).

**2** NVD less extensive than this standard, but accompanied by *any* vitreous or preretinal haemorrhage (Fig. 8.10).

**3** New vessels elsewhere (NVE), more than two disc areas in size, together with *any* vitreous or preretinal haemorrhage.

The incidence of severe visual loss with high-risk characteristics and the benefits of treatment are shown in Table 8.4.

**Table 8.3.** High-risk characteristics identified by the Diabetic Retinopathy Study [8, 9].

| | | |
|---|---|---|
| NVD | ≥ | DRS standard photo 10 A (Fig. 8.10) |
| NVD | < | Standard photo 10 A (Fig. 8.10) but with *any* vitreous/preretinal haemorrhage |
| NVE | ≥ | Two disc areas with any vitreous/preretinal haemorrhage |

NVD: optic disc new vessels; NVE: new vessels elsewhere.

**Table 8.4.** Outcome of patients with high-risk characteristics (from the Diabetic Retinopathy Study [8, 9]).

| | Percentage with severe visual loss |
|---|---|
| Without treatment | 25% at 2 years<br>50% at 5 years |
| With treatment | 11% at 2 years<br>26% at 5 years |

### *Photocoagulation treatment of preproliferative retinopathy*

It is not known whether photocoagulation should be given early, at the preproliferative stage, of deferred until high-risk characteristics develop. This question was not considered by the DRS but is currently being addressed by the ETDRS [1].

There are, however, theoretical advantages in treating preproliferative retinopathy. Treatment can be staged rather than rushed for fear of imminent vitreous haemorrhage, and pretreatment of existing macular oedema reduces the risk of its later exacerbation by pan-retinal photocoagulation. Moreover, there are indications that treating preproliferative retinopathy may often be curative, whereas treating established proliferative disease is frequently only palliative.

While awaiting the outcome of the ETDRS, it is the author's personal practice to treat the first eye of a patient with preproliferative retinopathy with pan-retinal photocoagulation [7, 20]. Any existing macular oedema is treated first (see below). If treatment is effective and there are no adverse effects, the other eye is then treated similarly.

Indications for laser photocoagulation of proliferative and preproliferative diabetic retinopathy are suggested in Table 8.5.

### *Photocoagulation treatment of macular oedema*

The ETDRS finished recruiting 3928 patients in 1985 [3]. Although the study was primarily designed to determine the appropriate timing and type of pan-retinal photocoagulation, its results to date have been confined to the photocoagulation of macular oedema [3, 6, 7]. Patients with macular oedema were either not treated or given photocoagulation on diagnosis, with focal treatment for discrete lesions and diffuse 'grid' treatment for widespread capillary leakage and non-perfusion. Any residual leakage was re-treated every 4

**Table 8.5.** Proliferative and preproliferative diabetic retinopathy. Indications for laser photocoagulation.

| Condition | Recommended action |
|---|---|
| NVD* | Pan-retinal photocoagulation before vitreous haemorrhage occurs |
| NVE* | Pan-retinal photocoagulation before retinal detachment occurs |
| Rubeosis* | Pan-retinal photocoagulation before neovascular glaucoma develops |
| Preproliferative | Pan-retinal photocoagulation, of first eye |
| Peroperative* | Pan-retinal endolaser photocoagulation of all attached retina |

NVD: optic disc new vessels; NVE: new vessels elsewhere; * benefit proven by Diabetic Retinopathy Study [8, 9].

months; follow-up treatment was commonly needed during the ETRDS study [4]. Case examples of focal treatment are illustrated in Figs 8.22–8.24, and of 'grid' photocoagulation in Fig. 8.26.

The outcome of photocoagulation treatment of clinically significant macular oedema in the ETDRS study is summarized in Table 8.6. Overall, the risk of severe visual loss in treated eyes was less than one-half of that in control eyes [3].

### Vitreo-retinal surgery

The ultimate blinding complications of proliferative diabetic retinopathy are severe vitreous haemorrhage and secondary retinal detachment. The latter is determined by certain important anatomical considerations [28]. In the normal eye, the vitreous is loosely applied to the entire retina, with firm bonds only at the optic disc, adjoining major retinal vessels and at the peripheral vitreous base (Fig. 8.27a). Neovascular tissue invading from the optic disc and elsewhere through the retina produces a fibro-vascular carpet spreading to line the vitreo-retinal interface. This carpet is 'nailed down' to the underlying retina by the original fibro-vascular ingrowths and is fused to the overlying cortical vitreous. Detachment of the posterior surface of the vitreous from the retina (Fig. 8.27b), which occurs normally in the elderly, will result in tractional forces being applied to the neovascular membrane. These tractional forces, combined with intrinsic contraction of the membrane itself, may result in vitreous haemorrhage

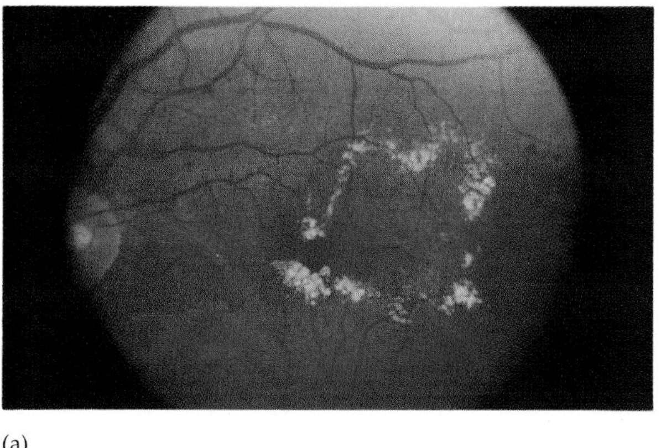

(a)

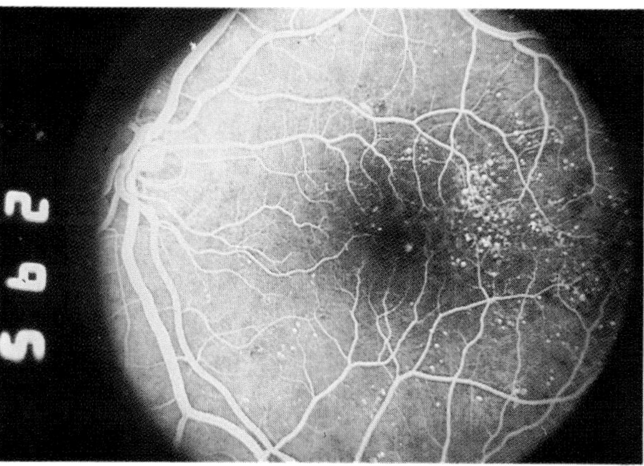

(b)

**Fig. 8.22.** Focal treatment of macular oedema. Pretreatment photograph (a) and matching angiogram (b) showing features of localized macular oedema.

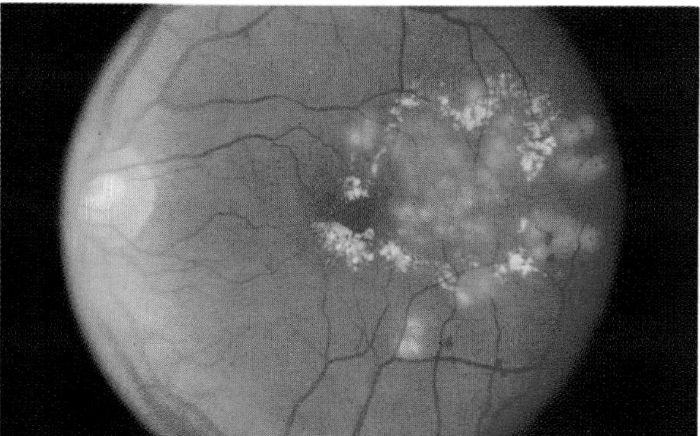

**Fig. 8.23.** Immediate posttreatment photograph of area shown in Fig. 8.22a.

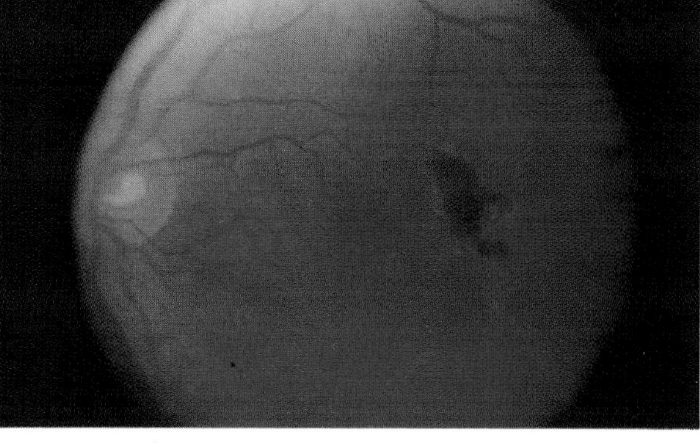

(a)

(b)

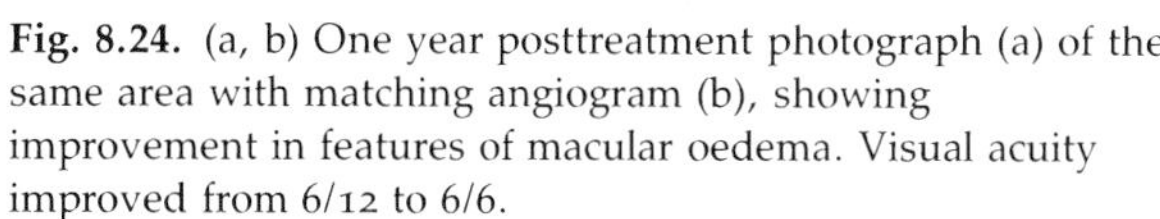

**Fig. 8.24.** (a, b) One year posttreatment photograph (a) of the same area with matching angiogram (b), showing improvement in features of macular oedema. Visual acuity improved from 6/12 to 6/6.

**Table 8.6.** Clinically significant macular oedema. Outcome of treatment at diagnosis compared with deferral of treatment on visual loss*. (Adapted from ETDRS — see text.)

| | Treated group (%) | Untreated group (%) |
|---|---|---|
| 1 year | 5 | 10 |
| 2 years | 8 | 21 |
| 3 years | 13 | 30 |

* Visual loss was defined as doubling of the initial visual angle, e.g. from 6/6 to 6/12, 6/36 to 6/60.

from shearing of the fragile new vessels, tractional retinal detachment and, if sufficient to tear a hole in the retina, in a combined rhegmatogenous and tractional retinal detachment (Figs 8.15–8.19). The role of the vitreous in the pathogenesis of these tractional complications is shown in Fig. 8.28.

Although vitrectomy can be performed electively for severe vitreous haemorrhage alone [11], urgent surgery is required for operable retinal detachment [12, 13, 17–19]. As mentioned above, the viability of the retina declines with increasing duration of detachment and in general, reattaching the macula

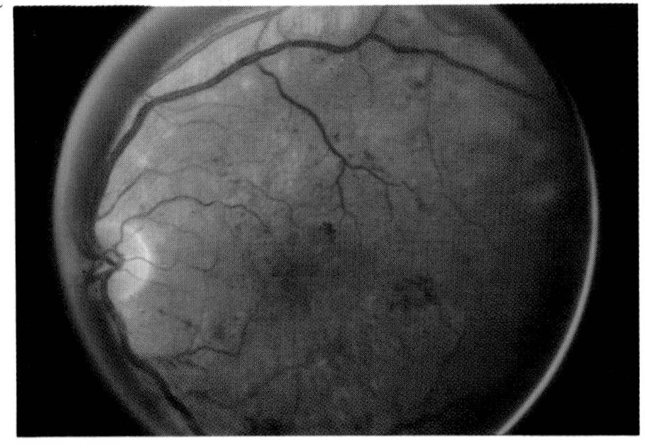

(a)

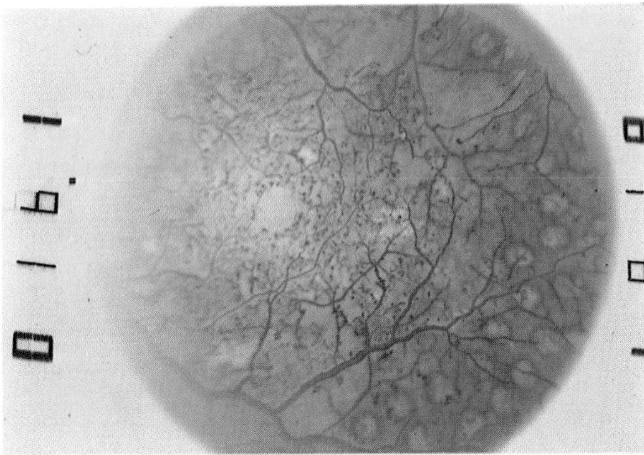

(b)

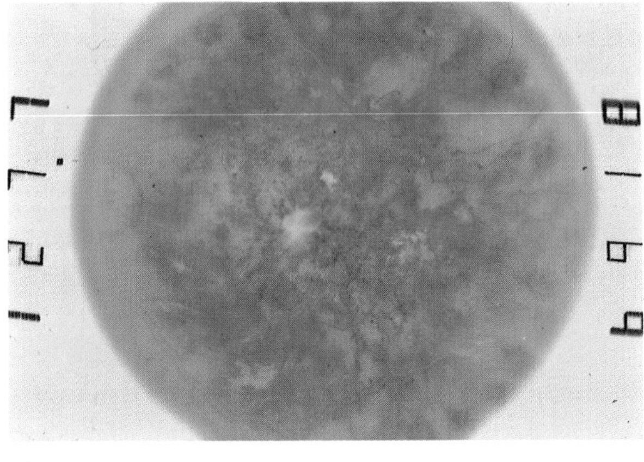

(c)

**Fig. 8.25.** (a) Pretreatment photograph of diffuse macular oedema. (b) Early-phase fluorescein angiogram of area in (a) showing extensive capillary non-perfusion. (c) Late-phase angiogram showing diffuse capillary leakage.

after 3 months will not usefully improve central vision.

All the techniques used in vitreo-retinal microsurgery require a closed intra-ocular approach [28]. The vitreous cavity can be entered safely

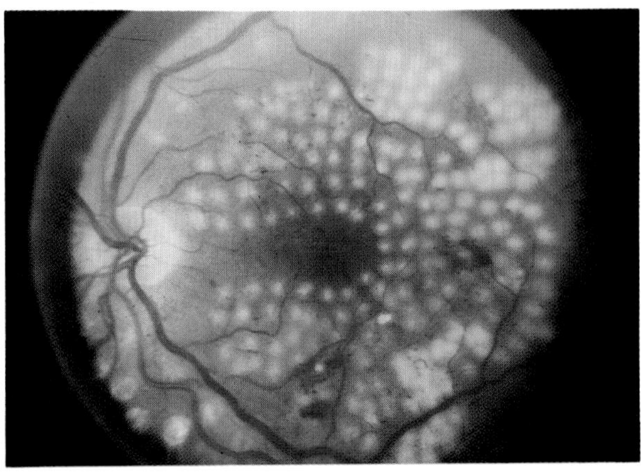

**Fig. 8.26.** Grid treatment of diffuse/ischaemic macular oedema, sparing the central macula and papillomacular bundle.

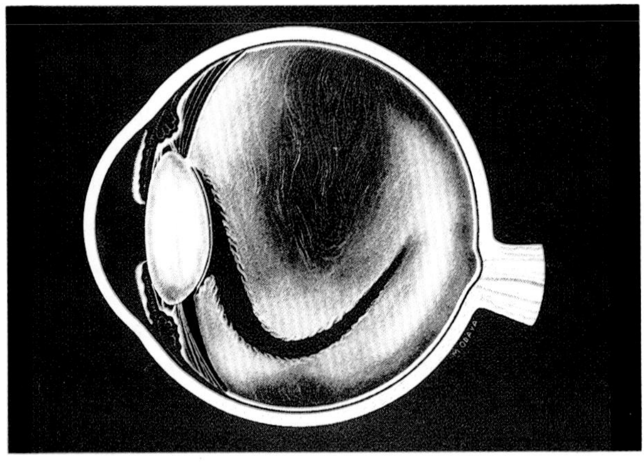

(a)

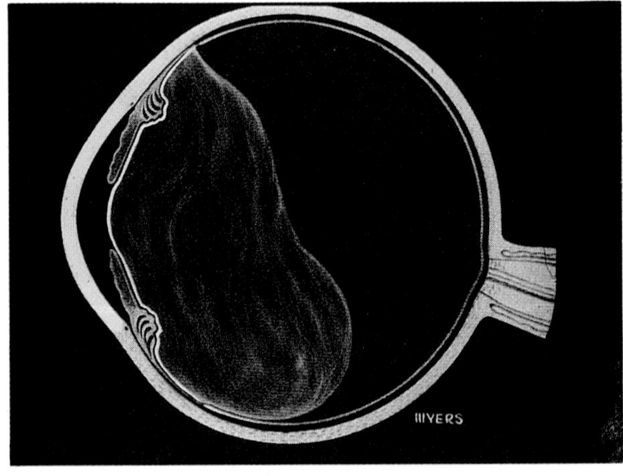

(b)

**Fig. 8.27.** (a) The normal vitreo-retinal relationships in a young person. The posterior surface of the vitreous is in total contact with the retina. (b) Complete posterior vitreous detachment from the retina occurs normally in the elderly.

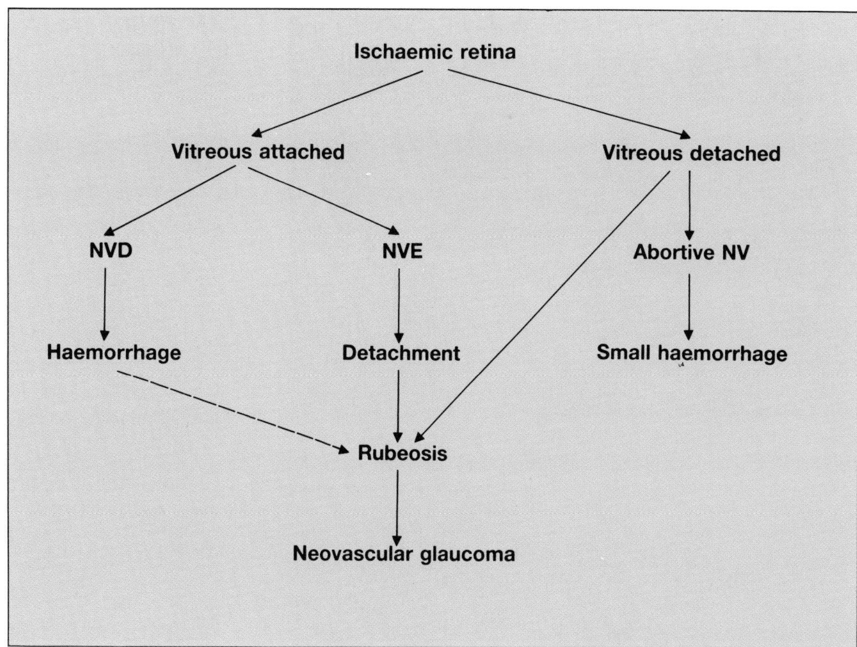


**Fig. 8.28.** The pathogenesis of diabetic blindness. NV: new vessels; NVD: on disc; NVE: elsewhere on retina.

through the *pars plana*, a 2-mm zone centred 4.5 mm lateral to the corneo-scleral junction which is sufficiently posterior to avoid damaging the crystalline lens and yet clear of the anterior edge of the retina (Fig. 8.29). Isotonic saline is infused into the ocular cavity through a cannula pushed through the pars plana, in order to maintain and control intra-ocular pressure. Operative instruments (cutters and aspirators) and a light source are introduced through two further sclerotomies; all instruments are common-gauge so that the sclerotomies are watertight. Using a corneal contact lens, the retina may be clearly seen and an operating microscope allows precise intra-ocular manipulation (Figs 8.30 and 8.31.) The vitreous and its contained haemorrhage are first removed, either with mechanical cutters or an yttrium–aluminium garnet (YAG) laser, and then replaced with infused saline. The retina can be physically re-attached to the choroid and is then treated peroperatively with endolaser photocoagulation to prevent both further detachment and subsequent neovascularization. Operative techniques are discussed in detail elsewhere [28–33].

Visual recovery can be both dramatic and sustained [11, 12, 17–19, 29], the pooled success rate for anatomical and functional success being around 65–70%. However, the principal complications of retinal detachment (either persistent or iatrogenic) and resultant neovascular glaucoma can result in an eye that is blind and painful; surgery is therefore not undertaken lightly.

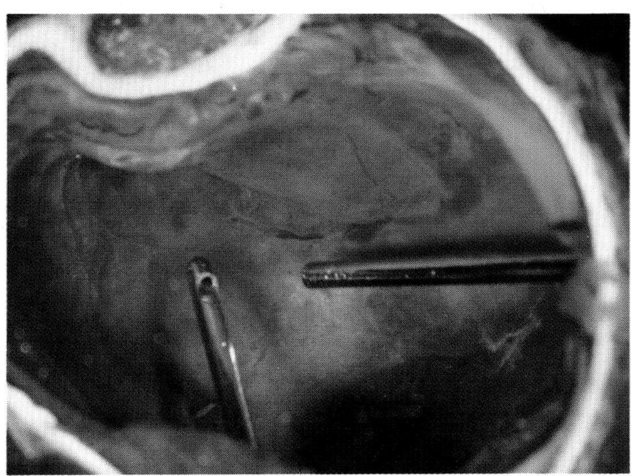

**Fig. 8.29.** Principles of vitreo-retinal surgery, illustrated by common-gauge instruments inserted through the pars plana of a transected cadaver eye.

The major indications for vitrectomy are shown in Table 8.7. Recent results from the Diabetic Retinopathy Vitrectomy Study (DRVS) indicate that early vitrectomy should be considered in eyes retaining useful vision but with advanced active proliferative retinopathy [12, 13]. In the author's experience, the most important factors in deciding whether to subject an eye to vitrectomy are the duration of macular detachment and the likelihood of achieving the surgical goals; failed surgery makes re-operation considerably more difficult.

The normal successful postoperative appearances are shown in Fig. 8.32. Most of the epiretinal

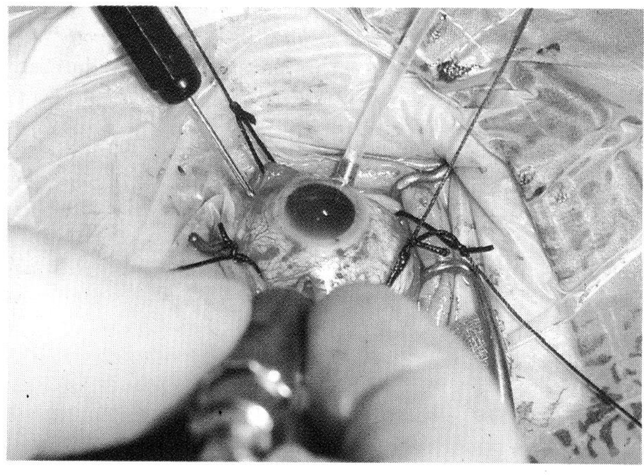

Fig. 8.30. Trans-pars plana vitrectomy with common-gauge instrumentation and infusion of saline to maintain intra-ocular pressure.

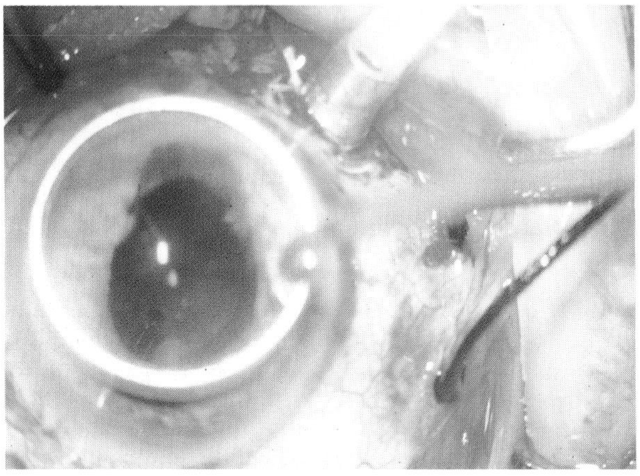

Fig. 8.31. Trans-pars plana vitrectomy. Peroperative view of retina through contact lens placed on cornea.

Table 8.7. Surgical indications for diabetic vitrectomy.

| |
|---|
| Long-standing severe vitreous haemorrhage (visual acuity worse than 6/60 for 6 months) |
| Recent tractional macular detachment |
| Combined rhegmatogenous/tractional detachment |
| Possibly in severe active proliferative retinopathy with good vision |
| Likelihood of achieving surgical goals |

membrane has been removed, leaving only minor residual islands of tissue, and the retina has remained re-attached for two years. Note the extensive laser scars and profound retinal ischaemia with avascular arterioles.

## Indications for ophthalmological referral

The need for vitrectomy in diabetic patients would largely disappear if adequate laser photocoagulation were applied promptly at an early stage. This can only be achieved if diabetic patients are regularly and effectively screened for ocular complications. The timing of eye examinations is outlined in Table 8.2, together with a schedule which is appropriate to a busy diabetic clinic. The indications for referral to an ophthalmologist are listed in Table 8.8, which also indicates the necessary urgency for each problem.

## Conclusions

Photocoagulation is now of indisputable value in treating two major threats to the vision of diabetic

Table 8.8. Indications for referring a diabetic patient to an ophthalmologist.

| Condition | Urgency |
|---|---|
| Cataract | Routine (few months) |
| Hard exudates: close to macula or numbers increasing<br>Retinal haemorrhages: numbers increasing<br>Preproliferative changes | Soon (few weeks) |
| Fall in visual acuity (two lines or more)<br>Visible maculopathy (oedema, exudates)<br>New vessels<br>Rubeosis iridis<br>Advanced diabetic eye disease, especially retinal detachment | Urgent (1 week) |
| Vitreous haemorrhage<br>Neovascular glaucoma | Immediate (same or next day) |

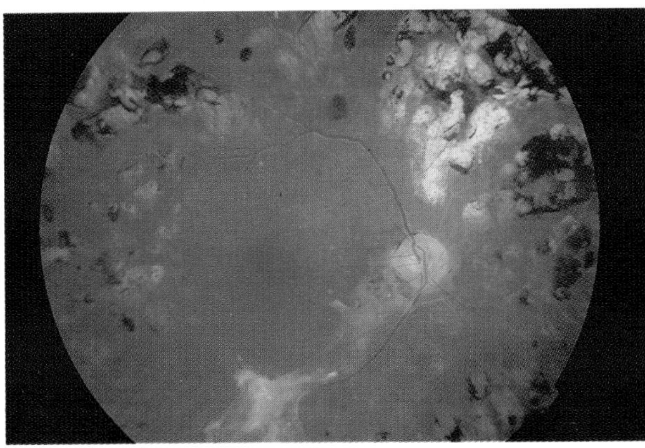

**Fig. 8.32.** Successful outcome of vitreo-retinal surgery, showing residual islands of epiretinal membrane (temporal to macula, nasal to disc, and on upper vascular arcade), retinal reattachment and laser photocoagulation scars. There is still profound retinal ischaemia. Visual acuity has been restored to 6/12 from 1/60 preoperatively.

patients, namely proliferative retinopathy and macular oedema. Moreover, intra-ocular microsurgery can restore vision to some eyes with blindness which, only a few years ago, would have been untreatable. It is obvious that photocoagulation and microsurgery services must be made available to all diabetic patients, but the immense importance of early detection of diabetic eye disease and its correct monitoring cannot be overemphasized. It is to be hoped that measures such as these will go a long way towards eliminating and preventing blindness in diabetes.

## Recent developments

Further results from the Early Treatment Diabetic Retinopathy Study Research Group and the Diabetic Retinopathy Vitrectomy Study Research Group have been published [34–45]. These report longer periods of follow-up and developments in assessing risk factors for the progression of retinopathy.

PETER J. BARRY

## References


1 Early Treatment Diabetic Retinopathy Study (ETDRS). *Manual of Operations*. Baltimore: ETDRS Coordinating Center, Department of Epidemiology and Preventive Medicine, University of Maryland, 1985.

2 Whitelocke RAF, Kearns M, Blach RK, Hamilton AM. The diabetic maculopathies. *Trans Ophthalmol Soc UK* 1979; **99**: 314–20.

3 Early Treatment Diabetic Retinopathy Study Research Group. Photocoagulation for diabetic macular edema. ETDRS Report No 1. *Arch Ophthalmol* 1985; **103**: 1796–1806.

4 Murphy RP, Ferris FL. The current status of the Early Treatment Diabetic Retinopathy Study. *Ophthalmic Forum* 1984; **2**: 149–52.

5 Early Treatment Diabetic Retinopathy Study Research Group. Treatment techniques and clinical guidelines for photocoagulation of diabetic macular oedema: ETDRS Report No 2. *Ophthalmology* 1987; **94**: 761–74.

6 Early Treatment Diabetic Retinopathy Study Research Group. Techniques for scatter and local photocoagulation treatment of diabetic retinopathy: ETDRS Report No 3. *Int Ophthalmol Clin* 1987; **27** (No 4): 254–64.

7 Early Treatment Diabetic Retinopathy Study Research Group. Photocoagulation for diabetic macular edema: ETDRS Report No 4. *Int Ophthalmol Clin* 1987; **27** (No 4): 265–333.

8 The Diabetic Retinopathy Study Research Group. Design, methods and baseline results. Report No 6. *Invest Ophthalmol Vis Sci* 1981; **21** (suppl 1) (part 2): 1–209.

9 The Diabetic Retinopathy Study Research Group. Photocoagulation treatment of proliferative diabetic retinopathy. Clinical application of DRS findings. Report No 8. *Ophthalmology* 1981; **88**: 583–600.

10 Diabetic Retinopathy Vitrectomy Study Research Group. Two year course of visual acuity in severe proliferative diabetic retinopathy with conservative management. Diabetic Retinopathy Vitrectomy Study (DRVS) Report No 1. *Ophthalmology* 1985; **92**: 492–502.

11 Diabetic Retinopathy Vitrectomy Study Research Group. Early vitrectomy for severe vitreous haemorrhage in diabetic retinopathy. Two-year results of randomized trial. DRVS Report No 2. *Arch Ophthalmol* 1985; **103**: 1644–52.

12 Diabetic Retinopathy Vitrectomy Study Research Group. Early vitrectomy for severe proliferative diabetic retinopathy in eyes with useful vision: Results of a randomized trial. DRVS Research Report No 3. *Ophthalmology* 1988; **95**: 1307–20.

13 Diabetic Retinopathy Vitrectomy Study Research Group. Early vitrectomy for severe proliferative diabetic retinopathy in eyes with useful vision: Clinical application of results of a randomized trial. DRVS Report No 4. *Ophthalmology* 1988; **95**: 1321–34.

14 British Multicentre Study Group. Photocoagulation for proliferative diabetic retinopathy: a randomized control clinical trial using the xenon arc. *Diabetologia* 1984; **26**: 109–15.

15 British Multicentre Study Group. Photocoagulation in the treatment of diabetic retinopathy. *Lancet* 1975; **ii**: 1110–13.

16 British Multicentre Study Group. Photocoagulation for diabetic maculopathy. *Diabetes* 1983; **32**: 1010–16.

17 Michels R. Vitrectomy for complications of diabetic retinopathy. *Arch Ophthalmol* 1978; **96**: 237–46.

18 Blankenship G, Machemer R. Pars plana vitrectomy for management of severe diabetic retinopathy. *Am J Ophthalmol* 1978: **85**: 553–62.

19 Mandelcorn MS, Blankenship G, Machemer R. Pars plana vitrectomy for the management of severe diabetic retinopathy. *Am J Ophthalmol* 1976; **81**: 561–70.

20 The Diabetic Retinopathy Study Research Group. Indications for photocoagulation treatment of diabetic retinopathy: Report No 14. *Int Ophthalmol Clin* 1987; **27** (suppl 4): 239–53.

21 Marshall J, Glover G, Rothery S. Some new findings on retinal irradiation by krypton and argon lasers. *Doc Ophthalmol* 1984; **36**: 21–37.

22 Weiter JJ, Zuckerman R. The influence of the photorecep-

tors — RPE complex on the inner retina; an explanation for the beneficial effects of photocoagulation. *Ophthalmology* 1980; **87**: 1133–9.

23 Glaser BM, Hayashi H, Krause WG. A protease inhibitor accumulates within the vitreous following panretinal photocoagulation (PRP) in primates: possible mechanisms for the effect of PRP on retinal neovascularization. *Invest Ophthalmol Vis Sci* 1988; **29** (suppl): 1180.

24 Glaser BM, D'Amore PA, Michels RG, Patz A, Fenselau A. Demonstration of vasoproliferative activity from mammalian retina. *J Cell Biol* 1980; **84**: 298–30.

25 Glaser BM, Campochiaro PA, Davis JL, Jerdan JA. Retinal pigment epithelial cells release inhibitors of neovascularization. *Ophthalmology* 1987; **94**: 780–4.

26 McDonald HR, Schatz E. Macular oedema following panretinal photocoagulation. *Retina* 1985: **5**: 5–10.

27 Edererer F, Hiller R. Clinical trials, diabetic retinopathy and photocoagulation. A reanalysis of 5 studies. *Survey Ophthalmol* 1975; **19**: 267–86.

28 Charles S. *Vitreous Microsurgery*, 2nd edn. Baltimore: Williams & Wilkins, 1987.

29 DeBustros S, Thompson JJ, Michels RG, Rice TA. Vitrectomy for progressive proliferative diabetic retinopathy. *Arch Ophthalmol* 1987; **105**: 196–9.

30 McLeod D, James CRH. Viscodelamination at the vitreoretinal juncture in severe diabetic eye disease. *Br J Ophthalmol* 1988; **72**: 413–19.

31 Barry PJ, Hiscott PS, Grierson I, Marshall J, McLeod D. Reparative epiretinal fibrosis after diabetic vitrectomy. *Trans Ophthalmol Soc UK* 1985: **104**: 285–96.

32 Acheson RW, Capon M, Cooling RJ, Leaver PK, Marshall J, McLeod D. Intraocular argon laser photocoagulation. *Eye* 1987; **1**: 97–105.

33 McLeod D. Silicone oil injection during closed microsurgery for diabetic retinal detachment. *Graefes Arch Klin Exp Ophthalmol* 1986; **224**: 55–9.

34 Diabetic Retinopathy Vitrectomy Study Research Group. Early vitrectomy for severe vitreous hemorrhage in diabetic retinopathy. Four-year results of a randomized trial: Diabetic Retinopathy Vitrectomy Study Report 5. *Arch Ophthalmol* 1990; **108**: 958–64.

35 Early Treatment Diabetic Retinopathy Study Research Group. Early Treatment Diabetic Retinopathy Study design and baseline patient characteristics. ETDRS Report No 7. *Ophthalmology* 1991; **98**: 741–56.

36 Early Treatment Diabetic Retinopathy Study Research Group. Effects of aspirin treatment treatment on diabetic retinopathy. ETDRS Report No 8. *Ophthalmology* 1991; **98**: 757–6.

37 Early Treatment Diabetic Retinopathy Study Research Group. Early photocoagulation for diabetic retinopathy. ETDRS Report No 9. *Ophthalmology* 1991; **98**: 766–85.

38 Early Treatment Diabetic Retinopathy Study Research Group. Grading diabetic retinopathy from stereoscopic color fundus photographs — an extension of the modified Airlie House classification. ETDRS Report No 10. *Ophthalmology* 1991; **98**: 786–806.

39 Early Treatment Diabetic Retinopathy Study Research Group. Classification of diabetic retinopathy from fluorescein angiograms. ETDRS Report No 11. *Ophthalmology* 1991; **98**: 807–22.

40 Early Treatment Diabetic Retinopathy Study Research Group. Fundus photographic risk factors for progression of diabetic retinopathy. ETDRS Report No 12. *Ophthalmology* 1991; **98**: 823–33.

41 Early Treatment Diabetic Retinopathy Study Research Group. Fluorescein angiographic risk factors for progression of diabetic retinopathy. ETDRS Report No 13. *Ophthalmology* 1991; **98**: 833–40.

42 ETDRS Investigators. Aspirin effects on mortality and morbidity in patients with diabetes mellitus. Early Treatment Diabetic Retinopathy Study Report 14. *J Am Med Ass* 1991; **268**: 1292–300.

43 Chew EY, Williams GA, Burton TC, Barton FB, Remaley NA, Ferris FL III. Early Treatment Diabetic Retinopathy Study Research Group. Aspirin effects on the development of cataracts in patients with diabetes mellitus. Early Treatment Diabetic Retinopathy Study Report 16. *Arch Ophthalmol* 1992; **110**: 339–42.

44 Flynn HW, Chew EY, Simons BD, Barton F, Remaley NA, Ferris FL. Early Treatment Diabetic Retinopathy Study Research Group. Pars plana vitrectomy in the Early Treatment Diabetic Retinopathy Study. ETDRS Report No. 17. *Ophthalmology* 1992; **99**: 1351–7.

45 Prior MJ, Prout T, Miller D, Ewart R, Kumar D, ETDRS Research Group. C-peptide and the classification of diabetes mellitus patients in the Early Treatment Diabetic Retinopathy Study. Report No 6. *Ann Epidemiol* 1993; **3**: 9–17.

# 9 Psychological, Social and Practical Aspects of Visual Handicap for the Diabetic Patient


**Summary**

- Diabetes is the commonest cause of visual loss in the British working population.
- 'Blindness' is defined as the inability to perform any task for which eyesight is essential, and 'partial sighted' as substantial and permanent visual loss.
- Loss of vision is psychologically devastating, often causing prolonged shock, denial, anxiety, anger and depression.
- Many blind people use 'mental mapping', a combination of tactile input and visual imagery, to find their way around and perform daily activities. This encourages mobility, independence and self-assurance.
- Many aids are available to help blind and partially sighted patients to draw up insulin accurately and measure their blood glucose concentration.
- It is essential to register blind or partially sighted patients immediately to activate the many social services and facilities available to them.


Loss of vision — which often implies loss of status, independence, self-confidence and income — is a devastating experience for anyone. As shown in Table 9.1, diabetes is the commonest cause of blindness in people of working age in the UK. For diabetic patients, who have to relearn how to manage their diabetes as well as a new way of life, loss of vision presents added difficulties. However, much can be done for the diabetic person under these circumstances and, indeed, helping the patient to overcome the practical difficulties of diabetic management can often accelerate his or her progress towards independence and greater self-esteem.

This section will first describe the psychological and social aspects of losing vision, including the process of 'mental mapping' by which many blind people find their way around. Finally, the practical management of the partially sighted or blind diabetic patient will be discussed, with emphasis on the services, benefits and aids available.

## Psychological and social aspects

As with all grieving processes, the psychological trauma associated with visual loss may comprise shock, denial, anxiety, anger and depression [1]. This is the usual response to loss of sight, and a process that all go through (to a variable extent) before they come to terms with their disability; there is a 'need to mourn the loss of vision before being able to accept the reality of blindness' [2]. The immediate shock following visual loss can last weeks or months and is followed by denial that this could happen and anxiety about how to cope with life and the future. Some may feel guilty and blame themselves for blindness, which is sometimes regarded as a punishment for past sins. Depression can last for a long time, even years. Some people lean heavily on their relatives, who may be overprotective, whereas others are determined to lead a normal life and soon become quite independent [2, 3] (Conyers, unpublished). The grieving process is influenced by personality, age, rapidity of visual loss and the quality of help available to the newly blind. Rapid visual loss in the young produces greater psychological trauma than gradually declining vision in the elderly who have more time to adjust to what is happening and possibly fewer expectations of life [2, 3].

*In the UK population as a whole*:
- 1.75 million people suffer from significant visual loss
- 78% of visual handicap registrations are in people over 65 years of age

*The role of diabetes*:
- The overall prevalence of retinopathy in the diabetic population is 26–35%, and of severe (proliferative or advanced) retinopathy is 9–11%
- Diabetic retinopathy is the major cause of blindness in people under 65 years of age (about 300 visual handicap registrations per year)
- In visually handicapped diabetic patients, diabetic eye disease is responsible in 44% of younger-onset patients, 22% of older-onset patients treated with insulin and 11% of older-onset patients not receiving insulin

**Table 9.1.** Current UK statistics concerning loss of vision and diabetes. (Sources: Office of Population Censuses and Surveys, 1989 and [6].)

It is essential to be honest with people who are losing their vision: to hold out false hopes only encourages the health workers, not the patient [2] (Conyers, unpublished). People able to accept blindness have much better psychological and social function [1, 2]. Allowing people to express their feelings of sadness, anger and fear may hasten the passing of depression [4, 5]. Another common problem, due partly to depression and partly to the loss of the close relationship between vision and sexual arousal, is decreased sexual activity and castration fears [2, 4]. Indirectly, visual loss can profoundly affect other family members, changing previous relationships and often imposing great strain on those who now have to care for the blind person. Nonetheless, rehabilitation is more difficult for those living alone than for those living within a family [2].

Rehabilitation, although essential, tends to segregate the disabled from normal society [6]. Many people feel anxious and uncomfortable when close to disability and need to recognize their prejudices, preconceptions and emotional reactions when dealing with blindness; 'the problem of the blind individual in dealing with the sighted may be greater than the problem of dealing with the blindness itself' [2]. It is easy to focus on the deficit of blindness, but vital not to overlook the person's other attributes which remain and may grow as he adjusts to his changed life.

## Mental imagery

Loss of vision promotes the use and heightens the sensitivity of the other senses, possibly because these are now essential for navigation and spatial awareness. Congenitally blind people employ 'haptic' navigation (i.e. using touch), whereas those who have lost sight retain visual imagery, which greatly improves their orientation and spatial skills [7–9]. These forms of imagery represent alternative forms of coding information; a distinction has been made between 'videation' (an image created using information from senses other than sight, including other people's observations) and a recreated visual image, generated by memory alone [10, 11].

Visual images draw attention to particular cues in the environment and their spatial relationships, and together with information gathered from experiences in navigation and problem solving, are used as a basis for mental mapping [12]. People who lose their vision relearn how to find their way around their home, to the local shops, and around the workplace and the houses of friends and relatives. Learning to make mental maps helps the individual to become mobile again, encouraging independence and self-assurance.

## Practical management of diabetes for the partially sighted and blind

Enabling the newly visually handicapped patient to take charge of his diabetic management again is often a significant first step in helping him to become generally independent.

### *Drawing up insulin*

For the partially sighted, a 1-ml plastic syringe graduated in black is the easiest to read, especially against a pale background in a good light. Several syringe magnifiers, designed to be fitted on to a plastic syringe barrel, are available. The Magniguide (Becton–Dickinson) is useful as it magnifies the whole length of the barrel (Fig. 9.1a); Monoject and Hypoguard produce smaller magnifiers. Another aid to drawing up the correct dose is the syringe guide (Terumo), consisting of a strip of plastic with a hole to take one of the wings of the syringe barrel (Fig. 9.1b). The strip is marked along its length in units corresponding to the syringe and is cut to the length corresponding to the dose by a sighted person. Insulin is then drawn up level to the end of the plastic strip. It is possible to have a different strip for each insulin dosage, which can be written in large black numbers on the back. 'Count a Dose' is a gadget which enables blind people to draw up a combination of insulins in a plastic syringe.

Blind diabetic patients can use two special types of glass syringe, which require no vision. The click-count syringe (Hypoguard) is a conventional glass syringe whose plunger is scored at unit intervals and clicks against a ratchet incorporated into the base of the syringe as the plunger is withdrawn (Fig. 9.1c). The dosage of insulin, including different preparations, can be drawn up simply by counting the clicks. Insulin must be drawn up slowly in order to count the clicks, so there is less chance of drawing up air. The preset syringe (Rand Rocket) is a glass syringe with a threaded plunger carrying two screws (Fig. 9.1d). A sighted person sets the screws at the correct dose and insulin is then drawn up until the screws prevent any further movement. It is more likely that air will be drawn up using this syringe, as people tend to pull the plunger down more rapidly. Many blind people prefer to use plastic syringes because of their finer needles and disposability; the Terumo syringe guide can be used with a plastic syringe by the blind if the dosage is marked in braille or with Hymark on the back of the guide.

Different types of insulin can be distinguished by placing sticky tape or rubber bands around the neck of long-acting insulin vials. The NovoPen (I or II) is a great help for the partially sighted or blind patient. This can be carried around very easily, and the dosage easily counted either by depressing the cap (= 2 units on NovoPen I) or 'dialing' the number of units (NovoPen II). The 'neutral' and 'primed' positions on the NovoPen II are also identified by palpable marks on the barrel. With the pen devices, it is possible to test if there is any insulin left by ejecting one unit over the palm of the hand or wrist.

### *Oral medication*

Taking oral hypoglycaemic agents and other tablets obviously presents fewer problems than injecting insulin, but may still be difficult. Various containers are available which are prefilled by a sighted person and distribute one batch of tablets at a time (Fig. 9.2). These devices, as well as large-print and braille labels, are available from the Royal National Institute for the Blind (see Table 9.4).

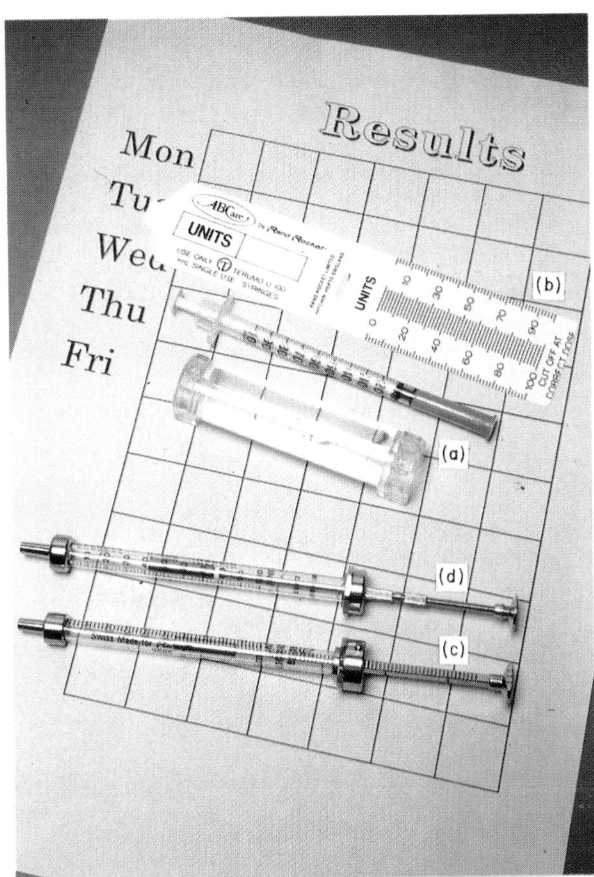


**Fig. 9.1.** A selection of useful gadgets: a large-print result sheet, magnifier and syringe guide. At the bottom is a click-count and preset syringe.

### *Home blood glucose monitoring*

Partially sighted and blind diabetic patients can be taught to measure their own blood glucose levels [13]. For the partially sighted, the standard Hypocount meter (BCL) with its large red LED display is very useful. Blind patients can use various specially adapted blood glucose meters which buzz, beep or speak the result. The buzzing Hypocount meter (BCL) gives the result as a series of buzzes (e.g. one buzz represents 0–3 mmol/l, two buzzes 4–7 mmol/l, and so on). The Glucochek SC (Ames) (Fig. 9.3) conveys more detailed information with a combination of different musical tones, whereas the 'talking' Hypocount meter

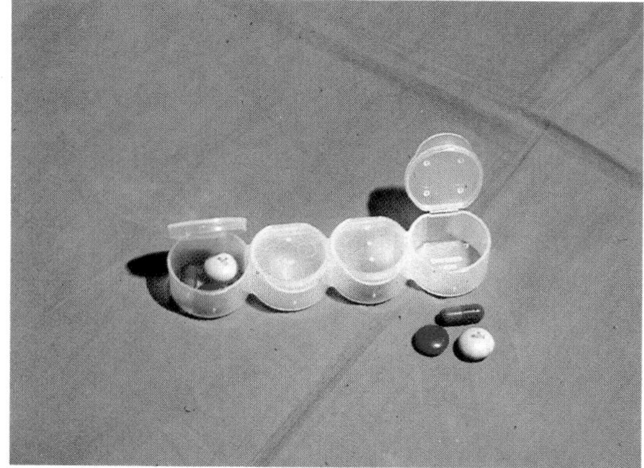

(a)

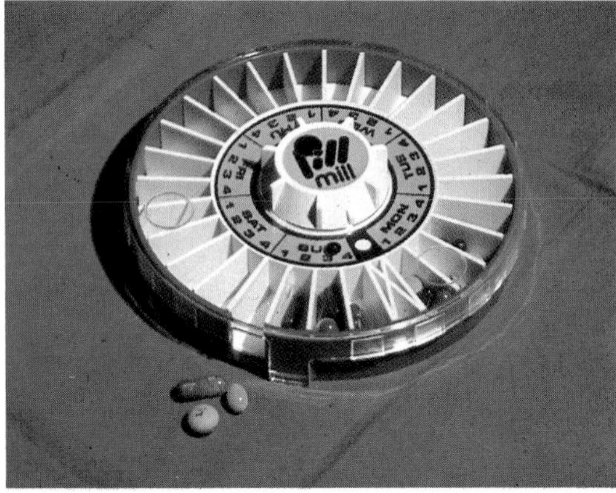


(b)

**Fig. 9.2.** (a) Daily pillminder, holding a day's supply of tablets. Compartments are differentiated by raised dots (not braille). (b) The Pillmill, a circular container with 28 compartments, holding one week's supply. The clear plastic top is turned to access successive doses. (Reproduced with permission from Mrs J. Williams, Fazakerley Hospital, Liverpool, and the Editors of *Practical Diabetes*.)

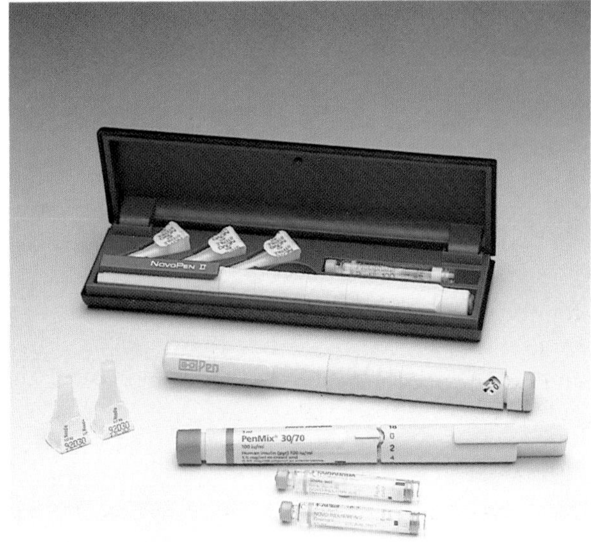


**Fig. 9.3.** Insulin pens and cartridges, which are particularly suitable for administering insulin in the visually-handicapped patient.

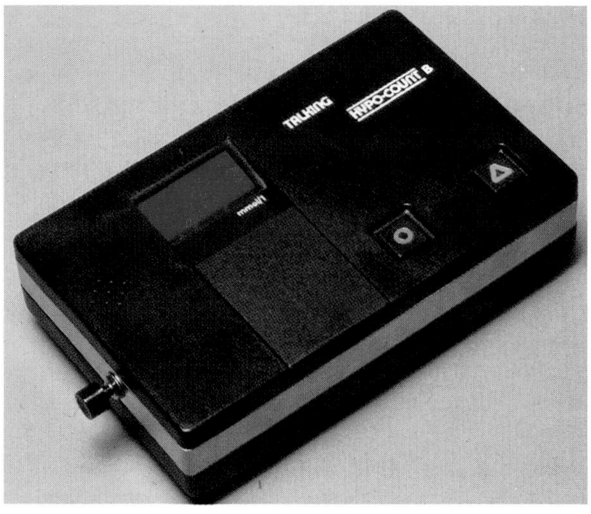


**Fig. 9.4.** The talking Hypocount meter. The large button on the left can be pressed at any time during the machine's sequence for the user to be told what is happening as well as speaking the result.

(Fig. 9.4) uses an electronically generated voice to give both instructions and the result. All of these machines are useful and patients enjoy using them.

There remains the problem of teaching someone with little or no vision to prick their finger and place a small drop of blood accurately on a reagent strip. Mental mapping can be exploited to produce an image of the finger, which has to be kept level to avoid losing the drop of blood. Orientating on the painful part of the finger which has been pricked, the reagent pad on the stick (identified with a fingernail) is then pressed against the finger so it can be felt just underneath the finger-prick site; the finger is then rolled on to the pad. Blank readings, where the drop of blood misses the stick completely, are quite common at first but with encouragement and perseverance, most people (except for those with severe sensory neuropathy, who cannot feel the needle) can learn this manoeuvre.

Results can be recorded by partially sighted patients on large-print, black-inked results sheets or on a tape recorder by the blind. The elderly are more difficult to teach than the young, chiefly because they have less confidence in their ability to learn new skills, and much patience and perseverence may be needed on the part of both the diabetic care team and the patient.

### Blind registration and social services

The definitions of 'partial sight' and 'blindness' for the purposes of registration are purely economic. Blindness is defined as the inability to perform any work for which eyesight is essential, and partial sight as substantial and permanent visual handicap. In the UK, the blind registration form (BD8) is completed by a consultant ophthalmologist and forwarded to the patient's local Social Services department, where it is passed to the social worker responsible for the handicapped. Different areas show considerable variation in the services available and the personnel who actually provide them. The social worker dealing with a disability is the 'gatekeeper' for both the official local services and for information concerning voluntary and other organizations specializing in support for that disability. The social worker who visits the visually handicapped offers emotional support, encouragement and practical help, as well as organizing local services. The various allowances and benefits for which blind diabetic patients may be eligible in the UK are shown in Table 9.2. Some local authorities also have technical officers who teach the blind person everyday tasks such as cooking, advise on special pieces of equipment and teach braille and typing. Mobility officers teach the newly blind long-cane training and help them to plan the layout of their surroundings. In many areas, these three disciplines are undertaken by one social worker. Other useful services are listed in Table 9.3, and a list of relevant addresses is provided in Table 9.4.

The Guide Dogs for the Blind Association arrange trials to assess an individual's suitability for a guide dog, which can give a greater degree of independence as well as a valuable companion. The RNIB residential centre at Torquay offers retraining for people wishing to return to work and a general, intensive rehabilitation course, with the aim of encouraging as much independence and self-confidence as possible. Most Job Centres have a Disability Resettlement Officer, to help and advise on retraining and employment.

**Table 9.2.** Allowances and benefits available*.

| Benefit | Amount (£/week) |
|---|---|
| Unemployment Benefit | 43.10 |
| Statutory Sick Pay: | |
| lower rate | 45.30 |
| higher rate | 52.30 |
| Sickness Benefit | 41.20 |
| Disability Living Allowance | |
| care component | 11.55–43.35 |
| mobility component | 30.30 |
| Invalidity Benefit | 54.15 |
| Allowance (age-dependent) | 3.60–11.50 |
| Invalidity Care Allowance | 32.55 |
| Attendance Allowance (65+ years) | |
| lower rate | 28.35 |
| higher rate | 43.35 |

* 1992 UK figures.

**Table 9.3.** Useful services and facilities in the UK for partially sighted and blind patients (addresses are given in Table 9.4).

*Talking books.* Giant cassette tapes and the machines for playing them are available from RNIB, British Talking Book Service for the Blind, Royal National Library for the Blind and Calibre Library

*Talking newspapers.* Some Sunday papers and monthly magazines are available on standard cassettes from the Talking Newspaper Association. Some local authorities provide local papers on cassette

*Library services.* Most libraries have large-print books and some have a service for housebound readers

*Residential establishments, courses, holiday homes and caravans* for the blind are organized by the RNIB

*Information and a wide range of aids to daily life* are available from the RNIB and the Partially Sighted Society

**Table 9.4.** Useful addresses for visually-handicapped people in the UK.

Royal National Institute for the Blind (RNIB), 224 Great Portland Street, London W1N 6AA, UK

Partially Sighted Society, c/o Royal London Society for the Blind, 105–109 Salisbury Road, London NW6 6RH, UK

London Association for the Blind, 14–16 Vernay Street, London SE16, UK

Guide Dogs for the Blind Association, Hillfield Burghfield Common, Reading, Berkshire RG7 3YG, UK,

Talking Newspaper Association of the UK, 10 Browning Road, Heathfield, East Sussex TN21 8DB, UK

## Recent developments

### *Drawing up insulin*

There is now a complete range of ready-mixed insulins available in many countries, with the proportions of short-acting and isophane insulin varying from 10:90 to 50:50. These are available in both vials and pen cartridges and are much simpler and more accurate than mixing in a syringe.

Insulin pens have become the easiest and most convenient way to self-administer insulin for the visually-handicapped. The NovoPen II delivers up to 36 units in 2-unit increments and the BD pen up to 30 units in single units. Both pens take 1.5-ml cartridges, holding 150 units of insulin. A disposable, preloaded pen capable of delivering up to 78 units at a time, and holding a 3-ml insulin cartridge of 300 units has also been made available recently.

### *Home blood glucose monitoring*

For the partially-sighted, blood glucose monitors that use newer, non-wipe strips are simple to use. In the UK, the Hypoguard Hypocount Supreme and BM Accutrend are examples of meters which are easy to use, and the Accutrend has a large display which is especially suitable for the partially-sighted.

JACQUELINE N. WILKINSON

## References


1 Keegan DL, Ash D, Greenough T. Adjustment to blindness. *Canad J Ophthalmol* 1976; **11** (suppl 2): 22–9.
2 Diffenburg RS. The psychology of blindness. *Geriatrics* 1967; **22**: 127–33.
3 Clark-Carter D. Psycho-social aspects of mobility training. *New Beacon* 1987; **71**: 217–19.
4 Fitzgerald RG. The newly blind, mental distress, somatic illness, disability and management. *EENT Monthly* 1973; **52**: 99–102.
5 Jones JN, Uccellari H. *Coping with Visual Loss*. British Diabetic Association, London, 1989.
6 Goffman E. *Stigma*. Englewood Cliffs, New Jersey: Spectrum Books, 1963: Chapter 3.
7 Herman JE. Cognitive mapping in blind people, acquisition of spatial relationships in a large scale environment. *J Vis Impair Blind* 1983; **77**: 161–6.
8 Sylvester RH. The mental imagery of the blind: discussion. *Psychol Bull* 1983; **10**: 210–11.
9 Finke RA. Mental imagery and the visual system. *Sci Am* 1986; **254**: 88–95.
10 Miller S. In: Gelder BD, ed. *The Problem of Imagery and Spatial Development. Knowledge and Representation*. London: Routledge & Kegan Paul, 1982.
11 Ryerson N. Using and creating visual images, a new task for rehabilitation. *J Vis Impair Blind* 1982; **76**: 421–3.
12 Dodds AG, Carter DDC. Memory of movement in blind children: the role of previous visual experience. *J Motor Behav* 1983; **15**: 343–52.
13 Prior JC, Alojado NC, Hunt JA, Begg IS. Use of tactile techniques for self-monitoring of blood glucose in visually impaired patients with diabetes mellitus. *Diabetes Care* 1984; **7**: 313–17.

# PART 3
# DIABETIC NEUROPATHY

# 10 Diabetic Neuropathy: Epidemiology and Pathogenesis


## Summary

- Diabetic neuropathy can be classified as either reversible (e.g. reduced nerve conduction velocity) or established (focal, multifocal, symmetric and mixed neuropathies).
- The epidemiology of diabetic neuropathy is unclear because of inconsistent definitions of what constitutes neuropathy — frequencies of 10–100% of patients affected have been reported.
- Nerve biopsies show axonal degeneration and regeneration, demyelination and remyelination and abnormalities of the vasa nervorum; capillary closure is correlated with the severity of neuropathy.
- Neurophysiological studies show reduced motor and sensory nerve conduction velocities and resistance to ischaemic conduction failure.
- The pathogenesis is still uncertain: metabolic factors may predominate in early disease and vascular factors at a later stage and in focal neuropathies.
- In experimental diabetic neuropathy, a possible metabolic mechanism involves hyperglycaemia-induced sorbitol accumulation, myonositol depletion, reduced $Na^+$–$K^+$–ATPase activity and an increase in intracellular $Na^+$ levels.
- The importance of non-enzymatic glycosylation of axonal proteins and changes in axoplasmic transport is uncertain.


A wide variety of disturbances of peripheral nerve function occur in relation to diabetes mellitus. Their precise classification is still not agreed, mainly because of persisting uncertainty as to their causation. In general, they can be divided into two categories (see Table 10.1). The first comprises rapidly reversible phenomena including distal paraesthesiae in the limbs and reduced nerve conduction velocity in newly diagnosed or poorly controlled diabetic subjects [1], and increased resistance to ischaemic conduction failure [2, 3]. The second category consists of more persistent phenomena ('established' neuropathy). These can be broadly subdivided into focal and multifocal neuropathies on one hand, and symmetric polyneuropathies on the other. Mixed syndromes are common.

This section considers the epidemiology, pathology, electrophysiology, pathogenesis and natural history of diabetic neuropathy.

## Epidemiology

Satisfactory information is not so far available for

**Table 10.1.** A classification of diabetic neuropathy.

| |
|---|
| *Rapidly reversible phenomena*: |
| Distal sensory symptoms |
| Reduced nerve conduction velocity |
| Resistance to ischaemic conduction failure |
| *'Established' neuropathy*: |
| Focal and multifocal neuropathies |
| • cranial mononeuropathies |
| • thoracoabdominal neuropathy |
| • focal limb neuropathies |
| • asymmetric proximal lower limb motor neuropathy (diabetic amyotrophy) |
| Symmetric neuropathies |
| • sensory/autonomic polyneuropathy |
| • proximal lower limb motor neuropathy |
| Mixed syndromes |

the incidence and prevalence of diabetic neuropathy, largely because of inconsistency in defining neuropathy. Ascertainment bias has also played a part. Currently available estimates of the frequency of diabetic neuropathy range between 10 and 100% [4], depending upon the criteria adopted. Those series reporting a prevalence of 100% have been based on the results of nerve conduction studies. Other series have given widely differing prevalences depending upon whether symptoms in the absence of signs, signs in the absence of symptoms, or the requirement that both should be present, have been taken as indicative of the presence of neuropathy. In a large prospective study of diabetic out-patients [5], the prevalence rose from 7.5% at the time of diagnosis of diabetes to 50% after 25 years. The prevalence after 20 years was over 40%. Yet in the prospective, community-based survey of Palumbo *et al*. [6], it was only half this value; this latter study, however, was a cohort analysis confined to NIDDM patients without neuropathy at entry. Attempts have recently been made [7] to define minimal criteria for the diagnosis of diabetic neuropathy and for staging the evolution of neuropathy. Future prospective studies employing such criteria are likely to yield more consistent information.

Neuropathy is uncommon in children with diabetes, the prevalence rate being in the region of 2% [8] Its prevalence increases progressively with age. The prospective study of Pirart [5] indicated that the risk of developing neuropathy is directly related to the duration of the diabetes so that the slopes for the increase in prevalence and annual incidence were approximately uniform (Fig. 10.1). The median time from the diagnosis of NIDDM to the development of neuropathy was found to be 9 years in one study [6].

There is no clear indication for any difference in liability to diabetic polyneuropathy between the sexes. Some series [5] have found a higher prevalence of males, but this was thought possibly to be related to confusion with other causes of neuropathy such as alcoholism. However, acute painful diabetic neuropathy and diabetic amyotrophy may be commoner in males. Little information is avail-

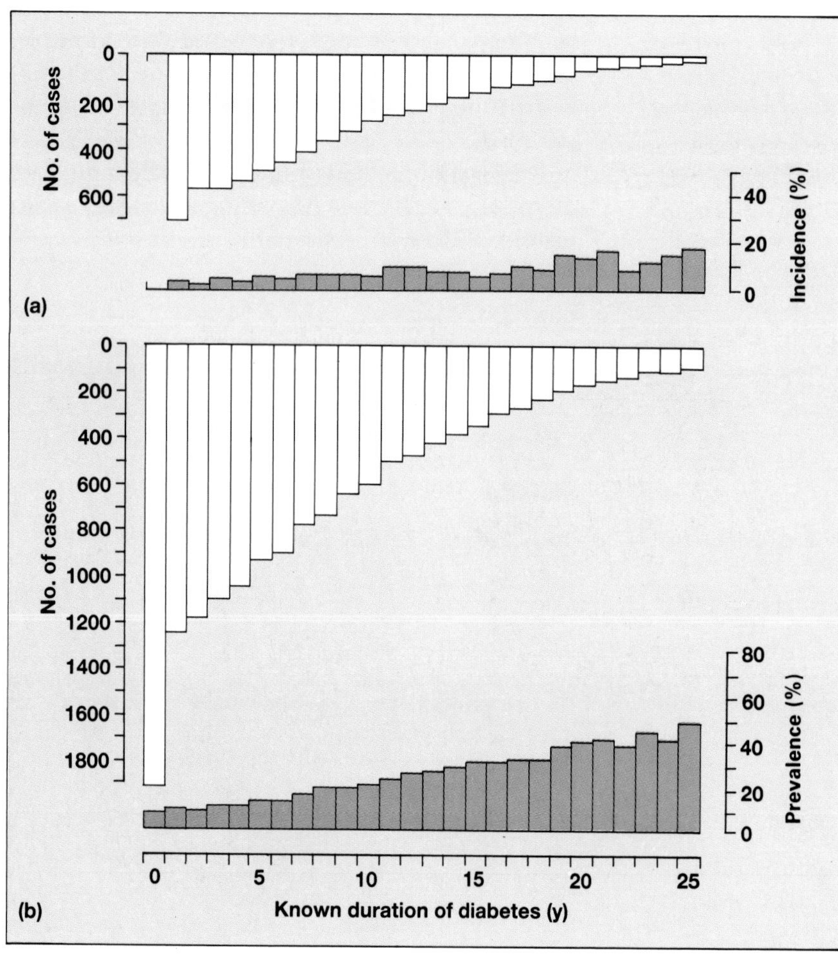


**Fig. 10.1.** Increase in the annual incidence and prevalence of diabetic neuropathy obtained from a prospective survey of 2795 cases observed from the time of diagnosis of diabetes. The suspended columns show the decrease in the number of subjects over time. (a) Incidence of neuropathy; (b) prevalence of neuropathy. (Redrawn with permission from [5].)

able for the relative prevalence in different racial groups or geographical areas. Most studies have been conducted in Europe, Scandinavia or North America; Osuntokun [9] reported a prevalence of 40% in Nigeria.

The possible contribution of genetic factors in susceptibility to neuropathy requires further investigation, and may help to explain why some individuals with poorly controlled diabetes never develop significant neuropathy whereas others with mild or well-controlled disease develop troublesome neuropathy. The possibility of genetic linkage to acetylator status has not been confirmed [10].

Neuropathy occurs both in IDDM and NIDDM. It has been noted that the prevalence of neuropathy is less in the former than the latter at the time of diagnosis, presumably because of the shorter duration of antecedent undiscovered diabetes. Thus Mincu [11] found a prevalence of neuropathy of 1.4% in newly diagnosed cases of IDDM and 14.1% for NIDDM.

There is general agreement that the commonest type of diabetic neuropathy in both IDDM and NIDDM is a symmetric sensory and autonomic polyneuropathy. Some series [12] have reported a high prevalence of asymmetric motor syndromes, probably because of selection bias. Focal neuropathies are accepted as being more common in patients with diabetes, although this has never been established by a community-based epidemiological study.

**Pathological changes**

Most information on the pathology of diabetic neuropathy has been derived from investigations on nerve biopsies, which sample a relatively small portion of the peripheral nervous system (PNS). Full autopsy studies to assess the distribution of the changes throughout the PNS are few in number. Patients with diabetic polyneuropathy show axonal loss which increases in severity distally, accompanied by moderate demyelination. In one biopsy study of untreated diabetic subjects [13], the predominant changes in patients without symptoms of neuropathy were segmental demyelination and remyelination; patients with symptomatic neuropathy showed the combination of demyelination and remyelination together with axonal degeneration. Finally, in treated cases, often with long-standing diabetes, axonal degeneration was the commonest abnormality. In painful diabetic neuropathy, predominant loss of small myelinated fibres and evidence of degeneration and regeneration of unmyelinated axons has been described [14]. Such examples of diabetic 'small fibre neuropathy' probably do not represent a separate group, but rather one end of a spectrum in which fibres of all sizes may be lost [15]. Prominent axonal regeneration (Fig. 10.2) is a conspicuous feature of diabetic neuropathy, except in advanced cases, where few axons may remain in distal sensory nerves. Some loss of dorsal root and autonomic ganglion cells and of anterior horn cells

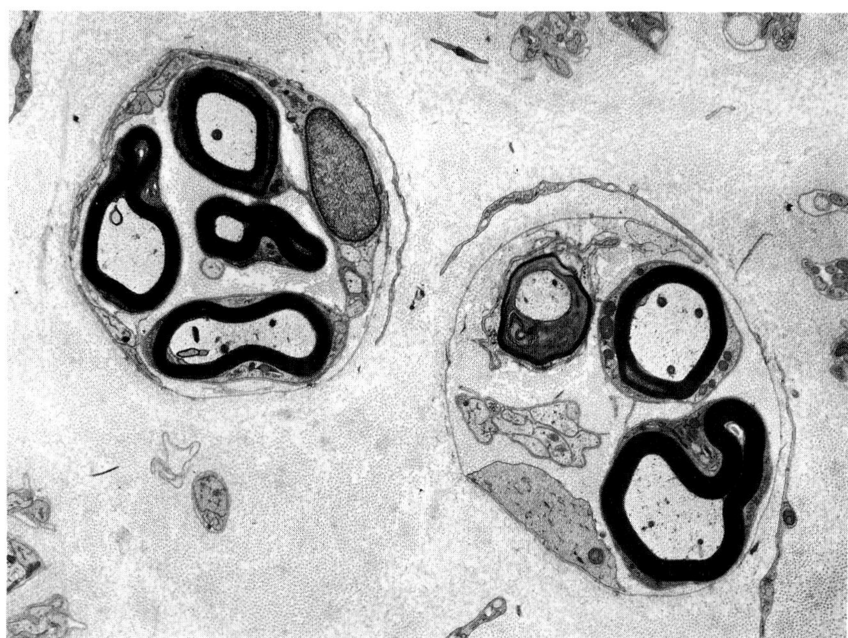

**Fig. 10.2.** Electron micrograph of transverse section of sural nerve biopsy from a patient with diabetic polyneuropathy, showing two regenerative clusters composed of groups of myelinated axons and associated Schwann cells.

occurs, but this is relatively modest. Degeneration of fibres is also detectable in the posterior columns of the spinal cord.

Fewer observations are available for patients with focal nerve lesions. In patients with third cranial nerve palsies, focal demyelination has been demonstrated in the nerve [16].

Attention to abnormalities of the vasa nervorum was drawn by Fagerberg [17] who found the walls of the endoneurial capillaries to be thickened by PAS-positive material. Electron microscopy showed this to be due to reduplication of the basal lamina (Fig. 10.3). Proliferation of endothelial cells, leading to narrowing of the vascular lumen has also been described, as have intraluminal deposits of fibrin. Dyck *et al.* [18] found that the numbers of closed capillaries in sural nerve biopsies were significantly greater than in age-matched control nerves and were positively correlated with the severity of the neuropathy (Fig. 10.4). More recently, however, Bradley *et al.* [19] have failed to confirm capillary closure in a series of younger patients with diabetic polyneuropathy.

### Neurophysiological changes

In asymptomatic diabetic patients, nerve conduction velocity, both motor and sensory, is frequently slightly reduced and sensory nerve action potentials are often of diminished amplitude, indicating subclinical neuropathy. Abnormalities may be detectable at common sites of compression or entrapment, reflecting an increased vulnerability of diabetic nerve to pressure damage [20]. The slight reduction of nerve conduction velocity which is present in newly diagnosed diabetic patients and which is rapidly reversed by institution of satisfactory glycaemic control [1] is of uncertain significance. It may reflect abnormalities of axolemmal function rather than indicating the presence of structural changes.

Diabetic nerves are abnormally resistant to the conduction failure normally caused by ischaemia, as can be demonstrated by electrophysiological means. Both evoked sensory nerve action potentials and conduction in motor fibres persist longer during ischaemia of a limb, produced by inflation of a pressure cuff above arterial pressure, than in normal subjects [3, 21].

In established diabetic polyneuropathy, the abnormalities are greater in sensory than motor fibres and are more prominent in the lower than in the upper limbs. The reduction in motor conduction velocity is mild or moderate, and severe slowing should raise the suspicion that the neuropathy has some other cause. Chronic inflammatory demyelinating polyneuropathy, hereditary motor and sensory neuropathy, and paraproteinaemic neuropathy are the three most important possibilities. Short-latency somatosensory evoked

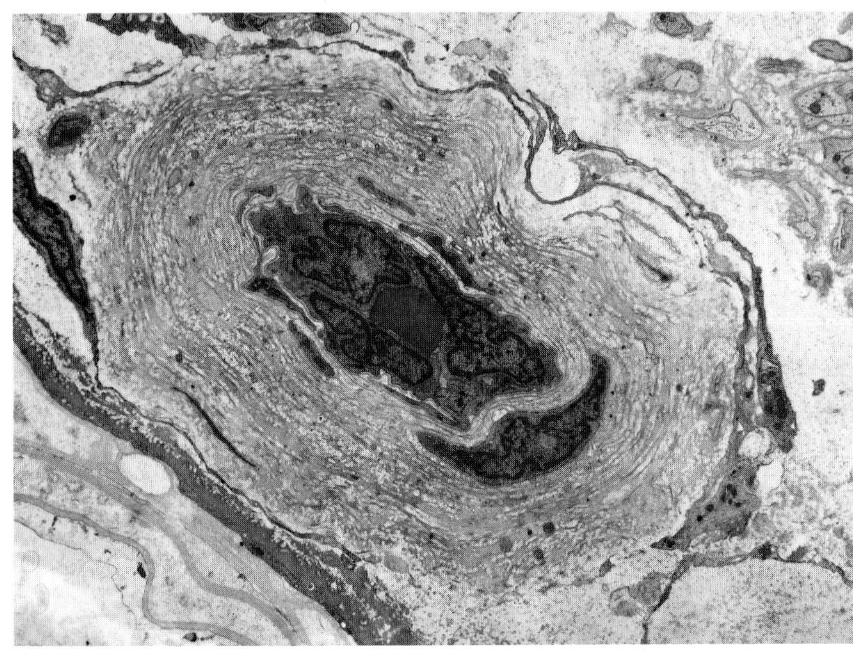

**Fig. 10.3.** Electron micrograph of endoneurial capillary from sural nerve biopsy from a patient with diabetic polyneuropathy, showing thickened surrounding zone composed of reduplicated basal lamina.

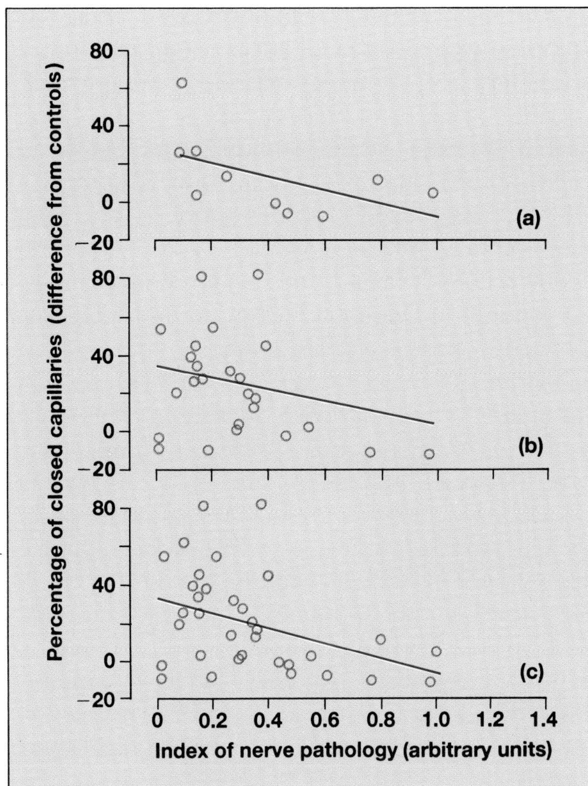


**Fig. 10.4.** Relationship between numbers of closed capillaries and the index of nerve pathology (IP) for sural nerve biopsies of patients with IDDM (a), NIDDM (b) and both combined (c). The number of closed capillaries is expressed as a percentage difference from controls. The IP combines the severity of loss of myelinated nerve fibres with abnormalities in surviving fibres. A higher IP value indicates less severe pathology. For all three groups, there is a significant negative slope, indicating a positive correlation between the numbers of closed capillaries and the severity of neuropathy. (Redrawn with permission from [18] and the publisher.)

responses may be delayed [22], indicating pathology in the spinal roots, dorsal columns, or both.

In patients with focal nerve lesions such as the carpal tunnel syndrome or ulnar neuropathy, localized abnormalities of nerve conduction are demonstrable. Similarly, conduction time may be prolonged in the femoral nerve in proximal lower limb motor neuropathy (diabetic amyotrophy).

Electromyography demonstrates denervation in affected muscles in patients with focal limb nerve lesions or proximal lower limb motor neuropathy. In the latter syndrome, denervation may be detectable in paraspinal muscles, suggesting involvement of spinal nerves as well as the lumbosacral plexus and femoral nerves. Some denervation may be present in distal muscles (sometimes only in the small foot muscles) in diabetic sensory/autonomic polyneuropathy, even in the absence of clinically demonstrable weakness.

## Pathogenesis

The causation of diabetic neuropathy is still not understood. Part of the difficulty stems from the fact that multiple abnormalities can be demonstrated in the PNS of human subjects with diabetes and in animals with experimentally induced or genetic diabetes. Identification of the causal chain of events leading to peripheral nerve damage is correspondingly difficult. Moreover, correlation does not imply causation. The major discussion concerns the relative contributions of metabolic and vascular factors.

### *Glycaemic control*

The question as to whether improved control of glycaemia can prevent or ameliorate diabetic neuropathy has recently been reviewed [23]. The balance of evidence favoured the conclusion that hyperglycaemia is an important determinant of neuropathy and that improved glycaemic control benefits nerve function. This was based on four lines of evidence. The first derives from several retrospective studies (which are defective in various respects) which concluded overall that neuropathy was commoner in poorly controlled individuals. Further evidence comes from assessments of neuropathy before and after starting diabetic treatment. Minor improvements in nerve conduction velocity and reversal of resistance to ischaemic conduction failure are well documented, but neither of these phenomena is known to be related to the later development of established neuropathy. Acute painful diabetic neuropathy has been reported to improve after the institution of tight glycaemic control [24] and painful neuropathy has also been found to be benefited by continuous subcutaneous insulin infusion (CSII) therapy [25]. Thirdly, untreated NIDDM patients show close correlations of nerve conduction velocity with plasma glucose and glycosylated haemoglobin levels [26]. Again, it is not yet clear whether such changes in nerve conduction velocity are a predictor for the later development of neuropathy. Finally, in a prospective randomized trial comparing standard and intensive diabetic (CSII) therapy [27], nerve conduction velocity and vibration sense threshold were found to improve after 8 months of CSII.

### *Polyol and myoinositol metabolism*

Brain, peripheral nerve and other tissues which do not depend upon insulin for the entry of glucose into their cells, have cytoplasmic glucose concentrations which reflect the degree of glycaemia. Aldose reductase, the rate-limiting enzyme of the polyol pathway (see Fig. 3.2), is present in peripheral nerve. Aldose reductase has a low affinity for its hexose sugar substrates, including glucose. At low glucose concentrations (during normoglycaemia), concentrations within nerves of its reaction product, the polyol sorbitol, are low. Sorbitol is converted to fructose by the enzyme sorbitol dehydrogenase. Hyperglycaemia results in greatly increased concentrations of glucose in peripheral nerve and, consequently, through increased activity of aldose reductase, leads to elevated concentrations of sorbitol and fructose. The original suggestion was that sorbitol accumulation itself could cause osmotic damage, but there is no histological evidence of this, either from animal or human nerves.

In the peripheral nerves of diabetic animals, the elevations of sorbitol and fructose are accompanied by a decrease in the concentration of another polyol, myoinositol [28]. Myoinositol concentrations are normally substantially greater in peripheral nerve than in plasma, as it is taken up by a sodium-dependent, energy-consuming active transport mechanism. Nerve conduction velocity can be improved by the administration of aldose reductase inhibitors to diabetic animals and also by dietary supplementation with myoinositol. From this it has been concluded that myoinositol depletion, rather than sorbitol accumulation, is responsible for the changes in nerve conduction velocity. These various experimental studies have been reviewed by Gillon *et al.* [29].

The activity of sodium–potassium-dependent adenosine triphosphatase ($Na^+$–$K^+$–ATPase) is known to be reduced in the peripheral nerves of diabetic rats and this can be corrected by the administration of aldose reductase inhibitors or dietary supplementation with myoinositol. It has been proposed that nerve $Na^+$–$K^+$–ATPase is controlled by membrane phosphoinositides, possibly via protein kinase C. The following chain of pathogenetic events has been proposed (Fig. 10.5) [30]. Reduced nerve myoinositol concentrations result in abnormal phosphoinositides, leading to reduced membrane $Na^+$–$K^+$–ATPase activity. Since myoinositol transport is dependent on this enzyme, a self-reinforcing cycle of reduced myoinositol uptake and $Na^+$–$K^+$–ATPase activity results, leading to increased intraaxonal $Na^+$ accumulation. This could affect nerve impulse generation, sodium-dependent amino acid uptake and other phenomena. It has been claimed [31] that intra-axonal accumulation of sodium in the paranodal region leads to axonal swelling and 'axoglial dysjunction', namely the separation of the terminations of the myelin lamellae from the axon, and further structural changes [31].

Although providing an attractive explanation for many of the phenomena observed in peripheral

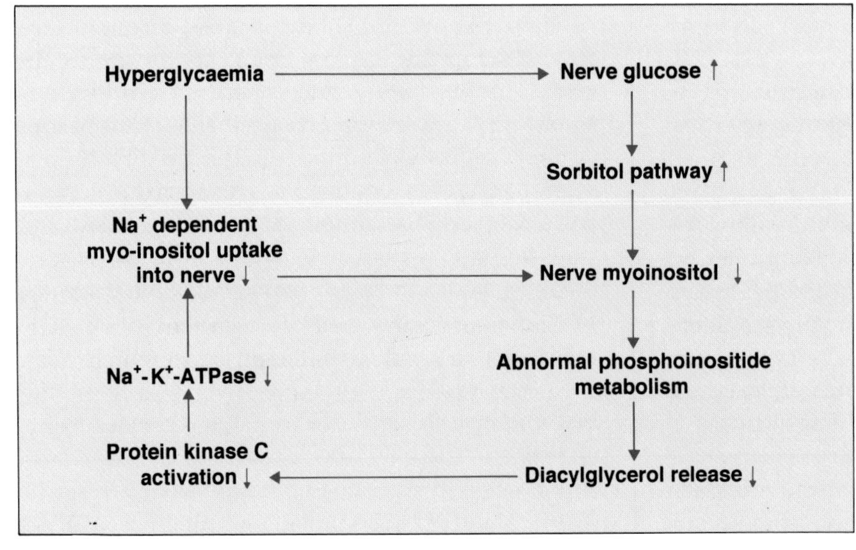


**Fig. 10.5.** Scheme summarizing proposed relationships between hyperglycaemia, sorbitol and myoinositol metabolism in peripheral nerve.

nerves in diabetic animals, it is difficult to transfer this hypothesis to the pathogenesis of human diabetic neuropathy. First, although sorbitol accumulates in peripheral nerves in human diabetes, reductions in nerve myoinositol concentrations have not been convincingly demonstrated [29, 32, 33]. Secondly, the morphological changes which characterize human diabetic neuropathy do not develop in the animal models so far studied. It has therefore not been possible to show that correction of nerve sorbitol, myoinositol and $Na^+-K^+-$ATPase activity in animals will prevent these changes. In man, aldose reductase inhibitors have so far been shown to improve nerve conduction velocity but produce no other convincing benefits. No definite benefit has been obtained by dietary myoinositol supplementation (see [29]). Finally, the results of recent observations on experimental galactose-induced neuropathy are important. Galactose is metabolized to galactitol by aldose reductase and accumulates in nerve. In this experimental model, in which nerve myoinositol is also reduced, $Na^+-Ka^+-$ATPase activity has been found to be *increased* rather than reduced [34]. There is thus no simple relationship between myoinositol metabolism and $Na^+-K^+-$ATPase activity.

### *Axonal transport*

Protein synthesis in neurons is effectively confined to the cell body. Materials such as enzymes, neurotransmitters and structural proteins must then be translocated down the axons in the fast and slow anterograde transport systems, following which degenerate material, together with substances such as growth factors taken up by nerve terminals, are taken back to the cell body in the retrograde transport system.

Fast anterograde transport in peripheral nerves remains normal in experimental diabetes, but there is a slight impairment of slow component 'a' (SCa), which can be correlated with the reduced axonal calibre found in this model. The SCa defect is not corrected either by myoinositol supplementation or by aldose reductase inhibitors, whereas impaired transport of the enzyme choline acetyl transferase, which is carried in SCb, is corrected by treatment with either agent. Retrograde axonal transport is also impaired in streptozotocin-induced diabetes in rats.

The relevance of these observations to human diabetic neuropathy is again uncertain. Acetyl cholinesterase and dopamine β-hydroxylase, both of which are fast-transported enzymes, have been reported to be reduced in human diabetic neuropathy whereas their transport is normal in the animal models.

The abnormalities of axonal transport in human and experimental diabetes have recently been reviewed by Sidenius and Jakobsen [35].

### *Non-enzymatic glycosylation of nerve proteins*

Abnormal glycosylation of axonal proteins has been demonstrated in experimental diabetes in animals [36]. The relevance of this to peripheral nerve function is so far uncertain. Non-enzymatic glycosylation of walls of the vasa nervorum and of the endoneurial connective tissue matrix [37] could also be important. Chronic changes in these tissues could eventually lead to ischaemic changes.

### *Ischaemia*

Clinical considerations suggest a vascular basis for diabetic mononeuropathies of acute onset, such as lesions of the third cranial nerve. There is some pathological support for this concept, although, as discussed earlier, further evidence is desirable.

One of the main points of current controversy regarding the pathogenesis of diabetic neuropathy is the possible role of vascular factors in the production of the diabetic polyneuropathies. Thus, multifocal lesions in proximal nerves have been found at autopsy [38–40] which may have summated to produce a symmetric distal polyneuropathy. The pathological changes also suggested the presence of diffuse fibre loss and, as these studies were performed on elderly patients, the superimposition of vascular lesions on a diffuse neuropathy of metabolic origin cannot be excluded. In another study, patchy fibre loss was found in sural nerve biopsies from a series of patients with diabetic neuropathy [41]. However, such patchy fibre loss is also a feature of neuropathies in which a vascular basis can be discounted [42]. Perhaps the most cogent morphological evidence so far is the correlation between the severity of the neuropathy and the number of 'closed' capillaries in sural nerve biopsies, to which reference has already been made [18], although this may only apply to older individuals. Intraneural recordings have also demonstrated reduced oxygen tension [43]. There is some supportive evidence from animal studies in that nerve blood flow has been shown to be reduced in streptozotocin-diabetic rats, in which intraneural oxygen tension is also reduced [44] (Fig. 10.6).

The weight of the current evidence favours a combination of metabolic factors, probably more important at the earlier stages in younger diabetic subjects, and vascular factors which become increasingly important with duration of diabetes and advancing age. It would appear difficult to attempt to explain the totality of diabetic neuropathy on a vascular basis. The features of diabetic polyneuropathy, with a predominance of sensory and autonomic features over motor involvement, differ in pattern from those observed in other neuropathies of ischaemic origin.

## Natural history

Few longitudinal surveys have been undertaken to follow the natural history of diabetic neuropathy. The more effective methods now available to quantify sensory, motor and autonomic deficits, together with nerve conduction studies, should make possible definitive observations on the evolution of the manifestations of the different types of peripheral nerve changes that occur. In general, these studies necessarily have to be of a long-term nature. Although some instances of diabetic sensory polyneuropathy have a relatively abrupt start, most have a slow and insidious onset. Acute painful diabetic neuropathy is an exception. This syndrome may be associated with precipitous weight loss. Following institution of glycaemic control and weight gain, the neuropathy resolves over some months [24] (Fig. 10.7). The same is true for the acute painful neuropathy which may follow the introduction of diabetic treatment or the establishment of euglycaemia in a previously poorly controlled patient [43]. It is general clinical experience that diabetic sensory polyneuropathy, once established, does not improve substantially, even with satisfactory glycaemic control. The Mayo Clinic CSII trial [27] documented only an improvement in nerve conduction velocity and vibration sensation without any change in symptoms over an 8-month period. Jakobsen *et al.* [46] have recently shown from studies employing quantitative sensory testing and assessment of autonomic function that over a 2-year period, in patients treated by CSII, neuropathy remained stable

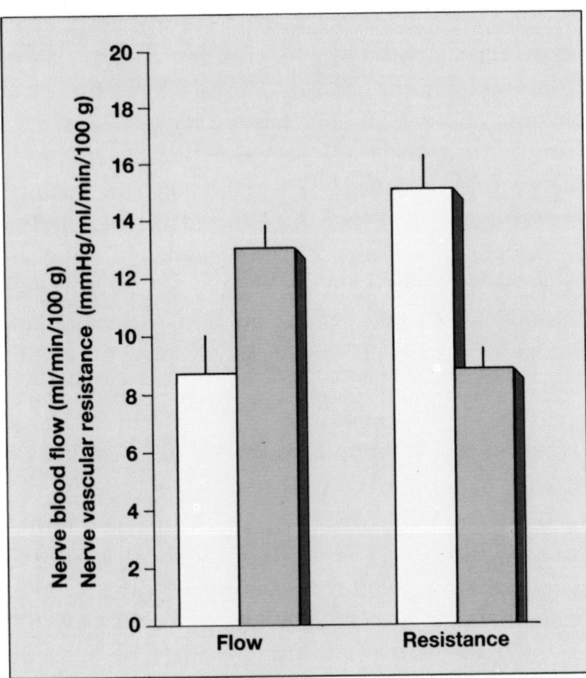


**Fig. 10.6.** Mean sciatic nerve blood flow and vascular resistance from seven streptozotocin-diabetic rats (yellow columns) and eight control rats (orange columns) showing reduced flow and increased vascular resistance in the diabetic animals. (Redrawn with permission from [42] and the Editor of *Brain*.)

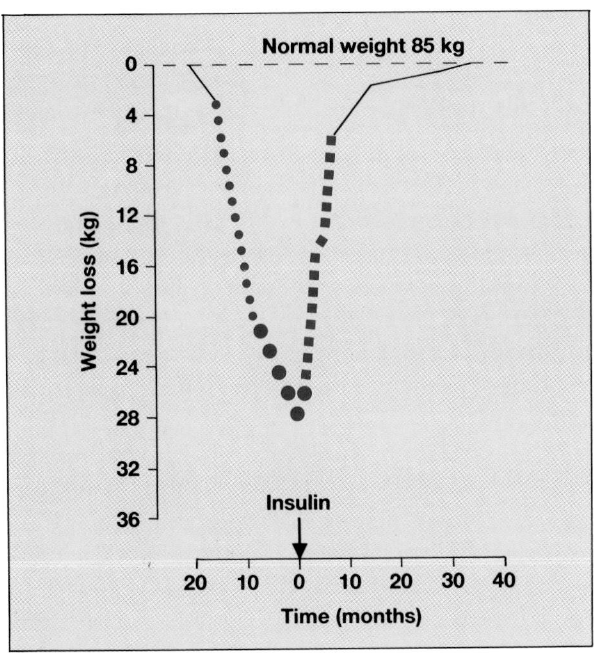


**Fig. 10.7.** Changes in body weight in a case of acute painful diabetic neuropathy. Initiation of treatment with insulin is indicated by the arrow, treatment before then having been with an oral hypoglycaemic agent. A precipitate loss of over 27 kg in weight is accompanied by the development of a mild (•) and then a severe (●) painful neuropathy. Restoration of body weight is associated with improvement (■) and then disappearance (——) of the neuropathy.

whereas in those receiving conventional insulin treatment it deteriorated.

Evidence of autonomic neuropathy may be present at the time of diagnosis of diabetes [47] or may appear within 1–2 years of diagnosis [48], but the precise relationship of autonomic dysfunction to duration of diabetes has not been established. Once symptomatic autonomic neuropathy is present, the prognosis for survival is substantially diminished. For a group of 73 patients followed prospectively for up to 5 years, mortality rates of 44% after 2.5 years and 56% after 5 years were found (see Fig. 12.3). Half of the deaths were from renal failure and the other half from causes which could be related to autonomic neuropathy [49].

For focal and multifocal neuropathies, the diabetic third cranial nerve lesions of acute onset characteristically recover satisfactorily. Proximal lower limb motor neuropathy (amyotrophy), particularly if of acute onset, may also recover in some cases. In one series of 12 cases [50], three recovered fully, four showed a good functional result and five continued with residual disability. In the experience of the writer, symptoms of the carpal tunnel syndrome tend not to respond as satisfactorily to surgical decompression in diabetic as in non-diabetic subjects.

## Recent developments

### *Epidemiology*

The prevalence of diabetic neuropathy was examined in a recent multicentre study in the UK involving 6425 hospital-treated patients with both IDDM and NIDDM [51]. Neuropathy was present in 28.3% of all patients and was positively correlated with age and duration of diabetes. In elderly patients with NIDDM, the prevalence reached 44%. Height and male sex were identified as additional risk factors by the American Diabetes Control and Complications Trial [52].

### *Pathogenesis*

The importance of strict glycaemic control has been emphasized by studies of patients treated by pancreatic transplantation [53] and CSII [54], both groups being followed over 2-year periods. Neuropathy in the treated cases stabilized whereas it deteriorated in conventionally-treated patients.

Observations on sural nerve biopsies from patients with diabetic neuropathy have failed to confirm the reduced myoinositol levels that characterize diabetic neuropathy in the rat [55]. Unless there is a small pool of myoinositol that controls phosphoinositide metabolism, this makes the myoinositol hypothesis less compelling. The same study established a positive correlation between the severity of neuropathy as judged by nerve-fibre density and the sorbitol concentrations in nerve. The possibility that the accumulation of sorbitol is implicated in the genesis of diabetic neuropathy is reinforced by the finding of increased nerve-fibre regeneration and remyelination in serial sural nerve biopsies taken before and after treatment with an aldose reductase inhibitor when compared with a placebo [56].

Recently, a possible role for essential fatty acids has been proposed. Dietary linoleic acid is converted to gamma-linolenic acid (GLA) and to further metabolites required for normal membrane structure and cell regulatory molecules. The conversion of linoleic acid to GLA is impaired in diabetes [57]. Motor nerve conduction velocity and abnormalities of axonal transport in streptozotocin-diabetic rats can be improved by GLA [58] and a preliminary controlled clinical trial has suggested that improvement may be obtained in human diabetic neuropathy [59].

### *Natural history*

The natural history of diabetic somatosensory and autonomic neuropathy was studied in patients with IDDM during the first 5 years after diagnosis by Ziegler *et al.* [60]. They showed that the development of subclinical and symptomatic somatosensory and autonomic neuropathy can be predicted by poor control.

Watkins [61] described his experience with the natural history of different clinical patterns of diabetic neuropathy and was able to subdivide these into reversible and substantially irreversible forms. Acute mononeuropathies, diabetic amyotrophy and acute painful diabetic neuropathy had a favourable prognosis, whereas diabetic sensory and autonomic polyneuropathies, once established, were persistent. Sampson *et al.* [62] reported on the evolution of patients with diabetic autonomic neuropathy and found that, in their series, the outlook was substantially better than in the series reported earlier by Ewing *et al.* [63].

P.K. THOMAS

## References


1 Ward JD, Barnes CG, Fisher DJ, Jessop JD, Baker RWR. Improvement in nerve conduction following treatment in newly diagnosed diabetics. *Lancet* 1971; **i**: 428–30.

2 Steiness IB. Vibratory perception in diabetics during arrested blood flow to the limb. *Acta Med Scand* 1959; **163**: 195–205.

3 Seneviratne KN, Peiris OA. The effect of ischaemia on the excitability of sensory nerves in diabetes mellitus. *J Neurol Neurosurg Psychiatr* 1968; **31**: 348–53.

4 Melton LJ, Dyck PJ. Epidemiology. In: Dyck PJ, Thomas PK, Asbury AK, Winegrad AI, Porte Jr D, eds. *Diabetic Neuropathy*. Philadelphia: WB Saunders, 1987: 27–35.

5 Pirart J. Diabetes mellitus and its degenerative complications: a prospective study of 4400 patients observed. *Diabetes Care* 1978; **1**: 168–88, 252–63.

6 Palumbo PJ, Elveback LR, Whisnant JP. Neurologic complications of diabetes mellitus: transient ischemic attack, stroke, and peripheral neuropathy. In: Schoenberg BS, ed. *Neurological Epidemiology: Principles and Clinical Applications*. New York: Raven Press, 1978: 593–601.

7 Dyck PJ, Karnes JL, Daube J, O'Brien P, Service FJ. Clinical and neuropathological criteria for the diagnosis and staging of diabetic polyneuropathy. *Brain* 1985; **108**: 861–80.

8 Hoffman J. Peripheral neuropathy in children with diabetes mellitus. *Acta Neurol Scand* 1964; **40** (suppl 8): 1–23.

9 Osuntokun BO. *The Neurology of Diabetes Mellitus in Nigerians*. MD Thesis. University of London, 1971.

10 Boulton AJM, Hardisty CA, Worth RC, Drury J, Wolfe E, Cudworth AG, Ward JD. Metabolic and genetic factors in diabetic neuropathy. *Diabetologia* 1984; **26**: 15–19.

11 Mincu I. Micro- and macroangiopathies and other chronic degenerative complications in newly detected diabetes mellitus. *Rev Rom Med Int* 1980; **18**: 155–64.

12 Sullivan JF. The neuropathies of diabetes. *Neurology (Minneap)* 1958; **8**: 243–9.

13 Dyck PJ, Sherman WR, Hallcher LM, Service FJ, O'Brien PC, Grina LA, Palumbo PJ, Swanson CJ. Human diabetic endoneurial sorbitol, fructose, and *myo*-inositol related to sural nerve morphometry. *Ann Neurol* 1980; **8**: 590–6.

14 Brown MJ, Martin JR, Asbury AK. Painful diabetic neuropathy: a morphometric study. *Arch Neurol* 1976; **33**: 164–71.

15 Dyck PJ, Lais A, Karnes JL, O'Brien P, Rizza R. Fiber loss is primary and multifocal in sural nerves in diabetic polyneuropathy. *Ann Neurol* 1986; **19**: 425–39.

16 Asbury AK, Aldridge H, Hershberg R, Fisher CM. Oculomotor palsy in diabetes mellitus: a clinico-pathological study. *Brain* 1970; **93**: 555–66.

17 Fagerberg SE. Diabetic neuropathy: a clinical and histological study on the significance of vascular affections. *Acta Med Scand* 1959; **164** (suppl 345): 1–80.

18 Dyck PJ, Hansen S, Karnes J, O'Brien P, Yasuda H, Windebank A, Zimmerman B. Capillary number and percentage closed in human diabetic sural nerve. *Proc Natl Acad Sci USA* 1985; **52**: 2513–17.

19 Bradley JL, King RHM, Llewelyn JG, Thomas PK. Is diabetic polyneuropathy a vascular disease? *J Neurol Neurosurg Psychiatr*, in press.

20 Mulder DW, Lambert EH, Bastron VA, Sprague RG. The neuropathies associated with diabetes mellitus: a clinical and electromyographic study of 103 unselected diabetic patients. *Neurology (Minneap)* 1961; **11**: 275–84.

21 Gregersen G. Diabetic neuropathy: influence of age, sex, metabolic control, and duration of diabetes on motor conduction velocity. *Neurology (Minneap)* 1967; **17**: 972–80.

22 Kuribayashi T, Kurihara T, Tanaka M, Tsuruta K, Araki S. Diabetic neuropathy and electrophysiological studies: evoked potentials, nerve conduction, and short latency SEP. In: Goto Y, Horuichi A, Kogure K, eds. *Diabetic Neuropathy*. Amsterdam: Excerpta Medica, 1982: 120–4.

23 Committee of Health Care Issues, American Neurological Association. Does improved control of glycemia prevent or ameliorate diabetic polyneuropathy? *Ann Neurol* 1986; **19**: 288–90.

24 Archer AG, Watkins PJ, Thomas PK, Sharma AK, Payan J. The natural history of acute painful diabetic neuropathy. *J Neurol Neurosurg Psychiatr* 1983; **46**: 491–9.

25 Boulton AJM, Drury J, Clarke B, Ward JD. Continuous subcutaneous insulin infusion in the management of painful diabetic neuropathy. *Diabetes Care* 1982; **5**: 386–91.

26 Porte D, Graf RJ, Halter JB, Pfeifer MA, Halar E. Diabetic neuropathy and plasma glucose control. *Am J Med* 1981; **70**: 195–200.

27 Service FJ, Rizza RA, Daube JR, O'Brien PC, Dyck PJ. Near normoglycaemia improves nerve conduction and vibration sensation in diabetic neuropathy. *Diabetologia* 1985; **28**: 722–7.

28 Greene DA, De Jesus PV Jr, Winegrad AI. Effects of insulin and dietary *myo*-inositol on impaired peripheral motor nerve conduction velocity in acute streptozotocin diabetes. *J Clin Invest* 1975; **55**: 1326–36.

29 Gillon KRW, King RHM, Thomas PK. The pathology of diabetic neuropathy and the effects of aldose reductase inhibitors. In: Watkins PJ, ed. *Long Term Complications of Diabetes. Clinics in Endocrinology and Metabolism*. Vol 15(4). London: WB Saunders, 1986: 837–54.

30 Greene DA, Lattimer SA, Sima AAF. Sorbitol, phosphoinositides, and sodium–potassium ATPase in the pathogenesis of diabetic complications. *N Engl J Med* 1987; **316**: 599–606.

31 Sima AAF, Nathaniel V, Bril V, McEwen TAJ, Greene DA. Histopathological heterogeneity of neuropathy in insulin-dependent and non-insulin-dependent diabetics and demonstration of axoglial dysjunction in human diabetic neuropathy. *J Clin Invest* 1988; **81**: 349–64.

32 Hale PJ, Nattrass M, Silverman SH, Sennit C, Perkins CM, Uden A, Sundkvist G. Peripheral nerve concentrations of glucose, fructose, sorbitol and myoinositol in diabetic and non-diabetic patients. *Diabetologia* 1987; **30**: 464–7.

33 Dyck PJ, Zimmerman BR, Vilen TH, Minnerath SR, Karnes JL, Yao JK, Poduslo JF. Nerve glucose, fructose, sorbitol, myo-inositol, and fiber degeneration and regeneration in diabetic neuropathy. *N Engl Med* 1988; **319**: 542–8.

34 Lambourne JE, Tomlinson DR, Brown AM, Willars GB. Opposite effects of diabetes and galactosaemia on adenosine triphosphatase activity in rat nervous tissue. *Diabetologia* 1987; **30**: 360–2.

35 Sidenius P, Jakobsen J. Axonal transport in human and experimental diabetes. In: Dyck PJ, Thomas PK, Asbury AK, Winegrad AI, Porte D Jr, eds. *Diabetic Neuropathy*. Philadelphia: WB Saunders, 1987: 260–5.

36 Williams SK, Howarth NL, Devenny JJ, Bitensky MW. Structural and functional consequences of increased tubulin glycosylation in diabetes mellitus. *Proc Natl Acad Sci USA* 1982; **79**: 6546–50.

37 Brownlee M, Cerami M, Vlassara H. Advanced glycosylation end products in tissue and the biochemical basis of diabetic complications. *N Engl J Med* 1988; **318**: 1315–21.

38 Sugimura K, Dyck PJ. Multifocal fiber loss in proximal sciatic nerve in symmetric distal diabetic neuropathy. *J*

*Neurol Sci* 1982; **53**: 501–9.

39 Dyck PJ, Karnes JL, O'Brien P, Okazaki H, Lais A, Engelstad J. The spatial distribution of fiber loss in diabetic polyneuropathy suggest ischemia. *Ann Neurol* 1986; **19**: 440–9.

40 Johnson PC, Doll SC, Cromer DW. Pathogenesis of diabetic neuropathy. *Ann Neurol* 1986; **19**: 450–7.

41 Dyck PJ, Lais A, Karnes JL, O'Brien P, Rizza R. Fiber loss is primary and multifocal in sural nerves in diabetic polyneuropathy. *Ann Neurol* 1986; **19**: 425–39.

42 Llewelyn JG, Thomas PK, Gilbey SG, Watkins PJ, Muddle JR. Pattern of myelinated fibre loss in the sural nerve in neuropathy related to Type 1 (insulin-dependent) diabetes. *Diabetologia* 1988; **31**: 162–7.

43 Newrick PG, Wilson AJ, Jakubowski J, Boulton AJM, Ward JD. Sural nerve oxygen tension in diabetes. *Br J Med* 1986; **293**: 1053–4.

44 Tuck RR, Schmelzer JD, Low PA. Endoneurial blood flow and oxygen tension in the sciatic nerves of rats with experimental diabetic neuropathy. *Brain* 1984; **107**: 935–50.

45 Llewelyn JG, Thomas PK, Fonseca V, King RHM, Dandona P. Acute painful diabetic neuropathy precipitated by strict glycaemic control. *Acta Neuropathol (Berl)* 1986; **72**: 157–63.

46 Jakobsen J, Christiansen JS, Kristoffersen I, Christensen CK, Hermansen K, Schmitz A, Mogensen CE. Autonomic and somatosensory nerve function after 2 years of continuous subcutaneous insulin infusion in Type I diabetes. *Diabetes* 1988; **37**: 452–5.

47 Fraser DM, Campbell IW, Ewing DJ, Murray J, Neilson JMM, Clarke BF. Peripheral and autonomic nerve function in newly diagnosed diabetes. *Diabetes* 1977; **26**: 546–50.

48 Pfeifer MA, Cook D, Brodsky J, Tice D, Reenan A, Swedine S, Halter JB, Porte D Jr. Quantitative evaluation of cardiac parasympathetic activity in normal and diabetic man. *Diabetes* 1982; **31**: 339–45.

49 Ewing DJ, Campbell IW, Clarke BF. The natural history of diabetic autonomic neuropathy. *Q J Med* 1980; **193**: 95–108.

50 Casey EB, Harrison MJG. Diabetic amyotrophy: a follow-up study. *Br J Med* 1972; **1**: 656–9.

51 Young MS, Boulton AJM, McLeod AF, Williams DDR, Sönksen PH. A multicentre study of the prevalence of diabetic peripheral neuropathy in the UK hospital clinic population. *Diabetologia* 1993; **36**: 150–4.

52 DCCT Research Group. Factors in development of diabetic neuropathy. Baseline analysis of neuropathy in feasibility phase of diabetes control and complications trial (DCCT). *Diabetologia* 1988; **37**: 476–3.

53 Kennedy WR, Navarro X, Goetz FC, Sutherland DE, Najarian JS. Effects of pancreatic transplantation on diabetic neuropathy. *N Eng J Med* 1990; **323**: 1031–7.

54 Jakobsen J, Christiansen JS, Kristoffersen I, Christensen CK, Hermansen K, Schmitz A, Mogensen CE. Autonomic and somatosensory nerve function after 2 years of continuous subcutaneous insulin infusion in type 1 diabetes. *Diabetes* 1988; **37**: 452–5.

55 Dyck PJ, Zimmerman BR, Vilen TH, Minnerath SR, Karnes JL, Yao JK, Poduslo JF. Nerve glucose, fructose, sorbitol, myo-inositol, and fiber degeneration and regeneration in diabetic neuropathy. *N Engl J Med* 1988; **319**: 542–8.

56 Sima AAF, Bril V, Nathaniel V, McEwen TAJ, Brown MB, Lattimer SA, Greene DA. Regeneration and repair of myelinated fibers in sural-nerve biopsy specimens from patients with diabetic neuropathy treated with sorbinil. *N Engl J Med* 1988; **319**: 548–55.

57 Horrobin DF, Carmichael HA. Essential fatty acids in relation to diabetes. In: Horrobin DF, ed. *Treatment of Diabetic Neuropathy. A New Approach*. Edinburgh, Churchill Livingstone, 1992, pp. 21–39.

58 Tomlinson DR, Robinson JP, Compton AM, Keen P. Essential fatty acid treatment-effects on nerve conduction, polyol pathway and axonal transport in streptozotocin diabetic rats. *Diabetologia* 1989; **32**: 655–9.

59 Jamal GA, Carmichael H. The effect of gamma-linolenic acid on human diabetic peripheral neuropathy: a double-blind, placebo-controlled trial. *Diabetic Medicine* 1990; **7**: 319–23.

60 Ziegler D, Mayer P, Mühlen H, Gries FA. The natural history of somatosensory and autonomic nerve function in relation to glycaemic control during the first 5 years after diagnosis of Type 1 (insulin-dependent) diabetes mellitus. *Diabetologia* 1991; **34**: 822–9.

61 Watkins PJ. Natural history of the diabetic neuropathies. *Q J Med* 1990; **77**: 1208–9.

62 Sampson MJ, Wilson S, Karagianis P, Edmunds M, Watkins PJ. Progression of diabetic autonomic neuropathy over a decade in insulin-dependent diabetics. *Q J Med* 1990; **75**: 635–46.

63 Ewing DJ, Campbell IW, Clarke BF. The natural history of diabetic autonomic neuropathy. *Q J Med* 1980; **49**: 95–100.

# 11 Clinical Aspects of Diabetic Somatic Neuropathy

**Summary**

• Diabetic peripheral neuropathy may present as several syndromes which often overlap.

• *Chronic insidious sensory neuropathy* causes progressive development of unpleasant sensations, often with pain, in the legs and feet. Muscle wasting and autonomic dysfunction are commonly associated. This form is common and usually unrelated to glycaemic control.

• *Acute painful neuropathy* and *diabetic amyotrophy* both cause sudden-onset pain in thighs and/or legs, usually unilateral in amyotrophy, associated with severe muscle wasting and occasionally profound weight loss; there is little objective sensory loss. These often begin during a period of hyperglycaemia and may improve with strict control.

• *Diffuse motor neuropathy* presents as severe, generalized muscle wasting and weakness, usually without pain or sensory loss. It commonly affects older NIDDM patients; recovery is usually poor.

• *Focal neuropathies* are probably due to *pressure damage* (especially the carpal tunnel syndrome, which usually responds poorly to surgical decompression) or *vascular damage* (e.g. third nerve palsy, which is often painful, sometimes associated with hyperglycaemia and may recover with improved control).

• Other coexistent and potentially treatable causes of peripheral neuropathy must always be excluded.

• Peripheral nerve function can be assessed adequately by routine physical examination. Specialized tests for diagnostic difficulties and research applications include electrophysiological measurements of sensory and motor nerve conduction, determinations of vibration and thermal discrimination thresholds, and sural nerve biopsy.

• Painful symptoms in diabetic neuropathy may respond to improved glycaemic control, simple analgesia and tricyclic drugs; other agents (e.g. phenytoin, carbamazepine, mexiletine) are sometimes effective.

Clinical experience suggests that about 10% of insulin-treated diabetic patients have symptoms of peripheral neuropathy and that a further 10% also show obviously abnormal physical signs [1]. As well as being common, peripheral nerve damage is important because of its major contribution to the problems of the diabetic foot (see Chapter 19) and male impotence (Chapter 25).

## Clinical presentations of diabetic neuropathy

Diabetic peripheral neuropathy has been subdivided on simple topographical grounds [2] into *symmetrical polyneuropathy* (comprising sensory, motor or combined forms) and *focal and multifocal neuropathies* (including damage to cranial, limb or trunk nerves, and proximal motor neuropathy) (see Chapter 10). In clinical terms, however, it is useful to describe the various ways in which neuropathic syndromes may present. Most patients with neuropathy have the symmetrical sensorimotor form with autonomic features, but several other syndromes and mixed patterns occur, firmly indicating that many aetiological factors must contribute to human diabetic neuropathy. Despite their classification as predominantly 'sensory' or 'motor' neuropathies, it will be appreciated from the descriptions below that many patients show evidence of sensory, motor and autonomic involvement. The major clinical presentations, summarized in Fig. 11.1, are:

1 Chronic insidious sensory neuropathy.
2 Acute painful neuropathy.
3 Proximal motor neuropathy.
4 Diffuse motor neuropathy.
5 Pressure neuropathies.
6 Focal vascular neuropathies.

### *Chronic insidious sensory neuropathy*

This is the commonest syndrome. The patient describes a slow, progressive build-up of unpleasant sensations consisting of tingling, burning, cramps and frank pain, often dramatically described as 'shooting', 'tearing' or 'excruciating'. Hyperaesthesia is common, and contact with clothing or bedclothes may cause great discomfort. The legs and feet are mainly affected; intriguingly, similar symptoms are very unusual in the arms and hands. For unknown reasons, all symptoms are much worse at night and often prevent sleep. This form of neuropathy usually develops gradually, with no clear-cut association with hyperglycaemia, and symptoms often persist after glycaemic control has been improved. Most sufferers report no improvement in symptoms 5 years after onset [3]. Understandably, depression often aggravates the situation.

Clinical examination reveals patchy sensory loss, predominantly distal ('stocking' and sometimes also 'glove' distribution), and affecting all modalities. Vibration sensation is usually markedly reduced, and proprioception may be so impaired as to cause Romberg's sign. Ankle and knee tendon reflexes are usually reduced or absent. Many patients show significant generalized muscular wasting, particularly of the small muscles of the hand, with variable degrees of weakness. Cardiovascular and other autonomic function tests (see Chapter 12) are frequently abnormal in these patients, and many males will also be impotent. Other features, attributable largely to sensory loss with or without associated autonomic damage, include neuropathic ulceration of the feet and Charcot arthropathy (Chapter 19).

### *Acute painful neuropathy*

This is a relatively uncommon presentation which is probably a variant of proximal motor neuropathy (see below). Severe pain appears suddenly, usually in the thighs, legs and feet, and has a particularly excruciating and distressing quality. Marked muscle wasting and weakness develop rapidly, often accompanied by weight loss ('neuropathic cachexia') and depression. Surprisingly, knee and ankle tendon reflexes may be preserved in some patients and there is often only little objective sensory deficit to be demonstrated. Certain subjects have very warm legs (with skin temperature sometimes approaching core temperature (Fig. 11.3)) and distended veins (Fig. 11.2), suggesting arterio-venous shunting of blood as has been described in the numb neuropathic foot ([5]; see Chapter 19).

This acute syndrome usually occurs in association with hyperglycaemia and improved control will result in symptomatic recovery in many cases, generally within a year or so. Rapidly developing pain is more likely to resolve than that which develops progressively over several months [6]. Acute painful neuropathy, with or without sensory loss, may also occasionally be precipitated by a sudden improvement in glycaemic control, which is usually the result of starting insulin treatment. It may last for some weeks or months and in most cases resolves spontaneously.

### *Proximal motor myopathy (amyotrophy)*

Garland [7] described *diabetic amyotrophy* as the sudden onset of severe pain in one thigh, accompanied by profound wasting of the quadriceps muscles, usually during a period of marked hyperglycaemia. Other leg muscles, especially the anterior tibial and peroneal muscles, may be involved, and the condition may be bilateral (Fig. 11.4). The tendon reflexes of affected muscles are reduced. An unexplained feature is the extensor plantar reflexes displayed by a few patients. Despite the prominence of pain, objective evidence of sensory loss is only rarely found.

The cause of proximal motor myopathy is unknown. The condition was previously regarded as a femoral neuropathy or radiculopathy, which is suggested by the focal, unilateral onset in many patients. However, the bilateral involvement in some cases argues against this, and many subjects show significant features of widespread neuropathy. The combination of focal features superimposed on a diffuse neuropathy may suggest a vascular event complicating generalized biochemical nerve damage.

| Syndrome | Chronic insidious sensory neuropathy | Acute painful neuropathy | Proximal motor myopathy | Diffuse motor neuropathy | Focal nerve palsies | |
|---|---|---|---|---|---|---|
| Pattern | 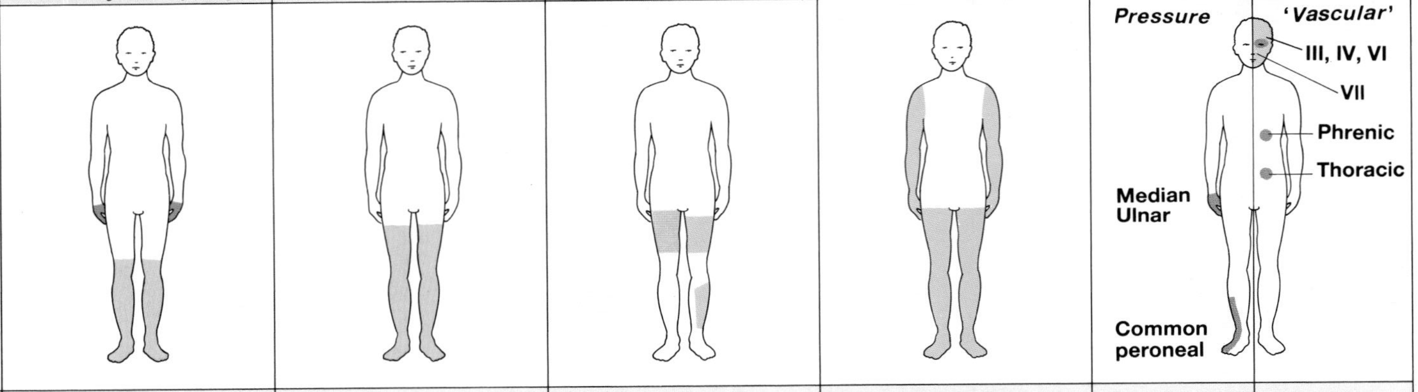 | | | | *Pressure*<br>Median<br>Ulnar<br>Common peroneal | *'Vascular'*<br>III, IV, VI<br>VII<br>Phrenic<br>Thoracic |
| Sensory loss | + → ++ | + | O | O → + | ++ | ++ |
| Pain | O → +++ | +++ | + → +++ | O | ++ | O → ++ |
| Tendon reflexes | ↓ | ↓ | ↓ | ↓ | + | + |
| Muscle wasting and weakness | O → ++ | + → ++ | +++ | ++ → +++ | + → ++ | O → ++ |
| Autonomic features | + → ++ | May be present | May be present | May be present | May be present | May be present |
| Prevalence and relationship to glycaemia | Common; usually unrelated to glycaemia | Relatively rare; onset often during hyperglycaemia | Relatively rare; onset often during hyperglycaemia | Relatively rare; generally unrelated to hyperglycaemia | Relatively rare; usually unrelated to hyperglycaemia | Relatively rare; sometimes related to hyperglycaemia |

**Fig. 11.1.** Clinical patterns of diabetic peripheral neuropathy.

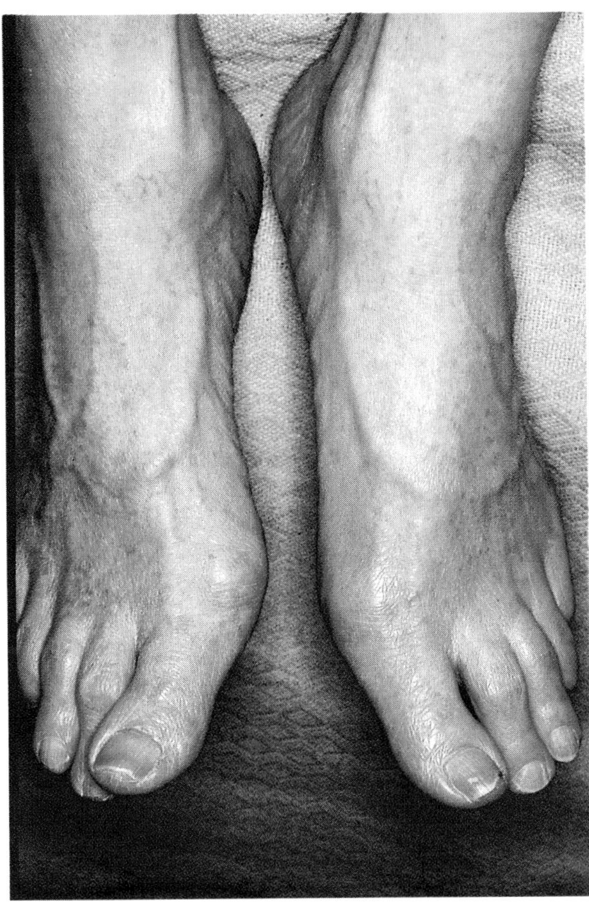

**Fig. 11.2.** Distended veins on the dorsum of the foot of a diabetic patient with painful peripheral neuropathy. (Reproduced by kind permission of Dr Geoff Gill, Walton Hospital, Liverpool.)

Many patients, but by no means all, recover spontaneously, especially after glycaemic control is improved; muscle wasting may persist and a few subjects become permanently disabled. In making the diagnosis, it is vitally important to exclude other causes of pain and muscle wasting in the legs — especially when the plantar responses are extensor — such as anterior disc protrusions or spinal tumours.

### *Diffuse motor neuropathy*

This is a condition of older patients, usually with NIDDM [8]. Over a 3–6 month period, severe generalized muscle wasting and weakness develop, often to an incapacitating degree, in the face of blood glucose and $HbA_1$ levels which are little above the non-diabetic range. Muscle wasting, often severe in the hands (Fig. 11.5), is accompanied by reduction or absence of reflexes and there is often some degree of sensory loss. Electrophysiological studies in these patients suggest diffuse nerve damage with significant focal involvement, perhaps indicating widespread vascular disease. Even with tightened glycaemic control, recovery is often poor. Rapidly progressing and severe generalized muscle wasting and weakness may occasionally be associated with hyperglycaemia, in which case there is usually a good response to insulin therapy.

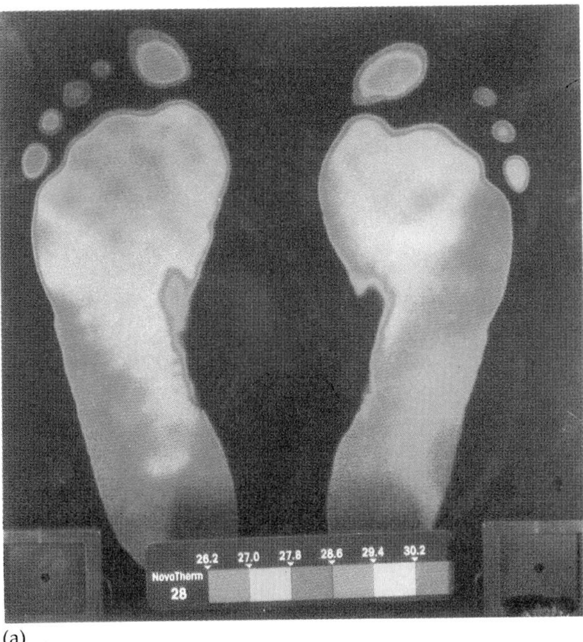


(a)

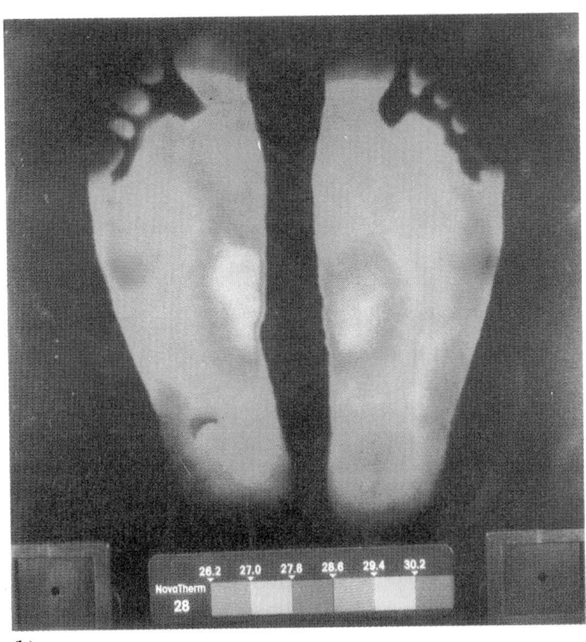


(b)

**Fig. 11.3.** Thermographs showing higher skin temperature in a diabetic patient with peripheral neuropathy (a) than in a non-diabetic subject (b). (Reproduced by kind permission of Dr Ah Wah Chan, Royal Liverpool Hospital.)

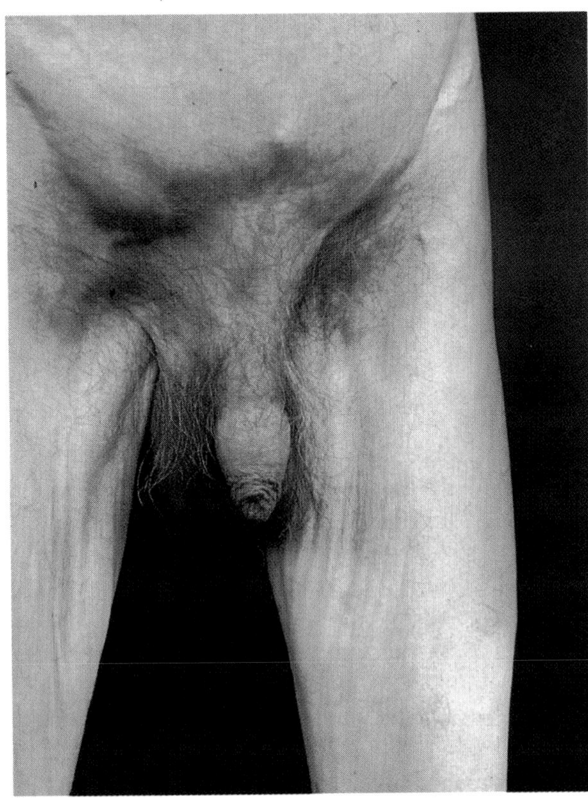

Fig. 11.4. Diabetic amyotrophy, showing marked wasting of both thighs.

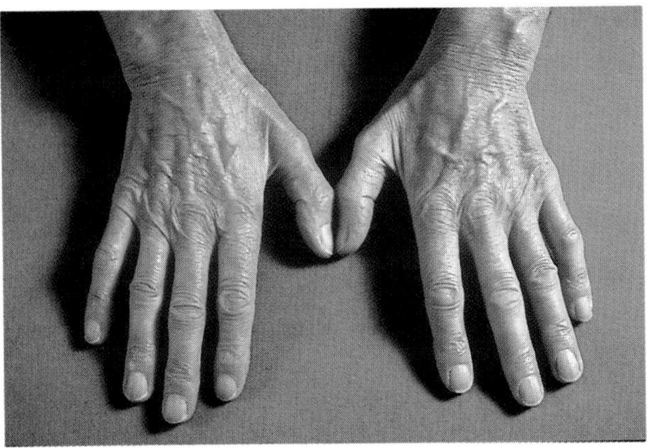

Fig. 11.5. Generalized wasting of small muscles of the hands due to diffuse motor neuropathy.

*Pressure neuropathies*

Diabetic nerves are particularly vulnerable to pressure damage. The commonest pressure palsy in diabetes involves the median nerve, producing a typical carpal tunnel syndrome. Characteristic symptoms include pain in the hands, which is worse at night and often radiates up the forearm. The hand may take up a stiffened posture, perhaps aggravated by the cheiroarthropathy of diabetes (Chapter 22), which can be mistakenly attributed to rheumatological disease. Surgical decompression is often performed to relieve the symptoms, but pain seems more likely to return in the diabetic patient than in the non-diabetic [9]. Other peripheral nerve palsies commonly seen in diabetic patients affect the ulnar and common peroneal nerves.

*Focal vascular neuropathies*

It is assumed that other focal lesions, where there is no reason to suspect pressure damage, are due to occlusion of intraneural vessels; indeed, one autopsy case supports this view [10]. Third cranial nerve palsy (Fig. 11.6) is by far the commonest and is usually accompanied by pain in the orbit, when other causes of painful third nerve palsies (aneurysm, tumour) must be considered in the differential diagnosis. However, the pupillary innervation is frequently unaffected in third nerve palsies due to diabetes, unlike those due to compression or invasion. This pupillary sparing may suggest that nerve damage is due to intraneural vascular occlusion [2]. Fourth, sixth and seventh cranial nerve palsies are well described in diabetic subjects and there are reports of intercostal and phrenic nerve lesions. These are all presumably of a similar aetiology, although pressure damage cannot be excluded.

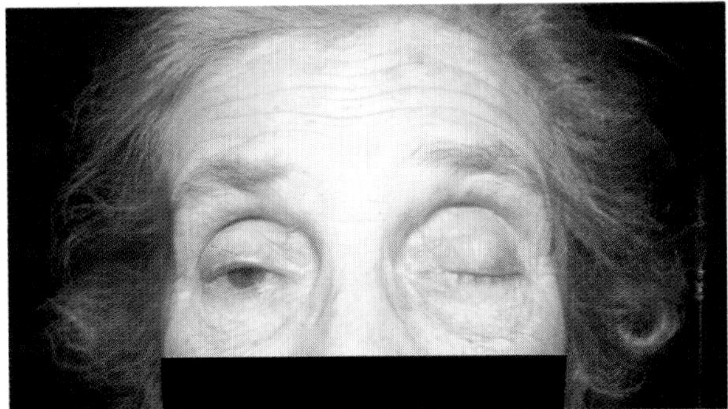

Fig. 11.6. Sudden onset of left ptosis (with diplopia) in a diabetic patient, due to third cranial nerve palsy. The patient complained of pain in the left orbit, and the left pupillary reactions were intact; pain and pupillary sparing are typical features of a third nerve palsy in diabetes.

### Assessment of nerve function

Clinical examination alone is usually adequate to assess a diabetic patient suspected of having neuropathy. An outline of the relevant tests is shown in Table 11.1. Certain specialized tests of nerve function may help to resolve difficult diagnostic problems, but it must be remembered that asymptomatic patients may have considerable functional impairment, and that results in an individual patient may be misleading. Quantitative tests of nerve function, which are essential in research applications, include electrophysiological measurements, determinations of vibration perception threshold and thermal discrimination threshold, and sural nerve biopsy.

#### *Electrophysiological measurements*

These investigations should preferably be performed by a specialist neurophysiologist. Measurement of motor and sensory conduction velocity are the most commonly used but only assess myelinated fibres which constitute about 25% of peripheral fibres. Conduction velocity is related to the ambient blood glucose at the time of testing, tending to improve as glycaemia improves [11, 12], and shows various abnormalities even in people without a distinct clinical problem. However, the tests do correlate in groups of patients with the presence of clinical neuropathy [13]. More sophisticated measurements include evoked sensory action potentials (which provide a measure of fibre number), and the Hoffman reflex and F-wave responses to assess the total sensorimotor arc [14]. The real significance of impaired conduction velocity is not yet known; for example, a similar improvement (3 m/s) in conduction velocity following improved glycaemic control has been observed in newly diagnosed patients *without* neuropathy as in a group of patients with chronic, unremitting, painful neuropathy treated with continuous subcutaneous insulin infusion (CSII) [15]. It is possible that part of the alteration in conduction velocity relates simply to the fluid and electrolyte content of the nerve at the time of measurement.

#### *Vibration perception threshold (VPT)*

This is a quantitative measure of large-fibre function using an electromechanical device which causes a tactor to vibrate at fixed frequency but variable amplitude [16]. A Biothesiometer or Somedic Vibrameter may be used, the latter standardizing the pressure with which the tactor is applied to the test site [17]. These devices are obviously superior to the traditional tuning-fork and results are reasonably reproducible, although there may be considerable and unpredictable variation between different sites, and between different times at a given site, in the same individual [18, 19]. Measurements are usually made on the tip of the big toe, the medial malleolus and on one finger, and values must be related to both site and the patient's age, as VPT increases significantly with age [16, 18, 20]. This very simple test is probably of use in epidemiological studies or large clinical studies but it remains to be seen whether it is sensitive enough for long-term prospective studies.

Since it has been demonstrated that significant impairment of VPT correlates with points of high pressure in the diabetic foot, which itself predisposes to ulcer formation, it has been suggested that VPT could be used to screen for subjects vulnerable to foot ulceration [21]. The measurement of VPT requires the shoes and socks to be removed, which in itself may be the most important act in screening for those at risk from foot ulcers.

#### *Temperature discrimination threshold (TDT)*

This index of small-fibre function can be measured by several different instruments, based on the Peltier thermocouple whose temperature rises or falls depending on the direction of the electrical current flowing through it [22]. Using a forced-choice technique, the patient responds to a rise or fall in the temperature of the thermocouple plate, which is altered in a random manner. This is more time-consuming than assessment of vibration sensitivity, but also seems to be a more sensitive measure as it is abnormal in many patients with normal VPT who may be at an earlier stage in the natural history of neuropathy [23].

#### *Sural nerve biopsy*

This is the ultimate test to assess changes in structure and composition of nerves. Histological examination can document features such as axonal loss, demyelination and the state of the microvasculature, and biochemical analyses can be performed [24, 25]. However, it rarely has a place in

**Table 11.1.** Assessment of peripheral nerve function.

| | Pathway | Modality | Clinical screen | Specialized tests | Comments |
|---|---|---|---|---|---|
| Sensory | Dorsal columns | Vibration | Tuning fork | VPT (Biothesiometer) | Tuning fork unreliable; VPT varies with age and site and may be poorly reproducible |
| | | Proprioception | Joint position, Romberg test | — | — |
| | | Light touch | Cotton wool | von Frey hairs | von Frey hairs still a research procedure and not widely available |
| | Spinothalamic | Temperature | — | TDT (Marstock thermode) | May be more sensitive than VPT; time-consuming |
| | | Pain | Pin-prick, deep pressure | Spring-loaded calipers to pinch skin; thermal pain threshold | Pain thresholds difficult to quantitate and poorly reproducible |
| | Single nerves | — | — | Electrophysiological measurements of sensory conduction velocity and action potential | Abnormalities early and common; include reduced conduction velocity and reduced amplitude with spreading of sensory action potential |
| Tendon reflexes | — | — | Ankles, knees (± reinforcement) | — | Ankle jerks often lost, but may be reduced or absent in elderly |
| Motor | — | — | Bulk, tone, power of limb muscles | — | Wasting of small hand muscles common in neuropathy, often with minimal weakness |
| | — | — | — | Electrophysiological measurements of motor conduction velocity | Motor nerve conduction velocity markedly reduced in clinical neuropathy, especially mixed forms |

VPT, vibration perception threshold; TDT, thermal discrimination threshold.

clinical management and should be reserved for carefully planned research projects.

### Staging of diabetic neuropathy

In routine clinical practice, it is quite sufficient to diagnose diabetic neuropathy and specify which neuropathic syndrome is present. However, if prospective studies of natural history or therapeutic intervention are to be carried out, it is essential to have some agreement as to the grade of neuropathy at the time of study. Most studies have wisely focused on the commonest neuropathy (chronic sensorimotor), and have avoided the acute syndromes which have a great potential for spontaneous fluctuation and recovery. It is now known that there is very reasonable correlation between symptoms and signs and functional neurophysiological investigations, although no single symptom or test is indicative of neuropathy in one individual. In a research setting, therefore, it is essential to perform electrophysiological tests on at least two nerves, as well as measurements of VPT and TDT. Assessment should also include a range of autonomic function tests (Chapter 12) and a very detailed quantitative assessment of symptoms and physical signs. Using this approach, P.J. Dyck [26] has proposed the following staging system:

0 — *No neuropathy*: No symptoms and fewer than two abnormalities of testing (including autonomic tests).

1 — *Asymptomatic neuropathy*: No symptoms but two or more abnormalities of functional testing.

2 — *Symptomatic neuropathy*: Symptoms of a lesser degree with two or more functional abnormalities.

3 — *Disabling neuropathy*: Disabling symptoms and two or more functional abnormalities.

Attempts such as this to standardize scores of both symptoms and neurophysiological measures should make it possible in the future to compare results between various studies.

### A diagnostic approach to the diabetic leg

Pain, discomfort or weakness in the legs of the diabetic patient are not necessarily due to peripheral diabetic neuropathy. Other forms of neuropathy should be considered, e.g. uraemia, nutritional deficiency, carcinoma, collagen–vascular diseases, amyloidosis and hereditary (see Fig. 11.7) and toxic neuropathies. Special consideration should be given to the role of alcohol, which despite conflicting evidence as to whether it is more commonly used by patients with diabetic neuropathy, probably plays a significant part in some clinical syndromes.

Intrinsic or extrinsic spinal cord disease (e.g. cauda equina tumour, spinal stenosis, anterior lumbar disc lesions) will occasionally present with pain and wasting in proximal leg muscles and may be confused particularly with diabetic amyotrophy.

The major diagnostic difficulty, however, is to evaluate the importance of peripheral vascular disease, which is commonly present in older patients. Clinical assessment of pulses in the legs and feet may be supplemented by the use of the Doppler ultrasound stethoscope to calculate the ankle pressure index (see Chapter 19) [27]. There is some evidence that the arterio-venous shunting

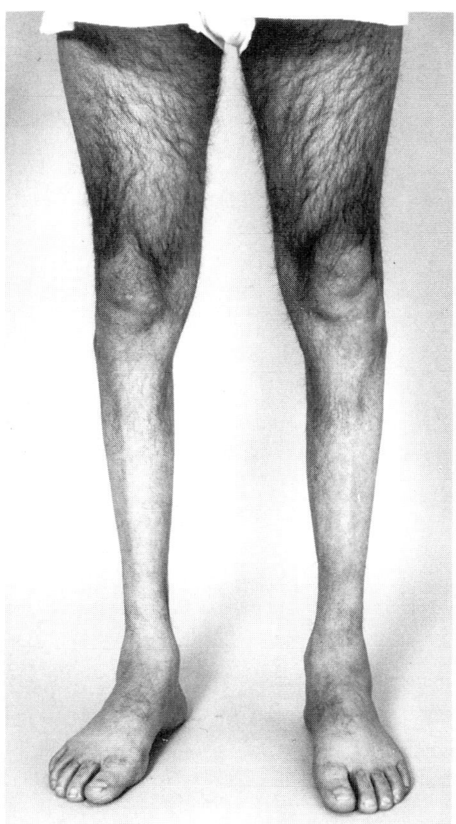

**Fig. 11.7.** Extreme muscular weakness with wasting in a 38-year-old man with diabetes for 11 years. Sensory loss was minimal and pain was absent. The 'inverted champagne bottle' pattern of wasting suggested the diagnosis of hereditary motor and sensory neuropathy Type 1 (Charcot–Marie–Tooth disease), which was confirmed by electrophysiological measurements.

seen in diabetic neuropathy may also cause discomfort, as the increased skin temperature and blood flow can be reversed by arterial occlusion, which surprisingly sometimes also relieves pain [5].

A good history may be diagnostic, especially if coupled with the characteristic physical signs described above. A totally anaesthetic foot may not cause complaint, but will show typical signs on examination. It is of interest that the totally numb neuropathic foot may also be the source of unpleasant tingling and burning sensations — the so-called 'painful–painless' foot.

## Management of diabetic neuropathy

The main indication for intervention in neuropathy is pain and other troublesome sensory symptoms. A suggested management scheme is outlined in Fig. 11.8.

As mentioned above, it is first essential to exclude other coexistent conditions which are potentially treatable. The next step is to try to achieve the best glycaemic control possible. Many neuropathic syndromes are related to hyperglycaemia and will improve, often rapidly, following tightened glycaemic control. There has been

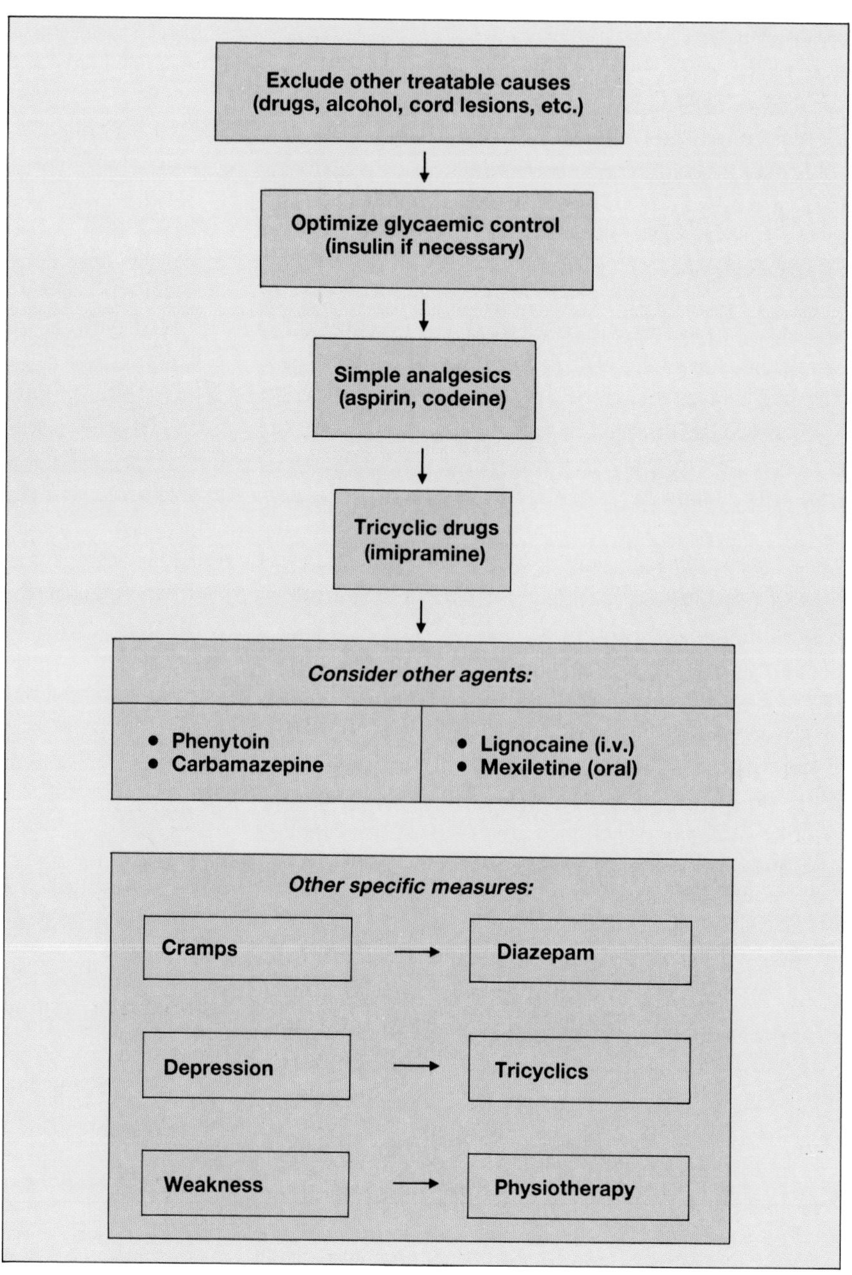


**Fig. 11.8.** Management of painful diabetic neuropathy.

controversy regarding the possible effects of the blood glucose concentration on pain perception: an initial report that the pain threshold was lower in non-diabetic subjects during glucose infusion [28] has been contradicted by a recent study [29].

Specific drug treatment should begin with simple analgesics (e.g. aspirin, codeine phosphate), with diazepam or quinine sulphate for troublesome muscle cramps. If there is no improvement after a few weeks of these general measures, a tricyclic drug such as imipramine should be used. These drugs do not apparently act centrally in this situation but probably are effective by modulating the activity of nociceptive C fibres and their receptors. None the less, depression accompanies any chronic painful condition, and their antidepressant effects may also contribute. The dosage range of 50–125 mg daily may induce drowsiness and in controlled trials, the addition of fluphenazine has been helpful [30–33]. Improvement, if it occurs, is usually seen within the first week or so. Sympathetic support of such patients is an important part of their management.

The use of local anaesthetic agents seems a logical way to approach discomfort due to peripheral nerve disease. Intravenous infusion of lignocaine is very effective in providing relief of symptoms which often persist for a period after withdrawal of the infusion [34]. Oral administration of a lignocaine analogue, mexiletine (200 mg thrice daily) has also been shown to be effective in double-blind clinical trials [35].

Other sedative agents have been variously reported to be of benefit and should be considered if improved blood glucose control, simple analgesics, tricyclics or mexiletine fail. Those with the best record of success (albeit with many failures) include phenytoin (200–300 mg daily) and carbamazepine (200 mg thrice daily). Motor symptoms are generally less troublesome in diabetic neuropathy, but physiotherapy and specific mechanical aids (such as ankle calipers or a toe spring for foot-drop) may be helpful in individual cases.

A number of other approaches may hold some hope for future therapy. Gangliosides — a complex of sialoglycolipids, found in high concentration in nervous tissue — are initiators of dendritogenesis and may stimulate nerve regeneration when administered after nerve damage. A few clinical trials have reported improvement in electrophysiological parameters and some symptomatic relief [36].

Aldose reductase inhibitors (ARI) are also currently under study. By preventing the vicious circle of sorbitol accumulation, myoinositol depletion and depression of $Na^+-K^+-$ATPase (see Chapter 10), these agents have immense theoretical potential, and in animal models, their use has been associated with improvements in both biochemical abnormalities and in structural and electrophysiological indices of nerve damage [37–39]. However, final proof of their possible efficacy in clinically significant diabetic neuropathy in man is not yet available. Of the several trials carried out in diabetic patients with symptomatic neuropathy [40–42], only one uncontrolled study [40] claimed to find any useful symptomatic improvement. There has been no consistent effect on various objective measurements of peripheral nerve function, in either symptomatic [40–42] or asymptomatic [43] patients, although improvements in certain electrophysiological indices and morphometric features in sural nerve biopsies have recently been reported following 12 months' treatment with sorbinil [44]. Supplementation of myoinositol is also ineffective [45]. The stage at which these agents (or others aiming to influence structure or function) are administered may be crucial. In symptomatic neuropathy, axon fall-out, demyelination and hypoxia of the nerve are already considerable (Chapter 10) and it may be too late to use agents which modify fundamental biochemical processes. The potential usefulness of these drugs may be to prevent nerve damage, and they will probably have most benefit when given at a much earlier stage in the natural history of nerve disease. Unfortunately, the 7–10 year prospective studies which will be necessary to prove efficacy pose obvious economic and organizational problems.

Supplementation of the diet of diabetic subjects with γ-linolenic acid has been shown to improve nerve conduction, perhaps by normalizing the metabolism of the long-chain essential fatty acids derived from linoleic acid [46]. However, no extensive clinical studies have yet been carried out with regard to symptoms.

### Prevention of diabetic neuropathy

The role of blood glucose control in preventing neuropathy must be stressed, although in many instances there is no clear-cut relationship between neuropathic manifestations and the degree of hyperglycaemia at the time of onset. Numerous studies have shown amelioration of various electrophysiological measures following improvement in glycaemia. In the Oslo study, the use of CSII to optimize blood glucose control resulted in better conduction velocities over a 3-year period [47], and a recent preliminary report found VPT to be lower in well-controlled than in poorly controlled young diabetic subjects [48]. In another group of adolescent diabetic subjects, impairment of motor conduction velocity at entry to the study was shown to predict the development of neuropathic symptoms 5 years later and that these subjects had higher glycosylated haemoglobin levels [49]. All this evidence, as with other complications of diabetes, obliges clinicians to help their patients to achieve the best possible blood glucose control at all times.

JOHN D. WARD

## References


1 Boulton AJM, Knight J, Drury J, Ward JD. The prevalence of symptomatic diabetic neuropathy in an insulin-treated population. *Diabetes Care* 1985; **8**: 125–8.

2 Thomas PK, Ward JD, Watkins PJ. Diabetic neuropathy. In: Keen H, Jarrett J, eds. *Complications of Diabetes*, 2nd edn. London: Edward Arnold, 1982: 109–36.

3 Boulton AJM, Armstrong WD, Scarpello JHB, Ward JD. The natural history of painful diabetic neuropathy — a 4-year study. *Postgrad Med J* 1983; **59**: 556–9.

4 Archer AG, Watkins PJ, Thomas PK, Sharma AK, Payan J. The natural history of acute painful neuropathy in diabetes mellitus. *J Neurol Neurosurg Psychiatr* 1983; **46**: 491–6.

5 Archer AG, Roberts VC, Watkins PJ. Blood flow patterns in painful diabetic neuropathy. *Diabetologia* 1984; **27**: 563–7.

6 Young RJ, Ewing DJ, Clarke BF. Chronic remitting painful diabetic polyneuropathy. *Diabetes Care* 1988; **11**: 34–40.

7 Garland H. Diabetic amyotrophy. *Br Med J* 1955; **2**: 1287–90.

8 Timperley WR, Boulton AJM, Davies-Jones GAB, Jarratt JA, Ward JD. Small vessel disease in progressive diabetic neuropathy associated with good metabolic control. *J Clin Pathol* 1985; **38**: 1030–8.

9 Clayburgh RH, Beckenbaugh RD, Dobyns JH. Carpal tunnel release in patients with diffuse peripheral neuropathy. *J Hand Surg* 1987; **12A**: 380–3.

10 Asbury AK, Aldredge H, Herschberg R, Fisher CM. Oculomotor palsy in diabetes mellitus: a clinicopathological study. *Brain* 1970; **93**: 555–7.

11 Gregerson G. Diabetic neuropathy: Influence of age, sex, metabolic control and duration of diabetes on motor conduction velocity. *Neurology* 1967; **17**: 972–6.

12 Service FJ, Rizza RA, Daube JR, O'Brien PC, Dyck PJ. Near normoglycaemia improved nerve conduction and vibration sensation in diabetic neuropathy. *Diabetologia* 1985; **28**: 722–7.

13 Dyck PJ, Karnes J, O'Brien PC. Diagnosis, staging and classification of diabetic neuropathy and associations with other complications. In: Dyck PJ, Thomas PK, Asbury AK, Winegrad AA, Porte D Jr, eds. *Diabetic Neuropathy*. Philadelphia: WB Saunders Co., 1987: 37–44.

14 Jarratt JA. The electrophysiological diagnosis of peripheral neuropathy. A brief review. *Bull Eur Physiopathol Res* 1987; **23** (suppl 11): 195–8.

15 Boulton AJM, Drury J, Clarke B, Ward JD. Continuous subcutaneous insulin infusion in the management of painful diabetic neuropathy. *Diabetes Care* 1982; **5**: 386–90.

16 Steiness IB. Vibratory perception in normal subjects. A biothesiometric study. *Acta Med Scand* 1957; **158**: 315–25.

17 Lowenthal LM, Hockaday TDR. Vibration sensory thresholds depend on pressure of applied stimulus. *Diabetes Care* 1987; **10**: 100–4.

18 Bertelsmann FW, Heimans JJ, van Rooy JC, Heine RJ, van der Veen EA. Reproducibility of vibratory perception thresholds in patients with diabetic neuropathy. *Diabetes Res* 1986; **3**: 463–6.

19 Fagius J, Wahren LK. Variability of sensory threshold determination in clinical use. *J Neurol Sci* 1981; **51**: 11–27.

20 Bloom S, Till S, Sönksen PH, Smith S. Use of a biothesiometer to measure individual vibration thresholds and their variation in 519 non-diabetic subjects. *Br Med J* 1984; **288**: 1793–5.

21 Boulton AJM, Hardisty CA, Betts RP, Franks CI, Worth RC, Ward JD, Duckworth T. Dynamic foot pressure and other studies as diagnostic and management aids in diabetic neuropathy. *Diabetes Care* 1983; **6**: 26–32.

22 Fowler CF, Carroll MB, Burns D, Howe N, Robinson K. A portable system for measuring cutaneous thresholds for warming and cooling. *J Neurol Neurosurg Psychiatr* 1987; **50**: 1211–15.

23 Guy RJC, Clark CA, Malcolm PN, Watkins PJ. Evaluation of thermal and vibration sensation in diabetic neuropathy. *Diabetologia* 1985; **28**: 131–7.

24 Dyck PJ, Sherman WR, Hallcher LM. Human diabetic endoneurial sorbitol, fructose and *myo*-inositol related to sural nerve morphometry. *Ann Neurol* 1980; **8**: 590–4.

25 Dyck PJ, Zimmerman BR, Vilen TH *et al*. Nerve glucose, fructose, sorbitol, *myo*-inositol, and fiber degeneration and regeneration in diabetic neuropathy. *N Engl J Med* 1988; **319**: 542–8.

26 Dyck PJ. Detection, characterization, and staging of polyneuropathy: Assessed in diabetics. *Muscle Nerve* 1988; **11**: 21–31.

27 Yao JST, Hobbs JT, Irvine WT. Ankle systolic pressure measurement in arterial disease affecting the lower extremities. *Br J Surg* 1969; **56**: 676–8.

28 Morley GK, Mooradian MD, Levine AL, Morley JE. Mechanisms of pain in diabetic peripheral neuropathy: effect of glucose on pain perception in humans. *Am J Med* 1984; **77**: 79–82.

29 Chan AW, MacFarlane IA, Bowsher DR *et al*. Does acute hyperglycaemia influence heat pain thresholds? *J Neurol Neurosurg Psychiatr* 1988; **51**: 688–90.

30 Kvinesdal BB, Molin J, Frøland A, Gram LF. Imipramine treatment of painful diabetic neuropathy. *J Am Med Ass* 1984; **251**: 1727–30.

31 Davis JL, Lewis SB, Gerich JE, Kaplan AR, Schultz TA, Wallin JD. Peripheral diabetic neuropathy treated with amitriptyline and fluphenazine. *J Am Med Ass* 1977; **238**: 2291–2.

32 Young RJ, Clarke BF. Pain relief in diabetic neuropathy: the effectiveness of imipramine and related drugs. *Diabetic Med* 1985; **2**: 363–6.

33 Gomez-Perez FJ, Rull JA, Dies H *et al*. Nortriptyline and fluphenazine in the symptomatic treatment of diabetic neuropathy. A double-blind cross-over study. *Pain* 1985; **23**: 395–400.

34 Kastrup J, Peterson P, Dejgård J, Hilsted J, Angelo HR. Treatment of chronic painful diabetic neuropathy with intravenous lidocaine infusion. *Br Med J* 1986; **292**: 173–6.

35 Dejgård J, Peterson P, Kastrup J. Mexiletine for treatment of painful diabetic neuropathy. *Lancet* 1987; **i**: 9–11.

36 Crepaldi G, Fedele D, Tiengo A *et al*. Ganglioside treatment in diabetic peripheral neuropathy. *Acta Diabetol Lat* 1983; **20**: 265–76.

37 Mayer JH, Tomlinson DR. Prevention of defects of axonal transport and nerve conduction velocity by oral administration of *myo*-inositol or an aldose reductase inhibitor in streptozotocin-diabetic rats. *Diabetologia* 1983; **25**: 433–8.

38 Greene DA, Lattimer SA. Action of sorbinil in diabetic peripheral nerve. Relationship of polyol (sorbitol) pathway inhibition to a *myo*-inositol-mediated defect in sodium–potassium ATPase activity. *Diabetes* 1984; **33**: 712–16.

39 Tomlinson DR, Townsend J, Fretten P. Prevention of defective axonal transport in streptozocin-diabetic rats by treatment with 'Statil' (ICI 128436), an aldose reductase inhibitor. *Diabetes* 1985; **34**: 970–2.

40 Jaspan J, Maselli R, Herold K, Bartkus C. Treatment of severely painful diabetic neuropathy with an aldose reductase inhibitor: relief of pain and improved somatic and autonomic nerve function. *Lancet* 1983; **ii**: 758–62.

41 Young RJ, Ewing DJ, Clarke BF. A controlled trial of sorbinil, an aldose reductase inhibitor, in chronic painful diabetic neuropathy. *Diabetes* 1983; **32**: 938–42.

42 Pitts NE, Vreeland F, Shaw GL *et al*. Clinical experience with sorbinil — an aldose reductase inhibitor. *Metabolism* **35** (suppl 1): 96–100.

43 Martyn CN, Reid W, Young RJ, Ewing DJ, Clarke BF. Six-month treatment with sorbinil in asymptomatic diabetic neuropathy. Failure to improve abnormal nerve function. *Diabetes* 1987; **36**: 987–90.

44 Sima AAF, Bril V, Nathaniel V, McEwen TAJ, Brown MB, Lattimer SA, Greene DA. Regeneration and repair of myelinated fibers in sural-nerve biopsy specimens from patients with diabetic neuropathy treated with sorbinil. *N Engl J Med* 1988; **319**: 548–55.

45 Gregerson G, Bertelsen B, Harbo H *et al*. Oral supplementation of myoinositol: effects on peripheral nerve function in human diabetics and on the concentration in plasma, erythrocytes, urine and muscle tissue in human diabetics and normals. *Acta Neurol Scand* 1983; **67**: 164–72.

46 Jamal GA, Carmichael H. The effect of gamma-linolenic acid on human diabetic peripheral neuropathy: a double-blind placebo-controlled. *Diabetic Med* 1990; **7**: 319–23.

47 Dahl-Jørgensen K, Bringhmann I, Hansen O, Hanssen KF, Ganes T, Kierul FP, Smeland E, Sandvik L. Effect of near normoglycaemia for two years on progression of early diabetic retinopathy, nephropathy and neuropathy: the Oslo Study. *Br Med J* 1986; **293**: 1195–9.

48 Frighi V, Loughnane JW, Pozzilli P, Tarn AC, Thomas JM, Taylor JE, Andreani D, Gale EAM. Early signs of neuropathy and microangiopathy in young Type 1 (insulin-dependent) diabetic patients: correlation with long-term metabolic control (abstract). *Diabetologia* 1987; **30**: 521A.

49 Young RJ, MacIntyre CCA, Ewing DJ, Prescott RJ. Prediction of neuropathy over 5 years in young insulin-dependent diabetic patients (abstract). *Diabetic Med* 1988: 5A.

# 12 Autonomic Neuropathy

**Summary**

- Up to 40% of diabetic patients show some evidence of autonomic dysfunction, but only a few have symptoms of autonomic neuropathy.
- Autonomic neuropathy may evolve through defects in thermoregulation and sweating in the legs, followed by impotence and bladder dysfunction, to cardiovascular reflex abnormalities. Late manifestations include generalized sweating disorders, postural hypotension, gastrointestinal problems and reduced awareness of hypoglycaemia.
- Symptomatic autonomic neuropathy carries a poor prognosis; death is usually due to associated diabetic complications (especially nephropathy) but is occasionally sudden and unexplained.
- Autonomic dysfunction is best diagnosed by evaluating the cardiovascular reflex responses to various stimuli: changes in heart rate to the Valsalva manoeuvre, deep breathing and standing up, and blood pressure changes following standing and sustained handgrip. These tests are simple, non-invasive and can be performed in the clinic within 30 min. Computer programs are available to analyse the results.
- Other tests include measurements of pupillary function and sweating.
- The most prominent symptom is postural hypotension, which is due to loss of mainly sympathetic reflexes. It is aggravated by antihypertensive agents, antidepressants and insulin and may respond to fludrocortisone treatment.
- Bladder dysfunction usually causes asymptomatic enlargement but may cause overflow incontinence and recurrent urinary tract infections.
- Erectile failure is common in diabetic men, but is not always due to autonomic neuropathy.

Diabetes mellitus commonly affects the autonomic nervous system, with up to 40% of diabetic patients demonstrating some autonomic abnormality [1]. Historically, autonomic nerve damage in diabetes has been classified as an aspect of peripheral neuropathy but it is now apparent that it affects far more patients than those showing the well-known 'glove and stocking' symmetrical polyneuropathy. In recent years, the original concept of dual parasympathetic and sympathetic systems has been replaced by one in which the autonomic nervous system exercises a key integrating role [2]. It is not surprising, therefore, that when autonomic damage occurs its effects can be detected all over the body. Some effects are readily apparent clinically, but others can only be identified by using sensitive tests (Fig. 12.1).

Terminology may cause some confusion. Autonomic damage is sometimes classified by systems, as cardiovascular neuropathy, genitourinary neuropathy, gastrointestinal neuropathy and so on. This approach neglects the widespread nature of autonomic nerve damage in diabetes, and the global terms 'autonomic neuropathy' and 'autonomic dysfunction' are preferable. For the purposes of this chapter, 'autonomic neuropathy' refers to suggestive clinical features of autonomic involvement combined with objective evidence of abnormal autonomic function which is usually based on cardiovascular tests (see below). The term 'autonomic dysfunction' describes abnormal tests in the absence of clinical symptoms.

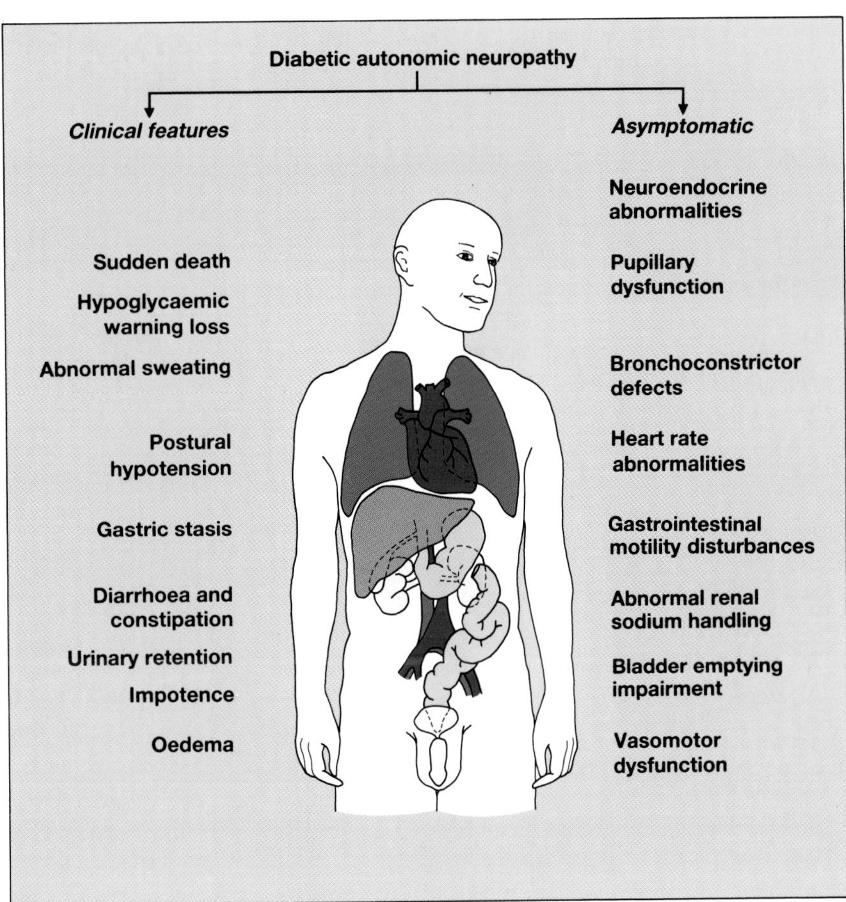


**Fig. 12.1.** Clinical features and asymptomatic effects of diabetic autonomic neuropathy.

## Epidemiology of autonomic neuropathy

The prevalence of autonomic damage in diabetes is not clear. Autonomic dysfunction has been demonstrated in 20% or more of diabetic patients, the exact percentages depending on the tests used and the population selected. In a recent series of 500 IDDM patients, abnormal cardiovascular reflexes were found in 17% overall, with more abnormalities in those aged 40–49 years and those with diabetes for more than 20 years [3]. Another study of 700 patients reported an overall prevalence of postural hypotension of 12%, predominantly in older patients and in those young subjects with a longer duration of diabetes [4]. There have been no satisfactory studies of the prevalence of autonomic symptoms. Widely variable figures have been reported in different series, possibly because of the often vague and non-specific nature of such symptoms. Impotence is relatively common in diabetic men (Chapter 25) and almost invariably accompanies other clinical features of autonomic neuropathy, but the relative contributions of autonomic neuropathy and of other causes are not known. Autonomic symptoms are uncommon in young diabetic patients, although there have been occasional case reports of severe symptomatic autonomic neuropathy [1].

## Aetiology of autonomic neuropathy

The prevalence of autonomic abnormalities is similar in IDDM and NIDDM, suggesting that the metabolic consequences of hyperglycaemia rather than the type of diabetes lead to autonomic nerve damage [5, 6]. The importance of hyperglycaemia was underlined by a recent prospective study of young IDDM patients, which demonstrated a clear relationship between deteriorating cardiovascular reflex tests and poor glycaemic control [7]. Moreover, patients whose metabolic control was improved for 2 years by continuous subcutaneous insulin infusion (CSII) have shown small but significant improvements in autonomic function [8]. There appears, therefore, to be a definite link between deteriorating autonomic function and hyperglycaemia, which may be partly reversed by improved metabolic control. The possible biochemical and pathophysiological basis of nerve damage in diabetes is discussed in Chapter 10.

No genetic factor has yet been implicated in the development of autonomic neuropathy. It has, however, been suggested that diabetic autonomic neuropathy is associated with iritis and that both might be caused by immunological damage [9], but this has been disputed [10].

## Relationship of autonomic neuropathy to other complications

Inevitably, as peripheral nerves contain both somatic and autonomic fibres, associations between somatic and autonomic neuropathy have been found [1]. Recently, this relationship was reexamined in diabetic subjects with various clinical manifestations of neuropathy [11] and in untreated NIDDM patients [12]. Both studies suggested that diffuse, symmetrical involvement of peripheral nerves occurred; selective damage to the various fibre types may account for the different clinical presentations.

It has traditionally been taught that diabetic nephropathy, retinopathy and neuropathy develop in parallel and that any patient with long-standing diabetes will have evidence of all three. However, the relationship between autonomic nerve damage and other diabetic complications is currently being reconsidered. Recent studies [13, 14] have suggested that autonomic damage itself may promote the development and progression of nephropathy and retinopathy, possibly through a direct effect of nerve damage on the microcirculation within these organs (Fig. 12.2).

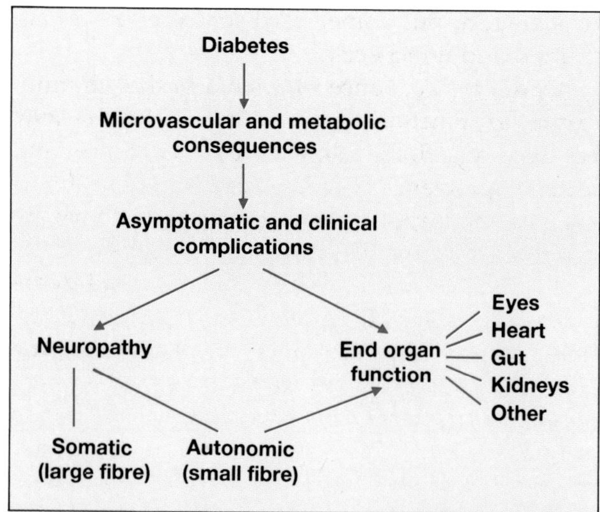


**Fig. 12.2.** Possible influence of autonomic nerve damage on other diabetic complications.

## Natural history

The natural history of autonomic involvement in diabetes is slowly being elucidated. Early autonomic dysfunction may in some cases progress to overt autonomic neuropathy. In one large series of patients assessed by cardiovascular reflex tests, approximately three-quarters had not deteriorated a few months to some years later, while the remaining quarter had developed new or additional autonomic symptoms and worsening autonomic function tests. Indices of autonomic function improved in only a very few [15]. In a 5-year prospective study of diabetic patients with abnormal cardiovascular reflexes and symptoms suggestive of autonomic neuropathy, the mortality rate was found to be 50% within 3 years (Fig. 12.3) [16]. Several other studies have now confirmed the poor prognosis of symptomatic autonomic neuropathy [17–19]. Many deaths are due to associated

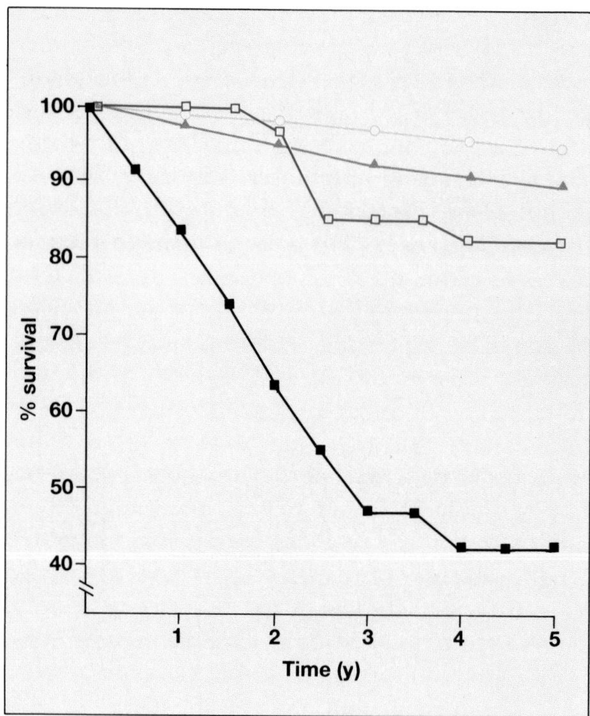


**Fig. 12.3.** Five-year survival curves for age- and sex-matched general population (○), age- and sex-matched diabetic population (▲), 33 diabetic patients with normal (□) and 40 diabetic patients with abnormal (■) autonomic function tests. (Redrawn with permission from [16].)

renal failure but some, as discussed below, are sudden and unexpected.

A possible sequence of events is that thermoregulatory function and sweating in the feet may be impaired first, followed by impotence and bladder problems. Cardiovascular reflex abnormalities then appear, and finally the late severe symptomatic manifestations of upper body sweating disturbance, reduced awareness of hypoglycaemia, postural hypotension and gastrointestinal problems (Fig. 12.4). It is not yet clear whether all diabetic patients inevitably progress through all these various stages, or whether some develop only a few early features and do not deteriorate further. Possible factors affecting autonomic nerves, and their consequences, are illustrated in Fig. 12.5.

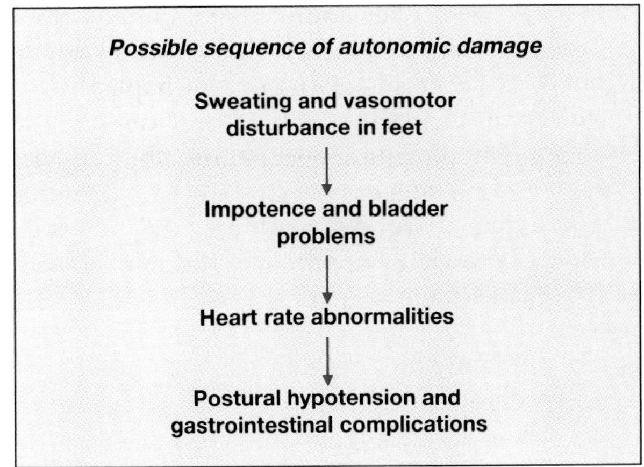


**Fig. 12.4.** Possible temporal sequence of the clinical progression of autonomic neuropathy in diabetes.

## Clinical features of autonomic neuropathy

Autonomic symptoms are often vague, remain unrecognized for some time and are of limited diagnostic value. However, severe autonomic neuropathy can present with a variable combination of postural hypotension, nocturnal diarrhoea, gastric problems, bladder symptoms, abnormal sweating, impotence in males, and a failure to recognize hypoglycaemia (Fig. 12.1). Most diabetic patients with severe symptomatic features also have advanced nephropathy, retinopathy and somatic neuropathy. Elsewhere in this book, gastrointestinal symptoms (Chapter 20), impotence (Chapter 25) and problems associated with the diabetic foot (Chapter 19) are covered in detail. Other clinical features are discussed below.

### *Postural hypotension*

Dizziness associated with a fall in blood pressure on standing up is the most obvious symptom of autonomic neuropathy, and is due to loss of predominantly sympathetically mediated reflexes. The patient may complain of postural weakness,

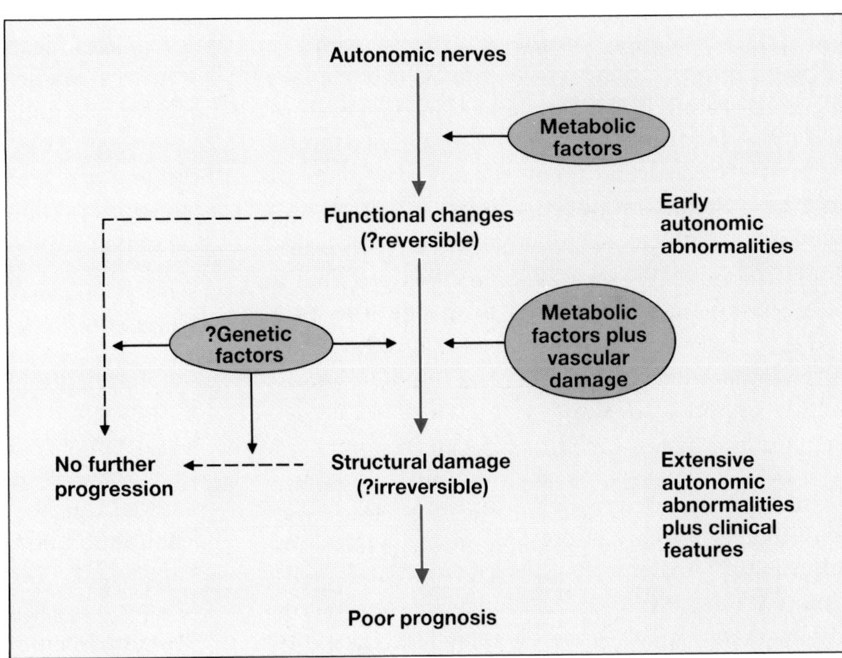


**Fig. 12.5.** Potential influences on autonomic nerves and their relation to the clinical progression of autonomic neuropathy in diabetes.

faintness, visual impairment or even loss of consciousness, symptoms which are sometimes wrongly attributed to hypoglycaemia. Many drugs, including antihypertensive agents, diuretics, tricyclic antidepressants, phenothiazines, vasodilators and nitrates worsen postural hypotension. Insulin treatment can also aggravate postural hypotension, possibly through a direct vasodilator action on peripheral blood vessels [20, 21]. Conversely, fluid retention, for example in cardiac failure or the nephrotic syndrome, may mask postural hypotension.

### *Sweating disturbances*

Diminished or absent sweating in the feet, extending in more severe cases to the whole leg and lower trunk, is a well-recognized clinical feature of diabetic autonomic neuropathy. Increased sweating over the upper part of the body is also common. Drenching sweats, sometimes mistaken for hypoglycaemic attacks, may affect the head and upper body, particularly in warm weather, during exercise or in bed. Gustatory sweating, starting within minutes of eating and provoked by certain foods, may also occur. It usually affects the forehead first and then spreads to the face, scalp and neck, and is often profuse [22].

### *Vasomotor problems, oedema and Charcot joints*

Autonomic damage impairs local microvascular reflexes which are mediated by vasoconstrictor and vasodilator fibres. Denervation and opening of arterio-venous anastomoses may cause shunting of blood into the skin, which could partly explain the high resting blood flow and skin temperature and dilated foot veins of some neuropathic patients [1, 23]. Paradoxically, they usually complain of cold feet. Peripheral oedema in patients with diabetic neuropathy is not uncommon and may also be related to increased arterio-venous shunting [1, 24]. Altered peripheral blood flow may also be a factor in the development of Charcot arthropathy (see Chapter 19).

### *Loss of hypoglycaemic warning symptoms*

So-called 'hypoglycaemic unawareness' has traditionally been associated with autonomic neuropathy. It is now clear, however, that diabetic patients without other evidence of autonomic involvement may also be affected, possibly because of failure of hypothalamic control mechanisms. Normally, hypoglycaemia first causes an asymptomatic parasympathetic response with bradycardia and mild hypotension, followed by sympathetic activation which usually produces easily recognizable symptoms. If these warning signs are absent, the first manifestation of hypoglycaemia may be neuroglycopenic symptoms with a rapid progression to unconsciousness. In clinical practice, less stringent glycaemic control may have to be accepted to avoid this problem.

### *Sudden unexpected death*

Some diabetic patients with autonomic neuropathy have died suddenly and unexpectedly. The reasons for this are unknown, but three possible explanations, none entirely convincing, have been suggested. Episodes of cardiorespiratory arrest have been observed in young diabetic patients with severe autonomic neuropathy [25], and it has been suggested that such subjects may not respond normally to hypoxia. However, laboratory studies of ventilatory control in diabetic patients have so far produced conflicting results [1]. Cardiac arrhythmias are a second possible explanation, but 24-h electrocardiogram monitoring has failed to demonstrate more frequent arrhythmias in diabetic patients than in normal subjects [26]. A third possibility is sleep apnoea, although patients with autonomic neuropathy do not appear to have abnormal breathing patterns during sleep [1, 27]. Failure of an as yet unidentified reflex mechanism under certain conditions may be responsible for unexpected deaths.

Any diabetic patient with autonomic neuropathy is a potential anaesthetic risk, and particular care needs to be taken during and after surgery to provide adequate oxygenation and appropriate monitoring. The same cautions apply to severe respiratory infections.

### *Bladder and erectile dysfunction*

Bladder dysfunction is a well-recognized feature of autonomic neuropathy, but usually remains asymptomatic until the late stages. Characteristically, there is an enlarged bladder and increased residual urine volume after micturition. As autonomic neuropathy progresses, there are lengthened intervals between micturition, an increase in the overnight urine volume, and a weakened or prolonged urinary stream with postmicturition dribbling. In advanced autonomic neuropathy, the bladder may become palpable, with overflow incontinence and rarely, acute retention of urine. Bladder stasis predisposes to urinary tract infection, which may in turn accelerate renal damage.

Impotence is invariably found in men with other features of autonomic neuropathy (see Chapter 25).

### *Asymptomatic abnormalities*

Diabetic patients have a higher resting heart rate than normal subjects (Figs 12.6 and 12.7), possibly due to autonomic damage [28]. A 'fixed' heart rate has also been described, although 24-h electrocardiographic monitoring has shown that very few diabetic patients have this abnormality and that most, including those with autonomic damage, have quite obvious diurnal heart rate variation [26].

Other asymptomatic abnormalities include defective pupillary responses and impaired bronchomotor function. The pupil shows a reduction in resting diameter [29] and loss of spontaneous oscillations ('hippus') [30, 31], and commonly fails to dilate quickly in the dark [30, 31]. Diminished bronchoconstriction in response to provocation tests such as breathing cold air has also been found [32, 33], but no specific clinical respiratory abnormality has yet been identified.

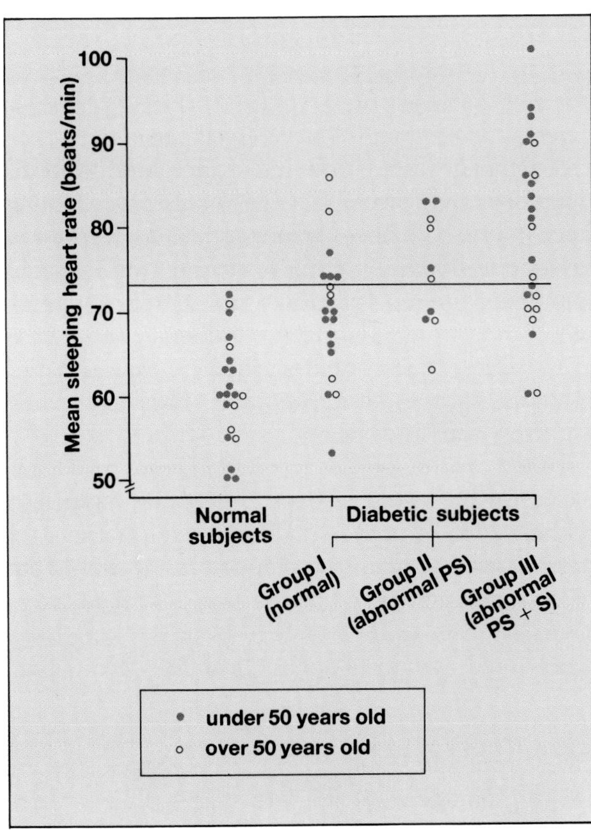


**Fig. 12.6.** Individual mean sleeping heart rates in normal subjects, diabetic patients with normal cardiovascular reflexes, with definite abnormalities (PS), and with severely abnormal cardiovascular reflexes (PS + S). The solid line represents two SDs above the group mean normal value. (Redrawn with permission from [26].)

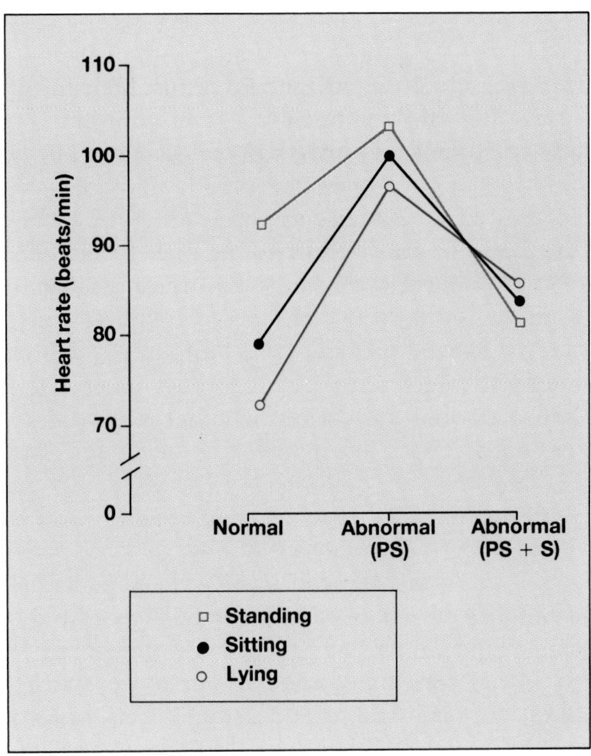


**Fig. 12.7.** Mean resting heart rates in three diabetic patients whose autonomic function changed with time from normal to definite (PS) and then severe (PS + S) damage. (Redrawn with permission from [28].)

### *Neuroendocrine changes*

Disturbances in the secretion of pancreatic polypeptide and other gastrointestinal hormones are increasingly being recognized in diabetic subjects with autonomic neuropathy. Abnormalities in the release of catecholamines and vasopressin and in the regulation of the renin–angiotensin system have also been described [1, 34]. The clinical consesequences of these and other neuroendocrine changes are not yet clear, although certain gastrointestinal symptoms associated with autonomic damage could, in part, be caused by abnormalities of gut regulatory peptides which have been demonstrated in experimental animals [35].

### *Central neuropathic damage*

The question of whether there is involvement of central neuronal pathways is a vexed one. The term 'diabetic encephalopathy' was coined in the 1950s [36] and certain degenerative pathological changes have subsequently been observed in the brains and spinal cords of young diabetic patients [37]. At a clinical level, there have been suggestions of subtle and selective defects of cognitive function in diabetic patients [38]. Profound and prolonged hypoglycaemia can severely damage the central nervous system but whether minor hypoglycaemia causes lesser effects is uncertain. The possible role of prolonged hyperglycaemia in central neuropathic damage is unknown.

The integrity of various central sensory pathways can be investigated using evoked potential techniques. Visual evoked potentials measure the latency and character of the electrical response of the visual cortex (recorded by electroencephalogram) to retinal stimulation using a checkerboard reversal pattern. The auditory pathways can similarly be investigated by the brain-stem auditory evoked potentials and conduction from the periphery to the sensory cortex by somatosensory evoked potentials. Results obtained in diabetic subjects have been conflicting [39, 40]. Some studies have suggested that central damage occurs early in the course of diabetes, while others have found no evidence at all of central involvement, even in patients with widespread complications.

## Diagnosis of autonomic neuropathy

The diagnosis of diabetic autonomic neuropathy was first based on symptoms but now depends on various objective reflex tests. There has been considerable debate as to what constitutes the 'best' diagnostic test or set of tests. Some, while useful for physiological studies, are impracticable for use in a diabetic clinic and others are too complex, 'invasive', inherently risky or poorly reproducible [41]. Cardiovascular tests have been best characterized and now allow objective assessment of autonomic function through a series of well-validated, non-invasive and relatively simple manoeuvres. Implicit in their use, however, is the assumption that cardiovascular reflex abnormalities reflect damage throughout the autonomic nervous system. Although this appears largely correct, early manifestations elsewhere may antedate certain cardiovascular reflex changes.

A consensus statement has recently been published to provide guidelines for the diagnosis and classification of diabetic neuropathy [42]. Recommendations relevant to the autonomic nervous system were that:

1 Symptoms, possibly reflecting autonomic neuropathy should not, by themselves, be considered markers for its presence.

2 Non-invasive validated measures of autonomic neural reflexes should be used as specific markers of autonomic neuropathy if end-organ failure is carefully ruled out and other important factors, such as concomitant illness, drug use, and age, are taken into account. An abnormality of more than one test on more than one occasion is desirable to establish the presence of autonomic dysfunction.

3 Independent tests of both parasympathetic and sympathetic function should be performed.

4 A battery of quantitative measures of autonomic reflexes should be used to monitor improvement or deterioration of autonomic nerve function, although their utility for monitoring patients over time has not clearly been established [42].

### *Cardiovascular tests*

Five simple, non-invasive tests using cardiovascular reflexes are now widely accepted for both diagnostic and research assessment of autonomic neuropathy [15]. These tests examine the responses to various stimuli of either heart rate (the Valsalva manoeuvre, deep breathing and standing up) or blood pressure (standing up and sustained handgrip). These tests are described below, and the range of normal, borderline and abnormal values are shown in Table 12.1.

Other cardiovascular tests sometimes used are based on the baroreflex responses, the heart rate responses to atropine and propanolol or the cold pressor test. None of these appear to be as reliable or as easily performed as the five described here. Two new tests, the heart rate responses to coughing and lying down, have not yet been fully evaluated.

#### HEART RATE RESPONSE TO THE VALSALVA MANOEUVRE

The Valsalva manoeuvre — forced expiration against resistance — causes complex reflex circulatory changes mediated by both parasympathetic and sympathetic pathways. While straining, the blood pressure normally falls and the heart rate rises. After release of the strain, the blood pressure

**Table 12.1.** Normal, borderline and abnormal values for cardiovascular autonomic function tests [15].

| | Normal | Borderline | Abnormal |
|---|---|---|---|
| *Heart rate tests* | | | |
| Heart rate response to Valsalva manoeuvre (Valsalva ratio) | ≥1.21 | – | ≤1.20 |
| Heart rate response to standing up (30 : 14 ratio) | ≥1.04 | 1.01–1.03 | ≤1.00 |
| Heart rate response to deep breathing (maximum minus minimum heart rate) | ≥15 beats/min | 11–14 beats/min | ≤10 beats/min |
| *Blood pressure tests* | | | |
| Blood pressure response to standing up (fall in systolic BP) | ≤10 mmHg | 11–29 mmHg | ≥30 mmHg |
| Blood pressure response to sustained handgrip (increase in diastolic BP) | ≥16 mmHg | 11–15 mmHg | ≤10 mmHg |

promptly rises and overshoots its resting value while the heart rate slows. With autonomic damage, the blood pressure falls during strain but only slowly returns to normal after release, with no overshoot; there is no change in heart rate. Heart rate is easily measured during and after the Valsalva manoeuvre, and gives a reliable guide to the overall integrity of the complex reflex pathways involved.

The test is performed by asking the subject to sit quietly and then to blow into a mouthpiece attached to an aneroid pressure gauge at a pressure of 40 mmHg for 15 s. Heart rate is recorded continuously using a standard electrocardiogram machine during and after the manoeuvre. The 'Valsalva ratio' is the ratio of the longest R–R interval found after (within about 20 beats of the end of the manoeuvre) to the shortest R–R interval during the manoeuvre. The result is taken as the mean ratio for three successive Valsalva manoeuvres. It is probably wise to avoid this test in diabetic patients with proliferative retinopathy because of the theoretical risk of provoking a retinal or vitreous haemorrhage. Subjects with cardiac failure may fail to show significant heart rate changes during the Valsalva manoeuvre.

### HEART RATE RESPONSE TO STANDING UP

Standing up from lying normally causes reflex alterations in heart rate which are mainly under parasympathetic control, with a small sympathetic component. Normally, there is an immediate increase in heart rate, maximal at about the 15th beat after standing, followed by relative bradycardia which is maximal around the 30th beat. Subjects with autonomic neuropathy show only a gradual increase, or no change in heart rate on standing.

For this test, the subject lies quietly on a couch and then stands up unaided. The electrocardiogram is recorded continuously. The heart rate response is best expressed as the '30 : 15 ratio', i.e. the ratio of the longest R–R interval (around the 30th beat after starting to stand up) to the shortest R–R interval (around the 15th beat). It is important to begin counting beats (by marking the ECG chart) when the subject *starts* to stand up, and not several seconds later when the postural change has been completed.

### HEART RATE RESPONSE TO DEEP BREATHING

In normal subjects, the heart rate continually varies, mostly in association with breathing. Heart rate increases during inspiration and decreases during expiration, with maximal variation at a respiratory rate of around six breaths/min. This so-called 'respiratory sinus arrhythmia' is under cardiac parasympathetic control. Autonomic neuropathy considerably reduces and may even abolish heart rate variation during breathing.

The test is conveniently performed by asking the patient to sit quietly and then breathe deeply and evenly at six breaths/min (i.e. 5 s in and 5 s out). The maximum and minimum heart rates during each 10-s breathing cycle are calculated from R–R intervals recorded by electrocardiogram. The mean of the differences during three successive breathing cycles gives the 'maximum–minimum heart rate'. An alternative way to express these changes is as a ratio of the heart rate at its slowest during expiration to that at its fastest during inspiration (the 'E:I ratio').

### BLOOD PRESSURE RESPONSE TO STANDING UP

On standing, blood pools in the legs and causes a fall in blood pressure which is normally rapidly corrected by a reflex combination of tachycardia and peripheral and splanchnic vasoconstriction. The cardiovascular reflexes concerned with postural homeostasis are complex and involve both sympathetic and parasympathetic pathways. Defective sympathetic reflexes impair splanchnic vasoconstriction, leading to postural hypotension.

Blood pressure is simply measured while the subject is lying down and again 1 min after standing up, and the difference in systolic blood pressure noted.

### BLOOD PRESSURE RESPONSE TO SUSTAINED HANDGRIP

During sustained handgrip, a sharp rise in blood pressure normally occurs due to a heart rate-dependent increase in cardiac output with unchanged peripheral vascular resistance. If the reflex pathways controlling this response are damaged, as in severe diabetic autonomic neuropathy, the blood pressure rise is attentuated.

The test is performed by asking the subject to squeeze a handgrip dynamometer as hard as possible for a few seconds and then to maintain steady pressure at 30% of that maximum for as long as possible, which is usually between 3–4 min. Blood pressure is measured each minute, and the difference between the diastolic blood pressure before starting and just before releasing handgrip is taken as the measure of response.

### PRACTICAL ASSESSMENT OF CARDIOVASCULAR AUTONOMIC FUNCTION

This battery of tests can be performed easily in the clinic. All that is needed are a sphygmomanometer, electrocardiogram machine, aneroid pressure gauge attached to a mouthpiece by a rigid or flexible tube, and a handgrip dynamometer (available from Tephcotronics Ltd, 5 Hillview Drive, Edinburgh EH12 8QW, UK). In practice, all the tests can be performed in a simple planned sequence within 15–20 min (Table 12.2). Data can be handled in two ways. Before the advent of the microcomputer, a ruler and electrocardiogram strip were adequate and are still sufficient where tests are only occasionally performed. However, a number of computer programs are now available which measure R–R intervals automatically, calculate the required ratios, and group the results. One package specifically designed for the five tests outlined above is the 'Autocaft' system (UnivEd Technologies Ltd, 16 Buccleuch Place, Edinburgh EH8 9LN, UK) which operates with BBC- or IBM PC-compatible microcomputers. It has the advantages of allowing blood pressure measurements to be entered and of automatically classifying the results as normal, borderline or abnormal.

The results from these five tests enable the severity of autonomic damage (Fig. 12.8) to be categorized according to a system derived from observations on large numbers of subjects over a number of years [15]. The categories are:

**1** Normal: all five tests normal, or one borderline.

**Table 12.2.** Flow-plan for performing cardiovascular autonomic function tests.

| Tests (performed in this order) | Position of subject | Approximate time of test (min) | Apparatus required |
|---|---|---|---|
| Heart rate response to Valsalva manoeuvre | Sitting | 5 | Aneroid manometer, electrocardiograph |
| Heart rate response to deep breathing | Sitting | 2 | Electrocardiograph |
| Blood pressure response to sustained handgrip | Sitting | 5 | Handgrip dynamometer, sphygmomanometer |
| Heart rate response to standing up | Lying, then standing | 3 | Electrocardiograph |
| Blood pressure response to standing up | | | Sphygmomanometer |

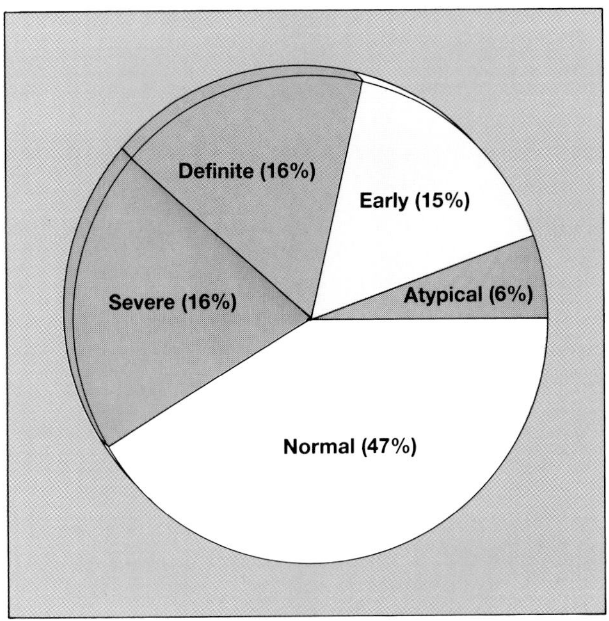


**Fig. 12.8.** Results of cardiovascular autonomic function tests in 1469 diabetic subjects, grouped according to the severity of autonomic damage.

**2** Early involvement: one of the three heart-rate tests abnormal or two borderline.
**3** Definite involvement: two or more of the heart-rate tests abnormal.
**4** Severe involvement: two or more of the heart-rate tests abnormal, plus one or both of the blood pressure tests abnormal, or both borderline.
**5** A typical pattern: any other combination of abnormal tests (only about 6% of diabetic subjects are 'atypical').

An alternative to this classification is to give each individual test a score of 0, 1 or 2 depending on whether it is normal, borderline or abnormal. An overall 'autonomic score' of 0–10 can then be obtained. Increasing scores from 0 to 10 correlate closely with the grades of severity given above [15]. Scoring of the tests in this way allows an 'atypical' pattern to be given a numerical value.

The classification proposed here avoids labelling the tests as specifically 'parasympathetic' or 'sympathetic', as the reflex pathways involved are extremely complex. The use of a single cardiovascular reflex test to assess autonomic function is misleading and should be avoided as it neglects the possible range of autonomic nerve damage.

### *Tests in other systems*

While cardiovascular reflex tests are generally accepted as the 'gold standard' for the assessment of autonomic dysfunction in diabetes, tests in other systems can sometimes be of value [1, 41]. However, most are more complex and are mentioned here only in outline.

#### GASTROINTESTINAL TESTS

Oesophageal function can be assessed by cineradiography after swallowing barium, by manometry, or by scintiscanning using solid and liquid meals labelled with $\gamma$-emitting isotopes (see Chapter 20). Abnormal motility and transit patterns have been found in diabetic autonomic neuropathy. Emptying of the stomach is a coordinated process involving both parasympathetic and sympathetic nerves. Gastric abnormalities in diabetic patients have been assessed by barium meal studies, by scintigraphic techniques, and by monitoring changes in gastric volume using electrical impedance measurements or ultrasonography [43, 44]. Within the small and large bowel there are no simple, reliable methods available to assess transit time or motor function, although certain marker techniques and breath hydrogen measurements have been used. Detailed studies of colonic motility have been reported, but such techniques are still research procedures.

#### BLADDER FUNCTION TESTS

Bladder function can be assessed using specialized cystometric and urodynamic methods, but these require expert interpretation. Three simpler tests are ultrasound imaging of the bladder to measure the approximate volume of residual urine, mictiography to quantitate urine flow time and volume, and intravenous pyelography. Their exact place in the non-invasive diagnosis and management of bladder involvement is, however, not yet established.

#### SWEAT TESTS

Sweating can be assessed roughly (and messily) by applying powders which change colour on contact with moisture. Two quantifiable tests have recently been described. The first uses a special 'cell' which stimulates local sweating by iontophoresis of acetylcholine — the so-called 'quantitative sudomotor axon reflex test' (or Q-SART) [45]. A second approach is to count the number of imprints made by sweat drops in a soft Silastic film applied to the skin, after stimulating sweating with pilocarpine [46].

#### PUPILLARY TESTS

Abnormalities of pupillary diameter are described above. Sophisticated pupillary analysis requires a costly infrared pupillometer, but two simple methods are available. The diameter of the dark-adapted pupil can be measured from a polaroid photograph of the eye, which provides a quantitative estimate of sympathetic pupillary innervation [47]. Pupil cycle time can also be measured. Regular oscillations of the pupil can normally be induced with a slit-lamp beam and are a sensitive indicator of parasympathetic function. In diabetic autonomic neuropathy, pupil cycle time is considerably prolonged [48].

#### NEUROENDOCRINE TESTS

These tests measure the stimulated levels of hormones whose secretion depends on sympathetic or parasympathetic pathways. The pancreatic polypeptide responses to hypoglycaemia and eating have been used to test vagal integrity, and changes in plasma catecholamine levels in response to various stimuli to indicate sympathetic activity [1, 34]. However, assay of the hormones and interpretation of the results can be difficult, thus limiting their practical usefulness.

## Management of autonomic neuropathy

### *General and preventative measures*

As mentioned above, diabetic patients with symptomatic autonomic neuropathy pose particular anaesthetic hazards and great care must be taken during the perioperative period. Hypoglycaemic warning symptoms may be lost and the possibility of relaxing glycaemic control should be considered in such patients. Neurogenic bladder problems may be helped by encouraging regular bladder emptying, if necessary by using manual suprapubic pressure every 3–4 h. Long-term single or cyclical chemotherapy may be indicated for recurrent or persistent urinary tract infections. Bladder neck resection may need to be considered in cases with large residual urine volumes, but may cause incontinence.

### *Symptomatic treatment*

Postural hypotension only needs treatment if it is symptomatic. Mild symptoms during the day can be treated by raising the head of the bed a few centimetres at night. In those with more marked symptoms, fludrocortisone is the drug of choice [49, 50] (Fig. 12.9). This acts directly to increase peripheral vascular tone and also increases blood volume [49]. Sometimes it is ineffective, when other drugs including pindolol, metoclopramide (either alone or in combination with flurbiprofen) and a combination of diphenhydramine and cimetidine can be tried. Antigravity suits and elastic tights are probably no longer necessary.

Profuse and socially embarrassing sweating may be limited by anticholinergic drugs such as propantheline hydrobromide or poldine methylsulphate. A prophylactic dose of either drug taken before a meal is often effective in preventing gustatory sweating. Side-effects, including urinary retention, often restrict the use of these agents.

### *Curative measures*

As yet, no way has been found to limit or reverse autonomic neuropathy. There have been some encouraging accounts of slight improvement in the reflex abnormalities with improved glycaemic control, particularly CSII [8]. Some reports have

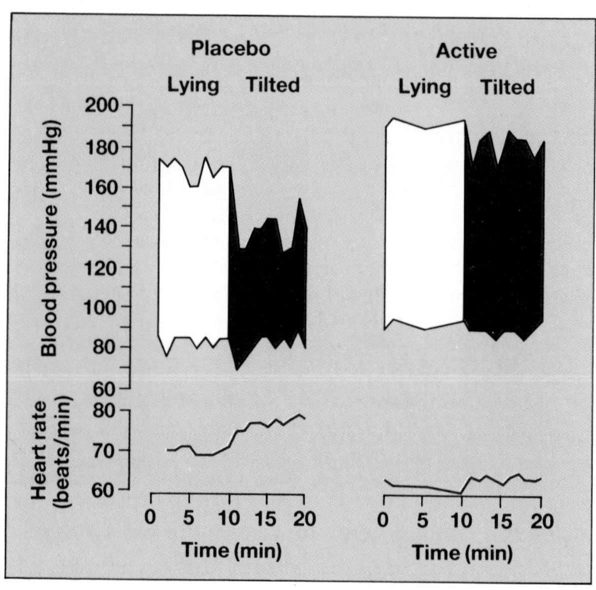


**Fig. 12.9.** Blood pressure and heart rate responses to tilting in a diabetic patient with autonomic neuropathy during placebo and fludrocortisone treatment periods. (Redrawn with permission from [49].)

suggested that treatment with the aldose reductase inhibitors may slightly improve certain cardiovascular test indices [51–54], but the clinical relevance of these results is uncertain. Such drugs administered long-term and before irreversible nerve damage has occurred may possibly prevent the morbid and mortal consequences of autonomic nerve damage.

## Recent developments

Some recent work in the field of diabetic autonomic neuropathy has been concerned with refining testing techniques, while others have examined different facets of clinical autonomic neuropathy. These advances are described in two recent reviews [55, 56].

DAVID J. EWING

## References


1 Ewing DJ, Clarke BF. Diabetic autonomic neuropathy: present insights and future prospects. *Diabetes Care* 1986; **9**: 648–65.

2 Bannister R. Introduction and classification. In: Bannister R, ed. *Autonomic Failure. A Textbook of Clinical Disorders of the Autonomic Nervous System*. Oxford: Oxford University Press, 1988: 1–20.

3 O'Brien IAD, O'Hare JP, Lewin IG, Corrall RJM. The prevalence of autonomic neuropathy in insulin-dependent diabetes mellitus: a controlled study based on heart rate variability. *Q J Med* 1986; **61**: 957–67.

4 Krolewski AS, Warram JH, Cupples A, Gorman CK, Szabo AJ, Christlieb AR. Hypertension, orthostatic hypotension and the microvascular complications of diabetes. *J Chronic Dis* 1985; **38**: 319–26.

5 Pfeifer MA, Weinberg CR, Cook DL, Reenan A, Halter JB, Ensinck JW *et al*. Autonomic neural dysfunction in recently diagnosed diabetic subjects. *Diabetes Care* 1984; **7**: 447–53.

6 Masaoka S, Lev-Ran A, Hill LR, Vakil G, Hon EHG. Heart rate variability in diabetes: relationship to age and duration of the disease. *Diabetes Care* 1985; **8**: 64–8.

7 Young RJ, MacIntyre CCA, Martyn CN, Prescott RJ, Ewing DJ, Smith AF *et al*. Progression of subclinical polyneuropathy in young patients with Type 1 (insulin-dependent) diabetes: associations with glycaemic control and microangiopathy (microvascular complications). *Diabetologia* 1986; **29**: 156–61.

8 Jakobsen J, Christiansen JS, Kristoffersen I, Christensen CK, Hermansen K, Schmitz A *et al*. Autonomic and somatosensory nerve function after 2 years of continuous subcutaneous insulin infusion in Type 1 diabetes. *Diabetes* 1988; **37**: 452–5.

9 Guy RJC, Richards F. Edmonds ME, Watkins PJ. Diabetic autonomic neuropathy and iritis: an association suggesting an immunological cause. *Br Med J* 1984; **289**: 343–5.

10 Martyn CN, Young RJ, Ewing DJ. Is there a link between iritis and diabetic autonomic neuropathy? *Br Med J* 1986; **292**: 934.

11 Young RJ, Zhou YQ, Rodriguez E, Prescott RJ, Ewing DJ, Clarke BF. Variable relationship between peripheral somatic and autonomic neuropathy in patients with different syndromes of diabetic polyneuropathy. *Diabetes* 1986; **35**: 192–7.

12 Pfeifer MA, Weinberg CR, Cook DL, Reenan A, Halar E, Halter JB *et al*. Correlations among autonomic, sensory, and motor neural function tests in untreated non-insulin-dependent diabetic individuals. *Diabetes Care* 1985; **8**: 576–84.

13 Lilja B, Nosslin B, Bergstrom B, Sundkvist G. Glomerular filtration rate, autonomic nerve function and orthostatic blood pressure in patients with diabetes mellitus. *Diabetes Res* 1985; **2**: 179–81.

14 Winocour PH, Dhar H, Anderson DC. The relationship between autonomic neuropathy and urinary sodium and albumin excretion in insulin-treated diabetics. *Diabetic Med* 1986; **3**: 436–40.

15 Ewing DJ, Martyn CN, Young RJ, Clarke BF. The value of cardiovascular autonomic function tests: 10 years experience in diabetes. *Diabetes Care* 1985; **8**: 491–8.

16 Ewing DJ, Campbell IW, Clarke BF. The natural history of diabetic autonomic neuropathy. *Q J Med* 1980; **49**: 95–108.

17 Watkins PJ, Mackay JD. Cardiac denervation in diabetic neuropathy. *Ann Intern Med* 1980; **92**: 304–7.

18 Sala JMV, Saez JMG, Esteve RI, Hosselbarth AF, Uriach CV, Bertran MM *et al*. Mortalidad en la neuropatia vegetativa cardiovascular de la diabetes mellitus. *Med Clin (Barc)* 1983; **81**: 794–6.

19 Hasslacher C, Bassler G. Prognose der kardialen autonomen Neuropathie bei Diabetikern. *Münch Med Wschr* 1983; **125**: 375–7.

20 Page MMcB, Watkins PJ. Provocation of postural hypotension by insulin. *Diabetes* 1976; **25**: 90–5.

21 Takata S, Yamamoto M, Yagi S, Noto Y, Ikeda T, Hattori N. Peripheral circulatory effects of insulin in diabetes. *Angiology* 1985; **36**: 110–15.

22 Watkins PJ. Facial sweating after food; a new sign of diabetic autonomic neuropathy. *Br Med J* 1973; **1**: 583–7.

23 Archer AG, Roberts VC, Watkins PJ. Blood flow patterns in painful diabetic neuropathy. *Diabetologia* 1984; **27**: 563–7.

24 Edmonds ME, Archer AG, Watkins PJ. Ephedrine: a new treatment for diabetic neuropathic oedema. *Lancet* 1983; **i**: 548–51.

25 Page MMcB, Watkins PJ. Cardiorespiratory arrest and diabetic autonomic neuropathy. *Lancet* 1978; **i**: 14–16.

26 Ewing DJ, Borsey DQ, Travis P, Bellavere F, Neilson JMM, Clarke BF. Abnormalities of ambulatory 24 hour heart rate in diabetes mellitus. *Diabetes* 1983; **32**: 101–5.

27 Catterall JR, Calverley PMA, Ewing DJ *et al*. Breathing, sleep and autonomic neuropathy. *Diabetes* 1984; **33**: 1025–7.

28 Ewing DJ, Campbell IW, Clarke BF. Heart rate changes in diabetes mellitus. *Lancet* 1981; **i**: 183–6.

29 Hreidarsson AB. Pupil size in insulin-dependent diabetes. Relationship to duration, metabolic control, and long-term complications. *Diabetes* 1982; **31**: 442–8.

30 Hreidarsson AB, Gundersen HJG. Reduced pupillary unrest. Autonomic nervous system abnormalities in diabetes mellitus. *Diabetes* 1988; **37**: 446–51.

31 Smith SE, Smith SA, Brown PM, Fox C, Sönksen PH. Pupillary signs in diabetic autonomic neuropathy. *Br Med J* 1978; **2**: 924–7.

32 Douglas NJ, Campbell IW, Ewing DJ, Clarke BF, Flenley DC. Reduced airway vagal tone in diabetic patients with autonomic neuropathy. *Clin Sci* 1981; **61**: 581–4.

33 Heaton RW, Guy RJC, Gray BJ, Watkins PJ, Costello JF. Diminished bronchial reactivity to cold air in diabetic

patients with autonomic neuropathy. *Br Med J* 1984; **289**: 149–51.

34 Kennedy FP, Go VLW, Cryer PE, Bolli GE, Gerich JE. Subnormal pancreatic polypeptide and epinephrine responses to insulin-induced hypoglycemia identify patients with insulin-dependent diabetes mellitus predisposed to develop overt autonomic neuropathy. *Ann Int Med* 1988; **108**: 54–8.

35 Ballmann M, Conlon JM. Changes in the somatostatin, substance P and vasoactive intestinal peptide contents of the gastrointestinal tract following streptozotocin-induced diabetes in the rat. *Diabetologia* 1985; **28**: 355–8.

36 De Jong RN. The nervous system complications in diabetes mellitus with special reference to cerebrovascular changes. *J Nerv Ment Dis* 1950; **111**: 181–206.

37 Reske-Nielson E, Lundbaek K, Gregersen G, Harmsen A. Pathological changes in central and peripheral nervous system of young long-term diabetics. *Diabetologia* 1970; **6**: 98–103.

38 Franceschi M, Cecchetto R, Minicucci F, Smirne S, Baio G, Canal N. Cognitive processes in insulin-dependent diabetes. *Diabetes Care* 1984; **7**: 228–31.

39 Pozzessere G, Rizzo PA, Valle E *et al*. Early detection of neurological involvement in IDDM and NIDDM. Multimodal evoked potentials versus metabolic control. *Diabetes Care* 1988; **11**: 473–80.

40 Collier A, Reid W, McInnes A, Cull RE, Ewing DJ, Clarke BF. Somatosensory and visual evoked potentials in insulin-dependent diabetics with mild peripheral neuropathy. *Diabetes Res Clin Pract* 1988; **5**: 171–5.

41 Ewing DJ. Practical bedside investigation of diabetic autonomic failure. In: Bannister R, ed. *Autonomic Failure. A Textbook of Clinical Disorders of the Autonomic Nervous System*. Oxford: Oxford University Press, 1983: 371–405.

42 Consensus statement. Report and recommendations of the San Antonio Conference on diabetic neuropathy. *Diabetes* 1988; **37**: 1000–4.

43 Gilbey SG, Watkins PJ. Measurement by epigastric impedance of gastric emptying in diabetic autonomic neuropathy. *Diabetic Med* 1987; **4**: 122–6.

44 Vogelberg KH, Rathmann W, Helbig G. Sonographic examination of gastric motility in diabetics with autonomic neuropathy. *Diabetes Res* 1987; **5**: 175–9.

45 Low PA, Caskey PE, Tuck RR, Fealey RD, Dyck PJ. Quantitative sudomotor axon reflex test in normal and neuropathic subjects. *Ann Neurol* 1983; **14**: 573–80.

46 Kennedy WR, Sakuda M, Sutherland D, Goetz FC. The sweating deficiency in diabetes mellitus: methods of quantitation and clinical correlation. *Neurology (Cleveland)* 1984; **34**: 758–63.

47 Smith SA, Dewhurst RR. A simple diagnostic test for pupillary abnormality in diabetic autonomic neuropathy. *Diabetic Med* 1986; **3**: 38–41.

48 Martyn CN, Ewing DJ. Pupil cycle time: a simple way of measuring an autonomic reflex. *J Neurol Neurosurg Psychiatr* 1986; **49**: 771–4.

49 Campbell IW, Ewing DJ, Clarke BF. 9-alpha-fluorohydrocortisone in the treatment of postural hypotension in diabetic autonomic neuropathy. *Diabetes* 1975; **24**: 381–4.

50 Campbell IW, Ewing DJ, Clarke BF. Therapeutic experience with fludrocortisone in diabetic postural hypotension. *Br Med J* 1976; **1**: 872–4.

51 Jaspan JB, Herold K, Bartkus C. Effects of sorbinil therapy in diabetic patients with painful peripheral neuropathy and autonomic neuropathy. *Am J Med* 1985; **79** (suppl 5A): 24–37.

52 Fagius J, Brattberg A, Jameson S, Berne C. Limited benefit of treatment of diabetic polyneuropathy with an aldose reductase inhibitor: a 24-week controlled trial. *Diabetologia* 1985; **28**: 323–9.

53 Sundkvist G, Lilja B, Rosen I, Agardh C-D. Autonomic and peripheral nerve function in early diabetic neuropathy. Possible influence of a novel aldose reductase inhibitor on autonomic function. *Acta Med Scand* 1987; **221**: 445–53.

54 Young RJ, Martyn CN, Ewing DJ, Clarke BF. Improvement of nerve function with Statil (ICI 128436) in asymptomatic diabetic neuropathy: a six week controlled study. *Diabetic Med* 1986; **3**: 589A.

55 Ewing DJ. Autonomic neuropathy. In: Alberti KGMM, Krall LP, eds. *The Diabetes Annual* 6. Amsterdam: Elsevier Science Publishers, 1991.

56 Ewing DJ. Analysis of heart rate variability and other non-invasive tests with special reference to diabetes mellitus. In: Bannister R, Mathias CJ, eds. *Autonomic Failures*, 3rd edn. Oxford: Oxford University Press, 1992: 312–33.

# PART 4
# DIABETIC NEPHROPATHY

# 13 Epidemiology and Natural History of Diabetic Nephropathy

**Summary**

• Diabetic nephropathy is defined by persistent albuminuria (albumin excretion rate (AER) >300 mg/day; Albustix-positive), declining glomerular filtration rate (GFR) and rising blood pressure.

• Established nephropathy follows several years of incipient nephropathy, characterized by worsening microalbuminuria (AER, 30–300 mg/day) which is Albustix-negative and detectable by, for instance, radioimmunoassay.

• The natural history of nephropathy differs between IDDM and NIDDM. In IDDM, nephropathy develops in about 35% of cases, especially in males and those whose diabetes presents before the age of 15 years. The incidence of nephropathy peaks after 15–16 years of diabetes and declines thereafter. In NIDDM, estimates of prevalence range from 3 to 16% and nephropathy often supervenes after a shorter known duration of diabetes than in IDDM.

• The incidence of diabetic nephropathy is falling, possibly due in part to improved diabetic management.

• GFR is often increased above normal ('hyperfiltration') from the onset of IDDM, due to increased renal blood flow, glomerular capillary hypertension and increased filtration surface area. The glomeruli are hypertrophied and the kidneys enlarged. These changes do not seem to occur in NIDDM.

• In both IDDM and NIDDM, GFR begins to decline irreversibly when AER has risen to 100–300 mg/day, at an average rate of 10 ml/min/1.73 $m^2$ per year. This is due to progressive reduction of the filtration surface area through mesangial expansion. Serum creatinine levels begin to rise when GFR falls below 50 ml/min/1.73 $m^2$ and end-stage renal failure follows after an average of 5 years.

• Blood pressure is normal at the onset of IDDM and generally remains so in patients with normoalbuminuria. In microalbuminuric subjects, however, blood pressure begins to rise when AER exceeds 50 mg/day.

• Albuminuria in diabetic nephropathy is due to glomerular capillary damage and reflects generalized damage to the microcirculation and large vessels. Nephropathic patients have an increased incidence of retinopathy and a tenfold increase in cardiovascular mortality which is the major cause of death in nephropathic NIDDM patients.

• Other concomitants of albuminuria include increased urinary IgG excretion, hyperlipidaemia and elevated fibrinogen levels.

• The rate of progression of incipient and established nephropathy can be slowed and the associated mortality reduced by aggressive antihypertensive treatment.

Diabetic nephropathy is an important complication of diabetes for a number of reasons. Firstly, it is relatively common, affecting about one in three of patients with IDDM. Secondly, the proteinuria which is its hallmark is only one consequence of widespread damage to small and large blood vessels, and is a marker for the cardiovascular disease which is a common cause of death in these patients. Thirdly, there is increasingly convincing and optimistic evidence that the progression of nephropathy and its associated mortality can be ameliorated by antihypertensive and other treatments if started at an early stage.

This section will describe the epidemiology and natural history of the condition and will set the scene for the detailed descriptions of the causes, pathological and clinical features, diagnosis and treatment of diabetic nephropathy in the following chapters.

## Definitions

*Diabetic nephropathy* is characterized by persistent proteinuria, decreasing glomerular filtration rate (GFR) and increasing blood pressure. Persistent proteinuria is defined as a urinary protein excretion of >0.5 g/day, a level detectable by routine dip-stick testing of random urine samples (e.g. with Albustix) in more than two consecutive urine samples in a diabetic patient without urinary infection, cardiac insufficiency or other renal diseases. The excretion of 0.5 g/day of total protein is equivalent to a urinary albumin excretion of about 300 mg/day or 200 μg/min. This stage is preceded by a long 'silent' phase of *incipient diabetic nephropathy* characterized by a subclinical increase in albumin excretion to above the normal range but below the limit defining diabetic nephropathy. This degree of albuminuria is known as *microalbuminuria* (30–300 mg/day or 20–200 μg/min) and, being below the threshold of detection by Albustix, must be measured by radioimmunoassay or other highly-sensitive methods (see Fig. 13.1).

The morphological changes seen in the diabetic kidney consist of diffuse and nodular glomerulosclerosis and arteriolohyalinosis. The term 'diabetic nephropathy' is not synonymous with glomerulosclerosis as diabetic glomerulosclerosis is found in almost all (>90%) IDDM patients after 10 years of diabetes [1], whereas diabetic nephropathy (with persistent proteinuria and declining renal function) will develop in only about 35–40% of diabetic patients [2, 3]. The correlation between morphological and functional abnormalities is therefore poor [4, 5] therefore the diagnosis of clinical diabetic nephropathy cannot be made by light microscopy of renal biopsies (see Chapter 15). However, morphometric measurements by electron microscopy have demonstrated a good correlation between urinary albumin excretion rate (AER) and glomerular basement membrane thickness and mesangial expansion in normo- and microalbuminuric patients.

## Prevalence and incidence

Diabetic nephropathy occurs in both IDDM and NIDDM but its natural history differs between the two. In IDDM, the prevalence of diabetic nephropathy is about 15–20% while a further 15–28% of patients are reported to show persistent microalbuminuria [6, 7]. The incidence of diabetic nephropathy reaches a peak of 3–5% of unaffected patients per year after about 15–16 years of diabetes. Thereafter, the incidence decreases and reaches a very low level after 35 years of diabetes (Figs 13.2 and 13.3) [2, 3, 8]. The incidence is higher in males than in females [2] and higher in patients who develop diabetes before the age of 15 than after this age [9]. The majority of IDDM patients, however, do not develop clinical nephropathy, the cumulative incidence being 35% after 40 years of diabetes [2, 3]. The incidence of diabetic nephropathy seems to depend to some extent upon the quality of metabolic control [3]. Improved dia-

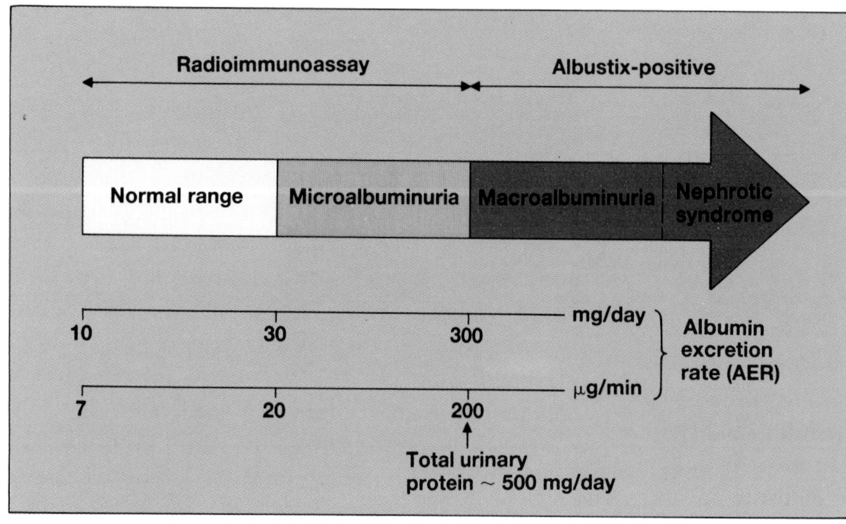


**Fig. 13.1.** Limits of normo-, micro- and macroalbuminuria.

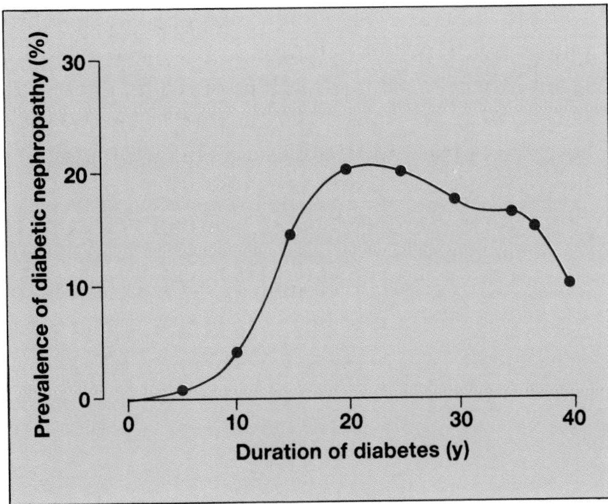


**Fig. 13.2.** Prevalence of diabetic nephropathy in IDDM. (Redrawn from [2].)

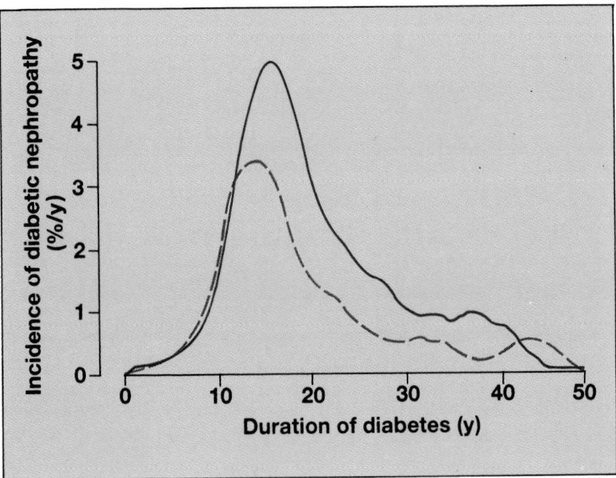


**Fig. 13.3.** Incidence of diabetic nephropathy in IDDM as a function of diabetes duration in women (blue), and men (red). (Redrawn from [8].)

betic care has been accompanied by and may have resulted in a 30% reduction in the incidence of diabetic nephropathy during the last 30 years [3, 9].

The epidemiology of diabetic nephropathy in NIDDM is less well-defined. The prevalence rates of clinical proteinuria reported in different studies vary from 3 to 16% [10, 11] and those of microalbuminuria from 15 to 59% [10, 12, 13]. The incidence of diabetic nephropathy in NIDDM is not known. The interval from the clinical onset of diabetes to the development of clinical nephropathy tends to be shorter in NIDDM than in IDDM, probably because the former may be present for some years before diagnosis.

## Natural history

The onset of persistent proteinuria is a late stage in a long-lasting process which in IDDM starts soon after the onset of diabetes. At this stage, when diabetes has been adequately controlled, urinary AER averages about 10 mg/day. In those patients who will later develop persistent proteinuria, AER increases at an exponential rate of about 20% per year (Fig. 13.4). This means that most of these patients will exceed the upper level of normoalbuminuria (about 30 mg/day) some 5 years after the onset of diabetes. Thereafter, AER continues to increase within the Albustix-negative, microalbuminuric range [14]. It must be appreciated that AER shows great variability and that repeated estimations may be required to characterize a given patient [15, 16]. AER also rises during exercise [17] in normoalbuminuric diabetic subjects and to a greater extent in those with microalbuminuria [18].

As discussed below, albuminuria is due to capillary lesions in the glomerulus and is a manifestation of widespread vascular damage. Patients with persistent microalbuminuria display other abnormalities, within and beyond the kidney. There is an increased urinary IgG excretion rate [19]. They also have a relatively raised blood pressure [20, 21] and the incidence of retinopathy is considerably increased [22]. Exchangeable sodium [23], LDL, VLDL, triglycerides and fibrinogen [24] are increased while serum albumin is decreased [23, 24]. The transcapillary escape rate

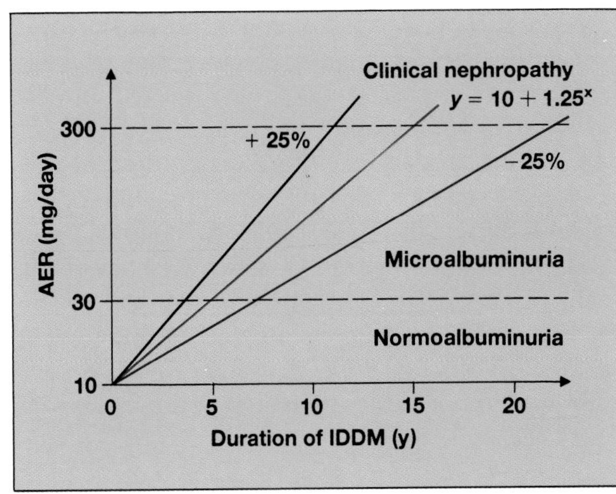


**Fig. 13.4.** Progression of microproteinuria and clinical nephropathy in IDDM, showing average rate and 25% confidence intervals for the increase in AER, plotted on a logarithmic scale. (Redrawn from [14].)

and the catabolic rate of fibrinogen and albumin are increased [25, 26]. In contrast to the glomerular defects, tubular function as assessed by urinary excretion of $\beta_2$-microglobulin or retinol-binding protein appears to be normal [19]. The cause of albuminuria is unknown but might be due to alterations in the metabolism of anionic compounds of the glomerular basement membrane (see Chapter 14).

### Evolution of changes in GFR

Glomerular filtration rate is significantly increased from the onset of IDDM [27, 28]. This 'hyperfiltration' is due to a combination of hyperperfusion (i.e. increased renal blood flow), glomerular hypertension and increased filtration surface area [29, 30]. Not only are individual glomeruli enlarged but overall kidney size is increased from the onset of IDDM [29, 31]. Glomerular hypertension and hyperperfusion probably play a role in the development of mesangial expansion. Hyperfiltrating IDDM patients seem to have a higher risk for development of clinical nephropathy than non-hyperfiltering normoalbuminuric diabetic patients [32–34]. The degree of hyperfiltration is considerably influenced by metabolic control and protein intake. As long as AER is normal, GFR remains elevated or normal in spite of long diabetes duration. In contrast to IDDM glomerular hyperfiltration and renal enlargement are less pronounced in NIDDM [35].

GFR starts to fall when AER is between 100 and 300 mg/day, at an average rate of about 10 ml/min/1.73 $m^2$ per year. This decline in GFR is caused by a reduction in the glomerular filtration surface area due to mesangial expansion [36]. Initially, mesangial expansion is compensated for by glomerular hypertrophy but in patients developing albuminuria, mesangial expansion becomes so marked that GFR cannot be maintained by this mechanism [37]. This results in an irreversible decline in GFR (Fig. 13.5). Once GFR is <50 ml/min/1.73 $m^2$, serum creatinine concentration begins to rise, and there is an inexorable decline towards end-stage renal failure at a rate which is quite constant for a given patient but highly variable between patients.

### Progression of hypertension

Blood pressure is normal or slightly elevated at the onset of IDDM and remains so in patients with

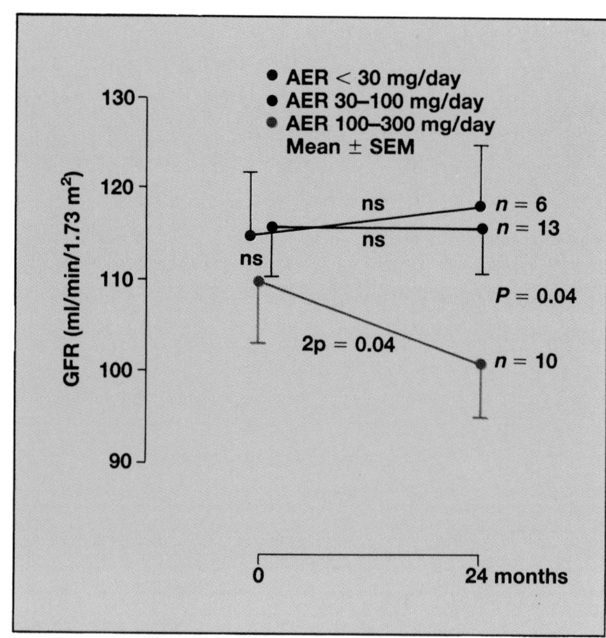


**Fig. 13.5.** GFR in IDDM. Patients who develop persistent albuminuria will demonstrate a decline in GFR after the onset of persistent microalbuminuria.

normal AER, despite chronic volume expansion and increased exchangeable sodium (see Chapter 18) [23]. In albuminuric patients, however, recent prospective studies have demonstrated that AER increases to about 50 mg/day before blood pressure begins to rise [21, 38]. The blood pressure increase in patients with persistent microalbuminuria seems to be of renal origin [23] and may be related to reduction in filtration capacity by mesangial expansion. Hypertension is associated with a further increase of extracellular sodium volume whereas plasma volume remains normal [23]. Plasma renin activity is low or normal and plasma aldosterone, angiotensin II and catecholamine concentrations are reduced [23].

### Prognosis of patients with albuminuria

Increased AER not only indicates renal disease, but reflects universal vascular damage affecting large and small vessels [39, 40]. In patients with persistent proteinuria, the incidence of coronary heart disease is significantly higher than in patients without proteinuria and their relative cardiovascular mortality is increased about ten-fold [40–43]. The incidence of proliferative retinopathy is also increased several-fold in proteinuric patients [22, 44, 45].

Without special care, about 50% of patients will die within 7 years of the onset of persistent proteinuria [2, 3]. The cause of death in these patients is not only uraemia but also cardiovascular diseases such as myocardial infarction, cardiac failure and cerebrovascular accidents [2, 43, 46, 47]. Among NIDDM patients with nephropathy, cardiovascular disease is the commonest cause of death, progression to end-stage renal failure being relatively unusual [48]. However, because NIDDM is more common than IDDM, nearly one-half of all diabetic patients receiving renal replacement therapy have NIDDM [48]. Indeed, most of the excess mortality among diabetic patients is associated with proteinuria [49]; those with normal AER have nearly normal survival. This consideration applies to both IDDM and NIDDM [12, 50, 51].

The prognosis of patients with incipient or established nephropathy can be altered by strict metabolic control and by effective antihypertensive therapy. Case-control studies have recently demonstrated that aggressive antihypertensive therapy can slow the rate of decline in GFR and postpone the onset of uraemia by many years [52]. Overall mortality is also reduced by such treatment [53, 54]. Furthermore the progression of incipient nephropathy to overt nephropathy can be halted by strict metabolic control and by keeping blood pressure below 140/90. The outlook for patients with diabetic nephropathy has therefore improved considerably in recent years.

## Conclusions and practical implications

Persistent albuminuria in diabetic patients not only indicates renal disease but also signifies generalized vascular damage and identifies those subjects at high risk of premature cardiovascular death [55]. However, the outcome of this condition is becoming less gloomy. The incidence of diabetic nephropathy has declined during recent years and this may be due to improved metabolic control; moreover, mortality in diabetic people with proteinuria can be reduced by effective antihypertensive therapy, which also retards the progression of nephropathy. These findings mean that the early identification of patients with incipient nephropathy (persistent microalbuminuria) is essential so that they can be offered appropriate therapy as soon as possible.

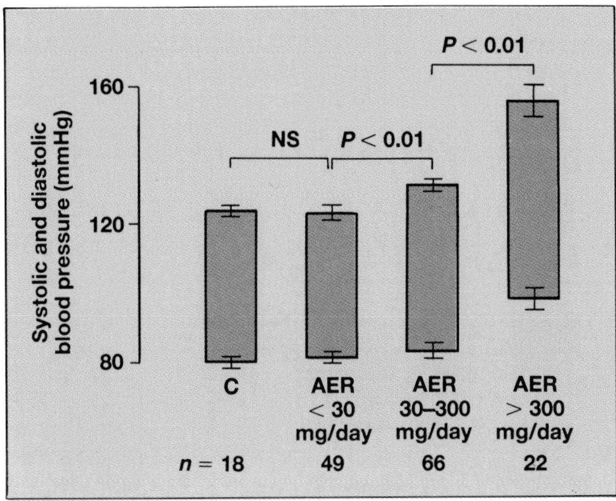


**Fig. 13.6.** Blood pressure among long-standing IDDM patients, showing progressively higher levels as AER increases. C: non-diabetic control population.

## Recent developments

Perhaps the most interesting development in this field has been the demonstration that electron microscopic measurements of glomerular basement membrane thickness and mesangial expansion in renal biopsies show good correlation with urinary albumin excretion rate, in normo- and microalbuminuric patients [56]. This represents a potential advance in the diagnosis of diabetic nephropathy, which in its early stages does not show any characteristic morphological changes on light microscopy. However, the subject remains controversial and the clinical implications of this are not yet clear; this topic is discussed further in Chapter 15.

TORSTEN DECKERT
KNUT BORCH-JOHNSEN
ANASUYA GRENFELL

## References

1 Thomsen AC. *The Kidney in Diabetes Mellitus*. PhD Thesis, Munksgaard, Copenhagen, 1965.
2 Andersen AR, Christiansen JS, Andersen JK, Kreiner S, Deckert T. Diabetic nephropathy in Type 1 (insulin-dependent) diabetes: An epidemiological study. *Diabetologia* 1983; **25**: 496–501.
3 Krolewski AS, Warram JH, Christleib AR *et al*. The changing natural history of nephropathy in type 1 diabetes. *Am J Med* 1985; **78**: 785–94.
4 Mauer SM, Steffes MW, Ellis EN, Sutherland DER, Brown DM, Goetz FC. Structural-functional relationship in diabetic nephropathy. *J Clin Invest* 1984; **74**: 1143–55.
5 Chavers BM, Bilous RW, Ellis EN, Steffes MW, Mauer SM. Glomerular lesions and urinary albumin excretion in type 1 diabetes without overt proteinuria. *N Engl J Med* 1989; **320**: 966–70.
6 Niazy S, Feldt-Rasmussen B, Deckert T. Microalbuminuria in insulin-dependent diabetes: Prevalence and practical consequences. *J Diabetic Compl* 1987: 76–80.

7 Parving H-H, Hommel E, Mathiesen E *et al*. Prevalence of microalbuminuria, arterial hypertension, retinopathy, and neuropathy in patients with insulin dependent diabetes. *Br Med J* 1986; **296**: 156–60.
8 Borch-Johnsen K, Andersen KP, Deckert T. The effect of proteinuria on relative mortality in Type 1 (insulin-dependent) diabetes mellitus. *Diabetologia* 1985; **28**: 590–6.
9 Kofoed-Enevoldsen A, Borch-Johnsen K, Kreiner S, Nerup J, Deckert T. Declining incidence of persistent proteinuria in type 1 (insulin-dependent) diabetic patients in Denmark. *Diabetes* 1987; **36**: 205–9.
10 Garancini P, Gallus G, Calori G *et al*. Microalbuminuria and its associated risk factors in a representative sample of Italian type II diabetics. *J Diabetic Compl* 1988; **2**: 12–15.
11 Fabré J, Balant LP, Dayer PG, Fox HM, Vernet AT. The kidney in maturity onset diabetes mellitus: A clinical study of 510 patients. *Kidney Int* 1982; **21**: 730–8.
12 Mogensen CE. Microalbuminuria predicts clinical proteinuria and early mortality in maturity onset diabetes. *N Engl J Med* 1984; **310**: 356–60.
13 Standl E, Rebell B, Steigler H *et al*. Prevalence and risk profile of incipient diabetic nephropathy in Type 2 (non-insulin dependent) diabetes mellitus. *Diabetologia* 1987; **30**: 584–5A.
14 Deckert T, Feldt-Rasmussen B, Borch-Johnsen K *et al*. Clinical assessment and prognosis of complications of diabetes. *Transplantation Proc* 1986; **18**: 1636–8.
15 Feldt-Rasmussen B, Mathiesen ER. Variability of urinary albumin excretion in incipient diabetic nephropathy. *Diabetic Nephropathy* 1984; **3**: 101–3.
16 Cohen DL, Close CF, Viberti GC. The variability of overnight urinary albumin excretion in insulin-dependent diabetic and normal subjects. *Diabetic Med* 1987; **4**: 437–40.
17 Viberti GC, Jarrett RJ, McCartney M, Keen H. Increased glomerular permeability to albumin induced by exercise in diabetic subjects. *Diabetologia* 1978; **14**: 293–300.
18 Feldt-Rasmussen B, Baker L, Deckert T. Exercise as a provocative test in early renal disease in Type 1 (insulin-dependent) diabetes: albuminuric, systemic, and renal haemodynamic responses. *Diabetologia* 1985; **28**: 389–96.
19 Deckert T, Feldt-Rasmussen B, Djurup R, Deckert M. Glomerular size and charge selectivity in insulin-dependent diabetes mellitus. *Kidney Int* 1988; **33**: 100–6.
20 Wiseman MJ, Viberti GC, Mackintosh D, Jarrett RJ, Keen H. Glycaemia, arterial pressure and microalbuminuria in Type 1 (insulin-dependent) diabetes mellitus. *Diabetologia* 1984; **26**: 401–5.
21 Mathiesen ER, Oxenbøll K, Johansen PAa, Svendsen PAå, Deckert T. Incipient nephropathy in Type 1 (insulin-dependent) diabetes. *Diabetologia* 1984; **26**: 406–10.
22 Barnett AH, Dallinger K, Jennings P *et al*. Microalbuminuria and diabetic retinopathy. *Lancet* 1985; **i**: 53–4.
23 Feldt-Rasmussen B, Mathiesen ER, Deckert T, Giese J, Christensen NJ, Bent-Hansen L, Nielsen MD. Central role for sodium in the pathogenesis of blood pressure changes independent of angiotensin, aldosterone and catecholamines in Type 1 (insulin-dependent) diabetes mellitus. *Diabetologia* 1987; **30**: 610–17.
24 Jensen T, Stender S, Deckert T. Abnormalities in plasma concentration of lipoproteins and fibrinogen in Type 1 (insulin-dependent) diabetic patients with increased urinary albumin excretion. *Diabetologia* 1988; **31**: 142–5.
25 Feldt-Rasmussen B. Increased transcapillary escape rate of albumin in Type 1 (insulin-dependent) diabetic patients with microalbuminuria. *Diabetologia* 1986; **29**: 282–6.
26 Bent-Hansen L, Deckert T. Metabolism of albumin and fibrinogen in type 1 (insulin-dependent) diabetes mellitus. *Diabetes Res* 1988; **7**: 159–64.
27 Christiansen JS, Gammelgaard J, Tronier B, Svendsen PA, Parving H-H. Kidney function and size in diabetics before and during initial insulin treatment. *Kidney Int* 1982; **21**: 683–8.
28 Wiseman MJ, Viberti GC, Keen H. Threshold effect of plasma glucose in the glomerular hyperfiltration of diabetes. *Nephron* 1984; **38**: 257–60.
29 Mogensen CE. Abnormal physiological processes in the kidney. In: Brownlee M, ed. *Handbook of Diabetes Mellitus*, 23–85. New York: Garland STMP Press, 1981.
30 Viberti GC, Wiseman MJ. The kidney in diabetes: significance of the early abnormalities. *Clin Endocrinol Metab* 1986; **15**: 753–82.
31 Wiseman MJ, Viberti GC. Glomerular filtration rate and kidney volume in Type 1 (insulin-dependent) diabetes mellitus revisited. *Diabetologia* 1982; **25**: 530.
32 Hostetter TH, Rennke HG, Brenner BM. The case for intrarenal hypertension in the initiation and progression of diabetic and other glomerulopathies. *Am J Med* 1982; **72**: 375–80.
33 Steffes MW, Brown DM, Mauer SM. Diabetic glomerulopathy following unilateral nephrectomy in the rat. *Diabetes* 1978; **27**: 35–41.
34 Mogensen CE. Early diabetic renal involvement and nephropathy. Can treatment modalities be predicted from identification of risk factors? *Diabetes Ann* 1987; **3**: 306–24.
35 Friedman EA, Sheih SD, Hirsch SR *et al*. No supranormal glomerular filtration (GFR) in type II (non-insulin-dependent) diabetes. *Am Soc Nephrol* 1981; **14**: 102A.
36 Ellis EN, Steffes MW, Goetz FC, Sutherland DER, Mauer SM. Glomerular filtration surface in type 1 diabetes mellitus. *Kidney Int* 1986; **29**: 889–94.
37 Østerby R, Gundersen HJG, Hørlyck A, Kroustrup JP, Nyberg G, Westberg G. Diabetic glomerulopathy. Structural characteristics of the early and advanced stages. *Diabetes* 1983; **32**: 79–82.
38 Mathiesen ER, Rønn B, Jensen T, Storm B, Deckert T. Relationship between blood pressure and urinary albumin excretion in development of microalbuminuria. *Diabetes* 1990; **39**: 245–9.
39 Gatling W, Mullee MA, Knight C, Hill RD. Microalbuminuria in diabetes. Relationship between urinary albumin excretion and diabetes related variables. *Diabetic Med* 1988; **5**: 348–51.
40 Jensen T, Borch-Johnsen K, Kofoed-Enevoldsen A, Deckert T. Coronary heart disease in young Type 1 (insulin-dependent) diabetic patients with and without diabetic nephropathy: Incidence and risk factors. *Diabetologia* 1987; **30**: 144–8.
41 Gonzalez-Carrillo M, Moloney A, Bewick M, Parsons V, Rudge CJ, Watkins PJ. Renal transplantation in diabetic nephropathy. *Br Med J* 1982; **285**: 1713–16.
42 Braun WE, Phillips DF, Vidt DG *et al*. Coronary artery disease in 100 diabetics with end stage renal failure. *Transplantation Proc* 1984; **16**: 603–7.
43 Borch-Johnsen K, Kreiner S. Proteinuria — a predictor of cardiovascular mortality in insulin dependent diabetes mellitus. *Br Med J* 1987; **294**: 1651–4.
44 Ramsay RC, Knobloch WH, Barbosa JJ, Sutherland DER, Kjellstrand CM, Najarian JS, Goetz FC. The visual status of diabetic patients after renal transplantation. *Am J Ophthalmol* 1979; **87**: 305–10.
45 Kofoed-Enevoldsen A, Jensen T, Borch-Johnsen K, Deckert T. Incidence of retinopathy in Type 1 (insulin-dependent)

diabetes: Association with clinical nephropathy. *J Diabetic Compl* 1987; **3**: 96–9.

46 Moloney A, Tunbridge WMG, Ireland JT, Watkins PJ. Mortality from diabetic nephropathy in the United Kingdom. *Diabetologia* 1983; **25**: 26–30.

47 Kussman MJ, Goldstein HH, Gleason RE. The clinical course of diabetic nephropathy. *J Am Med Ass* 1976; **236**: 1861–3.

48 Friedman EA. Diabetes with kidney failure. *Lancet* 1986; **i**: 1285.

49 Borch-Johnsen K, Andersen KP, Deckert T. The effect of proteinuria on relative mortality in Type 1 (insulin-dependent) diabetes mellitus. *Diabetologia* 1985; **28**: 590–6.

50 Schmitz A, Vaeth M. Microalbuminuria: A major risk factor in non-insulin-dependent diabetes. A 10-year follow-up study of 503 patients. *Diabetic Med* 1988; **5**: 126–34.

51 Jarrett RJ, Viberti GC, Argyropoulos A *et al.* Microalbuminuria predicts mortality in non-insulin dependent diabetes. *Diabetic Med* 1984; **1**: 17–19.

52 Parving H-H, Andersen AR, Smidt UM, Hommel E, Mathiesen ER, Svendsen PA. Effect of anti-hypertensive treatment on kidney function in diabetic nephropathy. *Br Med J* 1987; **294**: 1443–7.

53 Parving H-H, Hommel E. Prognosis in diabetic nephropathy. *Br Med J* 1989; **299**: 230–3.

54 Mathiesen ER, Borch-Johnsen K, Jensen DV, Deckert T. Improved survival in patients with diabetic nephropathy. *Diabetologia* 1989; **32**: 884–6.

55 Deckert T, Feldt-Rasmussen B, Borch-Johnsen K, Jensen T, Kofoed-Enevoldsen A. Albuminuria reflects widespread vascular damage. The Steno hypothesis. *Diabetologia* 1989; **32**: 219–26.

56 Walker JD, Close CL, Jones SL, Rafferty M, Keen H, Viberti GC, Østerby R. Glomerular structure in type 1 (insulin-dependent) diabetes with normo- and microalbuminuria. *Kidney Int* 1992; **41**: 741–8.

# 14 Aetiology and Pathogenesis of Diabetic Nephropathy: Clues from Early Functional Abnormalities


**Summary**

• Functional abnormalities which occur early in the natural history of diabetic nephropathy include microalbuminuria and glomerular hyperfiltration. These features may help to identify a subset of patients at risk of developing clinical nephropathy, defined by persistent proteinuria and a progressive decline in renal function.

• *Microalbuminuria* is a subclinical increase in urinary albumin excretion rate (AER) in the range 30–300 mg/day. This is below the detection threshold of conventional methods for measuring protein in urine and so is detectable only by highly sensitive techniques such as radioimmunoassay. Persistent albuminuria detectable by dip-stick methods corresponds to an AER of over 250–300 mg/day and is termed *macroalbuminuria* or *clinical albuminuria*.

• The ratio of albumin: creatinine concentrations in a first morning urine sample is a useful screening test: values exceeding 2.0 mg/mmol indicate microalbuminuria.

• Microalbuminuria is due to increased permeability of the glomerular capillaries, probably because of raised glomerular capillary pressure and loss of negative charge on the glomerular basement membrane. Clinical albuminuria develops with further loss of membrane charge and an increase in membrane pore size.

• IDDM subjects with microalbuminuria have a 20-fold greater risk of ultimately developing clinical nephropathy than those with normal albumin excretion. Microalbuminuria also predicts clinical nephropathy and increased mortality in NIDDM.

• Diabetic nephropathy is closely associated with hypertension. Arterial blood pressure is elevated (although usually below the conventional threshold defining hypertension) in patients with microalbuminuria. Hypertension accelerates the rates at which albuminuria increases and glomerular filtration rate declines.

• The tendency to develop nephropathy may be partly genetically determined, as cases tend to cluster within families. A genetic predisposition to hypertension is suggested by the finding of increased blood pressure in the parents of diabetic patients with nephropathy.

• Sodium–lithium countertransport activity in red blood cells — which reflects physiologically important cation exchange mechanisms — is increased in nephropathic patients and their parents; increased activity is a marker for essential hypertension.

• *Glomerular hyperfiltration* is an increase in glomerular filtration rate (GFR) above the normal range, which occurs early in 20–40% of IDDM patients. Possible causes of hyperfiltration include increased renal plasma flow and filtration surface area in the glomerulus. Hyperglycaemia and disturbances in the balance between vasodilating and vasoconstricting prostaglandins may contribute to hyperfiltration.

• The relationship of glomerular hyperfiltration to the subsequent development of clinical nephropathy is uncertain.

• Strict glycaemic control can reduce microalbuminuria and lower glomerular hyperfiltration into the normal range. Effective antihypertensive treatment and restriction of dietary protein intake (to 45 g/day) can both reduce urinary albumin excretion. Whether these interventions influence the ultimate progression to clinical nephropathy is not known.

The term *diabetic nephropathy* describes a clinical state in which there are persistent proteinuria and a progressive decline in renal function, accompanied by retinopathy and arterial hypertension. By definition, other causes of renal disease are excluded.

Diabetic nephropathy is a major diabetic complication whose impact varies considerably in different diabetic populations. Clinically progressive renal disease develops in approximately 30% of IDDM patients and in approximately 15% of NIDDM patients of European origin [1–3]. In IDDM, the incidence of nephropathy reaches a peak after about 15 years duration of diabetes. In NIDDM, the condition may be detected sooner after diagnosis and, although nephropathy is rarer than in IDDM, the larger number of patients with NIDDM results in the absolute numbers of patients with nephropathy being similar in both types of diabetes [2]. Nephropathy may be commoner in NIDDM subjects of certain ethnic origins, especially in Asian and Afro-Caribbean people resident in Britain [4–6], who accounted for 48% of all NIDDM patients receiving renal replacement therapy in a recent series from King's College Hospital in London [5]. On the other hand, the frequency of end-stage renal failure in the Pima Indians of Arizona, in whom NIDDM is particularly common, is similar to that in the general IDDM population in North America [7].

Diabetic nephropathy is therefore an important problem. Attempts to trace its genesis can be made by investigating the earliest functional abnormalities seen in diabetic patients and in animal models of diabetes. This may eventually enable us to identify a subset of diabetic subjects at special risk of developing nephropathy and help to target preventative and therapeutic measures.

## Microalbuminuria

Conventional methods for detecting protein in urine include the salicylsulphonic acid test and various acid–base colour-change indicators used in dip-stick methods such as Albustix. These methods are relatively insensitive and can reliably detect protein excretion rates in excess of about 250–300 mg/day. Albustix-positive proteinuria is termed *macroproteinuria*, or *clinical proteinuria*.

In 1963, a sensitive and specific radioimmunoassay was described which could detect human albumin at low concentrations in the urine [8]. This subclinical, Albustix-negative elevation in urinary albumin excretion has been termed *microalbuminuria*. The reported prevalence of microalbuminuria varies from 20% in a hospital clinic in Denmark to 5.7% in a community-based survey in England [9, 10].

### *Definition and measurement of microalbuminuria*

The albumin excretion rate (AER) in healthy, non-diabetic individuals ranges from 2.5 to 26.0 mg/day with a geometric mean of 9.5 mg/day; 92% of the values fall below 18 mg/day [11]. Albumin in these subjects represents 11% of total urinary protein. This range of AER is defined as *normoalbuminuria*. Albumin excretion rates of 30–300 mg/day are termed *microalbuminuria*, whereas persistent *macroalbuminuria* (Albustix-positive) corresponds to an AER exceeding 300 mg/day. Albumin in microalbuminuric patients represents about 22% of the total urinary protein and some 50% in patients with clinical proteinuria. These arbitrary terms of definition serve as a useful broad clinical classification (Table 14.1), although the cut-off levels separating the different categories very somewhat between centres.

Urinary albumin excretion in diabetic and non-diabetic subjects has an average day-to-day variation of 40–50% and is further influenced by urine flow, posture, exercise and diet [12–17]. It is higher during the day in the upright, ambulant position than at night in the recumbent position. In an attempt at standardization, the overnight urine collection has been suggested and adopted by many investigators [10, 18, 19]. Due to the wide intrinsic variation in AER, multiple collections are necessary in order to define accurately an individual's status; patients whose AER lies near one of the cut-off levels are likely to move into and out of different categories (Fig. 14.1).

Present evidence suggests that the albumin concentration in random urine samples has a linear relationship with the AER [19]. In order to improve precision in screening for an elevated AER, the urinary albumin : creatinine ratio (ACR) has been suggested [20–22]. An ACR of greater than 2.0 mg/mmol in a first morning urine sample has a sensitivity of 96% and a specificity of 100% for detecting an overnight AER of $>30\,\mu g/min$ [10].

Increasingly, clinical chemistry departments are able to offer routine urinary albumin concentration measurements as newer automated assays become more widely available [24]. Low concentrations of

**Table 14.1.** Characteristics of urinary albumin excretion in different phases of diabetic nephropathy. (a) Normoalbuminuria; (b) microalbuminuria; and (c) macroalbuminuria.

| | (a) | (b) | (c) |
|---|---|---|---|
| *AER*: | | | |
| mg/day | <30 | 30–300 | >300 |
| μg/min | <20 | 20–200 | >200 |
| *Albumin/total urinary protein* | 11% | 22% | 50% |
| *Albustix reaction* | – | – | + |

AER, albumin excretion rate.

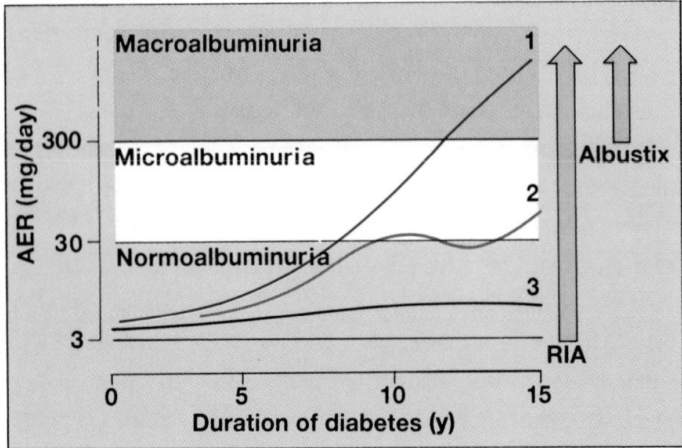


**Fig. 14.1.** Schematic time-courses of albumin excretion rate (AER) in IDDM patients, showing thresholds for normo-, micro- and macroalbuminuria and the detection limits of RIA and Albustix methods for measuring albumin concentrations in urine. About one-third of IDDM patients will ultimately develop clinical nephropathy with macroproteinuria (1). The remainder will stay within the microalbuminuric (2), or normoalbuminuric (3) ranges. Because of intrinsic variability in AER, individual subjects may move between one category and another.

urinary albumin can now be measured semi-quantitatively as a side-room test, e.g. Albusure (Cambridge Life Sciences) and Micro-bumintest (Ames). These sensitive, specific and rapid tests are suitable for screening purposes [20]. The latter is a modified protein-error-of-indicators method and detects albumin concentrations above about 40 μg/ml. Other methods under development include laser turbidometry.

### *The origins of microalbuminuria*

The barrier between the glomerular capillary and the urinary space of Bowman's capsule may be considered as a membrane perforated by pores of average size of 55 nm and coated with a negative electrical charge which is attributed to heparan sulphate and other proteoglycans [25]. Thus, both the size and charge of molecules will determine their passage across this membrane, in addition to the hydraulic and other dynamic forces controlling glomerular filtration. In early microalbuminuria, the clearances of albumin, a polyanion (pI 4.8, molecular weight 69 kDa) and IgG, a larger electrically neutral molecule (pI 7.5–7.8, molecular weight 160 kDa), are both increased. This is most likely to be due to an increase in the transglomerular pressure, which would favour increased filtration of proteins in general, irrespective of their charge [26]. As microalbuminuria increases, there is a disproportionate rise in albumin clearance and therefore a lower ratio of the clearances of IgG and albumin (the selectivity index). This may be due to loss of the electronegative glycosialoproteins and proteoglycans of the glomerular basement membrane, together with further haemodynamic abnormalities [26–28]. Subsequently, as the pore size enlarges, microalbuminuria progresses to macroalbuminuria and the GFR begins to decline as the glomerular filtration barrier loses its size-selectivity (Figs 14.2 and 14.3).

### *The prognostic significance of microalbuminuria*

Evidence is accumulating that microalbuminuria represents an early stage of diabetic renal disease which, in both IDDM and NIDDM, will tend to progress to clinically overt nephropathy (see Table 14.2). Three prospective studies in IDDM patients have identified a relationship between a raised AER and the subsequent development of clinical nephropathy [29–31]. IDDM subjects with an overnight or 24-h AER between 50 and 250 mg/day have a 20-fold greater risk of developing nephropathy than those with an AER below this level (Fig. 14.4) [29]. After initial stabilization of diabetes, microalbuminuria is found only rarely in the first 5 years of IDDM (see Fig. 14.1), suggesting that microalbuminuria may be a true sign of early disease rather than simply a marker of susceptibility [33].

In NIDDM patients, two studies have shown a raised AER to be associated with the later development of clinical proteinuria as well as increased mortality, especially from cardiovascular disease (Table 14.1) [3, 32]. The overall findings of these studies are remarkably similar and the different

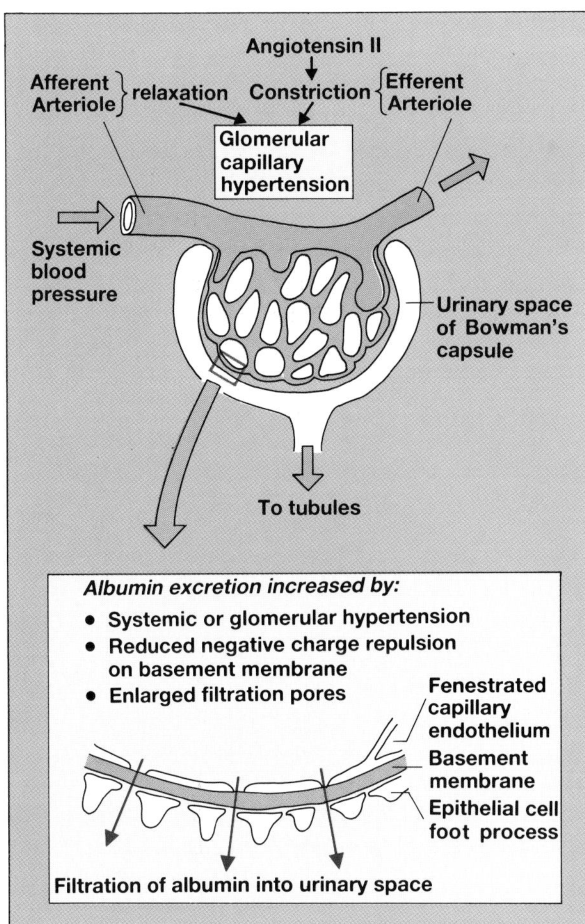


**Fig. 14.2.** Schematic diagram of glomerulus, indicating the main factors influencing excretion of albumin into the urine.

risk levels of AER quoted are likely to be due to different methods of urine collection and length of follow-up.

### *Concomitants of microalbuminuria*

The immediate causes of microalbuminuria are not known but a number of clinical and biochemical associations have been identified. These are summarized in Table 14.3.

#### BLOOD PRESSURE

The relationship between microalbuminuria and raised arterial blood pressure has aroused considerable interest. A positive, linear correlation exists between arterial pressure and AER [30, 34]. IDDM patients with microalbuminuria have mean systolic and diastolic blood pressures which are higher than those of a matched group of patients with normal AER, even though blood pressure generally remains within the 'normal' limits defined by WHO. As microalbuminuric patients have a normal or raised GFR (see below), it is improbable that the blood pressure elevation is simply a consequence of renal impairment. It is possible that hypertension *per se* causes microalbuminuria, which is found in non-diabetic hypertensive patients and is a predictor of cardio-

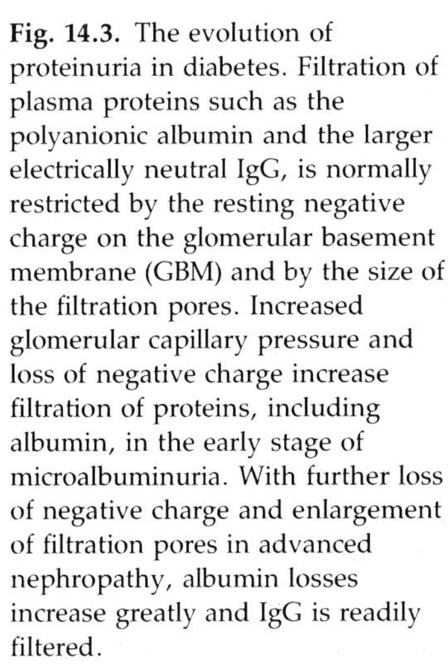

**Fig. 14.3.** The evolution of proteinuria in diabetes. Filtration of plasma proteins such as the polyanionic albumin and the larger electrically neutral IgG, is normally restricted by the resting negative charge on the glomerular basement membrane (GBM) and by the size of the filtration pores. Increased glomerular capillary pressure and loss of negative charge increase filtration of proteins, including albumin, in the early stage of microalbuminuria. With further loss of negative charge and enlargement of filtration pores in advanced nephropathy, albumin losses increase greatly and IgG is readily filtered.

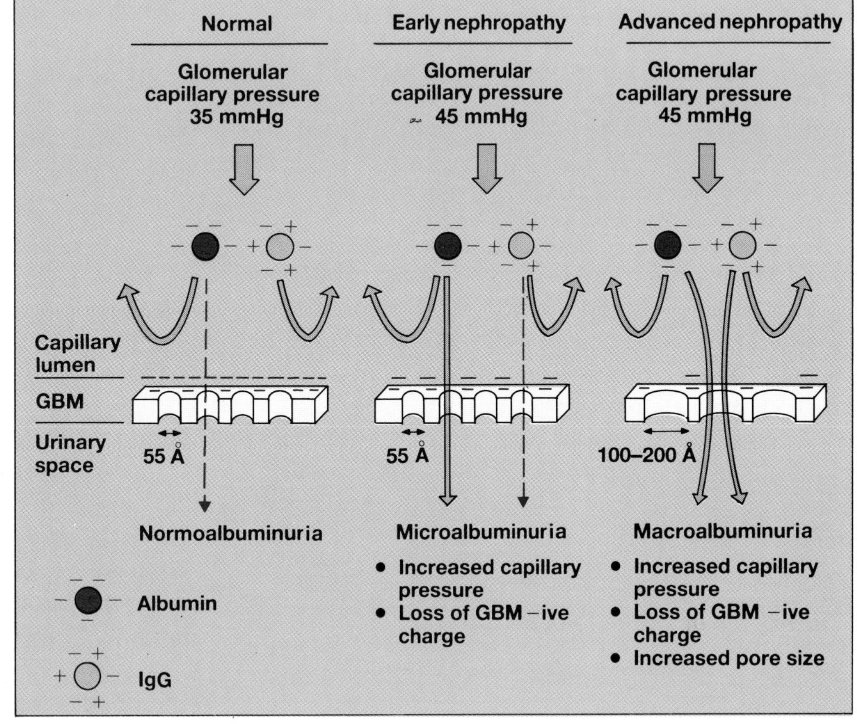

**Table 14.2.** Values of urinary albumin excretion (microalbuminuria) which predict the development of clinical nephropathy and/or mortality in diabetic patients.

| Group | Type of diabetes | Predictive AER level | Urine collection method | Duration of follow-up (y) | Reference |
|---|---|---|---|---|---|
| Guy's Hospital | IDDM | 30 μg/min | Overnight | 14 | 29 |
| Steno | IDDM | 70 μg/min | 24 h | 6 | 30 |
| Aarhus | IDDM | 15 μg/min | 1–2 h | 6–14 | 31 |
| Guy's Hospital | NIDDM | 10 μg/min* | Overnight | 14 | 32 |
| Aarhus | NIDDM | 30 μg/ml | Morning | 10 | 3 |

Note the different units for AER used by the Aarhus group [3].
* Predictive of increased mortality, predominantly from cardiovascular disease.

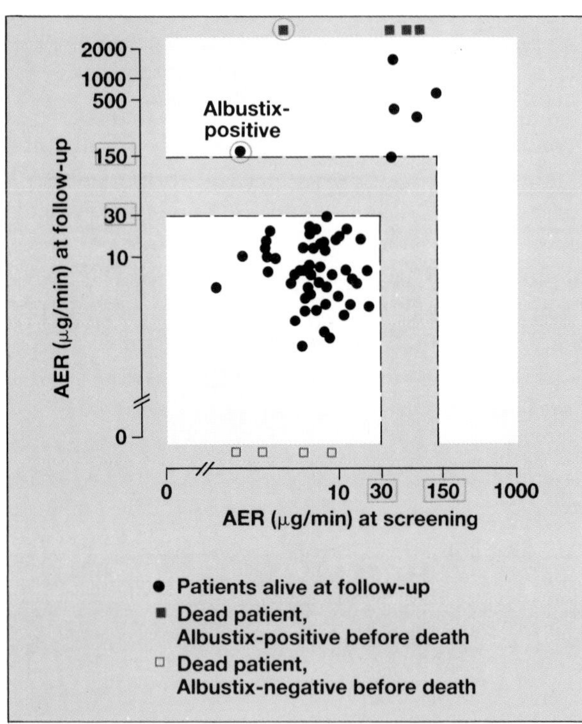


**Fig. 14.4.** Outcome in 63 IDDM patients with different levels of microalbuminuria at presentation, 55 of whom were followed up 14 years later. Only two cases with AER <30 μg/min at screening had developed Albustix-positive proteinuria (ringed symbols), whereas seven out of the eight with initial AER >30 μg/min had become clinically proteinuric. The outer shaded area shows the threshold for Albustix-positivity and the inner segregates the patients who did not progress. (Redrawn from [29] with kind permission.)

vascular disease in these subjects. An alternative hypothesis is that hypertension and microalbuminuria share a common determinant, which may be genetic. Recent evidence supports this possibility.

### *Possible genetic factors*

The tendency to hypertension in nephropathic patients may be partly inherited, as after careful matching for age, sex and body mass index, blood pressure was found to be higher in the parents of IDDM patients with proteinuria than in the parents of non-proteinuric patients (Fig. 14.5) [35]. There was also a correlation between blood pressure in the proteinuric IDDM patients and their parents. The clustering of cases of diabetic nephropathy within families is further evidence of a genetic predisposition in at least a proportion of patients [36, 37].

The activity of cation-exchange pumps in cell membranes, which are essential to many metabolic processes including electrolyte homeostasis may also be partly inherited. The pump most accessible to study is the sodium–lithium countertransport mechanism in red blood cell membranes. This is thought to reflect the physiological sodium–hydrogen ion antiporter, found in all cells, which regulates physiological functions such as cell growth and is also thought to be important in determining sodium reabsorption from the proximal renal tubular cell. It is apparently a marker for essential hypertension [38]. Sodium–lithium countertransport activity aggregates in families and is largely genetically determined, even though a number of environmental factors may further affect it [39–41].

Two recent studies [42, 43] have demonstrated that red-cell sodium–lithium countertransport activity is increased in IDDM patients with either macroproteinuria or microproteinuria (see Fig. 14.6). Moreover, direct measurements of the sodium–hydrogen ion antiporter in fibroblasts have shown increased activity and enhanced cell growth in nephropathic IDDM patients as com-

**Table 14.3.** Concomitants of microalbuminuria in IDDM.

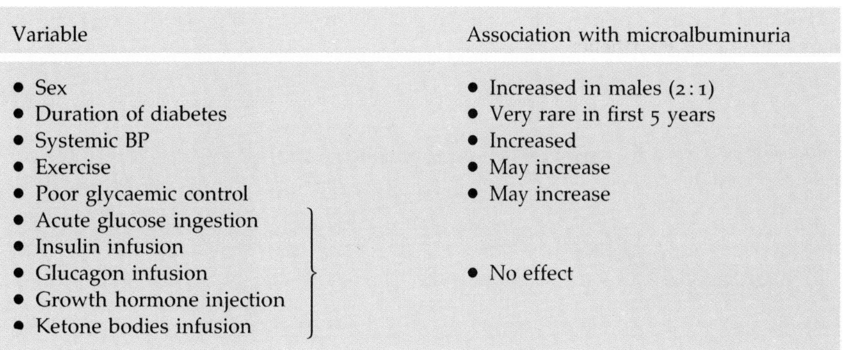

| Variable | Association with microalbuminuria |
|---|---|
| • Sex | • Increased in males (2:1) |
| • Duration of diabetes | • Very rare in first 5 years |
| • Systemic BP | • Increased |
| • Exercise | • May increase |
| • Poor glycaemic control | • May increase |
| • Acute glucose ingestion | |
| • Insulin infusion | |
| • Glucagon infusion | • No effect |
| • Growth hormone injection | |
| • Ketone bodies infusion | |

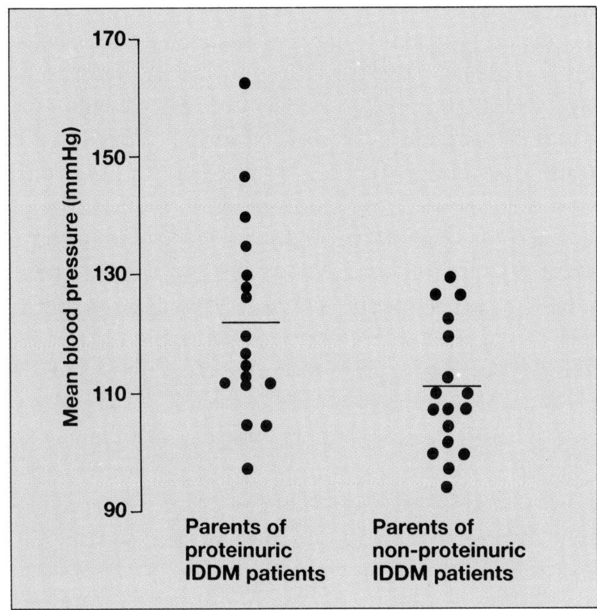


**Fig. 14.5.** Mean arterial blood pressure in the parents of proteinuric and non-proteinuric IDDM patients who were matched for age, sex and duration of diabetes. (Redrawn from [35], with permission of the Editor.)

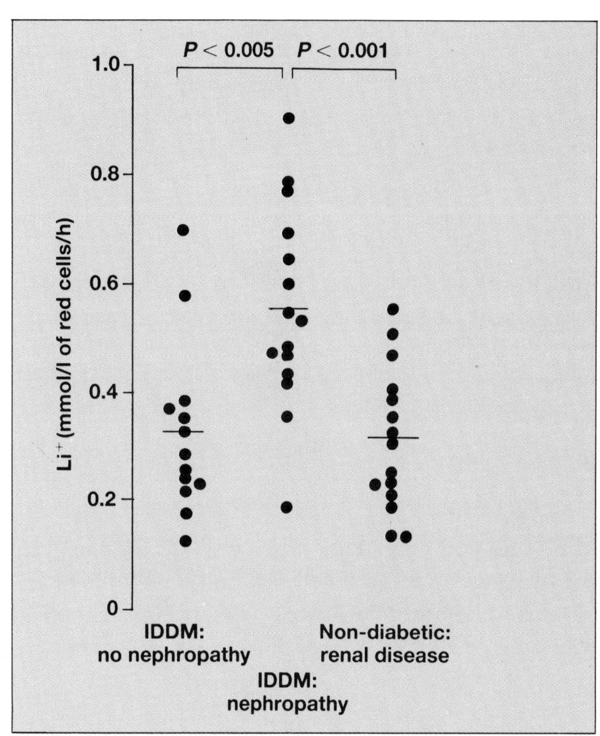


**Fig. 14.6.** Sodium–lithium countertransport activity in red blood cells of IDDM patients with nephropathy, compared with non-nephropathic IDDM patients and with non-diabetic subjects with other renal diseases. (Redrawn from [43], with kind permission of the Editor of the *New England Journal of Medicine*.)

pared with matched, normoalbuminuric control subjects [44]. Increased activity of this pump could be involved in the pathogenesis of diabetic nephropathy and may partly explain certain abnormalities, such as increased exchangeable sodium, previously demonstrated in IDDM patients with nephropathy [45].

As with hypertension, increased cation countertransport activity may be partly inherited. Red blood cell sodium–lithium countertransport activity in the parents of IDDM patients with proteinuria has been found to be greater than in parents of IDDM patients with normoalbuminuria [46]. Furthermore, there is a significant correlation in countertransport activity between parents and offspring. A familial element therefore contributes to the elevation of the sodium–lithium countertransport activity seen in diabetic nephropathy. Prospective studies in normo- and microalbuminuric patients with increased activities are needed to clarify the specificity and sensitivity of this possible genetic marker.

## Glomerular hyperfiltration

Abnormalities in GFR may precede microalbuminuria and may therefore be an even earlier indicator of diabetic renal disease. The theory that the GFR may be elevated in diabetes was first advanced in 1934 and current accurate measurements have shown that GFR is increased on average by 20–40% in children or adults with IDDM, compared with matched non-diabetic subjects (see Fig. 14.7) [47–49]. This abnormal increase in GFR is termed 'hyperfiltration'. Approximately 25% of insulin-dependent patients have a GFR exceeding the normal non-diabetic range (84–135 ml/min/1.73 $m^2$) and even those with a GFR within the normal range may have a higher value than would be predicted if they were not diabetic [50].

### *Factors leading to glomerular hyperfiltration*

GFR has four main determinants — renal plasma flow, glomerular transcapillary hydraulic pressure, afferent capillary oncotic pressure, and filtration surface area — which theoretically could contribute to hyperfiltration.

#### RENAL PLASMA FLOW (RPF)

RPF has been reported to be elevated in diabetes but in studies where both GFR and RPF have been measured simultaneously, the rise in RPF accounted for only 50–60% of that in GFR [50–52]. The finding of an increased filtration fraction (i.e. GFR/RPF) in IDDM has been taken to suggest that intraglomerular pressure may be elevated [53]. This proposition is supported by some, but not all, micropuncture studies in moderately hyperglycaemic diabetic rats which demonstrate an increase in the transglomerular pressure gradient [54–56]. This appears to be mediated by a reduction in total arteriolar resistance which is more marked at the afferent than efferent end of the arteriole [55]. In human diabetic subjects with glomerular hyperfiltration, a similar alteration in intraglomerular haemodynamics is indirectly suggested by the finding of a reduced renal vascular resistance [58]. Intraglomerular hypertension can be reduced and prevented, at least in diabetic rats, by angiotensin-converting enzyme (ACE) inhibitors. These may act by relaxing the efferent arterioles which are thought to be particularly sensitive to the vasoconstrictor action of angiotensin II. As discussed below, ACE inhibitors have been the subject of several clinical trials in diabetic patients at various stages of nephropathy [58].

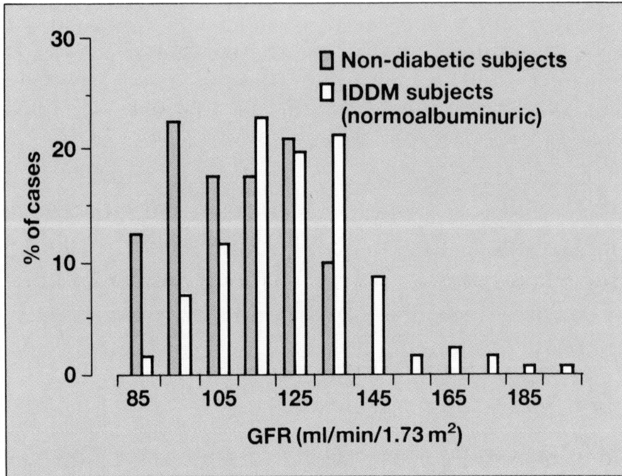


**Fig. 14.7.** Frequency histogram showing GFR in normoalbuminuric IDDM subjects and in age-matched non-diabetic controls (S.L. Jones, unpublished data).

#### OTHER FACTORS

Oncotic pressure is thought to be normal in diabetes. This suggests that increased intracapillary pressure accounts for a further proportion of the rise in GFR.

*Filtration surface area* is increased in IDDM patients in proportion to the rise in GFR [60, 61]. The kidneys may be enlarged in diabetic patients and in animal models of diabetes, mainly through increased glomerular volume. Renal volume is also related to various other determinants of the GFR [52, 61].

Overall, the elevated GFR found in some diabetic patients is probably mediated by a combination of structural and functional changes. The relative contributions of these, and the extent to which they may vary between individuals, remain to be established [59, 60].

### *Possible metabolic and endocrine determinants of hyperfiltration*

The principal metabolic and endocrine factors implicated in hyperfiltration are shown in Table 14.4.

**Table 14.4.** Possible metabolic and endocrine mediators of glomerular hyperfiltration.

| Mediator | Increase in GFR when administered experimentally | Comment |
|---|---|---|
| Glucose | 5–13% | • Only with moderate hyperglycaemia<br>• Threshold level of 14–16 mmol/l<br>• Effect more marked in hyperfiltering subjects |
| Ketone bodies | Up to 48% | • High physiological or pharmacological doses required |
| Glucagon | 6% | • Supraphysiological levels required |
| Growth hormone | 7% | • Requires several days of administration |
| Insulin | — | • Trivial effect at levels tested |
| Prostaglandins | ? | • Elevation of 6-keto $PGF_{1\alpha}$ associated with hyperfiltration |
| Renin–angiotensin axis | ? | • Controversial (see text) |
| Atrial natriuretic peptide | ? | • Controversial. Possibly higher in hyperfiltration |

### GLYCAEMIC CONTROL

Hyperfiltration only occurs under conditions of moderate hyperglycaemia (>14 mmol/l). Diabetic patients with glomerular hyperfiltration show a further increase in GFR (by 10–15%) following an intravenous glucose challenge [53, 62]; this response does not occur in subjects with a normal GFR. Acute reduction of blood glucose levels by insulin infusion reduces the GFR within 30–60 min, but only by about 5% [63].

### PROSTAGLANDINS

Prostaglandins affect many aspects of renal function and have a possible role in causing glomerular hyperfiltration. A recent study has found increased urinary excretion of 6-keto $PGF_{1\alpha}$ (a vasodilator prostaglandin derivative of vascular, possibly glomerular, origin) in hyperfiltering IDDM patients as compared with matched subjects whose GFR was normal. Urinary levels of $PGE_2$ (another vasodilator compound) and of thromboxane $B_2$ (a vasoconstrictor) were comparable in both diabetic groups and in non-diabetic subjects [64]. Another study found increased urinary excretion of both 6-keto $PGF_{1\alpha}$ and of $PGE_2$ in IDDM subjects [65]. Short-term improvements in blood glucose control which produce small reductions in GFR are accompanied by decreased urinary excretion of 6-keto $PGF_{1\alpha}$ and of $PGE_2$ [65, 66]. These findings suggest an imbalance between the vasodilating and vasoconstricting prostaglandins which could account for, or contribute towards, the hyperfiltration of diabetes.

### RENIN–ANGIOTENSIN–ALDOSTERONE AXIS

The renin–angiotensin–aldosterone axis has also been investigated as a possible mediator of glomerular hyperfiltration but conflicting results have so far been obtained, with either small elevations or decreases in plasma renin activity being described in hyperfiltering patients [67, 68].

## *The prognostic significance of renal haemodynamic changes*

Glomerular haemodynamic disturbances apparently influence the development of glomerular pathology in experimental models of diabetes [69]. In humans, the situation is less clear. Three studies, one retrospective [31] and two prospective, have attempted to address this question. Mogensen and colleagues [31] reported that patients with glomerular filtration showed a faster fall in GFR and that more progressed to clinical nephropathy than those whose GFR was initially normal. However, this finding may be difficult to interpret as some of the hyperfiltering patients also had microalbuminuria. The other two studies attempted to remove this confounding factor by investigating hyperfiltering patients with normal albumin excretion. In a 5-year prospective study, patients with glomerular hyperfiltration at the outset showed a faster fall in GFR than a matched group with initially normal GFR, although the number progressing to nephropathy (defined as the development of microalbuminuria) was not increased in the hyperfiltering group (S.L. Jones, unpublished observations). A recent 18-year follow-up study has also found no association between early glomerular hyperfiltration and follow-up AER [70].

On balance, glomerular hyperfiltration alone and in the absence of microalbuminuria does not appear at present to predict the later development of nephropathy.

## Correction of early renal abnormalities: implications for the prevention and treatment of diabetic nephropathy

A number of studies attempting to correct microalbuminuria and glomerular hyperfiltration have helped to clarify the pathophysiological basis of these abnormalities and have highlighted the possible benefits of treatment at these early stages of nephropathy. Several strategies have been investigated.

### *Improved glycaemic control*

Strict glycaemic control can reduce or normalize both microalbuminuria and glomerular hyperfiltration [71–73]. A 2-year randomized prospective study of patients with persistently elevated AER (30–300 mg/day) showed that improved metabolic control prevented a further rise in AER and the development of clinical proteinuria, but failed to lower albumin excretion [72]. A 4-year study involving patients with AER in the high normoalbuminuric range showed that a group treated with continuous subcutaneous insulin infusion (CSII) and obtaining a significant reduction in $HbA_1$ levels compared with a conventionally treated control group, reduced their AER during the treatment period. A group treated with multiple daily injections, achieving an $HbA_1$ level intermediate between the CSII group and the conventionally treated group, showed no reduction in AER, as was the case in the conventionally treated group [73]. The long-term significance of these results is still unclear but these preliminary findings suggest that strict glycaemic control may arrest or even reverse 'established' microalbuminuria and high-normal levels of albumin excretion.

The effects of improved glycaemic control on kidney size are less clear-cut. A reduction in renal volume has been reported after 3 months of insulin therapy and improved control in newly diagnosed IDDM subjects [74]. In another study, however, 6 months of improved glycaemic control had no effect on kidney volume in a group of hyperfiltering IDDM subjects, despite a reduction in GFR [75].

### *Antihypertensive treatment*

The close clinical association between hypertension and diabetic nephropathy is described in Chapter 16, and the possible pathogenic effects of hypertension within the glomerulus have been discussed above. There is considerable debate as to whether hypertension precedes microalbuminuria or vice versa and therefore as to which is likely to be the prime mover [76–78].

Whatever the basis of the relationship, there is now no doubt that effective antihypertensive treatment can retard the progression of established nephropathy [79, 80], and recent studies have suggested similar benefits in the microalbuminuric stage. Various drugs have been used. In initial long-term studies, marginal blood pressure elevations in microalbuminuric patients were treated with diuretics and β-blockers, and a reversal in the steady increase in AER through the microalbuminuric range was seen (Fig. 14.8) [81]. Recently, attention has focused on the ACE inhibitors, largely because of their beneficial effects in reducing both intraglomerular hypertension and proteinuria in streptozotocin-diabetic rats [58]. In diabetic patients with various degrees of clinical nephropathy and macroproteinuria, ACE inhibitors reduced blood pressure, decreased urinary protein losses and slowed the rate of fall of GFR [80, 82, 83]. ACE inhibitors may also have ben-

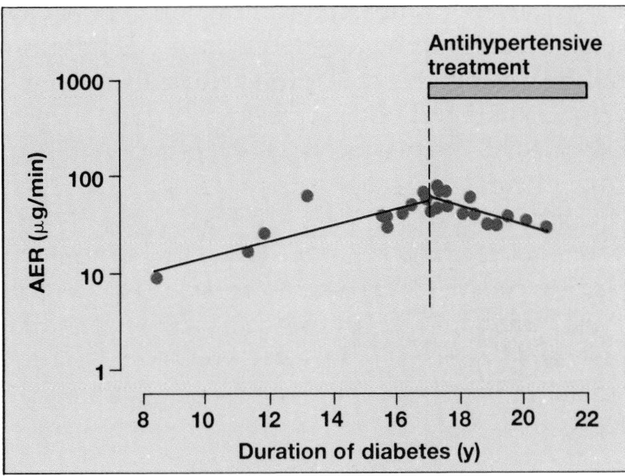


**Fig. 14.8.** Effect of antihypertensive treatment in reversing the steady increase in AER in an IDDM patient with microalbuminuria. (Redrawn from [81] with kind permission of the Editor of the *Journal of Diabetic Complications*.)

eficial effects in microalbuminuric patients, even when blood pressure is still below the accepted threshold for hypertension. In a small controlled trial, normotensive IDDM patients with microalbuminuria treated with enalapril showed a fall in AER and their blood pressure remained stable. By contrast, both AER and blood pressure rose in the untreated control group [84]. A reduction in the filtration fraction and fractional clearance of albumin in this study may suggest that these agents reduce intraglomerular pressure as well as systemic pressure, as in the animal model. However, the failure of enalapril to alter either GFR or RPF in a group of children with glomerular hyperfiltration, normal blood pressure and normal albumin excretion, may argue against this mechanism [85].

### *Dietary protein restriction*

Intake of dietary protein has been found to influence renal haemodynamics and filtration selectivity. Short-term (3-week) controlled studies in diabetic patients have shown that a diet restricted to 45 g of protein per day can significantly reduce microalbuminuria and GFR independently of changes in blood glucose concentration or blood pressure (Fig. 14.9) [17, 86]. These findings complement studies in diabetic animals, in which dietary protein restriction protects the kidney against hyperfiltration, intraglomerular hypertension, albuminuria and the subsequent development of histological lesions [69].

### *Other agents*

Preliminary reports have suggested that aldose reductase inhibitors given to diabetic rats cause a reduction in proteinuria [87]; results of controlled trials of these agents in man are awaited [88]. The recent discovery that the long-term deleterious effects of excessive glycosylation of structural membrane proteins may be prevented or even reversed by the administration of aminoguanidine (Chapter 3) opens up the possibility of influencing the biochemical steps which are thought responsible, at least in part, for the tissue damage of diabetes [89].

## Screening for diabetic nephropathy

From the preceding discussion, it is clear that microalbuminuria is, at present, the most reliable indicator of early diabetic renal disease. In view of the preliminary studies suggesting that certain interventions can reduce AER and thus potentially delay, prevent or even reverse established diabetic nephropathy, screening for microalbuminuria is of considerable value.

For screening purposes, measurement of the urinary albumin concentration or albumin : creatinine ratio in the first morning urine sample is sufficient. This should ideally be carried out annually after 5 years of diabetes in IDDM patients (or sooner, if hypertension or retinopathy develop), and from the time of diagnosis in NIDDM patients. An albumin concentration exceeding 15 mg/l or an ACR of >2 mg/mmol should prompt timed overnight urine collections (probably at least three) and appropriate investigations should be carried out to exclude other causes of proteinuria, such as urinary tract infection and cardiac failure. As mentioned above, microalbuminuria has been defined by several criteria; our working definition is an AER of greater than 30 mg/day in least two out of three timed overnight collections. If persistent microalbuminuria is confirmed in a given patient, the following options are available to the clinician:

### *Glycaemic control*

On the basis of present evidence, this should be optimized as far as possible.

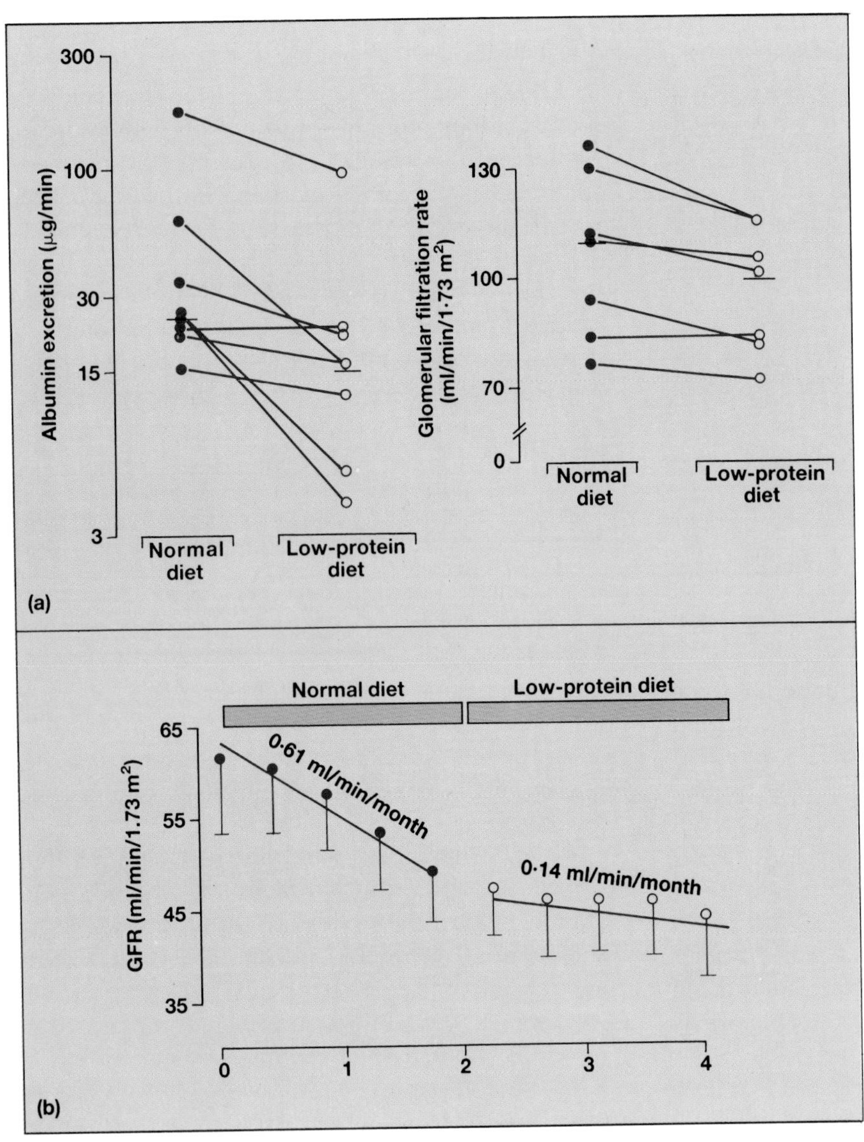


**Fig. 14.9.** (a) Effects of dietary protein restriction in microalbuminuric patients, showing falls in both albumin excretion rate and in GFR. (Redrawn from [17] with kind permission of the Editor.) In proteinuric IDDM patients, (b), a low-protein diet significantly reduced AER (not shown) and significantly slowed the rate of decline in GFR. (Redrawn from [86] with kind permission of the Editor).

### *Blood pressure control*

Centile charts of blood pressure (see Fig. 14.4) [90] may help to decide whether an individual has an acceptable blood pressure for his or her age. At present, there are no specific guidelines but the WHO criteria for the definition of hypertension are probably inadequate, given that many diabetic patients with microalbuminuria are young; the normal age- and sex-adjusted blood pressure may therefore be the appropriate treatment target. As discussed above, preliminary data suggest that ACE inhibitors reduce both blood pressure and AER and therefore may be of particular value in these patients. Treatment of hypertension is discussed further in Chapters 16 and 18.

### *Dietary protein*

A reduction in dietary protein intake can effectively reduce AER in microalbuminuric diabetic patients, but the diet is unpalatable to many people and unlikely to meet with compliance.

### *Reducing other cardiovascular risk factors*

Proteinuria is clearly the renal manifestation of a disease process affecting the entire vascular bed and is associated with both microvascular disease in other organs and macrovascular disease. The association with the latter, which may be attributable to lipid abnormalities, accounts for the fact that the additional mortality due to cardiovascular disease in diabetic patients is virtually confined to patients with proteinuria [91, 92, 93]. These patients must therefore be carefully screened for coronary heart and peripheral vascular disease, which may be significant but often remain subclinical. Other risk factors — particularly smoking and lipid abnormalities which may be exacerbated by certain antihypertensive drugs — must be identified and treated as vigorously as possible.

### *Management of established clinical nephropathy*

This is dealt with in detail in Chapter 16. The aim in this late phase is to retard the rate of decline of renal function. To date, the only therapies which are clearly established to slow the rate of decline in renal function are treatment of blood pressure and reduction in dietary protein intake.

## Conclusions

The last few years have witnessed a steady broadening of our understanding of the events leading to diabetic nephropathy and, with this, the growing conviction that early identification and treatment may help to slow, prevent or even reverse the disease process. The increasing availability of simple screening tests for microalbuminuria will allow this hypothesis to be tested on a large scale in the next few years.

## Recent developments

New insights into the predisposition to and the mechanisms of diabetic renal disease, and possibly the attendant cardiovascular disease, has come from recent studies of families and of cell-membrane cation transport systems. Earle *et al.* have recently demonstrated that, among patients with IDDM, a parental history of cardiovascular disease was associated with a 3-fold increased risk of developing nephropathy. Moreover, among the diabetic patients with nephropathy, those who had had a cardiovascular event were 6.2 times more likely to have a positive family history of cardiovascular disease than those who had not had such an event [94].

Rates of red cell sodium–lithium countertransport, a system in which the activity is largely genetically determined and which is associated with an increased risk of essential hypertension [95, 96], have been found to be higher in proteinuric diabetic patients and their parents than in matched, long-term normoalbuminuric controls [97–99]. The risk of nephropathy seems to be magnified by the combination of a previous history of poor glycaemic control and the possession of a high sodium–lithium countertransport [97]. Microalbuminuric diabetic patients, a group at increased risk of overt nephropathy, have also been found to have higher rates of sodium–lithium countertransport [100]. A relationship has been described between plasma lipoprotein levels and sodium–lithium countertransport activity in IDDM patients without persistent clinical proteinuria. Higher rates of sodium–lithium countertransport were associated with elevated LDL cholesterol, total and VLDL triglycerides and with reduced $HDL_2$ cholesterol concentrations [101]. The mechanisms of the association between sodium–lithium countertransport activity, hypertension and lipid abnormalities, in the context of susceptibility to diabetic renal and vascular disease, could be related to factors involved in the control of insulin sensitivity [102]. In a study of short-term, non-clinically-proteinuric diabetic patients with arterial hypertension (blood pressure greater than 140/90 mmHg), the hypertensive patients with higher rates of sodium–lithium countertransport were more insulin resistant, and had higher albumin excretion rates, increased total-body exchangeable sodium, enlarged kidneys and left ventricular hypertrophy [103]. These associations were independent of the actual level of blood pressure or the duration of arterial hypertension. These findings suggest that it is the diabetic hypertensive patient with high sodium–lithium countertransport who displays those features (albuminuria, left ventricular and renal hypertrophy, and insulin resistance) that have been related to renal and vascular injury [104–107]. The association between insulin resistance and elevated sodium–lithium countertransport seems to precede even the development of microalbuminuria and raised blood pressure, as has recently been described in normotensive, normoalbuminuric patients [108]. This combination of risk factors may not be confined to the diabetic population but may be a manifestation of a syndrome also described in the general population [109].

Sodium–lithium countertransport has close similarity with the physiological sodium–hydrogen antiport, a system crucial in the control of intracellular pH, cell growth and the renal reabsorption of sodium, and thus in the regulation of blood pressure [110]. Recently, leukocytes and cultured skin fibroblasts from IDDM patients with albuminuria have been reported to have elevated sodium–hydrogen antiport activity [111, 112]. Moreover, an increased [$^3$H]thymidine incorporation into DNA of skin fibroblasts of diabetic patients with nephropathy has been documented [111]. These findings are consistent with the view that cells of diabetic patients who develop nephropathy have an intrinsically-enhanced growth capacity and that this phenomenon is associated with high rates of sodium–hydrogen exchanger activity. Thus the activity of the sodium–hydrogen antiport seems to act as an indicator of some mechanism, possibly genetically determined, controlling cell growth and hypertrophy on the one hand, and intracellular sodium homeostasis on the other. The environmental changes brought about by diabetes could lead to dysregulation of these mechanisms in susceptible individuals, and induce cell hypertrophy and hyperplasia, contributing in the kidney to glomerular hypertrophy and mesangial expansion, as well as tubular hypertrophy and hyperplasia. An increased renal sodium reabsorption would augment systemic and renal perfusion pressure so as to maintain sodium balance. The increased perfusion pressure would be readily transmitted to the glomerular capillaries because of the general vasodilation present in diabetes [113]. This would be expected to lead to increased intraglomerular pressure which determines, at least in part, the increase in GFR, and may be responsible for the disruption of glomerular membrane permeability, thus generating proteinuria.

That early rises in arterial pressure are critical in the process leading to nephropathy, together with prior glycaemic control, has been recently confirmed by prospective studies in normoalbuminuric patients with both IDDM and NIDDM. In all these studies, the normoalbuminuric patients who progressed to microalbuminuria displayed higher values of initial blood pressure, albeit within the normal range, than those patients who remained normoalbuminuric over several years. Arterial pressure remained higher throughout the observation period and emerged as a significant independent determinant of microalbuminuria [114–116]. The crucial role of blood pressure has been further underscored by recent controlled, randomized trials of angiotensin-converting enzyme inhibitors (ACEI) in IDDM patients with microalbuminuria but without hypertension. Administration of an ACEI not only lowered albumin excretion rate but significantly prevented the development of persistent proteinuria and overt nephropathy. These effects appeared independent of changes in blood glucose control and other factors, such as protein intake, which could potentially affect the evolution of diabetic renal disease [117].

JAMES D. WALKER
GIAN CARLO VIBERTI

## References


1 Andersen AR, Sandahl Christiansen J, Andersen JK, Kreiner S, Deckert T. Diabetic nephropathy in Type 1 (insulin-dependent) diabetes. An epidemiological study. *Diabetologia* 1983; **25**: 496–501.
2 Rettig B, Teutsch SM. The incidence of end-stage renal disease in type I and type II diabetes mellitus. *Diabetic Nephropathy* 1984; **3**: 26–7.
3 Mogensen CE. Microalbuminuria predicts clinical proteinuria and early mortality in maturity-onset diabetes. *N Engl J Med* 1984; **310–356**: 356–60.
4 Grenfell A, Bewick M, Parsons V, Snowden S, Taube D, Watkins PJ. Non-insulin dependent diabetes and renal replacement therapy. *Diabetic Med* 1988; **5**: 172–6.
5 Allawi J, Rao PV, Gilbert R, Scott G, Jarrett RJ, Keen H, Viberti GC, Mather HM. Microalbuminuria in non-insulin-dependent diabetes: its prevalence in Indian compared with European patients. *Br Med J* 1988; **296**: 462–4.
6 Mather HM, Keen H. The Southall diabetes survey: prevalence of known diabetes in Asians and Europeans. *Br Med J* 1985; **291**: 1081–4.
7 Nelson RG, Newman JM, Knowler WC *et al.* Incidence of end-stage renal disease in Type 2 (non-insulin-dependent) diabetes mellitus in Pima Indians. *Diabetologia* 1988; **31**: 730–6.
8 Keen H, Chlouverakis C. An immunoassay for urinary albumin at low concentrations. *Lancet* 1963; **ii**: 913–16.
9 Parving HH, Hommel E, Mathiesen ER, Skott P, Edsberg B, Bahnser M *et al.* Prevalence of microalbuminuria, arterial hypertension, retinopathy and neuropathy in patients with insulin-dependent diabetes. *Br Med J* 1988; **296**: 156–60.
10 Gatling W, Knight C, Mullee MA, Hill RD. Microalbuminuria in diabetes: a population study of the prevalence and an assessment of three screening tests. *Diabetic Med* 1988; **5**: 343–97.
11 Viberti GC, Wiseman MJ, Redmond S. Microalbuminuria: its history and potential for prevention of clinical nephropathy in diabetes mellitus. *Diabetic Nephropathy* 1984; **3**: 70–82.
12 Cohen DL, Close CF, Viberti GC. The variability of overnight urinary albumin excretion in insulin-dependent diabetic and normal subjects. *Diabetic Med* 1987; **4**: 437–40.
13 Feldt-Rasmussen B, Mathiesen E. Variability of urinary albumin excretion in incipient diabetic nephropathy. *Diabetic Nephropathy* 1984; **3**: 101–3.
14 Viberti GC, Mackintosh D, Bilous RW, Pickup JC, Keen H. Proteinuria in diabetes mellitus: role of spontaneous and experimental variation of glycaemia. *Kidney Int* 1982; **21**: 714–20.
15 Viberti GC, Mogensen CE, Keen H *et al.* Urinary excretion of albumin in normal man: the effects of water loading. *Scand J Clin Lab Invest* 1982; **42**: 147–51.
16 Viberti GC, Jarrett RJ, McCartney M, Keen H. Increased

glomerular permeability to albumin induced by exercise in diabetic subjects. *Diabetologia* 1978; **14**: 293–300.

17 Cohen DL, Dodds R, Viberti GC. Effect of protein restriction in insulin dependent diabetics at risk of nephropathy. *Br Med J* 1987; **294**: 795–8.

18 Rowe DJF, Bagga H, Betts PB. Normal variations in rate of albumin excretion and albumin to creatinine ratios in overnight and daytime urine collections in non-diabetic children. *Br Med J* 1985; **291**: 693–4.

19 Hutchinson AS, Paterson KR. Collecting urine for microalbumin assay. *Diabetic Med* 1988; **5**: 527–32.

20 Gatling W, Knight C, Hill RD. Screening for early diabetic nephropathy: which sample to detect microalbuminuria? *Diabetic Med* 1985; **2**: 451–5.

21 Marshall SM, Alberti KGMM. Screening for early diabetic nephropathy. *Ann Clin Biochem* 1986; **23**: 195–7.

22 Grenfell A. Screening for at risk microalbuminuria in Type 1 (insulin-dependent) diabetes mellitus. *Diabetologia* 1987; **30**: 525A.

23 Viberti GC, Wiseman MJ. The kidney in diabetes: significance of the early abnormalities. In: Watkins PJ, ed. *Long-term Complications of Diabetes. Clin Endocrinol Metab* 1986; **15**: 753–82.

24 Close CF, Scott GS, Viberti GC. Rapid detection of urinary albumin at low concentration by an agglutination inhibition technique. *Diabetic Med* 1987; **4**: 491–2.

25 Myers BD, Winetz JA, Chui F, Michaels AS. Mechanisms of proteinuria in diabetic nephropathy: a study of glomerular barrier function. *Kidney Int* 1982; **21**: 633–41.

26 Viberti GC, Keen H. The patterns of proteinuria in diabetes mellitus. *Diabetes* 1984; **33**: 686–92.

27 Mogensen CE. Kidney function and glomerular permeability to macromolecules in early juvenile diabetes. *Scand J Clin Lab Invest* 1971; **28**: 79–90.

28 Partasarathy N, Spiro RG. Effect of diabetes on the glycosaminoglycan component of the human glomerular basement membrane. *Diabetes* 1982; **31**: 738–41.

29 Viberti GC, Hill RD, Jarrett RJ, Argyropoulos A, Mahmud U, Keen H. Microalbuminuria as a predictor of clinical nephropathy in insulin-dependent diabetes mellitus. *Lancet* 1982; **i**: 1430–2.

30 Mathiesen ER, Oxenbøll K, Johansen PAa, Svendsen PA, Deckert T. Incipient nephropathy in Type 1 (insulin-dependent) diabetes. *Diabetologia* 1984; **26**: 406–10.

31 Mogensen CE, Christensen CK. Predicting diabetic nephropathy in insulin-dependent patients. *N Engl J Med* 1984; **311**: 89–93.

32 Close CF, on behalf of the MCS Group. Sex, diabetes duration and microalbuminuria in Type 1 (insulin-dependent) diabetes mellitus. *Diabetologia* 1987; **30**: 508A.

33 Jarrett RJ, Viberti GC, Argyropoulos A *et al.* Microalbuminuria predicts mortality in non-insulin dependent diabetics. *Diabetic Med* 1984; **1**: 17–19.

34 Wiseman MJ, Viberti GC, Mackintosh D, Jarrett RJ, Keen H. Glycaemia, arterial pressure and microalbuminuria in Type 1 (insulin-dependent) diabetes mellitus. *Diabetologia* 1984; **26**: 401–5.

35 Viberti GC, Keen H, Wiseman M. Raised arterial pressure in parents of proteinuric insulin-dependent patients. *Br Med J* 1987; **295**: 515–17.

36 Seaquist ER, Goetz FC, Rich S, Barbosa J. Familial clustering of diabetic kidney disease. *N Engl J Med* 1989; **320**: 1161–5.

37 Pettitt DJ, Nelson RG, Saad MF, Knowler WC. Diabetic nephropathy in two generations of subjects with Type 2 diabetes mellitus (abstract). *Diabetes Res Clin Pract* 1988; **5**: 137.

38 Semplicini A, Mozato M-G, Sama B, Nosadini R, Fioretto P, Trevisan R *et al.* Na/H and Li/Na exchanger in red cells of normotensive and hypertensive patients with insulin-dependent diabetes mellitus. *Am J Hypertens* 1989; **2**: 174–7.

39 Boerwinkle E, Turner ST, Weinshilboum R, Johnson M, Richelson E, Sing CF. Analysis of the distribution of erythrocyte sodium–lithium countertransport in a sample representative of the general population. *Genet Epidemiol* 1986; **3**: 365–78.

40 Hilton PJ. Cellular sodium transport in essential hypertension. *N Engl J Med* 1986; **314**: 227–9.

41 Cooper R, Miller R, Trevisan M, Sempos C, Larbie E, Vestima H *et al.* Family history of hypertension and red cell cation transport in high school students. *J Hypertens* 1983; **1**: 145–52.

42 Krolewski AS, Canessa M, Rand LI, Warram JH, Christlieb AR, Knowler WC, Kahn CR. Genetic predisposition to hypertension as a major determinant of development of diabetic nephropathy. *N Engl J Med* 1988; **318**: 140–5.

43 Mangili R, Bending JJ, Scott GS, Li LK, Gupta A, Viberti GC. Increased sodium–lithium countertransport activity in red cells of patients with insulin-dependent diabetes and nephropathy. *N Engl J Med* 1988; **318**: 146–9.

44 Trevisan R, Li LK, Walker JD, Viberti GC. Overactivity of the Na/H antiport and enhanced cell growth in insulin-dependent patients with nephropathy. *Diabetologia* 1989; **32**: 549A.

45 Feldt-Rasmussen B, Mathiesen ER, Deckert T, Giese J, Christensen NJ, Bent-Hansen L *et al.* Central role for sodium in the pathogenesis of blood pressure changes independent of angiotensin, aldosterone and catecholamines in Type 1 (insulin-dependent) diabetes mellitus. *Diabetologia* 1987; **30**: 610–17.

46 Walker JD, Tariq T, Viberti GC. Sodium–lithium countertransport activity in parents of Type I (insulin-dependent) diabetics with nephropathy. *Diabetologia* 1989; **32**: 555A.

47 Cambier P. Application de la théorie de Remberg à l'étude clinique des affections rénales et du diabète. *Ann Méd* 1934; **35**: 273–99.

48 Ditzel J, Schwartz M. Abnormal glomerular filtration rate in short term insulin treated diabetic subjects. *Diabetes* 1967; **16**: 264–7.

49 Mogensen CE. Glomerular filtration rate and renal plasma flow in short term and long term juvenile diabetes mellitus. *Scand J Clin Lab Invest* 1971; **28**: 91–100.

50 Christiansen JS, Gammelgaard J, Frandsen M, Parving HH. Increased kidney size, glomerular filtration rate, and renal plasma flow in short-term insulin-dependent diabetics. *Diabetologia* 1981; **20**: 451–6.

51 Ditzel J, Junker K. Abnormal glomerular filtration rate, renal plasma flow and renal protein excretion in recent and short term diabetics. *Br Med J* 1972; **2**: 13–19.

52 Mogensen CE, Andersen MJF. Increased kidney size and glomerular filtration rate in early juvenile diabetics. *Diabetes* 1972; **22**: 706–12.

53 Mogensen CE. Renal function changes in diabetics. *Diabetes* 1976; **25**: 872–9.

54 Deen WM, Satvat B. Determinants of glomerular filtration of proteins. *Am J Physiol* 1981; **241**: F162–70.

55 Hostetter TH, Troy JC, Brenner BM. Glomerular haemodynamics in experimental diabetes mellitus. *Kidney Int* 1981; **19**: 410–15.

56 Michels LD, Davidman M, Keane WF. Determinants of glomerular filtration and plasma flow in experimental diabetic rats. *J Lab Clin Med* 1981; **98**: 869–85.

57 Wiseman MJ, Mangili R, Alberetto M, Keen H, Viberti GC. Mechanisms of the glomerular response to glycaemic changes in insulin-dependent diabetic subjects. *Kidney Int* 1987; **31**: 1012–18.
58 Zatz R, Dunn R, Meyer TW, Anderson S, Rennke HG, Brenner BM. Prevention of diabetic glomerulopathy by pharmacological amelioration of glomerular capillary hypertension. *J Clin Invest* 1986; **77**: 1925–30.
59 Hirose K, Tsuschida H, Østerby R, Gunderson HJG. A strong correlation between glomerular filtration rate and filtration surface in diabetic kidney hyperfunction. *J Lab Invest* 1980; **43**: 434–7.
60 Østerby R, Parving HH, Nyberg G, Hommel E, Jørgensen HE, Løkkegaard H *et al.* A strong correlation between glomerular filtration rate and filtration surface in diabetic nephropathy. *Diabetologia* 1988; **31**: 265–70.
61 Wiseman MJ, Viberti GC. Glomerular filtration rate and kidney volume in Type 1 (insulin-dependent) diabetes mellitus revisited. *Diabetologia* 1982; **25**: 530.
62 Wiseman MJ, Viberti GC, Keen H. Threshold effect of plasma glucose in the glomerular hyperfiltration of diabetes. *Nephron* 1984; **38**: 257–60.
63 Christiansen JS, Frandsen M, Parving HH. The effect of intravenous insulin infusion on kidney function in insulin-dependent diabetics. *Diabetologia* 1981; **20**: 199–204.
64 Viberti GC, Benigni A, Bognetti L, Remuzzi G, Wiseman MJ. Glomerular hyperfiltration and urinary prostaglandins in insulin-dependent diabetes mellitus. *Diabetic Med* 1989; **6**: 219–23.
65 Collier DA, Matthews DM, Bell G, Watson MC, Clarke BF. Increased urinary excretion of 6-keto $PGF_{1\alpha}$ and $PGE_2$ in male insulin dependent diabetics. *Diabetic Med* 1986; **3**: 358A.
66 Esmatjes E, Levy I, Gaya J, Rivera F. Renal excretion of prostaglandin $E_2$ and plasma renin activity in type 1 diabetes mellitus: relationship to normoglycemia achieved with artificial pancreas. *Diabetes Care* 1987; **10**: 428–31.
67 Esmatjes E, Fernandez MR, Halperin I *et al.* Renal hemodynamic abnormalities in patients with short-term insulin dependent diabetes mellitus: role of renal prostaglandins. *J Clin Endocrinol Metab* 1985; **60**: 1231–6.
68 Wiseman MJ, Drury PL, Keen H, Viberti GC. Plasma renin activity in insulin dependent diabetics with raised glomerular filtration rate. *Clin Endocrinol* 1984; **21**: 409–14.
69 Zatz R, Meyer TW, Rennke HG, Brenner BM. Predominance of hemodynamic rather than metabolic factors in the pathogenesis of diabetic glomerulopathy. *Proc Natl Acad Sci USA* 1985; **82**: 5963–7.
70 Lervang HH, Jensen S, Brochner-Mortensen J, Ditzel J. Early glomerular hyperfiltration and the development of late nephropathy in Type I (insulin-dependent) diabetes mellitus. *Diabetologia* 1988; **31**: 723–9.
71 The Kroc Collaborative Study Group. Blood glucose control and the evolution of diabetic retinopathy and albuminuria. *N Engl J Med* 1984; **311**: 365–72.
72 Feldt-Rasmussen B, Mathiesen ER, Deckert T. Effect of two years of strict metabolic control on progression of incipient nephropathy in insulin-dependent diabetics. *Lancet* 1986; **ii**: 1300–4.
73 Dahl-Jørgensen K, Hanssen KF, Kierulf P, Bjoro T, Sandvik L, Aageraes O. Reduction of urinary albumin excretion after 4 years of continuous subcutaneous insulin infusion in insulin-dependent diabetes mellitus. The Oslo study. *Acta Endocrinol (Copenhagen)* 1988; **117**: 19–25.
74 Mogensen CE, Andersen MJF. Increased kidney size and glomerular filtration rate in untreated juvenile diabetes: normalisation by insulin treatment. *Diabetologia* 1975; **11**: 221–4.
75 Wiseman MJ, Saunders AJ, Keen H, Viberti GC. Effect of blood glucose on glomerular filtration and kidney size in insulin-dependent diabetics. *N Engl J Med* 1985; **312**: 617–21.
76 Mathiesen ER, Ronn B, Jensen T, Storm B, Deckert T. Microalbuminuria precedes elevation in blood pressure in diabetic nephropathy. *Diabetologia* 1988; **31**: 519A.
77 Knowler WC, Bennett PH, Nelson RG, Saad MF, Pettit DJ. Blood pressure before the onset of diabetes predicts albuminuria in Type 2 (non-insulin-dependent) diabetes. *Diabetologia* 1988; **31**: 509A.
78 Jensen T, Borch-Johnsen K, Deckert T. Changes in blood pressure and renal function in patients with type 1 (insulin-dependent) diabetes prior to clinical diabetic nephropathy. *Diabetes Res* 1987; **4**: 159–62.
79 Parving HH, Andersen AR, Smidt VM, Hommel E, Mathiesen ER, Svendsen PA. Effect of antihypertensive treatment on kidney function in diabetic nephropathy. *Br Med J* 1987; **294**: 1443–7.
80 Parving HH, Hommel E, Smidt VM. Protection of kidney function and decrease in albuminuria by captopril in insulin-dependent diabetics with nephropathy. *Br Med J* 1988; **297**: 1086–91.
81 Christensen CK, Mogensen CE. Antihypertensive treatment: long-term reversal of pressure of albuminuria in incipient diabetic nephropathy. A longitudinal study of renal function. *J Diabetic Compl* 1987; **1**: 45–52.
82 Hommel E, Parving HH, Mathiesen E, Edsberg B, Neilsen MD, Giese J. Effect of captopril on kidney function in insulin-dependent diabetic patients with nephropathy. *Br Med J* 1986; **293**: 467–70.
83 Björck S, Nyberg G, Mulec H, Granerus G, Herlitz H, Aurell M. Beneficial effects of angiotensin converting enzyme inhibitors on renal function in patients with diabetic nephropathy. *Br Med J* 1986; **293**: 471–4.
84 Marre M, Chatellier G, Leblanc H, Guyene TJ, Menard J, Passa P. Prevention of diabetic nephropathy with enalapril in normotensive diabetics with microalbuminuria. *Br Med J* 1988; **297**: 1092–5.
85 Drummond K, Levy-Marchal C, Laborde K. Enalapril does not alter renal function in normotensive, normoalbuminuric, hyperfiltering Type 1 (insulin-dependent) diabetic children. *Diabetologia* 1989; **32**: 255–60.
86 Walker JD, Bending JJ, Dodds RA, Mattock MB, Murrells TJ, Keen H, Viberti GC. Restriction of dietary protein and progression of renal failure in diabetic nephropathy. *Lancet* 1989; **ii**: 1411–15.
87 Beyer-Mears A, Cruz E, Edelist T, Varagiannis E. Diminished proteinuria in diabetes mellitus by Sorbinil, an aldose reductase inhibitor. *Pharmacology* 1986; **32**: 52–60.
88 Beyer-Mears A. The polyol pathway, sorbinil and renal dysfunction. *Metabolism* 1986; **35**: 46–54.
89 Brownlee M, Vlassara H, Kooney A, Cerami A. Inhibition of glucose-derived protein cross-linking and prevention of early diabetic changes in glomerular basement membrane by aminoguanidine. *Diabetes* 1986; **35**: 42A.
90 Acheson RM. Blood pressure in a national sample of U.S. adults: percentile distribution by age, sex and race. *Int J Epidemiol* 1973; **2**: 293–301.
91 Winocour PH, Durrington PN, Ishola M, Anderson DC, Cohen H. Influence of proteinuria on vascular disease, blood pressure, and lipoproteins in insulin dependent diabetes mellitus. *Br Med J* 1987; **294**: 1648–51.

92 Borch-Johnsen K, Kreiner S. Proteinuria: value as predictor of cardiovascular mortality in insulin dependent diabetes mellitus. *Br Med J* 1987; **294**: 1651–4.

93 Deckert T, Feldt-Rasmussen B, Borch-Johnsen K, Jensen T, Kofoed-Enevoldsen A. Albuminuria reflects widespread vascular damage. The Steno hypothesis. *Diabetologia* 1989; **32**: 219–26.

94 Earle K, Walker J, Hill C, Viberti GC. Familial clustering of cardiovascular disease in patients with insulin-dependent diabetes and nephropathy. *N Engl J Med* 1992; **326**: 673–7.

95 Dadone MM, Hasstedt SJ, Hunt SC, Smith JB, Ash KO, Williams RR. Genetic analysis of sodium–lithium countertransport in ten hypertension-prone kindreds. *Am J Med* 1984; **17**: 565–77.

96 Boerwinkle E, Turner ST. Weinshilboum R, Johnson M, Richelson E, Sing CF. Analysis of the distribution of sodium–lithium countertransport in a sample representative of the general population. *Gen Epidemiol* 1986; **3**: 365–78.

97 Krolewski AS, Canessa M, Warram JM *et al*. Predisposition to hypertension and susceptibility to renal disease in insulin-dependent diabetes mellitus. *N Engl J Med* 1988; **318**: 140–5.

98 Mangili R, Bending JJ, Scott G, Li LK, Gupta A, Viberti GC. Increased sodium–lithium countertransport activity in red cells of patients with insulin-dependent diabetes and nephropathy. *N Engl J Med* 1988; **318**: 146–50.

99 Walker JD, Tariq T, Viberti GC. Sodium–lithium countertransport activity in red cells of patients with insulin dependent diabetes and nephropathy and their parents. *Br Med J* 1990; **301**: 635–8.

100 Jones SL, Trevisan R, Tariq T *et al*. Sodium–lithium counter transport in microalbuminuric insulin-dependent diabetic patients. *Hypertension* 1990; **15**: 570–5.

101 Jones SL, Faria J, Tariq T, Mattock MB, Viberti GC. Sodium–lithium countertransport activity and serum lipoproteins in insulin-dependent diabetic patients. *Diabetic Med* 1989; **6** (suppl 2): 28A.

102 Bunker CH, Mallinger AG. Sodium–lithium countertransport, obesity, insulin and blood pressure in healthy premenopausal women. *Circulation* 1985; **72** (S3): III-296.

103 Nosadini R, Viberti GC, Doria A *et al*. Increased $Na^+/H^+$ countertransport activity is associated with cardiac hypertrophy and insulin resistance in hypertensive type 1 (insulin-dependent) diabetic patients. *Diabetologia* 1989; **32**: 523A.

104 Chavers BM, Bilous RW, Ellis EN, Steffes MW, Mauer SM. Glomerular lesions and urinary albumin excretion in type 1 diabetes without overt proteinuria. *N Engl J Med* 1989; **320**: 966–70.

105 Foster DW. Insulin resistance — a secret killer? *N Engl J Med* 1989; **320**: 733–4.

106 Silberberg JS, Barre PE, Prichard SS, Sniderman AD. Impact of left ventricular hypertrophy on survival in end-stage renal disease. *Kidney Int* 1989; **36**: 286–90.

107 Sampson MJ, Chambers J, Sprigings D, Drury PL. Intraventricular septal hypertrophy in type 1 diabetic patients with microalbuminuria or early proteinuria. *Diabetic Med* 1990; **7**: 126–31.

108 Lopes de Faria JB, Jones SL, Macdonald F, Chambers J, Mattock MB, Viberti GC. Sodium–lithium countertransport activity and insulin resistance in normotensive IDDM patients. *Diabetes* 1992; **41**: 610–15.

109 Reaven GM, Hoffman BP. A role for insulin in the aetiology and course of hypertension? *Lancet* 1987; **ii**: 435–7.

110 Mahnensmith RL, Aronson PS. The plasma membrane sodium–hydrogen exchanger and its role in physiological and pathological processes. *Circulation Res* 1985; **56**: 773–88.

111 Li LK, Trevisan R, Walker JD, Viberti GC. Overactivity of $Na^+/H^+$ antiport and enhanced cell growth in fibroblasts of type 1 (insulin-dependent) diabetics with nephropathy. *Kidney Int* 1990; **37**: 199.

112 Ng LL, Simmons D, Frigh V, Garrido MC, Bomford J. Effect of protein kinase C modulators on the leucocyte $Na^+/H^+$ antiport in type 1 (insulin-dependent) diabetic subjects with albuminuria. *Diabetologia* 1990; **33**: 278–84.

113 Parving H-H, Viberti GC, Keen H, Christiansen JS, Lassen NA. Haemodynamic factors in the genesis of diabetic microangiopathy. *Metabolism* 1983; **32**: 943–9.

114 Microalbuminuria Collaborative Study Group, UK. Risk factors for development of microalbuminuria in insulin dependent diabetic patients: a cohort study. *Br Med J* 1993; **306**: 1235–9.

115 Nelson RG, Pettitt DJ, Baird HR *et al*. Pre-diabetic blood pressure predicts urinary albumin excretion after the onset of type 2 (non-insulin-dependent) diabetes mellitus in Pima Indians. *Diabetologia* 1993 (in press).

116 Haneda M, Kikkawa R, Togawa M *et al*. High blood pressure is a risk factor for the development of microalbuminuria in Japanese subjects with non-insulin-dependent diabetes mellitus. *J Diab Comp* 1992; **6**: 181–5.

117 Mathiesen ER, Hommel E, Giese J, Parving HH. Efficacy of captopril in postponing nephropathy in normotensive insulin dependent diabetic patients with microalbuminuria. *Br Med J* 1991; **303**: 81–7.

# 15 The Relationship between Structural and Functional Abnormalities in Diabetic Nephropathy

**Summary**

• The characteristic histopathological features of the diabetic kidney occur in the glomerulus.
• The major abnormalities are: increased glomerular volume secondary to basement membrane thickening and mesangial enlargement; hyaline deposits (of uncertain significance); and global glomerular sclerosis due to mesangial expansion or ischaemia, or both.
• GFR is closely correlated with the surface area of the glomerular capillary basement membrane (the filtration surface), itself determined by the number of glomeruli at diagnosis, the extent of mesangial expansion, the capacity for expansion and the number of sclerosed glomeruli.
• Urinary albumin excretion is related to the filtration slit pore length.
• Microalbuminuria is not always associated with abnormalities of glomerular structure.

The focus of microvascular injury in the kidney is the glomerulus and, accordingly, this has been the subject of intensive histological study. This chapter will briefly describe the pathological appearances of the glomerulus and other renal structures in diabetes, and will present the current understanding of the glomerular structural correlates of changes in glomerular filtration rate (GFR) and albuminuria. Finally, the indications for renal biopsy in diabetic patients will be discussed.

## Normal glomerular histology

The renal glomerulus comprises a tuft of 20–40 capillary loops arising from an afferent and drained by an efferent arteriole [1]. The loops are arranged in lobules (Fig. 15.1) which are supported by mesangial tissue which has both cellular and acellular (matrix) components. Electron microscopy has shown that each loop is made up of a basement membrane lined by a fenestrated endothelium and covered by parietal epithelium. These epithelial cells are highly specialized 'podocytes' which do not lie entirely on the basement membrane, but possess foot processes which interdigitate along the membrane, leaving small gaps — the filtration slits or pores — between them. No two adjacent foot processes arise from the same podocyte [2]. The basement membrane is an amorphous, acellular structure whose average width is 383 nm in normal men and 326 nm in women [3]. It has a central lamina densa sandwiched between the less electron dense lamina rara interna and externa. The lamina densa is continuous with the mesangial matrix and both contain Type IV collagen, proteoglycan, laminin and fibronectin. The glomerular tuft is enclosed by Bowman's capsule which is continuous with the tubular basement membrane and defines the urinary space. It is lined by flattened visceral epithelial cells. Filtration takes place from within the capillary, across the endothelium (probably via the fenestrae), the basement membrane, the epithelium (probably via the filtration slit pores), into the urinary space and thus into the proximal tubule.

## Pathology of the kidney in diabetes

### *Renal hypertrophy*

Enlargement of the whole kidney and of individual glomeruli has been recognized at diagnosis of

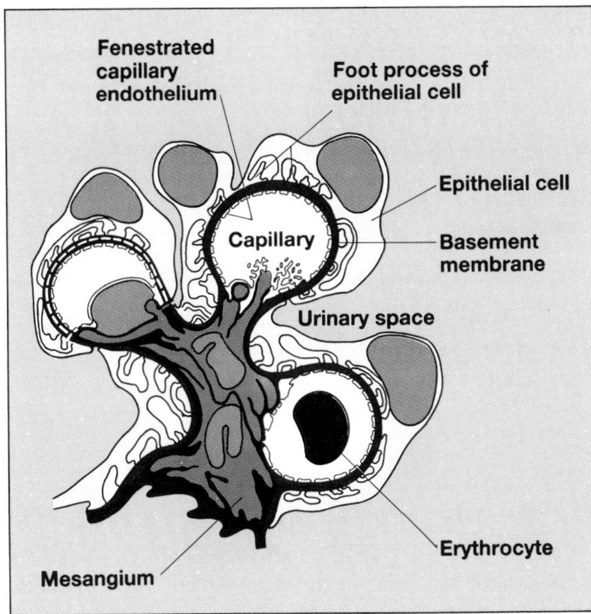


**Fig. 15.1.** Schematic representation of glomerular capillary tuft. Note continuity of glomerular basement membrane with mesangial matrix material (solid lines). (Adapted from [10] with permission of the *Journal of Clinical Investigation*.)

diabetes [4], and enlarged glomeruli have been described in many cases of advanced nephropathy [5]. The early increase in glomerular volume is probably secondary to an increase in production of basement membrane material and an enlargement of the filtration surface area [6]. Later glomerular enlargement may represent an accommodation of an expanding mesangium or a response to nephron loss from global sclerosis [6]. As the glomeruli represent only 1% of total renal volume, most of the observed increase in total kidney volume must be of tubular or interstitial origin [8].

### *Basement membrane*

Basement membrane thickening in diabetes was first described in 1959 and is considered one of the pathological hallmarks of the disease [9]. The membrane width is normal at diagnosis of diabetes, but significant thickening can be detected within 2 years [4], and after 10 years or more the vast majority of patients have marked thickening [10], irrespective of the severity of other diabetic complications (Fig. 15.2). Similar increases in basement membrane width have been demonstrated in normal kidneys transplanted into diabetic recipients [11]. It is thought that basement membrane is produced by the epithelium and metabolized by mesangial cells [12]; whether the observed increase in membrane width is due to overproduction, or impaired clearance, or both is not clear. The increased basement membrane thickness is mostly uniform both within and between glomeruli in the same patient, but thinner irregular segments have been described in some patients with established nephropathy and these may represent either new capillary growth or microaneurysm formation [13].

### *Mesangium*

Diffuse mesangial enlargement is a further pathological feature of diabetic glomerulosclerosis [14] (Fig. 15.2) and, like basement membrane thickening, can be detected after only 2 years of diabetes

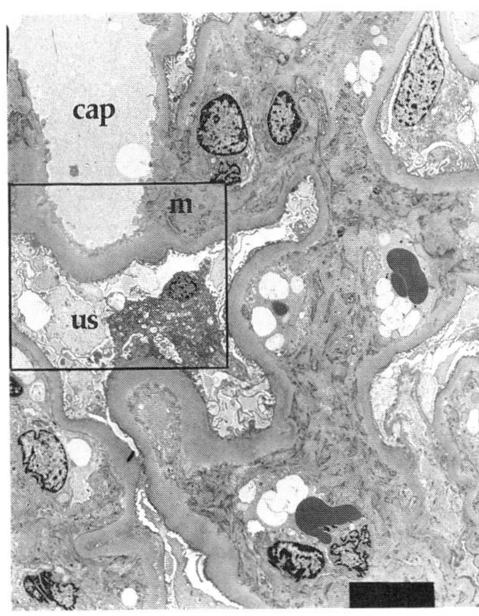


(a)

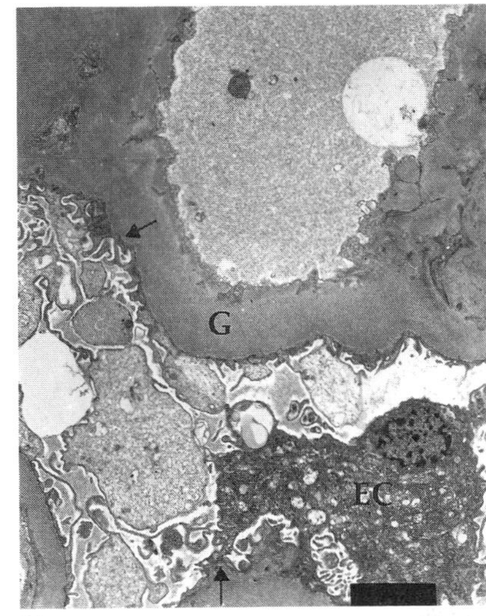


(b)

**Fig. 15.2.** Photomicrographs showing glomerular basement membrane thickening and mesangial expansion in the kidney of a diabetic patient. (a) × 1700; m: mesangial cell and matrix; us: urinary space; cap: capillary lumen. (b) × 4300, enlargement of boxed area in (a). G: glomerular basement membrane; EC: epithelial cell. Foot processes can be clearly seen (arrow). (Courtesy of Dr A. Morley, Department of Pathology, Medical School, University of Newcastle upon Tyne.)

[4]. However, in contrast to basement membrane thickening, careful study has shown that mesangial volume is by no means always increased and may be normal after 25 years of diabetes [10]. What is certain, however, is that patients with established nephropathy always have marked mesangial expansion [10]. Most of the enlargement is secondary to an increase in periodic acid–Schiff positive (PAS positive) matrix material, but cellular elements are also increased. Nodular lesions, which were the first glomerular changes to be described and are almost pathognomonic of diabetes [15], comprise ovoid accumulations of PAS-positive material which may be lamellated, and often occupy the central mesangium of a lobule (Fig. 15.3). They are by no means invariably present in patients with established nephropathy, and often coexist with diffuse changes [14]. Some workers consider that the nodules represent obliterated microaneurysms.

Electron microscopic studies in patients with nephropathy have suggested that the expanding mesangium gradually encroaches along the peripheral basement membrane, thus leading to a reduction in filtration surface area.

### *Hyaline lesions*

Collections of eosinophilic, acellular hyaline are characteristic but not specific for diabetes and their precise significance is unclear. They can occur on the inside of Bowman's capsule ('capsular drop'), or within a capillary loop between the endothelial cell and basement membrane ('fibrin cap'). Hyaline deposition in afferent arterioles is an extremely common and non-specific pathological finding, but efferent arteriolar hyaline is thought to be pathognomonic of diabetes [11].

### *Other glomerular changes*

Podocyte and endothelial structure are remarkably well preserved even in advanced nephropathy. Foot process width is probably increased, however, but not as markedly as in other nephropathies [16]. Abnormalities in endothelial fenestrae reported in diabetic animals have not yet been confirmed in man. Thickening and splitting of Bowman's capsule is a common feature of advanced nephropathy [14] and new capillary growth has been demonstrated within the thickened capsule. Global glomerular sclerosis or occlusion [5, 7, 10] due to either internal glomerular obliteration by unrestrained mesangial expansion, or ischaemia secondary to afferent arteriolar occlusion, is a feature of patients with a declining glomerular filtration rate (GFR). In support of the ischaemia hypothesis is the observation of clustering of occluded glomeruli in lines perpendicular to the surface of the kidney and parallel to the course of the interlobular arteries [17].

### *Tubular and interstitial changes*

The first renal pathological abnormality to be described in diabetic man was the Armanni–

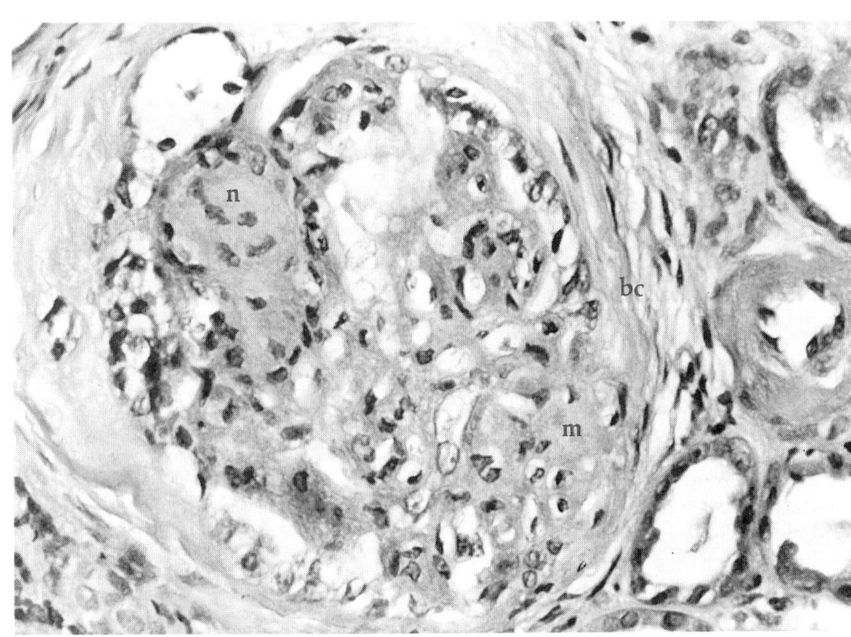


**Fig. 15.3.** Nodular glomerulosclerosis in a patient with diabetic nephropathy. Note thickened and split Bowman's capsule (bc) and obvious nodule (n). There is also a diffuse mesangial expansion (m) (× 6000). (Courtesy of Dr A. Morley, Department of Pathology, Medical School, University of Newcastle upon Tyne.)

Ebstein lesion of glycogen-containing vacuoles in the proximal tubular cells [15]. Since the advent of insulin treatment, this lesion is now rarely seen in man. Tubular basement membrane width also increases and parallels the changes seen in the glomerulus. Tubular atrophy and interstitial changes are probably secondary to glomerular occlusion, and not, as previously thought, to an increased incidence of pyelonephritis [10].

### *Immunopathology*

The immunopathological appearances are thought to represent secondary protein entrapment or accumulation in the basement membrane, rather than a primary cause of glomerulosclerosis. The most commonly described abnormality is a linear deposition of immunoglobulins and albumin, which is entirely non-specific [15].

## Glomerular structure and GFR

The surface area of the glomerular capillary basement membrane in diabetic patients (also called the filtration surface — see Fig. 15.1) is closely related to GFR, whether estimated by creatinine clearance [18] or by radioisotopic methods [7] (Fig. 15.4). However, there does not appear to be any strict relationship between basement membrane thickness and GFR.

The total filtering surface area per kidney is the product of the filtration surface per glomerulus and the number of glomeruli per kidney, and the filtration surface per glomerulus has been shown to be determined by the degree of mesangial expansion and the volume of the glomerular tuft in which it is accommodated [18]. Put simply, a larger glomerulus would accommodate a considerable increase in mesangial tissue before any appreciable loss of filtration surface occurs.

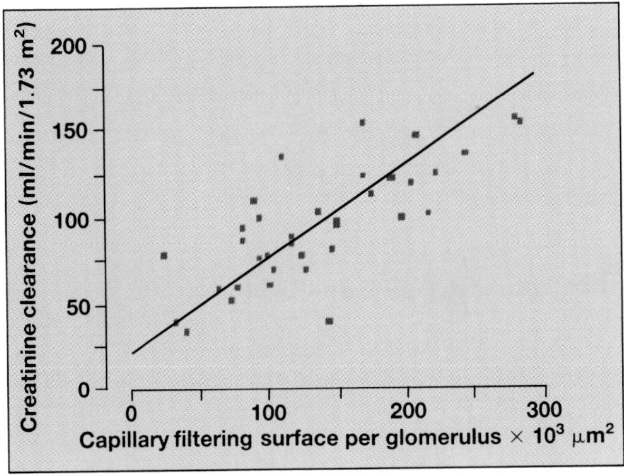


Fig. 15.4. Linear correlation ($r = 0.79$, $P < 0.01$) between GFR (in this case estimated by creatinine clearance) and filtration surface per glomerulus. Note wide range of filtration surface area for any given GFR reflecting the role of other factors such as glomerular number and per cent sclerosed glomeruli (see text). (Adapted from [7] with permission.)

Glomerular enlargement is known to be a feature of established nephropathy [5, 7, 10, 18] and we have shown that diabetic patients with nephropathy after 24–26 years of diabetes have larger glomeruli than those with nephropathy developing after 14–16 years [19]. Thus a capacity for glomerular enlargement may be a modifying factor of the rate of development of nephropathy in those patients destined to develop this complication. Glomerular number, on the other hand, is dependent upon the original number of glomeruli in the kidney (said to vary from 350 000 to 1100 000 between individuals) (Bendtsen and Nyengaard, personal communications) and the number of those obliterated by glomerulosclerosis. These various factors can all influence filtration surface area and thus GFR (Table 15.1) and it is perhaps not surprising that significant correlations have been described between GFR and mesangial volume [10] and the percentage of sclerosed glomeruli [7] in diabetic patients. Thus, the combination of fewer glomeruli at outset, the development of severe mesangial expansion and a limited capacity for glomerular enlargement with significant glomerular occlusion would lead to a rapidly declining GFR. Although it has yet to be shown that fewer or smaller glomeruli at diagnosis of diabetes represent risk factors for the later development of nephropathy, preliminary study of post-

**Table 15.1.** Renal structural factors affecting GFR in diabetes. *Positive*: positive effect on maintenance and preservation of GFR. *Negative*: negative effect on maintenance and preservation of GFR.

1 *Total number of glomeruli at diagnosis*: Probably genetically determined. *Positive*.

2 *Percentage of totally sclerosed glomeruli*: Secondary to factor 4, possible ischaemic component, ? both. *Negative*.

3 *Mean glomerular volume*: Probably genetically determined at diagnosis. May be influenced by glycaemic control. Late enlargement possibly secondary to factor 2. *Positive*.

4 *Mesangial volume for glomerulus*: Possibly related to glycaemic control or blood pressure. *Negative*.

mortem tissue has revealed fewer numbers of glomeruli in those patients dying with nephropathy compared with age- and duration-matched diabetic controls without clinical proteinuria (Bendtsen and Nyengaard, personal communication).

Near-normal glycaemic control can reverse glomerular and mesangial enlargement in diabetic animals [20], and pancreas transplantation might do the same in man [21]. There is, therefore, the intriguing possibility of baseline renal structure and glycaemic control operating as joint risk factors for the development of diabetic nephropathy.

## Glomerular structure and albuminuria

Heavy albuminuria is often associated with diminished GFR and thus severe glomerulosclerosis. Significant correlations between podocyte foot process width, filtration slit pore length per glomerulus and the extent of urinary albumin excretion rate (AER) over the normal to nephrotic range have been recently described [16]. These observations lend support to the hypothesis that filtration of macromolecules occurs mainly through the filtration slit pore. As with GFR, there is no significant relationship between AER and basement membrane width.

The intense interest in the phenomenon of microalbuminuria, variously defined as an AER of >30 μg/min [22], 40 mg/24 h [23], 70 μg/min [24] or 15 μg/min [25] depending upon the method of collection used, but always <300 mg/l, derives from the association between microalbuminuria and the later development of nephropathy (Chapters 13 and 14). Detailed morphometric analysis has, however, failed to show any correlation between glomerular structure and microalbuminuria (>20 mg/24 h) in patients with normal blood pressure and GFR [26]. However, if patients with an AER of 40–200 mg/24 h and hypertension are selected, a significant association with increased mesangial volume is observed [26]. Thus, microalbuminuric patients with hypertension probably have established, albeit early, nephropathy. However, microalbuminuria alone does not automatically imply a particular severity of glomerular lesion. Furthermore, analysis of glomeruli from patients with normal AER reveals a wide range of mesangial volumes, suggesting that normoalbuminuria does not exclude underlying glomerulopathy [26]. Prospective studies are necessary to determine the long-term significance of these glomerular lesions in normoalbuminuric patients.

## Indications for renal biopsy in diabetic patients

As diabetes is a common condition, the presence of non-diabetic causes of renal failure and proteinuria must always be borne in mind. If a patient has significant proteinuria or haematuria with normal retinal fundoscopy, then renal biopsy might reveal a potentially treatable glomerular disease [27], although many such patients will turn out to have diabetic glomerulosclerosis with a dissociation between renal and retinal complications [28]. Renal biopsy of diabetic patients is important and necessary from both clinical and research standpoints. The techniques for quantitative assessment of renal biopsy material are well described, provide reliable and reproducible data, and are relatively easy to perform [5, 10, 29, 30]. It is only when prospective studies of renal function are combined with renal biopsy, and the glomerular structural counterparts of the changes in GFR and AER are demonstrated, that the pathophysiology of this most serious complication of diabetes will be understood and rational interventions can be undertaken to prevent or modify its natural history.

## Recent developments

The importance of the study of kidney structure and its relationship to function was recognized by the award of the Camillo Golgi Lecture to Dr Ruth Østerby in 1991 [31], and has been emphasized by the first quantitative study in non-insulin-dependent patients showing similar relationships between glomerular structure and function to those which have been previously reported in IDDM [32].

### *Glomerular structure and GFR*

What has been learned recently about the four glomerular structural determinants of GFR listed in Table 15.1?

*Total number of glomeruli*. Normal mature human kidneys were found to contain on average 600 000 glomeruli [33]. This number was negatively correlated with age and positively correlated with kidney weight. Both insulin- and non-insulin-dependent patients have similar numbers of glomeruli. Diabetic patients with early proteinuria have not been found to have fewer glomeruli than non-proteinuric age- and duration-matched subjects [34]. These data therefore do not support the hypothesis that glomerular number at diagnosis is a risk factor for the subsequent development of nephropathy.

*Percentage of sclerosed glomeruli.* A strong correlation was found between the number of totally sclerosed glomeruli and both the degree of arteriolar hyalinosis and the mesangial volume fraction [35]. These data support the view that global sclerosis can occur secondarily to reduced blood flow, and that internal obliteration may be the result of an expanding mesangium. The former, but presumably not the latter, may be ameliorated by antihypertensive treatment, thus perhaps explaining the partial effectiveness of this therapy in the prevention of progression of nephropathy.

*Mean glomerular volume.* In normal humans, total glomerular volume correlates significantly with body surface area and, by inference, metabolic rate [33]. Glomerular volume in renal allografts increases within 6 months after transplantation into diabetic recipients and this does not seem to relate to the later development of glomerulopathy [36]. These data suggest that glomeruli can adapt to a new metabolic demand by increasing their size, which supports the view that increased volume may ameliorate and not accelerate the glomerulopathic process.

*Mesangial volume.* The relative constituents of the mesangium were estimated in a large series of biopsies from patients with a wide range of glomerulopathy. Both cellular and matrix components were increased in an approximate ratio of 1 : 2 but the matrix volume related best to glomerular function [37]. Mesangial expansion, particularly involving the matrix, correlated strongly with GFR.

### Glomerular structure and albuminuria

There remains controversy over the relationship of glomerular lesions to albuminuria. Glomerular basement membrane thickening, as well as mesangial matrix expansion, have both been shown to correlate with AER [37]. Using precise estimates of glomerular structure, a significant increase in mesangial volume was found in a small group of microalbuminuric IDDM patients compared with a group of age- and duration-matched normoalbuminuric subjects [38]. However, others have reported patients who have definite glomerulopathy but normal albumin excretion [39].

### Conclusions

The relationship between glomerular structure and GFR has been further clarified and the role of glomerular volume adaptation seems to be assuming greater importance. However, there is still a paucity of data on the long-term significance of glomerular lesions in the absence of increased protein excretion. There is an important shift of emphasis in nephropathy research to include structural analysis as a part of intervention studies, and the results of these prospective studies are eagerly awaited.

RUDOLF W. BILOUS

## References


1 Tisher CC. Anatomy of the kidney. In: Brenner BM, Rector FC, eds. *The Kidney*, Vol 11. Philadelphia: WB Saunders, 1981: 3–75.

2 Rodewald R, Karnovsky MJ. Porous substructure of the glomerular slit diaphragm in the rat and mouse. *J Cell Biol* 1974; **60**: 423–33.

3 Steffes MW, Barbosa J, Basgen JM, Sutherland DER, Najarian JS, Mauer SM. Quantitative glomerular morphology of the normal human kidney. *Lab Invest* 1983; **49**: 82–6.

4 Mogensen CE, Østerby R, Gundersen HJG. Early functional and morphologic vascular renal consequences of the diabetic state. *Diabetologia* 1979; **17**: 71–6.

5 Østerby R, Gundersen HJG, Nyberg G, Aurell M. Advanced diabetic glomerulopathy. Quantitative structural characterisation of non-occluded glomeruli. *Diabetes* 1987; **36**: 612–19.

6 Østerby R, Gundersen HJG. Fast accumulation of basement membrane material and the rate of morphological changes in acute experimental diabetic glomerular hypertrophy. *Diabetologia* 1980; **18**: 493–500.

7 Østerby R, Parving H-H, Nyberg G, Hommel E, Jørgensen HE, Løkkegaard H, Svalander C. A strong correlation between glomerular filtration rate and filtration surface in diabetic nephropathy. *Diabetologia* 1988; **31**: 265–70.

8 Seyer-Hansen K, Hansen J, Gundersen HJG. Renal hypertrophy in experimental diabetes. A morphometric study. *Diabetologia* 1980; **18**: 501–5.

9 Bergstrand A, Bucht H. The glomerular lesions of diabetes mellitus and their electron microscopic appearance. *J Pathol Bacteriol* 1959; **77**: 231–42.

10 Mauer SM, Steffes MW, Ellis EN, Sutherland DER, Brown DM, Goetz FC. Structural–functional relationships in diabetic nephropathy. *J Clin Invest* 1984; **74**: 1143–55.

11 Mauer SM, Barbosa J, Vernier RL, Kjellstand CM, Buselmeier TJ, Simmons RL, Najarian JS, Goetz FC. Development of diabetic vascular lesions in normal kidneys transplanted into patients with diabetes mellitus. *N Engl J Med* 1976; **295**: 916–20.

12 Walker F. The origin, turnover and removal of glomerular basement membrane. *J Pathol* 1973; **110**: 233–44.
13 Østerby R, Nyberg G. New vessel formation in the renal corpuscles in advanced diabetic glomerulopathy. *J Diabetic Comp* 1987; **1**: 122–7.
14 Gellman DD, Pirani CL, Soothill JF, Muehrke RC, Kark RM. Diabetic nephropathy: a clinical and pathological study based on renal biopsies. *Medicine (Baltimore)* 1959; **38**: 321–67.
15 Morley AR. Renal vascular disease in diabetes mellitus. *Histopathology* 1988; **12**: 343–58.
16 Ellis EN, Steffes MW, Chavers BM, Mauer SM. Observations of glomerular epithelial cell structure in patients with type 1 diabetes mellitus. *Kidney Int* 1987; **32**: 736–41.
17 Hørlyck A, Gundersen HJG, Østerby R. The cortical distribution pattern of diabetic glomerulopathy. *Diabetologia* 1986; **29**: 146–50.
18 Ellis EN, Steffes MW, Goetz FC, Sutherland DER, Mauer SM. Glomerular filtration surface in type 1 diabetes mellitus. *Kidney Int* 1986; **29**: 889–94.
19 Bilous RW, Mauer SM, Sutherland DER, Steffes MW. Mean glomerular volume and rate of development of diabetic nephropathy. *Diabetes* 1989; **38**: 1142–7.
20 Steffes MW, Brown DM, Basgen JM, Mauer SM. Amelioration of mesangial volume and surface alterations following islet transplantation in diabetic rats. *Diabetes* 1980; **29**: 509–15.
21 Bilous RW, Mauer SM, Sutherland DER, Najarian JS, Goetz FC, Steffes MW. The effects of pancreas tranplantation on the glomerular structure of renal allografts in patients with insulin-dependent diabetes. *N Engl J Med* 1989; **321**: 80–5.
22 Viberti GC, Jarrett RJ, Mahmud U, Hill RD, Argyropoulos A, Keen H. Microalbuminuria as a predictor of clinical nephropathy in insulin-dependent diabetes mellitus. *Lancet* 1982; **ii**: 1430–2.
23 Parving H-H, Oxenbøll B, Svendsen PAå, Christiansen JS, Andersen AR. Early detection of patients at risk of developing diabetic nephropathy. A longitudinal study of urinary albumin excretion. *Acta Endocrinol* 1982; **100**: 550–5.
24 Mathiesen ER, Oxenbøll B, Johansen K, Svendsen PAå, Deckert T. Incipient nephropathy in Type 1 (insulin-dependent) diabetes. *Diabetologia* 1984; **25**: 406–10.
25 Mogensen CE, Christensen CK. Predicting diabetic nephropathy in insulin-dependent patients. *N Engl J Med* 1984; **311**: 89–93.
26 Chavers BM, Bilous RW, Ellis EN, Steffes MW, Mauer SM. Glomerular lesions and urinary albumin excretion in type 1 diabetes without overt proteinuria. *N Engl J Med* 1989; **320**: 966–70.
27 Hommel E, Carstensen H, Skøtt P, Larsen P, Parving H-H. Prevalence and causes of microscopic haematuria in Type 1 (insulin-dependent) diabetic patients with persistent proteinuria. *Diabetologia* 1987; **30**: 627–30.
28 Bilous RW, Viberti GC, Sandahl-Christiansen J, Parving H-H, Keen H. Dissociation of diabetic complications in insulin-dependent diabetes: a clinical report. *Diabetic Nephr* 1985; **4**: 73–6.
29 Ellis EN, Basgen JM, Mauer SM, Steffes MW. Kidney biopsy technique and evaluation. In: Clarke WL, Larner J, Pohl Sl, eds. *Methods of Diabetes Research. Clinical Methods*, Vol. 11. New York: J Wiley and Sons, 1986: 633–47.
30 Gundersen HJG, Bagger P, Bendtsen TF *et al*. The new stereological tools: disector, fractionator, nucleator and point sampled intercepts and their use in pathological research and diagnosis. *Acta Pathol Microbiol Immunol Scand* 1988; **96**: 857–81.
31 Østerby R. Glomerular structural changes in Type 1 (insulin-dependent) diabetes mellitus: causes, consequences and prevention. *Diabetologia* 1992; **35**: 803–12.
32 Hayashi H, Karasawa R, Inn H *et al*. An electron microscopic study of glomeruli in Japanese patients with non-insulin dependent diabetes. *Kidney Int* 1992; **41**: 749–57.
33 Nyengaard JR, Bendtsen TF. Number and size of glomeruli, kidney weight and body surface area in normal human beings. *Anat Rec* 1992; **232**: 194–201.
34 Bendtsen TF, Nyengaard JR. The number of glomeruli in Type 1 (insulin-dependent) and Type 2 (non-insulin-dependent) diabetic patients. *Diabetologia* 1992; **35**: 844–50.
35 Harris RD, Steffes MW, Bilous RW, Sutherland DER, Mauer SM. Global glomerular sclerosis and glomerular arteriolar hyalinosis in insulin dependent diabetes. *Kidney Int* 1991; **40**: 107–14.
36 Østerby R, Nyberg G, Karlberg I, Svalander C. Glomerular volume in kidneys transplanted into diabetic and non-diabetic patients. *Diabetic Med* 1992; **9**: 144–9.
37 Steffes MW, Bilous RW, Sutherland DER, Mauer SM. Cell and matrix components of the glomerular mesangium in Type 1 diabetes. *Diabetes* 1992; **41**: 679–84.
38 Walker JD, Close CL, Jones SL, Rafftery M, Keen H, Viberti GC, Østerby R. Glomerular structure in type 1 (insulin-dependent) diabetes with normo- and microalbuminuria. *Kidney Int* 1992; **41**: 741–8.
39 Lane PH, Steffes MW, Mauer SM. Glomerular structure in IDDM women with low glomerular filtration rate and normal urinary albumin excretion. *Diabetes* 1992; **41**: 581–6.

# 16 Clinical Features and Management of Established Diabetic Nephropathy


**Summary**

• Proteinuria develops in 40% of IDDM patients, of whom two-thirds will develop renal failure. Nephropathy is rarer in NIDDM, but due to the relatively high prevalence of NIDDM, 50% of diabetic patients entering end-stage renal failure in Britain each year are non-insulin-dependent.

• Non-diabetic renal disease accounts for proteinuria in up to 8% of diabetic patients. Alternative diagnoses are suggested by acute renal impairment, absence of retinopathy, haematuria, or short duration of IDDM (<5 years), and must be excluded by renal biopsy.

• Blood pressure is generally above normal in the early microalbuminuric stage of nephropathy. Hypertension affects virtually all patients with persistent proteinuria and tends to worsen as renal function declines. Supine hypertension and orthostatic hypotension (due to autonomic neuropathy) may coexist.

• Early effective control of blood pressure may delay the advent of end-stage renal failure by over 20 years. Angiotensin-converting enzyme inhibitors may have an additional beneficial effect in reducing intraglomerular pressure.

• Extensive, severe cardiovascular disease develops early in diabetic patients with nephropathy. Coronary heart disease is often asymptomatic but electrocardiographic and angiographic abnormalities are common. Peripheral vascular disease includes widespread multisegmental atheromatous lesions and medial arterial calcification in hands and feet; digital ischaemia and gangrene are common.

• Neuropathic foot ulceration affects one-quarter of diabetic patients with nephropathy, but Charcot joints are relatively uncommon. Tests of sensory and autonomic function are abnormal in most patients. Symptoms vary considerably.

• Retinopathy is virtually always present in nephropathy and is proliferative in about 70% of cases. Untreated retinopathy often deteriorates together with renal function, possibly through worsening hypertension and fluid retention.

• GFR, serum creatinine, urea and electrolytes must be monitored regularly in proteinuric patients. The interval to end-stage renal failure may be estimated by linear extrapolation of plots of inverse creatinine or GFR. Urine must be cultured regularly to exclude infection, especially in patients with incomplete bladder emptying. Infection, dehydration and radiographic contrast media may precipitate acute-on-chronic renal failure.

• Insulin requirements fall (often by 50%) in renal failure due to reduced renal elimination of insulin. Metformin and most sulphonylureas are also cleared through the kidneys and accumulate in uraemia, causing hypoglycaemia and toxicity: transfer to insulin treatment is therefore recommended.

• Moderate dietary protein restriction (45 g/day) may slow the rate of decline in GFR if started early in diabetic nephropathy (before GFR falls below 15 ml/min).

• Renal replacement therapy — renal transplantation, haemodialysis or continuous ambulatory peritoneal dialysis (CAPD) — should be offered as freely to diabetic as to non-diabetic patients as their survival rates are now nearly comparable.

• Renal transplantation, ideally from a live related donor, is the treatment of choice in patients under 60 years of age. Transplantation is recommended when the serum creatinine reaches about 500 μmol/l. 5-year survival now exceeds 60% for cadaver grafts at most centres. Transplanted kidneys generally develop histological features of diabetic nephropathy but this is not known to have caused graft failure as yet.
• Chronic haemodialysis may be complicated in diabetic patients by difficult vascular access, postural hypotension and poor metabolic control and was previously associated with rapidly worsening retinopathy, causing blindness in 40% of cases. Haemodialysis may need to be started relatively early (serum creatinine 500–600 μmol/l) because of the tendency to fluid retention. 5-year survival is now about 45% and only 3% of cases now suffer visual loss; prognosis is poorer in patients over 60 years. Common causes of death are cardiovascular disease, sepsis and uraemia following withdrawal from dialysis.
• CAPD is inexpensive, avoids rapid volume fluctuations and allows patients to be independent. It is suitable for elderly patients and those with ischaemic heart disease, severe autonomic neuropathy or visual impairment. Insulin (at about twice the usual subcutaneous dose) can be added directly to the dialysis fluid and is absorbed into the portal system. Peritonitis is no more common than in non-diabetic patients. 3-year survival is now about 60%.
• Coexistent vascular disease, retinopathy and foot problems must be identified and treated if possible before undertaking renal replacement therapy, and carefully monitored thereafter. Coronary heart disease is the major cause of death in the first few years after starting renal replacement therapy, accounting for 50–65% of deaths (10 times the rate in non-diabetic patients); patients receiving haemodialysis are particularly at risk. Strokes, digital and limb gangrene are also common.

Proteinuria was first recognized in diabetic patients over 150 years ago but its true importance as indicating a severe and often fatal complication of diabetes was not realized until the 1930s [1]. Most of the excess mortality of diabetes occurs in patients with proteinuria (Fig. 16.1) [2, 3]. About 40% of IDDM patients will develop proteinuria; two-thirds of these will develop renal failure whereas the rest will die of cardiovascular disease (Table 16.1) [2–5]. Nephropathy also affects NIDDM patients and although most die from cardiovascular disease [6, 7], the relatively high prevalence of NIDDM means that nearly 50% of the diabetic patients entering end-stage renal failure are non-insulin-dependent [8–11].

Diabetic patients with renal failure are now accepted for renal replacement therapy in steadily increasing numbers (Fig. 16.2) [12], accounting for up to 25% of new patients in some countries [8, 13, 14]. In Britain, however, relatively few of the 600 diabetic patients estimated to develop end-stage renal failure each year enter renal replacement programmes [15], probably because of the outdated impression that diabetic patients fare badly with dialysis or transplantation [16, 17]. In fact, the results of renal replacement therapy in diabetic

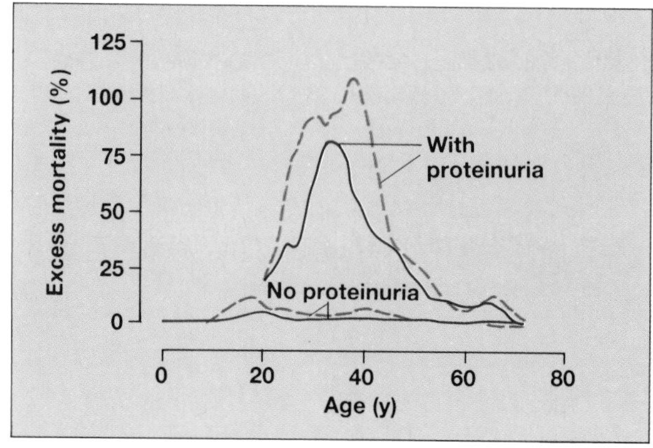


**Fig. 16.1.** Relative mortality of diabetic patients with and without persistent proteinuria, in men (——) and women (– – – – –) as a function of age. Mortality is greatly increased at all ages in proteinuric patients. (Redrawn from [2], with kind permission of the Editor of *Diabetologia*.)

**Table 16.1.** Causes of death in diabetic nephropathy.

| | UK study 1983 [5] | Steno [4] | Joslin [28] | UK study 1985 [92] |
|---|---|---|---|---|
| Renal failure | 60% | 66% | 59% | 50% |
| Cardiovascular disease | 25% | 24% | 36% | 25% |

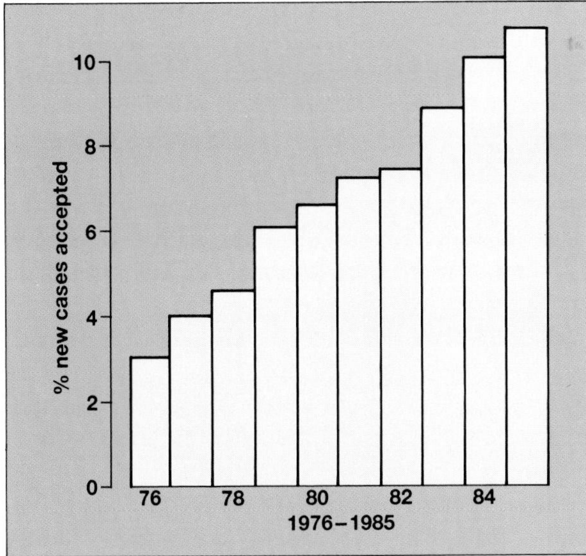


**Fig. 16.2.** Percentages of diabetic nephropathic patients entering end-stage renal failure who were accepted for renal replacement therapy in Europe in 1976–1985. (Redrawn from [12], with kind permission of Martinus Nijhoff Publishing, Boston.)

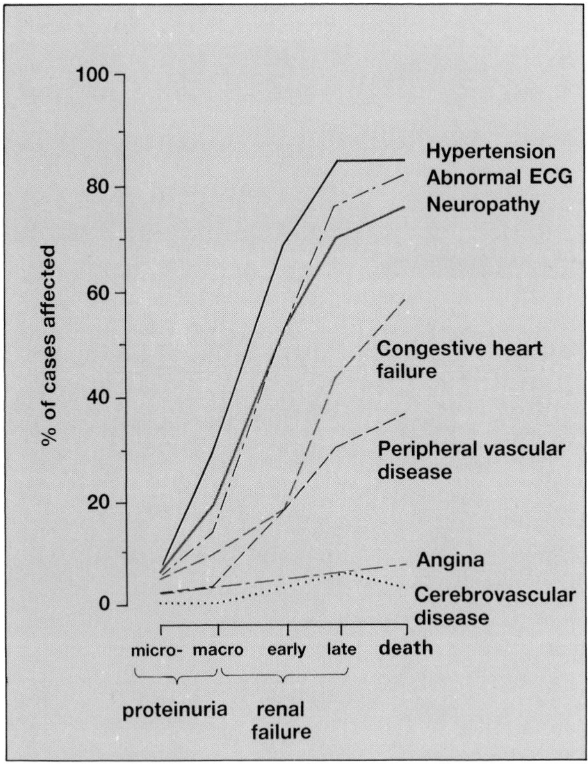


**Fig. 16.3.** Frequency of other diabetic complications at various stages of diabetic nephropathy. (Redrawn from [28], with kind permission of the Editor of the *Journal of the American Medical Association*.)

patients have improved considerably during the past 10 years and in some centres are now comparable with those in non-diabetic patients [18, 19].

Renal disease is often accompanied by widespread vascular disease, severe retinopathy and neuropathy (Fig. 16.3) [20], all complications which limit the success of renal replacement therapy. Successful management requires a joint approach by diabetes and renal specialist, with an understanding of the natural history of diabetic nephropathy.

This chapter will describe the clinical features and management of established diabetic nephropathy and end-stage renal failure.

## Clinical features of diabetic nephropathy

Proteinuria is usually the first manifestation of diabetic nephropathy and may be intermittent for many years before becoming persistent (see Chapter 13). Once persistent proteinuria has developed, renal function declines gradually but progressively, reaching end-stage renal failure on average within 7 years (see Figs 13.4 and 13.5) [4, 21]. Proteinuria increases as diabetic nephropathy progresses but only rarely reaches nephrotic proportions; however, fluid retention is common and occurs earlier than in non-diabetic patients [22].

Some elevation of blood pressure is usually present from the early, microalbuminuric stage of diabetic nephropathy (Fig. 16.4) [23–27], and almost all patients with persistent proteinuria have hypertension which continues to worsens as GFR falls (Figs 16.5 and 16.6). This may be masked by the postural hypotension of autonomic neuropathy, which is universal in such patients, if blood pressure is measured only in the sitting position; blood pressure must therefore be recorded both lying and standing to assess both the degree of hypertension and the effect of treatment. Hypertension in diabetic nephropathy is exquisitely volume-sensitive and this becomes more apparent as renal failure progresses.

Cardiovascular disease is common and extensive in diabetic nephropathy patients, even those in their 20s and 30s, but is often asymptomatic [28–30]. Angina is reported by only 10–20% of cases [5, 30, 31] and previous myocardial infarction is rare, but abnormal electrocardiograms are found in 50–70% of cases and radiographic evidence of cardiomegaly in 50% [28, 30, 32].

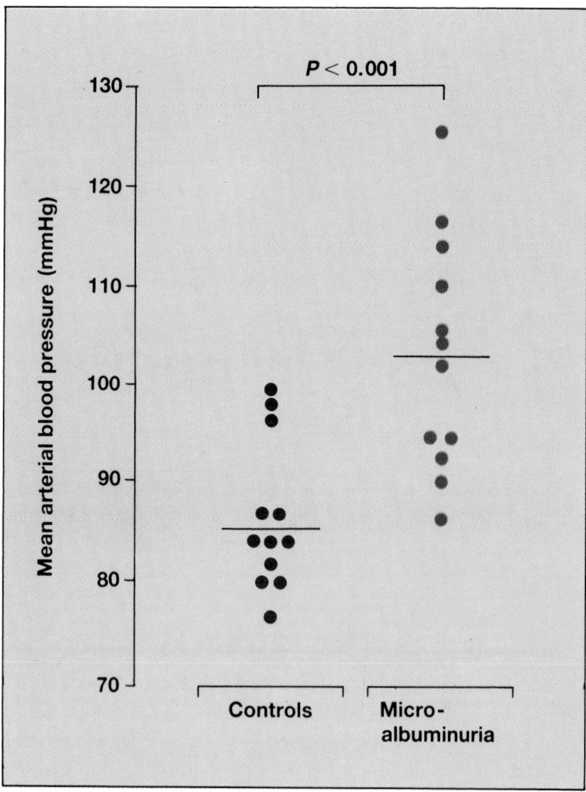


Fig. 16.4. Mean arterial blood pressure in IDDM patients with microalbuminuria (urinary albumin excretion 32–91 μg/min) and in matched diabetic patients with normal albumin excretion (2–10 μg/min). (Adapted from [25] with kind permission of the Editor of *Diabetologia*.)

Coronary angiography has shown the presence of significant coronary occlusive disease in 20–100% of patients, depending on selection and diagnostic criteria [29, 30, 33]. Even in the absence of significant coronary artery disease, diffuse myocardial dysfunction is frequent [34]. Left ventricular hypertrophy is common and usually severe in patients with advanced nephropathy (Fig. 16.7) [35, 36], probably reflecting long-standing and inadequately treated hypertension.

Peripheral vascular disease in patients with advanced nephropathy affects hands as well as feet, complicating vascular access for haemodialysis and leading to a high amputation rate especially after transplantation [37–41]. Among patients being considered for renal transplantation, 10–20% have absent foot pulses, claudication or gangrene and about 1–2% have had amputations [42, 43]. Atheromatous lesions in these patients are often multisegmental, bilateral and distal and involve the vessels below the knee [44]. Striking medial arterial calcification is frequently seen on radiographs and involves both large and small vessels, including the digital arteries of the hands and feet (Fig. 16.8) [32, 45]. This is partly related to the neuropathy which

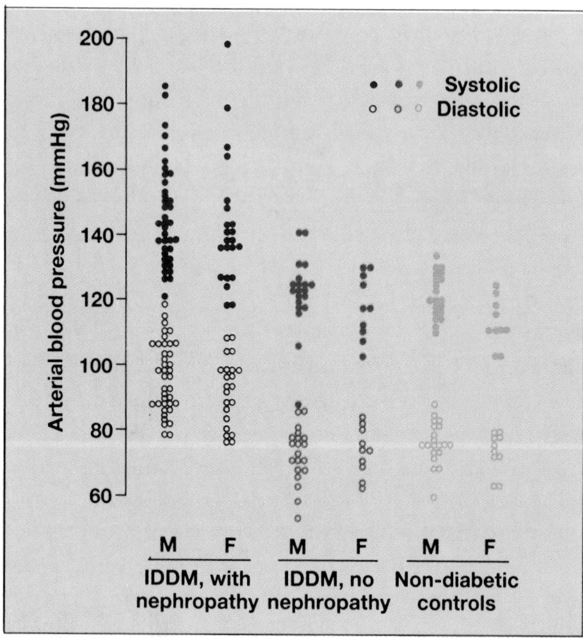


Fig. 16.5. Systolic and diastolic blood pressure in IDDM patients with and without nephropathy and in non-diabetic controls. All groups are age-matched. (Redrawn from [24] with kind permission of the Editor of *Diabetologia*.)

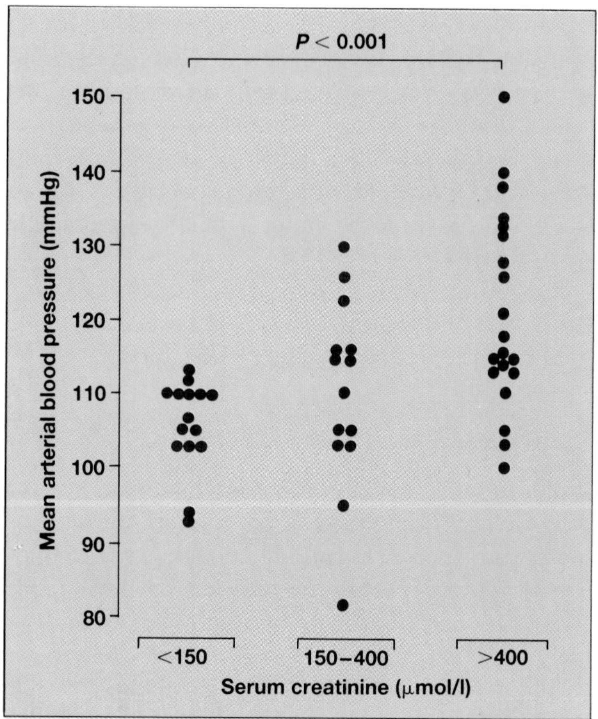


Fig. 16.6. Mean arterial blood pressure in three groups of diabetic nephropathic patients subdivided according to serum creatinine level (A. Grenfell, unpublished observations).

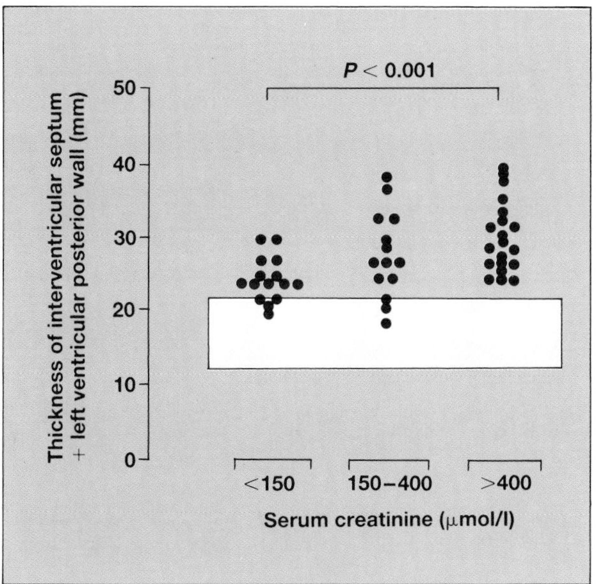


Fig. 16.7. Left ventricular wall thickness in patients with diabetic nephropathy subdivided according to serum creatinine level, showing increasing left ventricular hypertrophy with worsening renal impairment. Yellow area represents normal adult range. (Redrawn from [35] with kind permission of the Editor of *Diabetic Medicine*.)

affects these patients but is usually more extensive than in patients with neuropathy alone [46]. Digital arterial calcification is associated with the digital gangrene common in these patients (Fig. 16.9) but its precise aetiological role is uncertain [45].

Neuropathy affects most patients with advanced diabetic nephropathy to a variable extent [30, 32, 47], some being completely asymptomatic whereas others suffer severe features of somatic and autonomic neuropathy. Various reports suggest that 40–100% of patients receiving renal transplants have some degree of somatic neuropathy [30, 47, 48]. Neuropathic ulceration is the most important consequence, occurring in up to one-quarter of patients with diabetic nephropathy. Charcot joints are much rarer, affecting only 3% of a series of diabetic patients with renal failure at King's College Hospital (A. Grenfell, unpublished observations).

Autonomic neuropathy is almost invariable in those with established nephropathy, although symptoms are very variable. Postural hypotension is usually mild but may complicate antihypertensive therapy. Gustatory sweating and diarrhoea

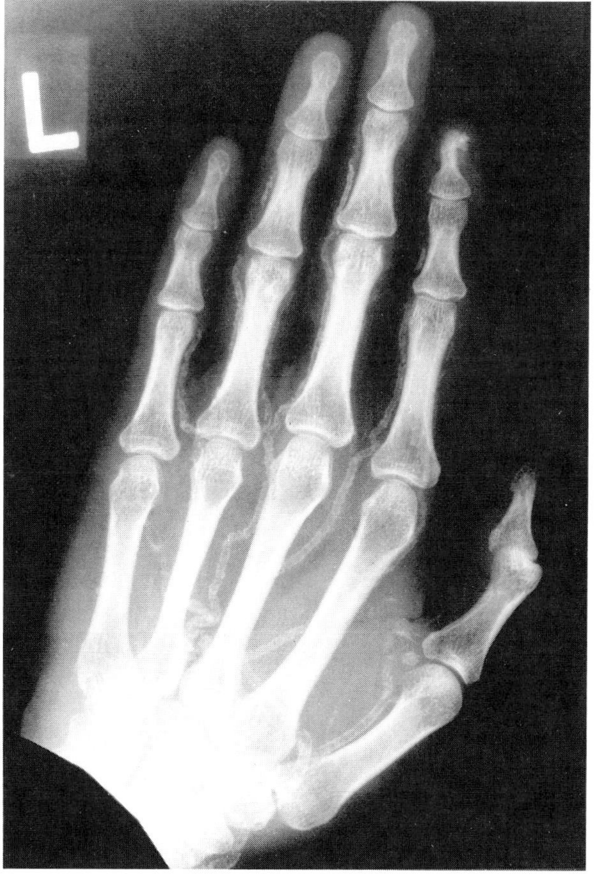


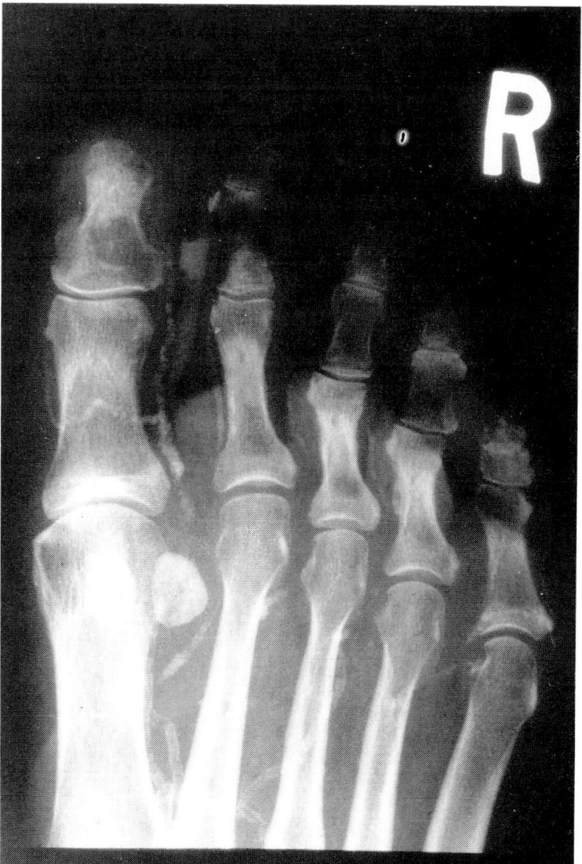


Fig. 16.8. Medial calcification of digital arteries of hands and feet in a patient with renal failure due to diabetic nephropathy.

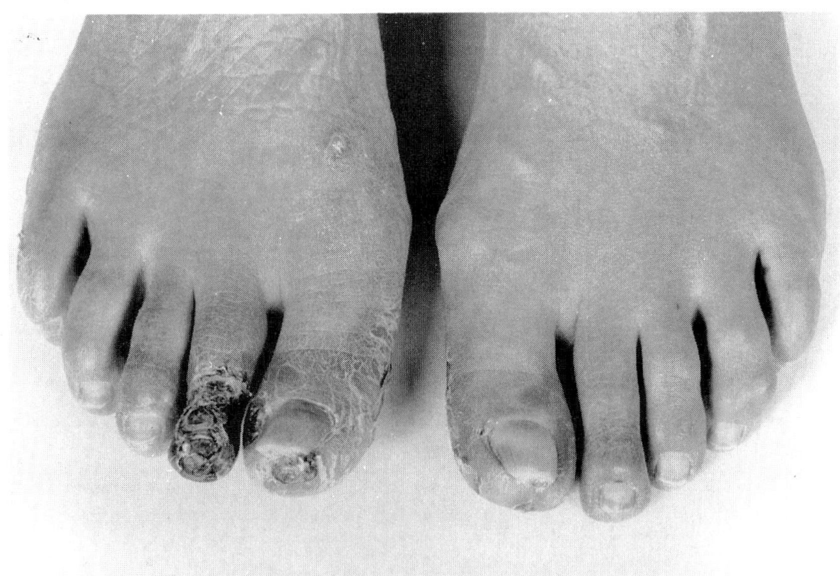

**Fig. 16.9.** Digital gangrene in a diabetic nephropathic patient with renal failure.

are relatively common and occur in about 50% of patients. Incomplete bladder emptying is rare: only 10% of patients assessed with micturating cystography at King's College Hospital had a significant residual urine volume (>50 ml). Vomiting due to gastroparesis is rare but can be devastating and refractory to treatment. Vomiting is difficult to assess in uraemic patients: a barium meal is often unhelpful and more sophisticated tests of stomach emptying may be required [49] (see Chapter 20). Respiratory arrests associated with sedative drugs or anaesthesia occur in occasional patients with autonomic neuropathy [50].

Retinopathy is virtually always present in established diabetic nephropathy [20, 51]; its absence suggests that the renal disease is not due to diabetes. Proliferative retinopathy is reported in 70% of cases, with roughly one-third registered blind and another one-third having severely impaired vision [32, 42, 48]. As renal failure develops, retinopathy tends to deteriorate, probably due to a combination of hypertension and fluid retention, especially if previously untreated [52].

## Diagnosis of diabetic nephropathy

Renal disease other than diabetic nephropathy may occur in diabetic patients [53, 54] and may account for proteinuria in 3–8% of cases [4, 55]. Of the 163 patients treated at King's College Hospital, 17% had a non-diabetic renal disease, being found more often among NIDDM (27%) than IDDM patients (10%). The distinction is crucial as other renal diseases may need specific treatment and may carry a different prognosis.

The diagnosis of diabetic nephropathy is straightforward in the presence of a typical history and clinical features. Proteinuria developing in an IDDM patient of 10–20 years standing who has other complications, especially retinopathy, needs few investigations. Urine should be examined for red cells and casts, and cultured to exclude infection. Ultrasound examination is important to demonstrate renal size. This is usually normal or even large in diabetic nephropathy [56], although biopsy-proven glomerulosclerosis has been observed in small kidneys [57]. Bladder ultrasound examination will exclude obstruction and urinary retention due to a neuropathic bladder. Immunological tests to exclude systemic lupus erythematosus and other glomerulonephritides should be performed as indicated.

Features suggestive of an alternative diagnosis (Table 16.2) [58] include a rapid deterioration in renal function from normal, sudden development of nephrotic syndrome, absence of retinopathy, the presence of haematuria [59] (although red cell casts occur rarely in diabetic nephropathy [60]),

**Table 16.2.** Features suggesting an alternative cause of renal impairment in diabetic patients.

- Rapid deterioration in renal function from normal
- Sudden development of nephrotic syndrome
- Presence of haematuria
- Short duration (<5 years) of IDDM

and short duration of otherwise uncomplicated IDDM. Renal biopsy should be performed if there is any doubt as to the diagnosis.

### Monitoring renal function

Renal function must be monitored in patients with diabetic nephropathy, both to estimate the time to end-stage renal failure and to determine the effects of intervention. Serum creatinine concentration does not reflect glomerular filtration rate (GFR) in the early stages of nephropathy and only rises when GFR is reduced by 50–70% (Fig. 16.10). GFR should therefore be measured, ideally using isotopic methods, during the early stages (Fig. 16.11). Serial plots of inverse creatinine (1000/creatinine in μmol/l) generally show a linear decline which, if extrapolated, may predict when end-stage renal failure is likely to occur (Fig. 16.12); this method is only useful when the serum creatinine concentration exceeds 200 μmol/l [61]. The quantity of proteinuria and serum albumin levels should also be monitored. Urine should be cultured to detect infection.

Certain circumstances, notably sepsis and dehydration, may cause an acute deterioration in patients with diabetic nephropathy [62]. Diabetic patients are particularly prone to septicaemia, especially arising from urinary tract infections, and to the serious complication of papillary necrosis [63]. Urinary retention due to autonomic neuropathy is rare but must be actively excluded; it is usually asymptomatic and commonly leads to recurrent urinary tract infections which aggravate renal impairment [64].

Radiographic contrast media should be avoided if possible, especially in patients whose serum creatinine exceeds 200 μmol/l, as renal function often declines acutely [65]; newer contrast agents with lower osmolarity are less nephrotoxic. Essential investigations (e.g. coronary angiography)

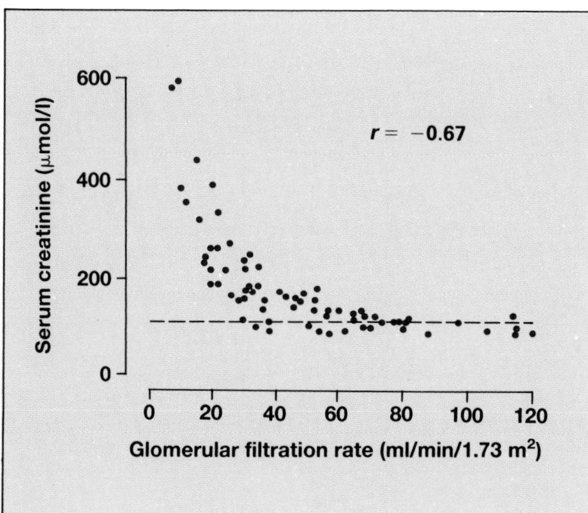


**Fig. 16.10.** Glomerular filtration rate (GFR) measured by $^{51}$Cr-EDTA clearance, plotted against serum creatinine concentration in 73 subjects at various stages of diabetic nephropathy. Dashed line represents upper limit of normal serum creatinine concentration. (Redrawn from [61] with kind permission of the Editor of the *American Journal of Medicine*.)

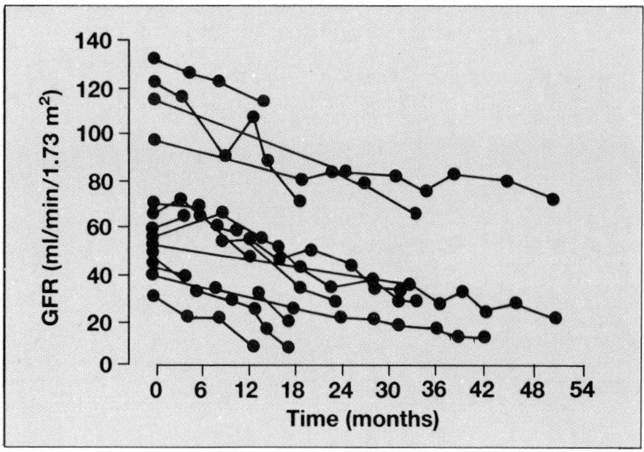


**Fig. 16.11.** Progressive and generally linear decline in GFR (measured by $^{51}$Cr-EDTA clearance) in 13 diabetic patients with nephropathy. (Redrawn from [61] with kind permission of the Editor of the *American Journal of Medicine*.)

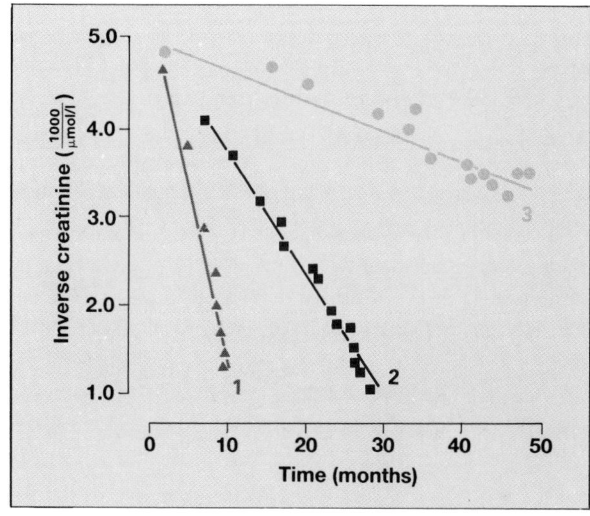


**Fig. 16.12.** Serial plots of inverse creatinine values (1000/serum creatinine concentration in μmol/l) in three representative diabetic nephropathic patients. Inverse serum creatinine declines linearly with time, at a fixed rate for each individual patient — fastest for patient 1 (▲) and slowest for patient 3 (●). (Adapted from Jones *et al. Lancet* 1979; i: 1105–6, with kind permission of the Editor.)

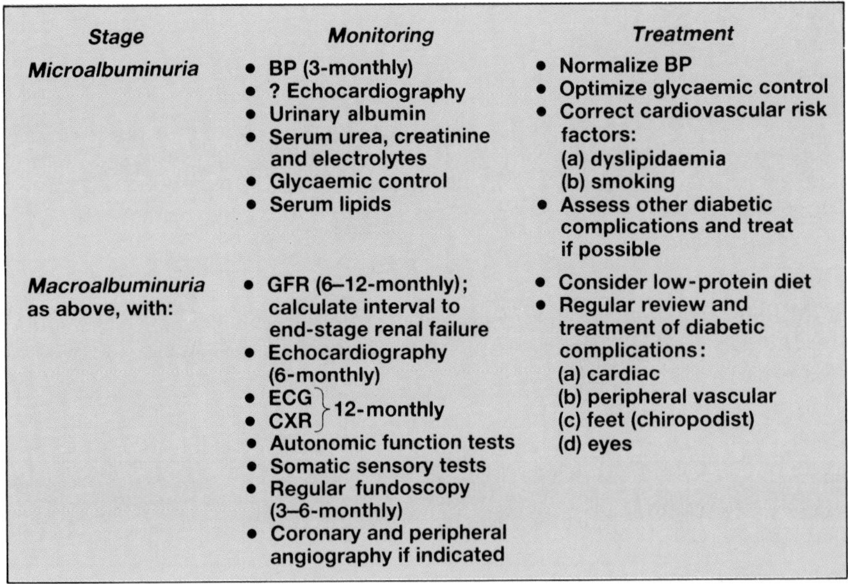


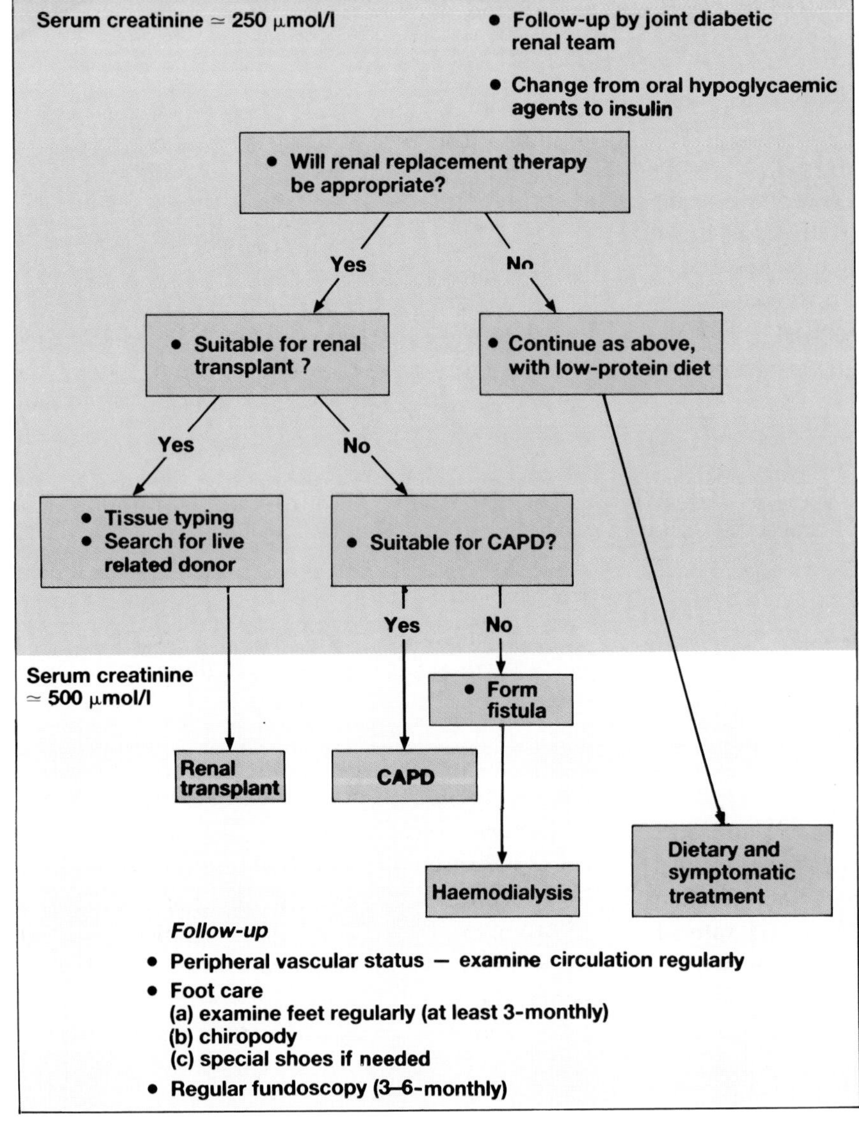


**Fig. 16.13.** Flow-chart illustrating the management of patients with diabetic nephropathy, before the onset of renal failure (upper panel) and with renal failure (lower panel).

should ideally be performed as early as possible and the patient should be well hydrated with intravenous fluids and mannitol [66]. Patients with significant renal impairment are best established on dialysis before investigation. Other nephrotoxic drugs (such as aminoglycosides, especially if used concurrently with loop diuretics) should similarly be avoided.

## Management of established diabetic nephropathy

Patients with persistent proteinuria should be followed up at least 3-monthly and every effort made to achieve good glycaemic control and a normal blood pressure and to correct any other risk factors (particularly smoking and dyslipidaemia) for the cardiovascular disease which will remain a serious threat to their lives.

Renal function should be monitored as above and, after GFR has been falling for some months, its rate of decline should be calculated and the likely interval to end-stage renal failure estimated. Once serum creatinine has reached 250 μmol/l, the patient is best managed by a joint team of diabetologist, renal physician and transplant surgeon, together with the diabetes specialist nurse, dietitian, and ultimately the renal replacement specialist nurse. Current policy in many centres is to aim for renal transplantation or long-term dialysis before the serum creatinine is much over 500 μmol/l; many preparations (e.g. tissue typing and searching for an appropriate live related donor) will need to be made before then. Patients with symptomatic uraemia will need to be seen at least every 1–3 months, and should have access to specialist advice in case of acute complications. A suggested management flow chart is shown in Fig. 16.13. The treatment of specific problems is described below.

### *Control of hypertension*

In 1976, Mogensen first demonstrated a positive correlation between diastolic blood pressure and the rate of decline of GFR [23]. Several studies have subsequently demonstrated that effective antihypertensive therapy can reduce the rate of decline, sometimes to less than one-fifth of pretreatment values (Fig. 16.14) [67–71]. The most favourable results suggest that the progression from normal GFR to end-stage renal failure may take up to 30 years, rather than the average of 7

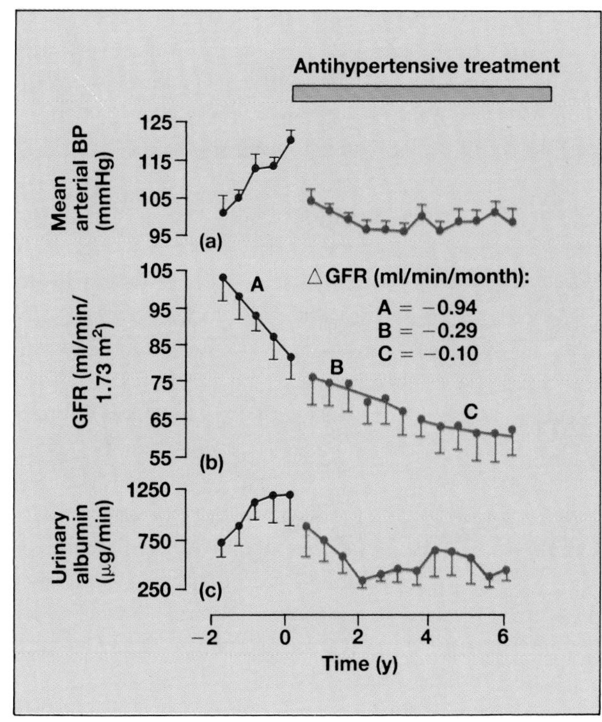


**Fig. 16.14.** Effects of antihypertensive treatment on mean arterial blood pressure (a), GFR (b) and urinary albumin excretion (c) in IDDM patients with nephropathy. Rate of decline in GFR and albumin excretion were both significantly reduced. Error bars are SEM. (Reproduced from [68] with kind permission of the Editor of the *British Medical Journal*.)

years in inadequately treated patients. Hypertension must therefore be discovered and treated early; all too often, lack of effective treatment initially may lead to a loss in GFR of several ml/min.

The optimal blood pressure and therapeutic target in nephropathic patients are uncertain (see Chapter 18). The WHO criteria may be too lax for this relatively young population and a more appropriate target may be the age-related norms (see Fig. 18.4) [72]. However, higher supine levels may have to be accepted if postural hypotension is a problem.

Many drugs, particularly β-blockers and diuretics, have been used to control blood pressure in patients with diabetic nephropathy but have not been adequately compared in controlled studies. Accordingly, no specific drug or combination of drugs can be regarded as first choice, although certain recommendations can be made. The aim should be to reduce blood pressure satisfactorily using drugs and other means acceptable to the patient (see Chapter 18), and in most cases this can be achieved. Important features of the main antihypertensive drugs used are shown in Table 18.3.

A diuretic is usually necessary and a rational choice as exchangeable sodium is increased in diabetic patients [73, 74] and oedema is a common problem. Blood pressure appears to be particularly volume-sensitive, especially when serum creatinine concentrations start to rise; loop diuretics may be needed at this stage. Selective $\beta_1$-adrenoceptor blockers are also useful despite their potential problems, notably delayed recovery from and impaired awareness of hypoglycaemia, exacerbation of lipid abnormalities and possibly hyperglycaemia. Most of these are probably of limited practical importance, as is suggested by their widespread and successful use. Calcium channel blockers such as nifedipine are often poorly tolerated by diabetic nephropathy patients as they often cause troublesome peripheral oedema. Vasodilators, and prazosin, have been used as second-line agents in diabetic patients but commonly exacerbate postural hypotension.

Angiotensin-converting enzyme (ACE) inhibitors are now promoted as first-line agents for treating diabetic nephropathy. As well as their systemic hypotensive action, these drugs are thought to reduce intraglomerular pressure by specifically relaxing efferent glomerular arterioles and so may further help to preserve renal function in the diabetic patient [75]. ACE inhibitors undoubtedly reduce the rate of decline of renal function in diabetic nephropathy [69]; whether this simply reflects effective blood pressure control or a specific action on glomerular haemodynamics is undetermined, as alternative antihypertensive drugs have achieved similar results. ACE inhibitors are well tolerated by diabetic patients and are useful first- or second-line agents when other drugs are unsuitable or blood pressure control is inadequate.

### *Glycaemic control*

The importance of hyperglycaemia in the progression of established diabetic nephropathy has been addressed by several studies [76–78] but remains unclear. Two controlled studies from Guy's Hospital showed no influence of strict metabolic control (imposed by CSII) on the rate of decline of GFR or fractional clearance of protein in diabetic patients with persistent or intermittent proteinuria [76, 77]. Both studies can be criticized for their small size (six patients in each group), inadequate control of hypertension (which is probably a more important factor than hyperglycaemia), and the fact that metabolic control may have been suboptimal. In patients with established nephropathy and tightly controlled blood pressure, progression of GFR has been reported to relate to the degree of metabolic control as assessed by $HbA_1$ [78].

As renal failure progresses, insulin clearance and degradation by the kidneys decreases and insulin requirements gradually fall in most patients, often by up to 50%. Frequent home blood glucose monitoring is therefore essential to direct any changes in the insulin regimen.

Most of the oral hypoglycaemic agents, particularly chlorpropamide, glibenclamide, tolbutamide and metformin, are normally metabolized or cleared by the kidneys and so accumulate in uraemic patients, increasing the risks of hypoglycaemia and toxicity. Some second-generation sulphonylureas such as gliclazide are cleared predominantly through the liver and may be relatively safer in renal failure. However, many specialist centres prefer to transfer all patients receiving oral agents to insulin when serum creatinine concentration reaches 250 μmol/l.

### *Dietary protein intake*

Dietary protein intake is known to influence renal function [79] and a low-protein diet prevents the progression of both experimental and human chronic renal failure [80, 81]. In diabetic renal failure, low-protein diets (20–30 g/day) were used initially to relieve the symptoms of advanced uraemia but did not apparently delay the progression to end-stage renal failure [82]. A cross-sectional study of IDDM patients found no correlation between protein intake and the presence of nephropathy or its rate of decline [83].

Studies of moderate protein restriction in early diabetic renal failure have yielded inconclusive and conflicting results [83–86]. In a study from Guy's Hospital [84], one year of treatment with a low protein diet slowed the rate of decline of GFR and reduced total urinary protein excretion in a group of 20 IDDM patients as a whole (see Fig. 14.9). However, individual responses varied considerably, GFR remaining stable or declining less rapidly in one half of the subjects but continuing to decline at the same rate in the rest. Equivocal results are also reported in a separate but similar study from the same centre [85]. By contrast, an Italian study found that a low-protein, low-phosphate diet supplemented with essential amino acids and ketoanalogues apparently slowed the fall in creatinine clearance and urinary protein excretion in all eight patients studied during a 17-month period [86].

Longer-term, larger-scale controlled studies are needed to clarify the role of dietary protein, although some sensible suggestions can be made [87]. Severe protein restriction (20–25 g/day) is inadvisable because it runs the risk of malnutrition and is unacceptable to most patients. Moderate protein restriction (45 g/day, 0.5–0.6 g/kg/day) if started before renal impairment is too advanced (GFR > 15 ml/min) may be useful and is nutritionally adequate for long periods. However, such diets are unpalatable for many patients and long-term compliance is likely to be poor.

In the past, carbohydrate-restricted diabetic diets have had a high protein content which may have had a deleterious effect on the kidneys. Pending clearer evidence regarding protein restriction, diabetic patients should be advised to eat more unrefined carbohydrate and therefore less protein, in line with recent guidelines [88].

### Assessment and management of other diabetic complications

Complications which commonly accompany diabetic nephropathy should be assessed carefully and at an early stage, in order to pre-empt the problems which in the past have placed diabetic patients with end-stage renal failure at such a high risk.

Cardiovascular examination is mandatory early in the course of diabetic nephropathy. Hypertension must be treated energetically, especially if causing left ventricular hypertrophy. This can be measured accurately and monitored using echocardiography, which should probably be performed at the microalbuminuric stage and then repeated every 3–6 months; effective antihypertensive therapy will reverse left ventricular hypertrophy.

Coronary angiography may be required, as non-invasive methods such as thallium stress testing do not seem to provide adequate information on myocardial status [89]. Future work will establish whether coronary angiography helps to select patients for renal replacement and whether coronary artery bypass or angioplasty will influence its outcome.

Peripheral vascular disease must be assessed and treated as necessary. The absence of foot pulses predicts poor healing of foot lesions which are common in these patients [90]. Plain radiography of the hands and feet will demonstrate medial arterial calcification (Fig. 16.8), which causes spuriously high systolic pressures. Arteriography should be performed to resolve any doubts about the circulation. Angioplasty is used increasingly and may accelerate the healing of foot lesions, but amputation should be considered for widespread vascular disease, particularly if complicated by infection or non-healing foot lesions and especially if transplantation is being considered.

Testing vibration perception threshold and thermal discrimination may identify feet at risk of neuropathic ulceration and this should be repeated regularly as sensation may only become impaired later in the course of nephropathy. Autonomic function tests are abnormal in virtually all nephropathic patients, but symptoms are very variable. The important manifestations are postural hypotension (which may complicate antihypertensive therapy) and incomplete bladder emptying. The latter should be assessed with ultrasound scanning or micturating cystography and may require regular self-catheterization.

Foot care is critical to the management of patients with diabetic nephropathy before, during and after renal replacement therapy and demands close liaison between chiropodist, shoe fitter, physician and surgeon [90]. Removal of callus and provision of special shoes to off-load weight-bearing areas avoids many problems but infection must be treated promptly and vigorously, with intravenous antibiotics if cellulitis is suspected. Early surgical drainage of abscesses and removal of necrotic tissue may prevent osteomyelitis or gangrene; limited ray amputation often successfully treats these complications [91].

Retinopathy, usually proliferative, almost always accompanies diabetic nephropathy and tends to deteriorate as renal failure progresses. With early regular ophthalmological review and prompt treatment as necessary, fewer patients should become blind before renal failure develops.

### Renal replacement therapy

Dialysis and renal transplantation are now accepted as appropriate for diabetic patients. In Europe the proportion of diabetic patients entering end-stage renal failure who were offered renal replacement therapy increased steadily from only

3% in 1976 to 10.7% in 1985 and reached 30% in some Scandinavian countries (see Fig. 16.2) [12]; in the UK in 1985, the proportion was 11.4% [15], indicating a considerable shortfall in treatment. A recent British survey showed that, despite increasing use of renal replacement therapy for diabetic renal failure, one-third of these patients died without receiving renal support, half of whom died directly from renal failure [92]. In Britain, diabetes accounts for some 20–25% of cases requiring renal replacement [93]. The patient populations accepted for renal replacement differ considerably between countries, IDDM patients being treated virtually exclusively in Sweden, Finland and Norway and those with NIDDM predominating in Austria, Denmark and the Federal Republic of Germany [94]. About 20% of British diabetic patients treated for renal failure are non-insulin-dependent. These different patterns may be partly explained by the high frequency of IDDM in Sweden, Finland and Norway and possibly by an accelerated progression of the disease in these countries.

The methods of renal replacement therapy chosen for diabetic patients differ from those for other primary renal diseases (Fig. 16.15) and also show geographical variation. Peritoneal dialysis, especially continuous ambulatory peritoneal dialysis (CAPD), is a relatively common initial and maintenance treatment for diabetic patients [94]. Renal transplantation is chosen more commonly as first-line treatment for IDDM patients than for those with NIDDM or other primary renal diseases. In Scandinavia particularly, many IDDM patients receive renal transplantation whereas surgeons in France and Germany still apparently resist transplanting patients with diabetic nephropathy (Fig. 16.16). In the UK in 1985, 46% of diabetic patients alive on renal replacement therapy were treated with CAPD while 34% had had a renal transplant [12].

### *Selection criteria*

Selection policies for renal replacement therapy vary considerably but until recently were stricter for diabetic than for non-diabetic patients. Older and more complicated diabetic patients are now being treated.

Age is an important selection criterion for renal replacement. Older patients (>60 years) have a much poorer prognosis [95] and therefore tend to be treated by dialysis alone and not referred for transplantation. However, age restrictions have recently been relaxed considerably, as is shown by the increasing number and greater age of NIDDM patients treated [10, 96].

Cardiovascular disease is probably the most important factor to consider in selecting patients for renal replacement therapy. Patients with severe symptomatic coronary artery disease, severe cardiac failure and/or marked cardiomegaly generally fare badly [43] and should probably be referred for

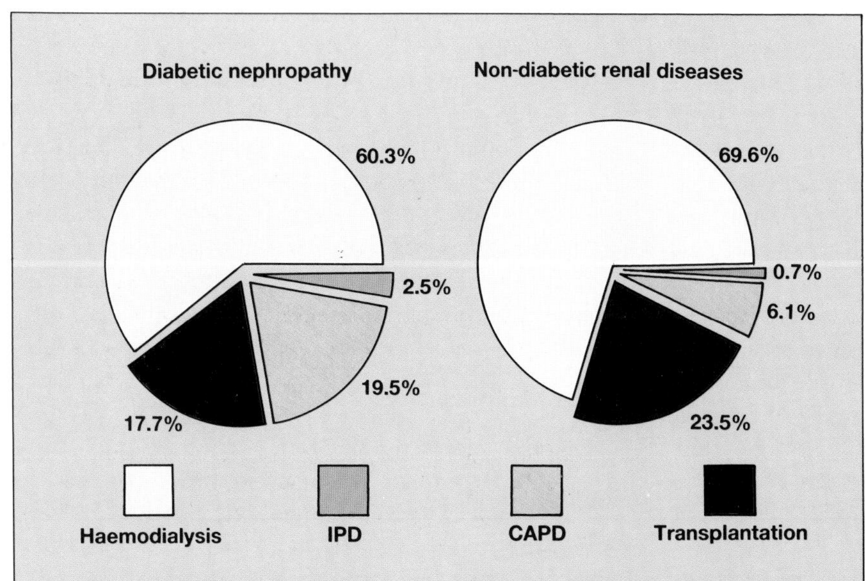


**Fig. 16.15.** Methods of renal replacement used to treat patients with diabetic nephropathy and other primary renal diseases throughout Europe in 1985. IPD and CAPD: intermittent and continuous ambulatory peritoneal dialysis respectively. (Redrawn from [12] with kind permission of Martinus Nijhoff Publishing, Boston.)

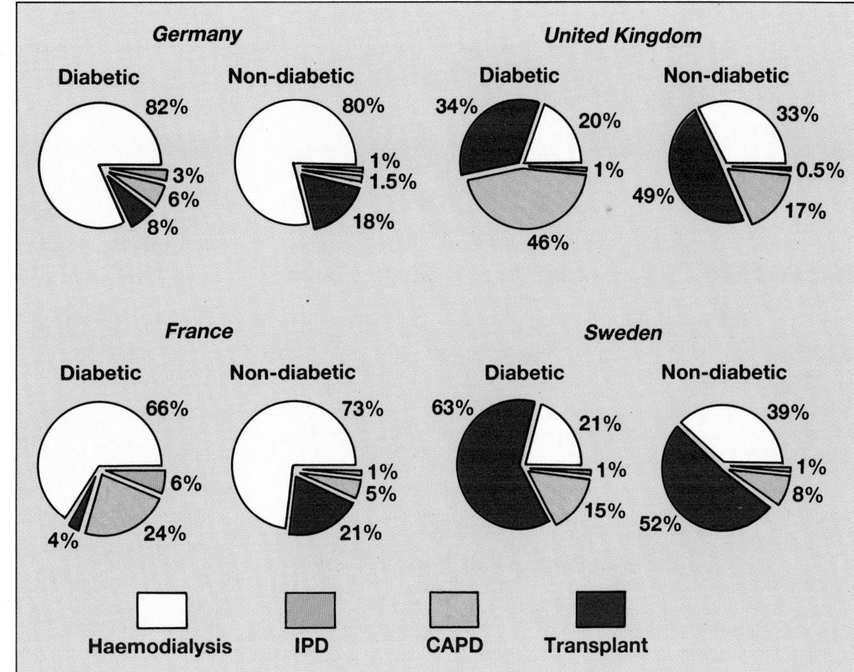


**Fig. 16.16.** Methods of renal replacement used to treat patients with diabetic nephropathy and other primary renal diseases in four different European countries in 1985. (Redrawn from [12] with kind permission of Martinus Nijhoff Publishing, Boston.)

dialysis rather than transplantation. Peripheral vascular disease does not contraindicate treatment but may limit vascular access for haemodialysis. Incipient or established gangrene and sepsis are contraindications for transplantation because of the risks of infection during immunosuppression.

Autonomic neuropathy may exacerbate hypotension during haemodialysis whereas a neuropathic bladder is a relative contraindication to transplantation. The presence of retinopathy should not influence decisions about renal replacement therapy. Deterioration of vision during haemodialysis is now rare with better treatment of hypertension and fluid overload and with early and more effective laser treatment. Blind patients usually manage well with all forms of treatment, including CAPD [97].

### *Timing of renal replacement*

Previously, diabetic patients were often referred very late or treated according to the criteria used for non-diabetic patients. However, diabetic patients are now recognized to have symptoms (especially of fluid overload) at lower creatinine levels than non-diabetic subjects. Earlier treatment is therefore now recommended. In Minneapolis, for example, transplantation is advised when serum creatinine levels reach about 500 μmol/l, an approach made possible by a large number of live related donors [19]. However, a period of uraemia is thought to help to prevent rejection by inducing a degree of immunosuppression; transplantation should therefore not be performed too early. Aggressive treatment of hypertension and fluid overload may make this compromise possible.

### *Transplantation*

Renal transplantation has been available as a rouine treatment for diabetic patients with end-stage renal failure in some centres for over 15 years and is considered by many to be the treatment of choice. The criteria identifying patients suitable for transplantation are outlined in Table 16.3.

The early results of renal transplantation in diabetic patients [16, 17, 43], although not as good as for non-diabetic patients, were considerably better than for chronic haemodialysis [98, 99]. Subsequent reports emphasized the value of renal transplantation for diabetic patients with renal failure [30, 38, 42, 47] and their considerably improved survival (Fig. 16.17). At some centres, the survival of diabetic patients who receive grafts from living donors is now the same as for non-diabetic subjects [18, 19]. Results of cadaver transplantation are less favourable but have nonetheless improved markedly. Factors underlying these

**Table 16.3.** Criteria for renal transplantation.

- Age <65 years
- Absence of severe cardiac disease
- Absence of sepsis
- Suitable donor available

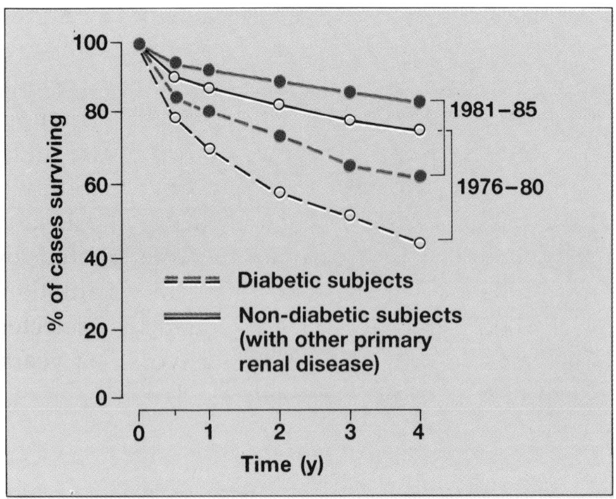


**Fig. 16.17.** Patient survival after first cadaver graft, for diabetic subjects and patients with other primary renal diseases, showing the improved survival of diabetic patients transplanted in 1981–1985 (●) as compared with 1976–1980 (○). (Adapted from [12] with kind permission of Martinus Nijhoff Publishing, Boston.)

improved results include the use of pretransplant blood transfusions, earlier acceptance and treatment of diabetic patients, better pretransplant management of hypertension and fluid overload, improved immunosuppression regimens with cyclosporin and lower steroid dosages, and better management of diabetes using intensive insulin regimens.

Preparation of the diabetic patient for transplantation is similar to that for non-diabetic subjects but also requires the careful assessment and treatment of diabetic complications. Transplantation, if possible, should be performed before dialysis is needed, especially in patients with live related donors.

Careful diabetic control during and after transplantation is important. Perioperatively, all patients should be treated with continuous intravenous insulin infusion until able to eat and drink (usually within 24 h). The use of steroids following transplantation usually demands an increase in insulin dose (often exceeding 50%) in IDDM patients and transfer to insulin in NIDDM patients. A regimen of soluble insulin before each meal and an intermediate-acting insulin before bed is suitable immediately postoperatively while insulin requirements are being established. Intravenous methylprednisolone for treating rejection episodes always causes severe hyperglycaemia which is best treated with a continuous intravenous insulin infusion started with the first pulse of steroid [100]. Increased oral steroids can usually be covered by increased doses of subcutaneous insulin.

Excellent rehabilitation is possible for diabetic patients following renal transplantation [13, 42]. At King's College Hospital, 80% of diabetic transplant patients were fit (although only half of these were in full-time work) and 20% of those transplanted between 1974 and 1987 have survived for longer than 5 years (range, 6–14 years) with good rehabilitation; the Minneapolis group have reported 26 patients surviving for over 10 years [101].

Histological changes compatible with diabetic nephropathy can be detected in most transplanted kidneys after about 4 years [102, 103] but vary considerably from minimal to severe changes. No transplanted kidney has yet been reported to have failed due to diabetic nephropathy *per se*.

### *Haemodialysis*

Despite the high transplant rates of some renal units and some countries, dialysis is the only treatment available for most patients [12, 92, 104]. Dialysis is indicated in patients unsuitable for transplantation, while awaiting transplantation or following graft failures. They early results of chronic haemodialysis in diabetic patients were very poor, with 2-year survival rates of only 20–40% and a high morbidity rate [105, 106]. Improved dialysis techniques and earlier dialysis, together with effective management of hypertension, metabolic state and nutrition, have made dialysis a viable long-term treatment option for the diabetic patient [40, 107].

Diabetic patients need careful preparation for haemodialysis. Dialysis may need to be started at lower serum creatinine levels (about 500 μmol/l) than in non-diabetic subjects because of the tendency to fluid retention and volume-dependent hypertension. Haemodialysis poses special problems in diabetic patients (Table 16.4). Vascular access should be created 3–6 months in advance,

**Table 16.4.** Problems of haemodialysis in diabetic patients.

| |
|---|
| • Difficult vascular access and failure of A–V fistulae |
| • Haemodynamic instability |
| • Erratic glycaemic control |
| • Progression of retinopathy |
| • Poor rehabilitation |

as technical problems due to arteriosclerosis and medial calcification are commoner and maturation of fistulae slower than in non-diabetic patients.

Arteriovenous fistulae also tend to fail prematurely: about 67% remain functional at 1 year compared with 83% in non-diabetic patients [108]. Bovine or PTFE grafts appear to survive better. Distal ischaemia causing pain and/or digital necrosis may supervene, sometimes requiring closure of the fistula or graft and occasionally amputation [109].

Satisfactory metabolic control during dialysis may be hard to achieve [110]. It is often difficult to impose fluid restriction on patients with thirst due to hyperglycaemia and to maintain adequate nutrition. Dialysate containing glucose (5–8 mmol/l) should be used to prevent hypoglycaemia and minimize protein catabolism and ketone body production. Insulin requirements may be very variable, depending on the patient's appetite, physical activity and other medical problems. With worsening renal failure, insulin requirements generally fall due to reduced renal clearance of insulin. On starting dialysis, insulin requirements increase, often to twice the predialysis level.

Chronic haemodialysis in diabetic patients was previously associated with rapid progression of retinopathy, leading to blindness in 40% of cases [111]. With earlier dialysis, improved treatment of hypertension and fluid overload and above all, active treatment of diabetic eye disease before beginning dialysis, only 3% of cases now suffer visual loss [40]. Indeed, vision may improve after starting dialysis due to loss of retinal oedema.

Significant postural hypotension due to autonomic neuropathy may make it impossible to remove enough fluid at haemodialysis to achieve the patient's optimal 'dry' weight, which is an important factor in the successful control of hypertension. Certain antihypertensive drugs aggravate the problem but can often be omitted while excess body fluid is gradually decreased over several weeks by progressive ultrafiltration. If blood pressure falls during dialysis before optimum weight has been achieved, it may be better to use hypertonic rather than normal saline to expand the intravascular volume as smaller volumes of fluid are required.

The prognosis of diabetic patients receiving haemodialysis has improved dramatically during the past 20 years. The 1- and 5-year survival figures of 85 and 45% respectively are now similar to those for cadaver transplants and many patients have survived for over a decade [107, 112]. In those over the age of 60 years, however, survival is much poorer. An important cause of death is withdrawal from dialysis by patients [107]. Prognosis and rehabilitation are worse in patients treated by haemodialysis than following transplantation, partly because older, high-risk patients are selected for dialysis [107]. Long-term survivors (>4 years) seem to have better rehabilitation [104].

### *Peritoneal dialysis*

Peritoneal dialysis, and particularly continuous ambulatory peritoneal dialysis (CAPD), offers specific benefits to the diabetic patient as well as its general advantages of independence and low cost (Table 16.5). Vascular access is not required. Extracellular fluid volume and blood pressure do not fluctuate rapidly, which benefits patients with ischaemic heart disease or severe autonomic neuropathy. Another major advantage of CAPD is that insulin may be administered intraperitoneally, which can provide a simple, physiological and very effective method of metabolic control. Intraperitoneal insulin is absorbed mainly by diffusion across the visceral peritoneum into the portal venous circulation and directly through the capsule of the liver, thereby acting preferentially on the liver and avoiding peripheral hyperinsulinaemia. Insulin is absorbed fastest when administered into an empty peritoneal cavity but most patients add insulin to their peritoneal dialy-

**Table 16.5.** Advantages of continuous ambulatory peritoneal dialysis (CAPD).

| |
|---|
| • Vascular access not required |
| • Haemodynamic instability rare |
| • Good metabolic control with intraperitoneal insulin |
| • Better rehabilitation |

sis bags, which produces peak insulin levels 90–120 min later [113]. Insulin absorption continues throughout the dwell time (6–8 h) but amounts only to about 50% of the total insulin administered. As peritoneal dialysis fluid contains glucose as an osmotic agent, which is partly absorbed and further increases insulin requirements, the daily intraperitoneal insulin dose is usually about twice the previous subcutaneous dose. The estimated daily requirement should be divided equally between the number of dialysis bags used (usually four); a reduced dose may be needed in the overnight bag to avoid nocturnal hypoglycaemia. Higher insulin doses, often double those used in isosmotic ('weak') bags, are required when hypertonic ('strong') bags of higher glucose concentration are used. CAPD exchanges containing insulin should be timed for 30–40 min before meals to match peak insulin action with food absorption and so minimize postprandial glycaemic swings. Excellent control can be achieved and insulin requirements often remain remarkably stable [114, 115].

Visual impairment is not a contraindication to CAPD [93]. With good education and support, blind patients can achieve excellent results [97]. Injection aids are available, or insulin can be injected into the dialysis bag by a nurse or partner up to 24 h before use without significant absorption of the insulin on to the plastic bags [116]. Blood glucose monitors and other equipment designed for visually impaired patients are described in Chapter 9.

The most important complication of CAPD is peritonitis, occurring at very similar rates (1–2 episodes per patient per year) in non-diabetic and diabetic patients [93, 14, 117]. The commonest organisms causing peritonitis in both groups of patients are skin bacteria, notably *Staphylococcus epidermidis*, accounting for about 40% of bacterial peritonitis. Other organisms isolated include *Staphylococcus aureus*, *Streptococcus viridans*, Gram-negative enteric organisms and very rarely anaerobic organisms. Peritonitis is occasionally caused by fungi. Treatment is the same for both diabetic and non-diabetic patients. Most episodes are mild and can be treated at home by the patient injecting antibiotics into the dialysis bags. Occasional severe episodes require hospital admission and parenteral antibiotics. The majority recover without complications but occasionally the dialysis catheter has to be removed due to persistent infection. Recurrent infections require a period of about a month off CAPD, when temporary haemodialysis is needed. During episodes of peritonitis, insulin requirements are usually increased [118]. The inflamed peritoneum increases absorption of both insulin and glucose, and the latter may lead to fluid retention, requiring additional exchanges or more frequent use of hypertonic dialysis fluid.

Long-term survival with CAPD is possible (Table 16.6) [93, 119]. Although experience is still limited, the outcome is probably somewhat worse for patients with diabetic nephropathy than with non-diabetic renal disease.

## Progression of complications following renal replacement therapy

Following renal replacement therapy, diabetic patients have a higher mortality (especially from cardiovascular disease) and morbidity than non-diabetic patients, because of coexistent diabetic complications.

Cardiovascular disease is the major determinant of outcome during renal replacement in both diabetic and non-diabetic subjects. Most early deaths in diabetic patients treated with dialysis or transplantation are due to pre-existing cardiovascular disease [107]. Long-term survivors tend to be relatively free of cardiovascular disease at the time of starting renal replacement therapy [112], but this remains the most important cause of morbidity and mortality: of those surviving for over 10 years after transplantation by the Minneapolis group, 20% have suffered myocardial infarcts and 15% strokes [101]. Of the 163 patients treated at King's College Hospital between 1974 and 1987, 15% suffered new cardiac events; three-quarters of these have died, most from myocardial infarction. Patients receiving haemodialysis appear to have the highest cardiovascular mortality (50–65%),

**Table 16.6.** Actuarial survival (%) of diabetic patients treated by CAPD.

| Study | Year | Years of CAPD 1 | 2 | 3 |
|---|---|---|---|---|
| Legrain *et al.* [41] | 1984 | 85 | 68 | 62 |
| Rottembourg *et al.* [118] | 1985 | 85 | 63 | 58 |
| Grefberg *et al.* [119] | 1984 | 80 | 57 | — |
| Amair *et al.* [114] | 1982 | 92 | 81 | — |
| Berisa *et al.* [93] | 1988 | 88 | 71 | 47 |

although this may largely reflect selection bias [40, 112].

Amputation is disturbingly common in diabetic patients receiving renal replacement. The higher rate after renal transplantation [37, 47] may be because many dialysis patients die before the need for amputation arises. The Minneapolis group have reported that following renal transplantation, 17% of diabetic patients underwent amputations (mostly of the lower limb), of whom two-thirds had more than one amputation [37]; 70% of amputations occurred 2 years or more after transplantation and 30% of patients surviving for over 10 years had undergone amputation [101]. Overall amputation rates reported by other groups range from 7% at King's College Hospital (A. Grenfell, unpublished observations) to 25% in Scandinavia [13]. Digital gangrene is particularly common and in some cases may be related to difficulties with vascular access. Patients receiving either CAPD or haemodialysis apparently have amputation rates of about 5–10% [40, 93, 95].

Neuropathic ulceration is a considerable problem during renal replacement therapy, affecting up to 20–25% of patients. Sepsis may spread rapidly to threaten the limb, especially in immunosuppressed patients, and may ultimately require ray excision or extensive amputation. Motor and sensory nerve conduction measurements show little change 1–2 years after transplantation [120], which is in contrast to reports of striking improvement in muscle weakness following transplantation [30, 47, 120]. Patients with severe somatic neuropathy show little symptomatic improvement after transplantation [47], but some autonomic symptoms may improve, notably gustatory sweating [32], postural hypotension [13], vomiting and diarrhoea.

As mentioned above, modern practice generally prevents significant deterioration in retinopathy and visual acuity often remains stable, especially in those with good vision before treatment [30, 47]. The frequency of blindness during haemodialysis has fallen dramatically [95], for the reasons discussed above rather than due to changes in heparinization [121], and is now comparable with that in transplanted patients [122]. However, retinopathy does progress: one-third of patients with background retinopathy at transplantation subsequently developed proliferative retinopathy [122]. About 30% of patients are blind 3–10 years after starting treatment, although most had been blind before renal replacement therapy: only one of the 26 patients surviving longer than 10 years after renal transplantation by the Minneapolis group became blind during this period [101].

Recent advances in laser therapy and microsurgery (see Chapter 8), together with more effective treatment of hypertension, should mean that fewer diabetic patients with nephropathy will become blind in the future, either before or after renal replacement therapy. Regular fundoscopy and testing of visual acuity are crucial.

Rehabilitation is obviously affected by severe visual impairment or blindness, but there is no evidence that the outcome of renal replacement therapy is adversely affected. One report suggesting that visually impaired patients had a poor prognosis following renal transplantation is probably explicable by the association with severe cardiac disease [43].

### Causes of death following renal replacement therapy

Cardiovascular disease and sepsis are the commonest causes of death in patients undergoing renal replacement therapy, whether diabetic or not. Among diabetic patients, cardiovascular deaths are particularly frequent, accounting for 50–65% of deaths [30–32, 40, 41, 43, 93, 107]. Fatal coronary heart disease is about 10 times commoner in young diabetic patients receiving renal replacement therapy than in comparable patients with other diseases. Cerebrovascular disease is also common: strokes account for about 10–12% of deaths in dialysed patients and for somewhat fewer in transplant recipients (6%).

Sepsis, sometimes arising from gangrenous lesions, is a common and serious complication responsible for between 30 and 50% of deaths [123]. Fatal sepsis is about twice as frequent in transplanted patients as in those receiving dialysis (presumably because of immunosuppressive treatment in the former), but relatively high rates are reported with increasing duration of dialysis [112].

Withdrawal from treatment may account for as many as 24% of deaths in diabetic dialysis patients [40, 112]. Patients with diabetes withdraw from dialysis about 4–5 times more commonly than non-diabetic patients, probably because of coexistent severe medical complications [124].

## Conclusions

The last decade has seen many improvements in the management of diabetic nephropathy. The conviction is now growing that the evolution of the early stages of the disease, which can now be identified relatively easily, can be favourably modified by effective antihypertensive therapy and perhaps by other measures including a moderately restricted protein intake.

There is now no doubt that renal replacement therapy by transplantation, haemodialysis or CAPD is virtually as successful in diabetic as in non-diabetic people; it is no longer acceptable to regard end-stage diabetic nephropathy as untreatable.

## Recent developments

### *Non-insulin-dependent diabetes*

Two main features have become apparent in recent years. Firstly, it is now recognized that NIDDM patients make a major contribution to those receiving renal replacement therapy and in many centres account for well over 50% of new patients [125–128]. Secondly, ethnic origin is of considerable importance, with non-Caucasian NIDDM patients having a high prevalence of both diabetes and nephropathy. The cumulative risk of persistent proteinuria is very similar in IDDM and NIDDM patients [127, 129, 130], although progression to end-stage renal failure (ESRF) is variable in different reports [131, 132]. These discrepancies result from a variety of factors [127, 133]. Non-Caucasian NIDDM have a much higher prevalence of both proteinuria [134–137] and microalbuminuria [138, 139]. ESRF is also much more common [140–142].

The diagnosis of diabetic nephropathy may not be straightforward in NIDDM. Retinopathy is not invariable and non-diabetic renal disease more common [143, 144]. Those without retinopathy should undergo renal biopsy, as about 50% will be found to have a non-diabetic renal disease [143].

### *Hypertension*

Blood pressure is raised at an early stage in diabetic nephropathy and plays a central role in progression of the disease. Nocturnal blood pressure fails to show its normal fall in patients with diabetic nephropathy [145–148] and 24-h ambulatory blood pressure profiles show a much better correlation with albumin excretion rate [149] and left ventricular mass [150, 151] than casual measurements of blood pressure and thus may be a better guide to treatment [152]. Aggressive antihypertensive therapy is now accepted as the mainstay of treatment and not only reduces the rate of decline of GFR [153] but also improves survival from 30 or 50% [154, 155] to 80% [156, 157] after 10 years of proteinuria.

The question as to whether ACE-inhibitors have a specific renal protective effect independent of any effect on systemic blood pressure remains unsolved [158]. Concern has been voiced over the use of diuretics which appear to accelerate progression of renal disease [159] and increase mortality in patients with diabetes [160, 161]. These issues are discussed in further detail in Chapter 18.

### *Haematuria*

Microscopic haematuria is relatively common but its significance is uncertain [162, 163]. It may be of little help in distinguishing diabetic nephropathy from other diseases [163] but, together with red cell casts, which are uncommon [164] and/or unusual clinical features, it is an indication for renal biopsy.

### *Low-protein diets*

The beneficial effects of such diets in slowing the rate of decline of GFR have been confirmed in a long-term prospective study [165]. In addition, it has been suggested that vegetarian diets of normal protein content may have the same beneficial effects [166].

ANASUYA GRENFELL

## References


1 Joslin EP, Root HF, White P, Marble A. *The Treatment of Diabetes Mellitus*. Philadelphia: Lea & Febiger, 1959.

2 Borch-Johnsen K, Andersen PK, Deckert T. The effect of proteinuria on relative mortality in Type 1 (insulin-dependent) diabetes mellitus. *Diabetologia* 1985; **28**: 590–6.

3 Borch-Johnsen K, Kreiner S. Proteinuria: value as predictor of cardiovascular mortality in insulin dependent diabetes mellitus. *Br Med J* 1987; **294**: 1651–4.

4 Andersen AR, Christiansen JS, Andersen JK, Kreiner S, Deckert T. Diabetic nephropathy in Type 1 (insulin dependent) diabetes: An epidemiological study. *Diabetologia* 1983; **25**: 496–501.

5 Moloney A, Tunbridge WMG, Ireland JT, Watkins PJ. Mortality from diabetic nephropathy in the United King-

dom. *Diabetologia* 1983; **25**: 26–30.
6 Mogensen CE. Microalbuminuria predicts clinical proteinuria and early mortality in maturity-onset diabetes. *N Engl J Med* 1984; **310**: 356–60.
7 Jarrett RJ, Viberti GC, Argyropoulos A, Hill RD, Mahmud U, Murrels TJ. Microalbuminuria predicts mortality in non-insulin dependent diabetes. *Diabetic Med* 1984; **2**: 17–19.
8 Rettig B, Teutsch SM. The incidence of end-stage renal disease in type I and type II diabetes mellitus. *Diabetic Nephropathy* 1984; **3**: 26–7.
9 Grenfell A, Bewick M, Parsons V, Snowden S, Taube D, Watkins PJ. Non-insulin dependent diabetes and renal replacement therapy. *Diabetic Med* 1988; **5**: 172–6.
10 Cameron JS, Challah S. Treatment of end-stage renal failure due to diabetes in the United Kingdom 1975–1984. *Lancet* 1986; **ii**: 962–6.
11 Ordonez JD, Hiatt RA. Comparison of type II and type I diabetics treated for end-stage renal disease in a large prepaid health plan population. *Nephron* 1989; **51**: 524–9.
12 Challah S, Brunner FP, Wing AJ. Evolution of the treatment of patients with diabetic nephropathy by renal replacement therapy in Europe over a decade: Data from the EDTA registry. In: Mogensen CE, ed. *The Kidney and Hypertension in Diabetes Mellitus*. Boston: Martinus Nijhoff Publishing, 1988: 365–77.
13 Jervell J, Dahl BO, Fauchold P *et al*. Clinical results of renal transplantation in diabetic patients. *Transplant Proc* 1984; **16**: 599–602.
14 Shyh T-P, Beyer MM, Friedman EA. Treatment of the uremic diabetic. *Nephron* 1985; **40**: 129–38.
15 Working Party Report. Renal failure in diabetics in the UK: Deficient provision of care in 1985. *Diabetic Med* 1988; **5**: 79–84.
16 Barnes BA, Bergan JJ, Braun WE *et al*. The 12th report of the human renal transplant registry. Prepared by the Advisory Committee to the Renal Transplant Registry. *J Am Med Ass* 1975; **233**: 787–96.
17 Kjellstrand CM, Simmons RL, Goetz FC *et al*. Renal transplantation in patients with insulin dependent diabetes. *Lancet* 1973; **ii**: 4–8.
18 Brynger H, Nyberg G, Larsson O. Renal transplantation, the optimal treatment for renal failure in diabetic patients. *Transplant Proc* 1986; **18**: 1713–14.
19 Sutherland DER, Canafax DM, Goetz FC, Najarian JS. Renal transplantation in diabetic patients: the treatment of choice. In: Mogensen CE, ed. *The Kidney and Hypertension in Diabetes Mellitus*. Boston: Martinus Nijhoff Publishing, 1988: 341–7.
20 Grenfell A, Watkins PJ. Clinical diabetic nephropathy. Natural history and complications. *Clin Endocrinol Metab* 1986; **15**: 783–805.
21 Krowleski AS, Warram JH, Christleib AR *et al*. The changing natural history of nephropathy in type 1 diabetes. *Am J Med* 1985; **78**: 785–94.
22 Viberti GC, Keen H. The patterns of proteinuria in diabetes mellitus. *Diabetes* 1984; **33**: 686–92.
23 Mogensen CE. High blood pressure as a factor in the progression of diabetic nephropathy. *Acta Med Scand* 1976; **602** (suppl): 29–32.
24 Parving H-H, Andersen AR, Smidt VM, Oxenbøll B, Edsberg B, Christiansen JS. Diabetic nephropathy and arterial hypertension. *Diabetologia* 1983; **24**: 10–12.
25 Wiseman M, Viberti GC, Mackintosh D, Jarrett RJ, Keen H. Glycaemia, arterial pressure, and microalbuminuria in Type 1 (insulin-dependent) diabetes mellitus. *Diabetologia* 1984; **26**: 401–5.
26 Mathiesen ER, Oxenbøll K, Johansen PAa, Svendsen PA, Deckert T. Incipient nephropathy in Type 1 (insulin-dependent) diabetes. *Diabetologia* 1984; **26**: 406–10.
27 Sampson MJ, Chambers J, Spriggings D, Drury PJ. Echocardiographic evidence of relative left ventricular hypertrophy in Type I (insulin-dependent) diabetic patients with microalbuminuria. *Diabetologia* 1988; **31**: 539A.
28 Knussman MJ, Goldstein HH, Gleason RE. The clinical course of diabetic nephropathy. *J Am Med Assoc* 1976; **236**: 1861–3.
29 Bennett WM, Kloster F, Rosch J, Barry J, Porter GA. Natural history of asymptomatic coronary arteriographic lesions in diabetic patients with end-stage renal disease. *Am J Med* 1978; **65**: 779–84.
30 Libertino JA, Zinman L, Salerno R, D'Elia J, Kaldany A, Weinrauch LA. Diabetic renal transplantation. *J Urol* 1980; **124**: 593–5.
31 Rohrer RJ, Madras PN, Sahyoun AI, Monaco AP. Renal transplantation in the diabetic. *World J Surg* 1986; **10**: 397–403.
32 Gonzalez-Carrillo M, Moloney A, Bewick M, Parsons V, Rudge CJ, Watkins PJ. Renal transplantation in diabetic nephropathy. *Br Med J* 1982; **285**: 1713–16.
33 Braun WE, Phillips DF, Vidt DG *et al*. Coronary artery disease in 100 diabetics with end-stage renal failure. *Transplant Proc* 1984; **16**: 603–7.
34 D'Elia JA, Weinrauch LA, Healy RN, Libertino JA, Bradley RF, Leland OS. Myocardial dysfunction without coronary artery disease in diabetic renal failure. *Am J Cardiol* 1979; **43**: 193–9.
35 Grenfell A, Monaghan M, Watkins PJ, McCleod AA. Left ventricular hypertrophy in diabetic nephropathy: An echocardiographic study. *Diabetic Med* 1988; **5**: 840–4.
36 Shapiro LM. A prospective study of heart disease in diabetes mellitus. *Q J Med* 1984; **209**: 55–68.
37 Peters C, Sutherland DER, Simmons RL, Fryd DS, Najarian JS. Patient and graft survival in amputated versus non-amputated diabetic primary renal allograft recipients. *Transplantation* 1981; **32**: 498–503.
38 Wilczek H, Gunnarsson R, Lundgren G, Ost L. Improved results of renal transplantation in diabetic nephropathy. *Transplant Proc* 1984; **16**: 623–7.
39 Rao VK, Andersen RC. The impact of diabetes on vascular complications following cadaver renal transplantation. *Transplantation* 1987; **43**: 193–7.
40 Shapiro FL. Haemodialysis in diabetic patients. In: Keen H, Legrain M, eds. *Prevention and Treatment of Diabetic Nephropathy*. Lancaster: MTP Press, 1983: 247–59.
41 Legrain M, Rottembourg J, Bentchikou A *et al*. Dialysis treatment of insulin dependent diabetic patients: ten year experience. *Clin Nephrol* 1984; **21**: 72–81.
42 Najarian JS, Sutherland DER, Simmons RL *et al*. Ten year experience with renal transplantation in juvenile onset diabetics. *Ann Surg* 1979; **190**: 487–500.
43 Jervell J, Dahl BO, Flatmark A *et al*. Renal transplantation in insulin dependent diabetics. A joint Scandinavian report. *Lancet* 1978; **ii**: 915–17.
44 Strandness DE Jr, Priest RE, Gibbons GE. Combined clinical and pathological study of diabetic and non-diabetic peripheral arterial disease. *Diabetes* 1964; **13**: 366–72.
45 Gilbey SG, Grenfell A, Edmonds ME, Archer A, Watkins PJ. Vascular calcification, autonomic neuropathy, and peripheral blood flow in patients with diabetic nephropathy. *Diabetic Med* 1989; **6**: 37–42.
46 Edmonds ME, Morrison N, Laws JW, Watkins PJ. Medial

arterial calcification and diabetic neuropathy. *Br Med J* 1982; **284**: 928–30.
47 Khauli RB, Novick AC, Braun WE *et al*. Improved results of cadaver renal transplantation in the diabetic patient. *J Urol* 1983; **130**: 867–70.
48 Traeger J, Dubenard JM, Bosie E *et al*. Patient selection and risk factors in organ transplantation in diabetics: experience with kidney and pancreas. *Transplant Proc* 1984; **16**: 577–82.
49 Horowitz M, Collins PJ, Shearman DJC. Disorders of gastric emptying in humans and the use of radionuclide techniques. *Arch Intern Med* 1985; **145**: 1467–72.
50 Page MMcB, Watkins PJ. Cardiorespiratory arrest and diabetic autonomic neuropathy. *Lancet* 1978; **i**: 14–16.
51 Ramsay RC, Knoblach WH, Barbosa JJ, Sutherland DER, Kjellstrand CM, Najarian JS *et al*. The visual status of diabetic patients after renal transplantation. *Am J Ophthalmol* 1979; **87**: 305–10.
52 Kohner E, Chahal PS. Retinopathy in diabetic nephropathy (a preliminary report) In: Keen M, Legrain M, eds. *Prevention and Treatment of Diabetic Nephropathy*. Lancaster: MTP Press, 1983: 191–6.
53 Kasinath BS, Mujais SK, Spargo BH, Katz AI. Non-diabetic renal disease in patients with diabetes mellitus. *Am J Med* 1983; **75**: 613–17.
54 Yum M, Maxwell DR, Hamburger R, Kleit SA. Primary glomerulonephritis complicating diabetic nephropathy: a report of 7 cases and review of the literature. *Hum Pathol* 1984; **15**: 921–7.
55 Fabre J, Balant LP, Dayer PG, Fox HM, Vernet AT. The kidney in maturity onset diabetes mellitus: a clinical study of 510 patients. *Kidney Int* 1982; **21**: 730–8.
56 Ellis EN, Steffes MW, Goetz FC, Sutherland DER, Mauer SM. Relationship of renal size to nephropathy in Type 1 (insulin-dependent) diabetes. *Diabetologia* 1985; **28**: 12–15.
57 Etz J, Ritz E, Hasslacher C, Gotz R. Renal size in diabetics with endstage renal failure. *Diabetic Nephropathy* 1985; **4**: 77–9.
58 Wass JAH, Watkins PJ, Dische FE, Parsons V. Renal failure, glomerular disease and diabetes mellitus. *Nephron* 1978; **21**: 289–96.
59 Hommel E, Carstensen H, Skøtt P *et al*. Prevalence and causes of microscopic haematuria in Type 1 (insulin-dependent) diabetic patients with persistent proteinuria. *Diabetologia* 1987; **30**: 627–30.
60 O'Neill WM, Wallim JD, Walker PD. Hematuria and red cell casts in typical diabetic nephropathy. *Am J Med* 1983; **74**: 381–95.
61 Viberti GC, Bilous RW, Mackintosh D, Keen H. Monitoring glomerular function in diabetic nephropathy. A prospective study. *Am J Med* 1983; **74**: 256–64.
62 Grenfell A. Acute renal failure in diabetics. In: Mogensen CE, ed. *The Kidney and Hypertension in Diabetes Mellitus*. Boston: Martinus Nijhoff Publishing, 1988: 243–50.
63 Eknoyan G. Renal papillary necrosis in diabetic patients. In: Mogensen CE, ed. *The Kidney and Hypertension in Diabetes Mellitus*. Boston: Martinus Nijhoff Publishing, 1988: 259–67.
64 Medina M, Tomasula JR, Cohen LS, Laugani GB, Butt KMH, Friedman EA. Diabetic cystopathy. In: Mogensen CE, ed. *The Kidney and Hypertension in Diabetes Mellitus*. Boston: Martinus Nijhoff Publishing, 1988: 269–81.
65 Manis T, Friedman EA. Contrast media induced nephropathy in diabetic nephropathy. In: Mogensen CE, ed. *The Kidney and Hypertension in Diabetes Mellitus*. Boston: Martinus Nijhoff Publishing, 1988: 251–8.
66 Anto HR, Chou SY, Porush JG, Schapiro WB. Infusion intravenous pyelography and renal function: effects of hypertonic mannitol in patients with chronic renal insufficiency. *Arch Intern Med* 1981; **141**: 1652–6.
67 Mogensen CE. Long term anti-hypertensive treatment inhibiting progression of diabetic nephropathy. *Br Med J* 1982; **285**: 685–8.
68 Parving H-H, Andersen AR, Smidt UM, Hommel E, Mathiesen ER, Svendsen PAå. Effect of anti-hypertensive treatment on kidney function in diabetic nephropathy. *Br Med J* 1987; **294**: 1443–7.
69 Björck S, Nyberg G, Mulec H, Granerus G, Herlitz H, Aurell M. Beneficial effects of angiotensin converting enzyme inhibition on renal function in patients with diabetic nephropathy. *Br Med J* 1986; **293**: 471–4.
70 Christensen CK, Mogensen CE. Antihypertensive treatment: long term reversal of progression of albuminuria in incipient diabetic nephropathy. A longitudinal study of renal function. *J Diabetic Compl* 1987; **1**: 45–52.
71 Marre M, Chatellier G, Leblanc H *et al*. Prevention of diabetic nephropathy with enalapril in normotensive diabetics with microalbuminuria. *Br Med J* 1988; **297**: 1092–5.
72 Acheson RM. Blood pressure in a national sample of US adults: percentile distribution by age, sex, and race. *Int J Epidemiol* 1973; **2**: 293–301.
73 Weidman P, Beretta-Piccoli C, Keusch G *et al*. Sodium-volume factor, cardiovascular reactivity and hypotensive mechanism of diuretic therapy in mild hypertension associated with diabetes mellitus. *Am J Med* 1979; **67**: 779–84.
74 O'Hare JA, Ferriss JB, Brady D, Twomey B, O'Sullivan DJ. Exchangeable sodium and renin in hypertensive diabetic patients with and without nephropathy. *Hypertension* 1985; **7** (suppl 2): II43–7.
75 Anderson S, Brenner BM. Pathogenesis of diabetic glomerulopathy: Haemodynamic considerations. *Diab Metab Rev* 1988; **4**: 163–77.
76 Viberti GC, Bilous RW, Mackintosh D, Bending JJ, Keen H. Long term correction of hyperglycaemia and progression of renal failure in insulin dependent diabetes. *Br Med J* 1983; **286**: 598–602.
77 Bending JJ, Viberti GC, Watkins PJ, Keen H. Intermittent clinical proteinuria and renal function in diabetes: evolution and the effect of glycaemic control. *Br Med J* 1986; **292**: 83–6.
78 Nyberg G, Blohme G, Norden G. Impact of metabolic control in progression of clinical diabetic nephropathy. *Diabetologia* 1987; **3**: 82–6.
79 Brenner BM, Meyer TW, Hostetter TH. Dietery protein intake and the progressive nature of kidney disease. *N Engl J Med* 1982; **307**: 652–60.
80 Hostetter TH, Meyer TW, Rennke HG, Brenner BM. Chronic effects of dietary protein in the rat with intact and reduced renal mass. *Kidney Int* 1986; **30**: 509–17.
81 Rosman JB, Ter Wee PM, Meyer S, Piers-Becht TPM, Sluiter WJ, Dohker AJM. Prospective randomised trial of early dietary protein restriction in chronic renal failure. *Lancet* 1984; **ii**: 1291–6.
82 Attman PO, Bucht H, Larsson O, Uddebom G. Protein reduced diet in diabetic renal failure. *Clin Nephrol* 1983; **19**: 217–20.
83 Nyberg G, Norden G, Attman PO *et al*. Diabetic nephropathy: is dietary protein harmful? *J Diabetic Compl* 1987; **1**: 37–40.
84 Bending JJ, Dodds R, Keen H, Viberti GC. Lowering protein

intake and progression of diabetic renal failure. *Diabetologia* 1986; **29**: 516A.

85 Walker JD, Bending JJ, Dodds RA, Mattock MB, Murrell TJ, Keen H, Viberti GC. Restriction of dietary protein and progression of renal failure in diabetic nephropathy. *Lancet* 1989; **ii**: 1411–15.

86 Barsotti G, Ciardella F, Morelli E, Cupisti A, Mantovanelli A, Giovanetti S. Nutritional treatment of renal failure in type 1 diabetic nephropathy. *Clin Nephrol* 1988; **29**: 280–7.

87 Levine SE, D'Elia JA, Bistrian B *et al*. Protein-restricted diets in diabetic nephropathy. *Nephron* 1989; **52**: 55–61.

88 Nutrition Sub-Committee of the Medical Advisory Committee of the British Diabetic Association. *Dietary Recommendation for Diabetics in the* 1980s. The British Diabetic Association, London, 1982.

89 Morrow CE, Schwartz JS, Sutherland DER *et al*. Predictive value of thallium stress testing for coronary and cardiovascular events in uremic diabetic patients before renal transplantation. *Am J Surg* 1983; **146**: 331–5.

90 Edmonds ME, Blundell MP, Morris HE *et al*. Improved survival of the diabetic foot: the role of a special foot clinic. *Q J Med* 1986; **232**: 763–71.

91 Edmonds ME. The diabetic foot: pathophysiology and treatment. *Clin Endocrinol Metab* 1986; **15**: 889–916.

92 Joint Working Party on Diabetic Renal Failure of the British Diabetic Association, Renal Association and the Research Unit of the Royal College of Physicians. Treatment of and mortality from diabetic renal failure in patients identified in the 1985 United Kingdom Survey. *Br Med J* 1989; **299**: 1135–6.

93 Berisa F, McGonigle R, Beaman M, Adu D, Michael J. The treatment of diabetic renal failure by continuous ambulatory peritoneal dialysis. *Diabetic Med* 1989; **6**: 67–70.

94 Brunner FP, Brynger H, Challah S *et al*. Renal replacement therapy in patients with diabetic nephropathy 1980–1985. Report from the European Dialysis and Transplant Association Registry. *Nephrol Dial Transplant* 1988; **3**: 585–95.

95 Whitley KY, Shapiro FL. Hemodialysis for end-stage diabetic nephropathy. In: Friedman EA, L'Esperance FA, eds. *Diabetic Renal–Retinal Syndrome 3*. New York: Grune & Stratton 1986: 349–62.

96 Cowie CC, Port FK, Wolfe RA, Savage PJ, Moll PP, Hawthorne VM. Disparities in incidence of diabetic end-stage renal disease according to race and type of diabetes. *N Engl J Med* 1989; **321**: 1074–9.

97 Flynn CT. Why blind diabetics with renal failure should be offered treatment. *Br Med J* 1983; **287**: 1177–8.

98 Totten MA, Izenstein B, Gleason RE, Kassissieh SD, Libertino JA, D'Elia JA. Chronic renal failure in diabetes: survival with hemodialysis versus transplantation. *Kidney Int* 1977; **12**: 492A.

99 Kjellstrand CM. Cadaver transplantation versus hemodialysis. *Trans Am Soc Artif Intern Organs* 1980; **26**: 611–24.

100 O'Donovan R, Devlin P, Bennet-Jones D, Parsons V, Bewick M, Weston M *et al*. The use of intravenous insulin in the treatment of diabetes during rejection episodes. *Transplant Proc* 1984; **16**: 643–4.

101 Sutherland DER, Bentley FR, Mauer SM *et al*. A report of 26 diabetic renal allograft recipients alive with functioning grafts at 10 or more years after primary transplantation. *Diabetic Nephropathy* 1984; **3**: 39–43.

102 Mauer SM, Goetz FC, McHugh LE, Sutherland DER, Barbosa J, Najarian JS *et al*. Long term study of normal kidneys transplanted into patients with type-1 diabetes. *Diabetes* 1989; **38**: 516–23.

103 Bohman S-O, Wilczek H, Jaremko G, Tyden G. Recurrence of diabetic nephropathy in renal transplants. In: Mogensen CE, ed. *The Kidney and Hypertension in Diabetes Mellitus*. Boston: Martinus Nijhoff Publishing, 1988: 395–402.

104 Jacobson SH, Fryd D, Sutherland DER, Kjellstrand CM. Treatment of the diabetic patient with end-stage renal failure. *Diabetes Metab Rev* 1988; **4**: 191–200.

105 Ghavamian M, Gutch C, Kopp F, Kolff WJ. The sad truth about hemodialysis in diabetic nephropathy. *J Am Med Ass* 1972; **222**: 1386–9.

106 Shapiro FL, Leonard A, Comty CM. Mortality, morbidity, and rehabilitation. Results in regularly dialysed patients with diabetes mellitus. *Kidney Int* 1974; **6**: (suppl 1): 8–14.

107 Matson M, Kjellstrand CM. Long-term follow-up of 369 diabetic patients undergoing dialysis. *Arch Intern Med* 1988; **148**: 600–4.

108 Aman LC, Levin NW, Smith DW. Hemodialysis access site morbidity. *Proc Clin Dial Transplant Forum* 1980; **10**: 277–82.

109 Buselmeier TJ, Najarian JS, Simmons RL. A–V fistulas and the diabetic: ischemia and gangrene may result in amputation. *Trans Am Soc Artif Intern Organs* 1973; **19**: 49–52.

110 Levitz CS, Hirsch S, Ross JM *et al*. Lack of blood glucose control in hemodialyzed and renal transplantation diabetics. *Trans Am Soc Artif Intern Organs* 1980; **26**: 362–5.

111 Leonard A, Comty C, Raij L. The natural history of regularly dialysed diabetics. *Trans Am Soc Artif Intern Organs* 1973; **19**: 282–6.

112 Kjellstrand CM, Lins L-E. Hemodialysis in type 1 and type 2 diabetic patients with end-stage renal failure. In: Mogensen CE, ed. *The Kidney and Hypertension in Diabetes Mellitus*. Boston: Martinus Nijhoff Publishing, 1988: 323–30.

113 Schade DS, Eaton RP, Davis T *et al*. The kinetics of peritoneal insulin absorption. *Metabolism* 1981; **30**: 149–55.

114 Amair P, Khanna R, Leibel B *et al*. Continuous ambulatory peritoneal dialysis in diabetics with end-stage renal disease. *N Engl J Med* 1982; **306**: 625–30.

115 Madden MA, Zimmerman SW, Simpson DP. CAPD in diabetes mellitus: the risks and benefits of intraperitoneal insulin. *Am J Nephrol* 1982; **2**: 133–9.

116 Twardowski ZJ, Nolph KD, McGary TJ, Moore HL. Influence of temperature and time on insulin absorption to plastic bags. *Am J Hosp Pharm* 1983; **40**: 583–6.

117 *Report of the National CAPD registry*. A publication of the National CAPD Registry of the National Institute of Arthritis, Diabetes and Digestive and Kidney Disease. Bethesda MD, 1986: 25–36.

118 Rottembourg J, Remaoun M, Maiga K *et al*. Continuous ambulatory peritoneal dialysis in diabetic patients. *Diab Hypertens* 1985; **7** (suppl 11): 125–30.

119 Grefberg N, Danielson BG, Nilsson P. Continuous ambulatory peritoneal dialysis in the treatment of end-stage diabetic nephropathy. *Acta Med Scand* 1984; **215**: 427–34.

120 Barbosa J, Burke B, Busselmeier TJ *et al*. Neuropathy, retinopathy, and biopsy findings in transplanted kidney in diabetic patients. *Kidney Int* 1974; **6** (suppl 1): S32–6.

121 Diaz-Buxo JA, Burgess WP, Greenman M. Visual function in diabetics undergoing dialysis: comparison of peritoneal and hemodialysis. *Int J Artif Organs* 1984; **7**: 257–62.

122 Ramsay RC, Knobloch WH, Cantrill HL *et al*. Visual status in transplanted and dialysed diabetic patients. In: Friedman EA, L'Espérance FA, eds. *Diabetic Renal–Retinal Syndrome 2*. New York: Grune & Stratton, 1982: 427–35.

123 Sagalowsky AI, Gailiunas P, Helderman JH *et al*. Renal

transplantation in diabetic patients: the end result does justify the means. *J Urol* 1983; **129**: 253–5.
124 Neu S, Kjellstrand CM. Stopping long-term dialysis. *N Engl J Med* 1986; **314**: 14–20.
125 Friedman EA. Diabetics with kidney failure. *Lancet* 1986; **3**: 1285.
126 Pugh JA. The epidemiology of diabetic nephropathy. *Diab Metab Rev* 1989; **5**: 531–46.
127 Ritz ERN, Fliser D, Kock M, Tschöpe W. Type II diabetes mellitus: Is the renal risk adequately appreciated? *Nephrol Dial Transplant* 1991; **6**: 679–82.
128 Grenfell A, Bewick M, Snowden S, Watkins PJ, Parsons VP. Renal replacement for diabetic patients: Experience at King's College Hospital between 1980–1989. *Q J Med* 1992; **85**: 861–74.
129 Ballard DJ, Humphrey LL, Metton JJ *et al*. Epidemiology of persistent proteinuria in type II diabetes mellitus. Population-based study in Rochester, Minnesota. *Diabetes* 1988; **37**: 405–12.
130 Hasslacher C, Ritz E, Wahl P, Michael C. Similar risks of nephropathy in patients with type 1 or type 2 diabetes mellitus. *Nephrol Dial Transplant* 1989; **4**: 859–63.
131 Fabre J, Balant LP, Dayer PG, Fox HM, Vernet AT. The kidney in maturity onset diabetes mellitus: a clinical study of 510 patients. *Kidney Int* 1982; **21**: 730–8.
132 Humphrey LL, Ballard DJ, Frohnest PP, Chu C-P, O'Fallon M, Pallumbo PJ. Chronic renal failure in non-insulin-dependent diabetes mellitus. *Ann Int Med* 1989; **111**: 788–96.
133 Catalano C, Marshall SM. Epidemiology of end-stage renal disease in patients with diabetes mellitus: from the dark ages to the middle ages. *Nephrol Dial Transplant* 1992; **7**: 181–90.
134 Cowie CC, Port FK, Wolfe RA, Savage PJ, Moll PP, Hawthorne VM. Disparities in incidence of diabetic end-stage renal disease according to race and type of diabetes. *N Engl J Med* 1989; **321**: 1074–9.
135 Haffner SM, Mitchell BD, Pugh JA *et al*. Proteinuria in Mexican Americans and non-Hispanic whites with NIDD. *Diabetes Care* 1989; **12**: 530–6.
136 Collins VR, Dowse GK, Finch CF, Zimmett PZ, Linnane AW. Prevalence and risk factors for micro- and macro-albuminuria in diabetic subjects and entire population in Naura. *Diabetes* 1989; **38**: 602–10.
137 Samanta A, Burden AC, Feehally J, Walls J. Diabetic renal disease: differences between Asians and white patients. *Br Med J* 1986; **293**: 366–7.
138 Allawi J, Rao PV, Gilbert R *et al*. Microalbuminuria in non-insulin dependent diabetes: its prevalence in Indian compared to Europid subjects. *Br Med J* 1988; **296**: 462–4.
139 West P, Tindall H, Lester E. Screening for microalbuminuria in a mixed ethnic diabetic clinic. *Ann Clin Biochem* 1993; **30**: 104–5.
140 Pugh JA, Stern MP, Haffner SM, Eifler CW, Zapata M. Excess incidence of treatment of end-stage renal disease in Mexican Americans. *Am J Epidemiol* 1988; **127**: 135–44.
141 Rostand SG, Kirk KA, Rutsky EA, Park BA. Racial differences in the incidence of treatment for end-stage renal disease. *N Engl J Med* 1982; **306**: 1276–9.
142 Burden A, McNally P, Feehally J, Walls J. Increased incidence of end-stage renal failure secondary to diabetes mellitus in Asian ethnic groups in the United Kingdom. Diabetic Med 1992; **9**: 641–5.
143 Parving H-H, Gall M-A, Skott P *et al*. Prevalence and causes of albuminuria in non-insulin dependent diabetic patients. *Kidney Int* 1992; **41**: 758–62.
144 Amoah E, Glickman JL, Malchoff CD, Steergill BC, Kaiser DL, Bolton WK. Clinical identification of non-diabetic renal disease in diabetic patients with Type 1 and Type 11 disease presenting with renal dysfunction. *Am J Nephrol* 1988; **8**: 204–11.
145 Hansen KW, Christensen CK, Andersen PH, Pedersen MM, Christiansen JS, Mogensen CE. Ambulatory blood pressure in microalbuminuric type 1 diabetic patients. *Kidney Int* 1992; **41**: 847–54.
146 Hansen KW, MauPedersen M, Marshall SM, Christiansen JS, Mogensen CE. Circadian variation of blood pressure in patients with diabetic nephropathy. *Diabetologia* 1992; **35**: 1074–9.
147 Moore WV, Donaldson DL, Chonko AM, Ideus P, Wiegman TB. Ambulatory blood pressure in Type 1 diabetes mellitus. Comparison to presence of incipient nephropathy in adolescents and young adults. *Diabetes* 1992; **41**: 1035–41.
148 Nielsen FS, Rossing P, Gall M-A, Parving H-H. Impaired nocturnal decline in arterial blood pressure in type 2 (non-insulin dependent) diabetic patients with nephropathy. *Diabetologia* 1992; **35** (suppl. 1): A48.
149 Opsahl J, Abraham PA, Halstenson CE, Keane WF. Correlation of office and ambulatory blood pressure measurements with urinary albumin and *N*-acetyl-β-D-glucosaminidase excretions in essential hypertension. *Am J Hypertens* 1988; **1** (suppl): 117s–120s.
150 Verdecchia P, Schillaci G, Guerieri M. Circadian blood pressure changes and left ventricular hypertrophy in essential hypertension. *Circulation* 1990; **81**: 528–36.
151 Devereux RB, Pickering TG. Relationship between ambulatory or exercise blood pressure and left ventricular structure: prognostic implications. *J Hypertens* 1990; **8**: (suppl. 6): S125–34.
152 Wiegman TB, Herron KG, Chonko AM, MacDougall ML, Moore WV. Recognition of hypertension and abnormal blood pressure burden with ambulatory blood pressure recordings in type 1 diabetes mellitus. *Diabetes* 1990; **39**: 1556–60.
153 Parving H-H, Andersen AR, Smidt UM, Hommel E, Mathiesen ER, Svendsen PA. Effect of antihypertensive treatment on kidney function in diabetic nephropathy. *Br Med J* 1987; **294**: 1443–7.
154 Andersen AR, Sandahl Christiansen J, Andersen JK, Kreiner S, Deckert T. Diabetic nephropathy in type 1 (insulin-dependent) diabetes: an epidemiological study. *Diabetologia* 1983; **25**: 496–501.
155 Krolewski AS, Warram JH, Christlieb AR. The changing natural history of nephropathy in type 1 diabetes. *Am J Med* 1985; **78**: 785–94.
156 Parving H-H, Hommel E. Prognosis in diabetic nephropathy. *Br Med J* 1989; **299**: 230–3.
157 Mathiesen ER, Borch Johnsen K, Jensen DV, Deckert T. Improved survival in patients with diabetic nephropathy. *Diabetologia* 1989; **32**: 884–6.
158 Mogensen CE, Hansen KW, Osterby R, Damsgaard EM. Blood pressure elevation versus abnormal albuminuria in the genesis and prediction of renal disease in diabetes. *Diabetes Care* 1992; **15** (9): 1192–204.
159 Walker WG, Herman J, Yin D, Murphy RP, Patz A. Diuretics accelerate diabetic nephropathy in hypertensive insulin dependent and non-insulin dependent subjects. *Trans Assoc Am Phys* 1987: C305–15.
160 Klein R, Moss SE, Klein BEK, DLD. Relation of ocular and systemic factors to survival in diabetes. *Arch Intern Med* 1989; **149**: 266–72.
161 Warram JH, Laffel LMB, Valsania P, Christlieb RA,

Krolewski AS. Excess mortality associated with diuretic therapy in diabetes mellitus. *Arch Intern Med* 1991; **151**: 1350–6.

162 Hommel E, Carstensen H, Skott P, Larsen S, Parving H-H. Prevalence and causes of microscopic haematuria in type 1 (insulin-dependent) diabetic patients with persistent proteinuria. *Diabetologia* 1987; **30**: 627–30.

163 Taft JL, Billson VR, Nankerris A, Kincaid-Smith P, Martin FJR. A clinical-histological study of individuals with diabetes mellitus and proteinuria. *Diabetic Med* 1990; **7**: 215–21.

164 Kincaid-Smith P, Whitworth JA. *Haematuria and Diabetic Nephropathy*. Boston: Martin Nijhoff Publishing, 1988: 81–9.

165 Zeller K, Whittaker E, Sullivan L, Raskin P, Jacobson HR. Effect of restricting dietary protein on the progression of renal failure in patients with insulin-dependent diabetes mellitus. *N Engl J Med* 1991; **324**: 78–84.

166 Kontessis PS, Dodds RA, Jones SL, Pinto JR, Trevisan R, Viberti GC. Renal, metabolic and hormonal responses to ingestion of protein of different sources in normal man. *Kidney Int* 1989; **35**: 470.

# PART 5
# MACROVASCULAR AND HEART DISEASE IN DIABETES MELLITUS

# 17 The Heart and Macrovascular Disease in Diabetes Mellitus


**Summary**

- Deaths from cardiovascular disease predominate in patients with diabetes of over 30 years' duration and in those diagnosed after 40 years of age. Patients with proteinuria have a greatly increased risk of fatal cardiovascular disease.
- The frequency of coronary heart disease (CHD) in diabetes is related to that in the background population (e.g. it is low in diabetic patients in China and Japan).
- General risk factors for cardiovascular disease include smoking, obesity, hyperlipidaemia, hypertension, insulin resistance, haemostatic and platelet abnormalities, lack of exercise and a positive family history. Specific diabetes-related risk factors may include hyperglycaemia (especially for peripheral vascular disease) and hyperinsulinaemia.
- CHD in diabetic patients is associated with increased plasma cholesterol levels, with reduced HDL-cholesterol in NIDDM patients, and possibly with increased triglyceride levels.
- The most common lipid abnormality in diabetes is raised triglyceride levels due to excess VLDL concentrations, caused by reduced clearance via the insulin-sensitive enzyme lipoprotein lipase and (in NIDDM) by increased VLDL production. Triglyceride levels often fall with intensified insulin treatment.
- LDL levels are also increased in poor metabolic control, due to decreased clearance by LDL receptors which are stimulated by insulin and have a lower affinity for glycosylated apoprotein B.
- HDL levels are reduced in NIDDM, in proportion to increased triglyceride and VLDL levels, but are relatively normal in IDDM; glycosylated HDL may be cleared more rapidly from the circulation.
- Hyperlipidaemia can be assessed from measurements of fasting plasma total cholesterol, HDL-cholesterol and triglyceride levels and calculation of LDL-cholesterol.
- Hyperlipidaemia is managed by improving metabolic control, dietary modification, stopping smoking and specific lipid-lowering drugs.
- A high-carbohydrate, low-fat (20–30% of total calories, 50% being unsaturated fat), low-cholesterol diet may lower cholesterol levels in IDDM. In NIDDM, weight reduction frequently lowers triglyceride concentrations and raises HDL.
- Lipid-lowering drugs suitable for use in diabetes include the fibrates (bezafibrate, gemfibrozil) for hypertriglyceridaemia or mixed hyperlipidaemia, and the resins (e.g. cholestyramine) and HMG CoA reductase inhibitors ('statins', e.g. simvastatin) for hypercholesterolaemia.
- Mortality from CHD in diabetic patients is increased about two and four times respectively for males and females, compared with the non-diabetic population.
- Acute myocardial infarction carries twice the mortality of that in the general population. Contributory factors may include coexistent diabetic cardiomyopathy, blunting of cardiac reflexes by autonomic neuropathy, and adverse cardiac and metabolic effects of increased non-esterified fatty acid levels.
- Acute myocardial infarction in diabetic patients should be managed with tight control of blood glucose and potassium levels and

**Table 17.1.** Percentage cause of death according to age at diagnosis and duration of diabetes. (Modified from [2].)

| Age at onset: | <20 | | | | 20–39 | | | | 40–59 | | | | ≥60 | | | |
|---|---|---|---|---|---|---|---|---|---|---|---|---|---|---|---|---|
| Duration (years): | <10 | 10–19 | 20–29 | ≥30 | <10 | 10–19 | 20–29 | ≥30 | <10 | 10–19 | 20–29 | ≥30 | <10 | 10–19 | 20–29 | ≥30 |
| *Cause of death* | | | | | | | | | | | | | | | | |
| Macrovascular (total) | 13 | 17 | 29 | 56 | 30 | 51 | 66 | 74 | 62 | 73 | 75 | 73 | 69 | 75 | 74 | 75 |
| Cardiac | 3 | 15 | 23 | 46 | 23 | 44 | 58 | 61 | 52 | 58 | 57 | 49 | 51 | 52 | 46 | 75 |
| Cerebral | 10 | 2 | 5 | 9 | 2 | 5 | 7 | 9 | 8 | 12 | 15 | 19 | 14 | 18 | 17 | — |
| Other | — | — | 1 | 1 | 5 | 2 | 1 | 3 | 2 | 3 | 3 | 5 | 4 | 5 | 11 | — |
| Nephropathy | 5 | 55 | 46 | 22 | 3 | 17 | 10 | 4 | 1 | 3 | 2 | — | 1 | 1 | 1 | — |
| Other causes | 82 | 28 | 25 | 22 | 67 | 32 | 24 | 22 | 37 | 24 | 23 | 27 | 30 | 24 | 25 | 25 |
| All causes | 100 | 100 | 100 | 100 | 100 | 100 | 100 | 100 | 100 | 100 | 100 | 100 | 100 | 100 | 100 | 100 |

prompt treatment of cardiac failure; the role of thrombolytic drugs is not yet established and they should be avoided in proliferative retinopathy.

- The symptoms of angina may be masked in diabetes by autonomic neuropathy.
- Angina may be treated by nitrates, calcium channel antagonists or β-blockers; other diabetic complications may influence the choice of drug.
- Coronary artery atherosclerosis may be more diffuse and severe than in non-diabetic subjects but the frequency of inoperable vessels is no higher, and the results and survival after coronary artery bypass grafting are now comparable with those in the general population. Coronary artery surgery or angioplasty should therefore be considered if medical treatment of angina is ineffective.
- Breathlessness and exercise intolerance in a diabetic patient is often due to heart failure, in which physical examination and chest X-ray may be normal. Possible causes include diabetic cardiomyopathy with microvascular disease and interstitial fibrosis and defective myosin and actinomyosin ATPases; autonomic neuropathy may also contribute.
- Management of cardiac failure involves improved glycaemic control, treatment of hypertension and the use of nitrates, calcium channel antagonists, loop diuretics and angiotensin converting enzyme inhibitors.
- Half of all lower-limb amputations are performed in diabetic patients. However, proximal and distal bypass grafting now often achieve good results.

Microvascular disease is an important cause of morbidity in diabetes, but diseases of the larger arteries and the heart are responsible for well over half of all deaths in diabetic patients. There is an association between micro- and macrovascular disease, as is demonstrated by the large excess of cardiovascular deaths in patients with proteinuria [1]. Although small vessel disease is specific to diabetes, arterial and cardiac diseases are also the commonest cause of death in the general population; the increased risk associated with diabetes is shared by those with impaired glucose tolerance (IGT).

## Epidemiology

Atherosclerotic arterial disease may be manifested clinically as coronary heart disease (CHD), cerebrovascular disease or peripheral vascular disease. The effect of diabetes on atherosclerosis is different at each of these sites. The relative risk of arterial disease also varies widely with gender, age, geographical location, type and duration of diabetes.

Mortality data from the Joslin Clinic [2] have been analysed according to age of onset and duration of diabetes (Table 17.1). In those diagnosed before the age of 20 years, there is a preponderance of renal deaths during the second and third decades of diabetes, but beyond 30 years from diagnosis, cardiovascular deaths predominate. In those diagnosed over the age of 40 years, renal disease only accounts for 1–2% of all deaths, and cardiovascular disease for 50–75%. In this group, the proportion of deaths attributable to CHD, but not to cerebral or peripheral arterial disease, is not related to the duration of diabetes.

These figures underline important differences between IDDM and NIDDM, which are often considered together in epidemiological studies. NIDDM, which predominates in the age group where cardiovascular disease is common, accounts for most of the differences described below.

### *Coronary heart disease*

In population studies, male diabetic patients have about twice, and females about 4 times, the CHD mortality rate of age- and sex-matched controls [3]. The mortality ratio is higher in young women: premenopausal non-diabetic females are at relatively low risk of CHD compared with males, but this protection is lost in diabetes. Non-fatal manifestations follow a similar pattern.

The Whitehall study of male civil servants has demonstrated twice the control rate of CHD mortality in subjects whose blood glucose concentration 2 h after a 50-g oral glucose load exceeded the 95th centile for the population (5.4 mmol/l) [4]. There was no trend in mortality at lower blood glucose levels, and the suggestion of a threshold effect for glucose has been supported by a number of other studies [3].

The frequency of CHD in diabetes depends on its frequency in the background population. In Japan and China, where the overall prevalence of CHD is low, angina and electrocardiographic (ECG) abnormalities are also uncommon in diabetic patients, although still commoner than in the background population [5]. Japanese migrants to Hawaii have a much higher CHD mortality than in Japan (presumably due to dietary differences), which is higher still in diabetic migrants [6]. If changes in diet can raise the risk of CHD, then the high risk in Western populations should be amenable to reduction by dietary manipulation.

In parts of Africa, large vessel disease is extremely rare in Black diabetic patients [7] despite a high prevalence of hypertension. This is not explicable by differences in serum lipid levels or adiposity [8], and is not restricted to malnutrition-associated diabetes.

### *Cerebrovascular disease*

Cerebrovascular mortality is increased about two- to fourfold in diabetes in Western populations, and here sex differences in relative mortality are less marked than in CHD [9]. In Japan, where cerebrovascular disease is the most frequent cardiovascular cause of death, strokes are predominantly haemorrhagic. Only a slight excess mortality is conferred by diabetes, the risk ratio being 1.15 [5], but the proportion of occlusive strokes is higher, suggesting an increased thrombotic tendency. The Whitehall study [10] again showed evidence of a threshold effect of blood glucose, with the relative risk of strokes, like myocardial infarction, being higher in the group above the 95th centile of the glucose distribution.

### *Peripheral vascular disease*

Diabetes confers a particularly high relative risk of peripheral vascular disease: about half of all lower limb amputations performed are on diabetic patients. The relative risk of amputation is highest below age 45, although the absolute risk increases with age [11]. These amputation figures include patients with microvascular disease and neuropathy, but in the 20-year Framingham study, the incidence of intermittent claudication was increased 3.8-fold in men and sixfold in women with diabetes as compared with non-diabetic subjects [12]. Loss of arterial foot pulses, unlike the manifestations of CHD, appears to be related to the duration of diabetes in both NIDDM and IDDM [9].

## Risk factors and prevention

The high prevalence of arterial disease in diabetes is partly explained by the increased frequency of conventional risk factors together with some additional interrelated factors associated with diabetes (Table 17.2). In practice, the important factors are those whose correction can be shown to reduce cardiovascular risk. This section will discuss the role of the various risk factors, and highlight the possible scope for their prevention (Table 17.2). Hypertension is discussed in full elsewhere (Chapter 18).

#### SMOKING

This seems to influence atherosclerosis similarly in diabetic and non-diabetic subjects [13], and little difference has been reported in smoking habits between the two groups [14]. The direct advice of a doctor is the most important single factor in motivating smokers to stop, and this should be a routine part of diabetic education.

#### OBESITY

Obesity adversely affects blood pressure, insulin sensitivity, blood glucose control and lipoprotein

**Table 17.2.** Risk factors and reductions for coronary heart disease.

| (a) Risk factors for coronary heart disease General | Diabetes-related |
|---|---|
| Smoking | Hyperglycaemia |
| Hypertension | Hyperinsulinaemia |
| Hyperlipidaemia | Proteinuria |
| Hypercoagulability | Microalbuminuria |
| Obesity | Both sexes affected equally |
| Lack of exercise | |
| Male sex | |
| Family history | |
| Oestrogen treatment | |

| (b) Approaches to risk reduction |
|---|
| Stop smoking |
| Optimize diabetic control |
| Seek and treat hypertension |
| Seek and treat hyperlipidaemia |
| Give dietary advice |
| • optimizing control |
| • maintaining ideal body weight |
| • lowering lipids |
| Encourage aerobic exercise |

patterns, and weight reduction is an important aspect of diabetic treatment. However, epidemiological studies relating obesity to cardiovascular risk in diabetes have yielded conflicting results, with some finding a positive association [13], and others finding no link [9, 15].

### EXERCISE

No direct information is available about the effects of physical exercise on the development of atherosclerosis in diabetes. However, aerobic exercise reduces obesity and plasma insulin levels and increases high-density lipoprotein (HDL) cholesterol, all of which are theoretically beneficial. Cardiovascular status and the presence of other complications should be considered when giving advice about exercise.

### HAEMOSTATIC FUNCTION

Haemostatic abnormalities, particularly raised fibrinogen and factor VII levels, are strongly predictive of CHD in non-diabetic subjects [16]. Preliminary evidence suggests that similar associations also apply in diabetes [17]. Fibrinogen levels are raised in both IDDM and NIDDM, and are higher in those with cardiovascular complications. Fibrinolytic activity is lower in NIDDM than IDDM and may be associated with ECG abnormalities However, factor VII levels are highest in diabetic patients with retinopathy and nephropathy, and have not been shown to be associated with large-vessel disease. Clotting factors may nonetheless be an important link between large- and small-vessel complications.

In addition to their role in thrombus formation, platelets are involved in atherogenesis through their release of platelet-derived growth factor and chemotactic factors which stimulate cellular proliferation in the atheromatous plaque. Measurements of platelet activity in diabetes have sometimes yielded conflicting results [18]. However, *in vitro* aggregation of platelets in response to ADP and collagen is increased in diabetes and is highest in those with complications. *In vivo* platelet activity, assessed from plasma levels of β-thromboglobulin and platelet factor 4, is elevated in non-diabetic subjects with vascular disease and in uncomplicated diabetes, and is further raised in those with retinopathy. Thromboxane production is increased in non-diabetic subjects with CHD; amongst diabetic patients, it is also highest in those with macrovascular complications.

The relationship between diabetic control and haemostatic function is not yet clear. Continuous subcutaneous insulin infusion has not led to consistent improvements in clotting factors or measures of platelet function in several studies in IDDM. However, fibrinolytic activity may improve after initiation of treatment for NIDDM [19]. Hypoglycaemia increases platelet activity through the action of catecholamines released as a counter-regulatory response, and this may partly account for the variable results obtained in studies of the effect of improved control on platelet function. Sulphonylureas appear to reduce platelet activity, but whether this is attributable to the improved blood glucose control or the drugs themselves is subject to debate.

#### BLOOD INSULIN LEVELS

Diabetic patients with arterial disease have higher fasting levels of C peptide, and higher circulating insulin levels (both fasting and after oral glucose challenge) than those without [20]. In non-diabetic subjects, exaggerated insulin responses to oral glucose are seen in subjects with cerebral, peripheral and coronary artery disease, and some prospective epidemiological studies have found significant associations between blood insulin concentration and subsequent development of ischaemic heart disease [21]. This association may partly be explained by the interactions between hyperinsulinaemia and hypertension, obesity and hypertriglyceridaemia, which may be related to insulin resistance. However, insulin stimulates proliferation of arterial smooth muscle cells *in vitro*, and lipid synthesis in the arterial wall in animals [20], suggesting that insulin could be directly involved in atherogenesis. High circulating insulin levels are seen both in NIDDM and in treated IDDM, and levels can be reduced by avoidance of obesity and by regular physical exercise. The relationship between hyperinsulinaemia and hypertension is discussed further in Chapter 18.

#### BLOOD GLUCOSE LEVELS

In a large study of several diabetic populations [22], no relationship was found between fasting glycaemia and ECG abnormalities, but there was a weak association with stroke and a strong association with peripheral vascular disease (especially amputation). A similar pattern was seen when duration of diabetes was considered in the same population. Further work is needed to examine IDDM specifically.

#### ADVANCED GLYCOSYLATION END-PRODUCTS

Prolonged exposure of proteins to glucose leads to reversible non-enzymatic glycosylation of amino groups, and subsequent covalent cross-linking of the proteins by complex modification of the glucose-derived groups (see Chapter 3) [23]. Collagen modified in this way shows increased binding of low-density lipoprotein (LDL) *in vitro* [24]. Modification of the structural proteins of the vessel wall and basement membrane may in itself contribute to luminal narrowing [23]. Moreover, macrophages recognizing modified proteins release various cytokines, which promote cellular proliferation [25]. These observations may provide a link between large- and small-vessel disease.

#### TREATMENT EFFECTS

Oral hypoglycaemic agents were found to be associated with increased cardiovascular mortality in the University Group Diabetes Program trial, which compared different treatment regimens [26]. These findings have been reviewed in the light of other data [9] and have not been confirmed.

### *Lipoprotein abnormalities*

The major lipoprotein classes can be separated by ultracentrifugation, and their characteristics and effects on atheroma are outlined in Table 17.3. Each comprises a hydrophobic core of triglycerides and cholesterol esters, surrounded by a coat containing polar phospholipids, free cholesterol and apoproteins. Their major metabolic pathways are outlined in Figs 17.1–17.3.

Data from the Framingham study suggest that plasma cholesterol has a similar influence on CHD in diabetic as in non-diabetic subjects [13]. A number of cross-sectional studies have demonstrated an inverse relationship between HDL-cholesterol and arterial disease in NIDDM, but reports in IDDM have been inconsistent [9]. Raised triglyceride levels have also been associated with CHD in cross-sectional studies [22]. The impact of lipid-lowering therapy on CHD in non-diabetic subjects is well established [27–29], and detection and treatment of hyperlipidaemia should be a key part of the routine management of cardiovascular risk factors (Table 17.2).

#### EFFECTS OF DIABETES ON LIPOPROTEINS

The commonest abnormality in diabetes is hypertriglyceridaemia due to an excess of very low density lipoprotein (VLDL) [30]. Lipoprotein lipase depends for its full activity on insulin (Fig. 17.1), and VLDL clearance is reduced in poorly controlled

**Table 17.3.** Lipoprotein classification.

| | Chylomicrons | VLDL | IDL | LDL | HDL |
|---|---|---|---|---|---|
| Diameter (nm) | 80–500 | 30–80 | 25–35 | 20 | 10 |
| Electrophoresis | Origin | Pre-beta | Broad beta | Beta | Alpha |
| Principal core lipid | Exogenous triglyceride | Triglyceride<br>Cholesterol esters | Cholesterol esters<br>Triglyceride | Cholesterol esters<br>Triglyceride | Cholesterol esters |
| Effect on atheroma | Nil | + | ++ | +++ | Protects |
| Major apoproteins | AI and II<br>B48<br>CII and III<br>E | B100<br>CII and III<br>E | B100<br>E | B100 | AI and II<br>CIII |
| Dietary and drug treatment | Diet<br>Drugs ineffective | Fibrates<br>Nicotinic acid<br>ω-3 (N-3) fish oils | Fibrates<br>Nicotinic acid | Resins<br>Nicotinic acid<br>Fibrates<br>Probucol | Fibrates<br>Nicotinic acid<br>ω-3 (N-3) fish oils<br>Resins raise HDL<br>Probucol lowers HDL |

HDL: high-density lipoproteins; IDL: intermediate density; LDL: low-density; VLDL: very low density. +, ++, +++: moderate, strong and very strong associations.

patients with IDDM. In NIDDM patients, there is also overproduction of VLDL and apoprotein (apo) B. Insulin deficiency or resistance increases production of non-esterified fatty acids from adipose tissue by the action of hormone-sensitive lipase, and these provide a substrate for hepatic triglyceride synthesis. Hypertriglyceridaemia in diabetes therefore usually responds to intensified insulin treatment.

LDL levels are also raised in association with poor glycaemic control, but a substantial improvement in blood glucose is required to lower LDL [31]. Insulin stimulates LDL receptor activity (Fig. 17.2) [32], increasing LDL clearance, while non-enzymatic glycosylation of apo B reduces its affinity for the receptor, thereby slowing LDL removal [33].

HDL levels vary inversely with VLDL, since reduced lipoprotein lipase activity impairs catabolism of VLDL and hence transfer of lipids and apoproteins to HDL (Fig. 17.3). In NIDDM, HDL levels are low, especially in association with hypertriglyceridaemia, whereas in IDDM the levels are normal. Glycosylation of HDL occurs *in vivo*, and in animal studies glycosylated HDL is removed faster from the circulation [34].

### ASSESSMENT

Initial screening is by measurement of plasma cholesterol, triglyceride and HDL cholesterol after a 12-h overnight fast. The LDL cholesterol can then be calculated (in mmol/l) from the Friedewald formula [35]:

$$\text{LDL cholesterol} = \text{total cholesterol} - \text{HDL cholesterol} - \left(\frac{\text{triglyceride}}{2.19}\right)$$

(This should not be used when the triglyceride level is over 5 mmol/l.)

Cholesterol levels are not significantly changed postprandially, but triglycerides may rise. A non-fasting sample may therefore be used for screening, but should be repeated fasting if the triglycerides are elevated.

### MANAGEMENT

The European Atherosclerosis Society has recently published guidelines for management of hyperlipidaemia which are outlined in Table 17.4 [36]. The same therapeutic goals are recommended in diabetes, but management should be guided by the fact that diabetes itself puts the patient into a high-risk group and therefore demands aggressive

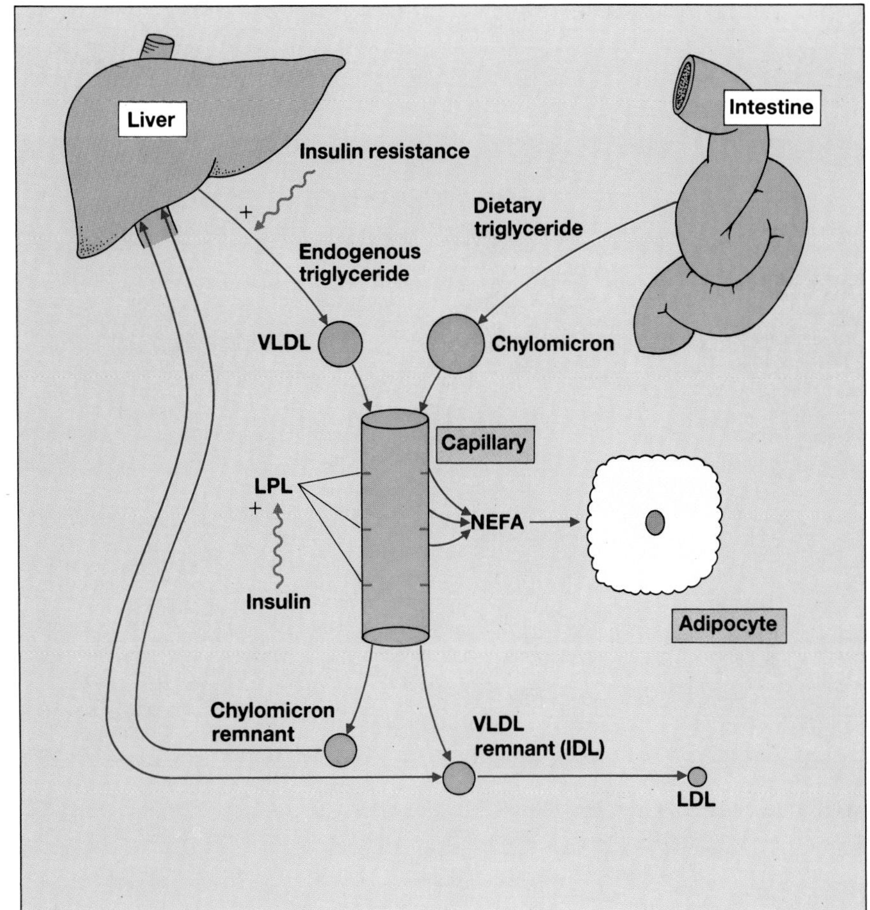


**Fig. 17.1.** Very low density lipoprotein (VLDL), containing endogenous triglyceride, and chylomicrons, containing dietary triglyceride, are catabolized by the endothelial enzyme lipoprotein lipase (LPL), releasing non-esterified fatty acids (NEFA) for use as fuel or storage in adipose tissue. The resulting remnant particles may be taken up by the liver, and the VLDL remnant (intermediate-density lipoprotein or IDL), containing all its original cholesterol, may be further catabolized to produce low-density lipoprotein (LDL).

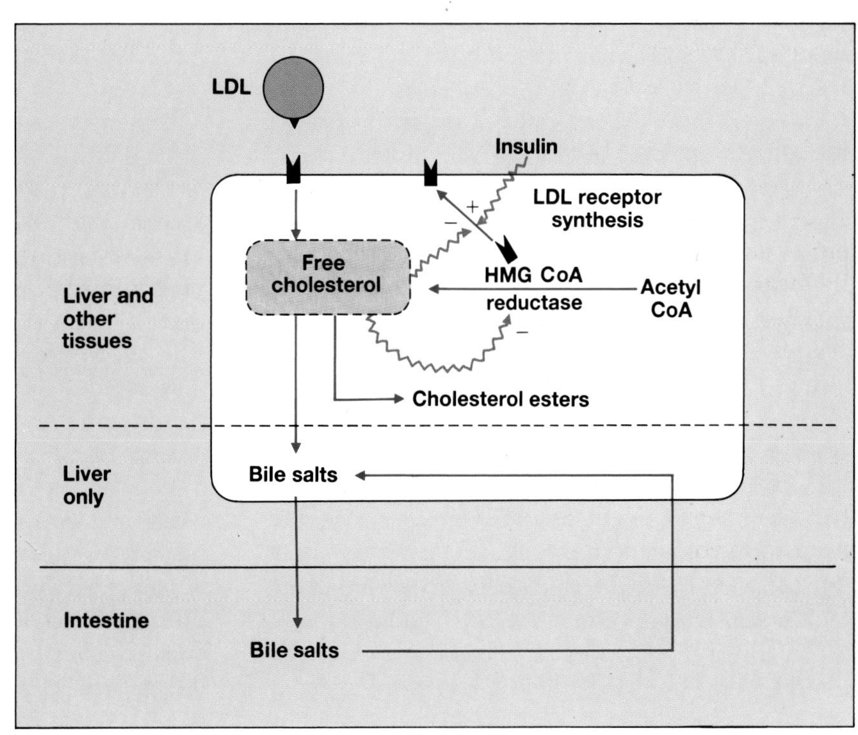


**Fig. 17.2.** Low-density lipoprotein (LDL) is taken up predominantly via a receptor recognizing apoprotein B100. Free cholesterol is released into the cytoplasmic pool, which also receives endogenously synthesized cholesterol. The cholesterol is used in membrane and bile-salt synthesis or stored as cholesterol ester. The free cholesterol inhibits both LDL receptor synthesis and the activity of HMG CoA reductase, the rate-limiting enzyme in cholesterol synthesis, thus regulating its own concentration.

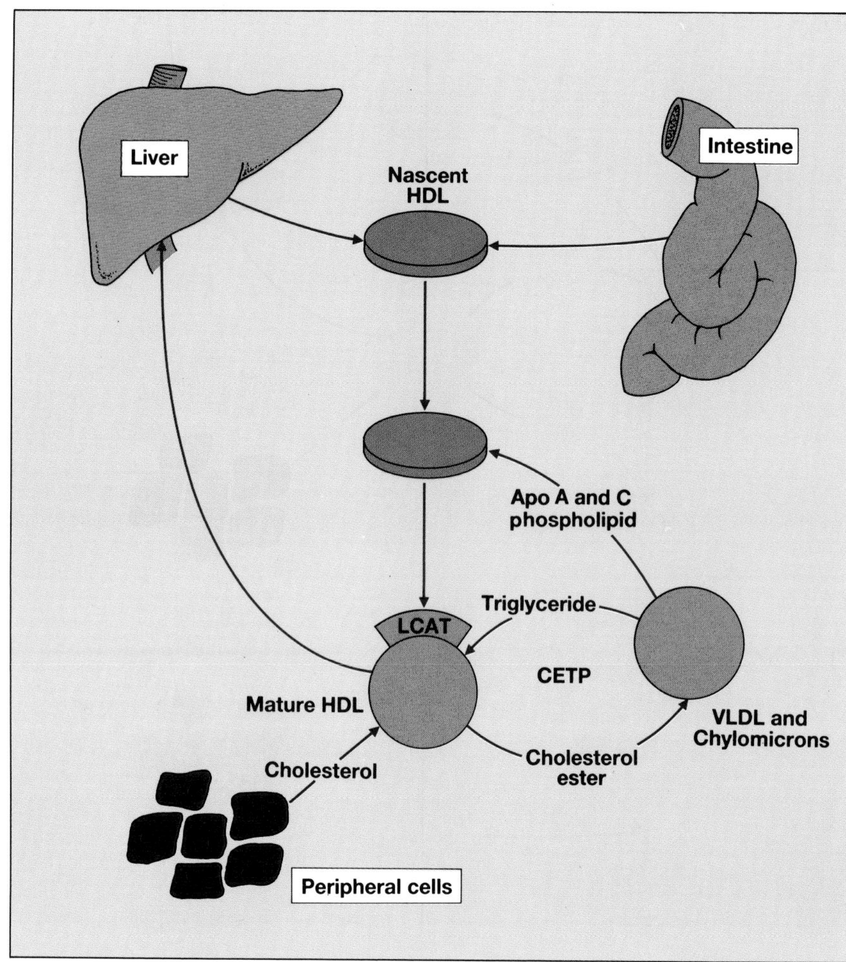


**Fig. 17.3.** High-density lipoprotein (HDL) is produced as a lipid-poor disc. It receives apoproteins and phospholipids from triglyceride-rich lipoproteins, and the enzyme lecithin : cholesterol acyltransferase (LCAT) is activated by apo AI. It can then receive cholesterol from peripheral cells, esterify it and transport it to the liver either directly or by transferring it to other lipoproteins via cholesterol ester transfer protein (CETP).

treatment. A management scheme is suggested in Fig. 17.4.

Initial treatment is by optimizing body weight and glucose control, and by dietary adjustment. In IDDM, a high-carbohydrate, low-saturated fat, low-cholesterol diet has been shown to lower cholesterol without a deterioration in glucose control or triglyceride levels [37], and the diet currently recommended for diabetes provides about 35% of energy as fat, with partial substitution of polyunsaturated for saturated fats [38]. The American Heart Association has published dietary recommendations for the treatment of hyperlipidaemia [39], with gradual introduction of the phases in Table 17.5; phase I is most commonly used in the UK.

In NIDDM, weight reduction is accompanied by a fall in triglycerides and a rise in HDL-cholesterol. A lowering of LDL depends on the dietary fat composition, but does not result from weight reduction alone. Dietary fibre, especially soluble gums and pectins found in pulses and legumes, is also important in lowering cholesterol.

Patients unresponsive to diet and intensified control may have an underlying primary hyperlipidaemia or another cause of secondary hyperlipidaemia (Table 17.6). They should be reassessed for these and dietary compliance checked before proceeding to drug treatment.

### DRUG THERAPY

In *hypertriglyceridaemia* or *combined hyperlipidaemia*, bezafibrate and gemfibrozil are the drugs of choice. They elevate HDL, which may have an additional protective effect [29]. Bezafibrate [40] may also improve glycaemic control. Nicotinic acid is also effective, but frequently causes flushing, pruritus and gastrointestinal side-effects. Its newer analogues such as acipimox are better tolerated.

For *hypercholesterolaemia*, the bile-acid sequestering resins, cholestyramine and colestipol, are

**Table 17.4.** Guidelines for management of hyperlipidaemia. Adapted from the guidelines of the European Atherosclerosis Society [36].

| Group | Lipid level (mmol/l) | Assessment | Treatment |
|---|---|---|---|
| A | Cholesterol 5.2–6.5<br>Triglyceride <2.3 | Assess overall risk of CHD | Restrict food energy if overweight; give nutritional advice and correct other risk factors. If high risk, monitor as in B |
| B | Cholesterol 6.5–7.8<br>Triglyceride <2.3 | Assess overall risk of CHD | Restrict food energy if overweight; prescribe lipid-lowering diet and monitor response and compliance. If cholesterol remains high, consider lipid-lowering drugs |
| C | Cholesterol <5.2<br>Triglyceride 2.3–5.6 | Seek underlying cause | Restrict food energy if overweight; treat underlying causes if present. Prescribe and monitor lipid-lowering diet. Monitor response and compliance |
| D | Cholesterol 5.2–7.8<br>Triglyceride 2.3–5.6 | Assess overall risk of CHD<br>Seek underlying cause | Proceed as for group C above. If response is inadequate and overall CHD risk is high, consider lipid-lowering drugs |
| E | Cholesterol >7.8, or<br>Triglyceride >5.6 | Make full diagnosis | Consider referral to lipid clinic or specialized physician for investigation and treatment |

**Table 17.5.** American Heart Association lipid-lowering dietary phases [39].

| | |
|---|---|
| Phase I | 30% calories as fat; equal proportions of saturated, monounsaturated and polyunsaturated; under 300 mg cholesterol |
| Phase II | 25% calories as fat; equal proportions of fatty acid types; 200–250 mg cholesterol |
| Phase III | 20% calories as fat; equal proportions of fatty acid types; 100–150 mg cholesterol |

**Table 17.6.** Causes of secondary hyperlipidaemia.

| | |
|---|---|
| Dietary | Alcohol |
| Hypothyroidism | Drugs: |
| Obesity | • thiazide diuretics |
| Chronic renal failure | • β-blockers |
| Nephrotic syndrome | • oral contraceptives |
| Dysglobulinaemia | • isotretinoin |

effective [27, 28], although unpleasant to swallow and subject to gastrointestinal side-effects. By preventing the enterohepatic recirculation of bile, these agents cause the hepatocyte to synthesize more bile acids from cholesterol and to increase the number of cell-surface LDL receptors to keep pace with the increased demand (Fig. 17.2). They may worsen any coexisting hypertriglyceridaemia because of a compensatory increase in hepatic VLDL secretion. Combined therapy with a fibrate and a resin avoids the adverse rise in triglycerides and has an additional cholesterol-lowering effect.

The inhibitors of 3-hydroxymethyl 3-glutaryl coenzyme A (HMG CoA) reductase, now known as statins (Fig. 17.2), are very effective cholesterol-lowering agents and the first of these, lovastatin, is available in the US. It inhibits intracellular cholesterol synthesis at its rate-limiting step, reducing the cytoplasmic pool of cholesterol, and thereby stimulating production of more LDL receptors. It has recently been shown to be effective in diabetes [41]. Pravastatin and simvastatin, two related drugs, are now available in the UK.

## Heart disease

The major clinical manifestations of CHD are heart failure, angina pectoris and myocardial infarction. The following discussion emphasizes their management in diabetes.

### *Heart failure*

#### PATHOPHYSIOLOGY

The origin of heart failure in diabetes is multifactorial. In a series of patients dying of heart failure of unknown cause [42], most were diabetic and showed multiple non-transmural infarcts at post-mortem examination. Non-invasive studies of resting left ventricular function have demonstrated abnormalities both of contraction and relaxation of the ventricle in diabetic patients without ischaemic heart disease or hypertension. About a quarter of such patients were affected in one study [43], the majority having evidence of microvascular disease (retinopathy of nephropathy). These findings have supported the concept of a specific diabetes-associated cardiomyopathy. In the dia-

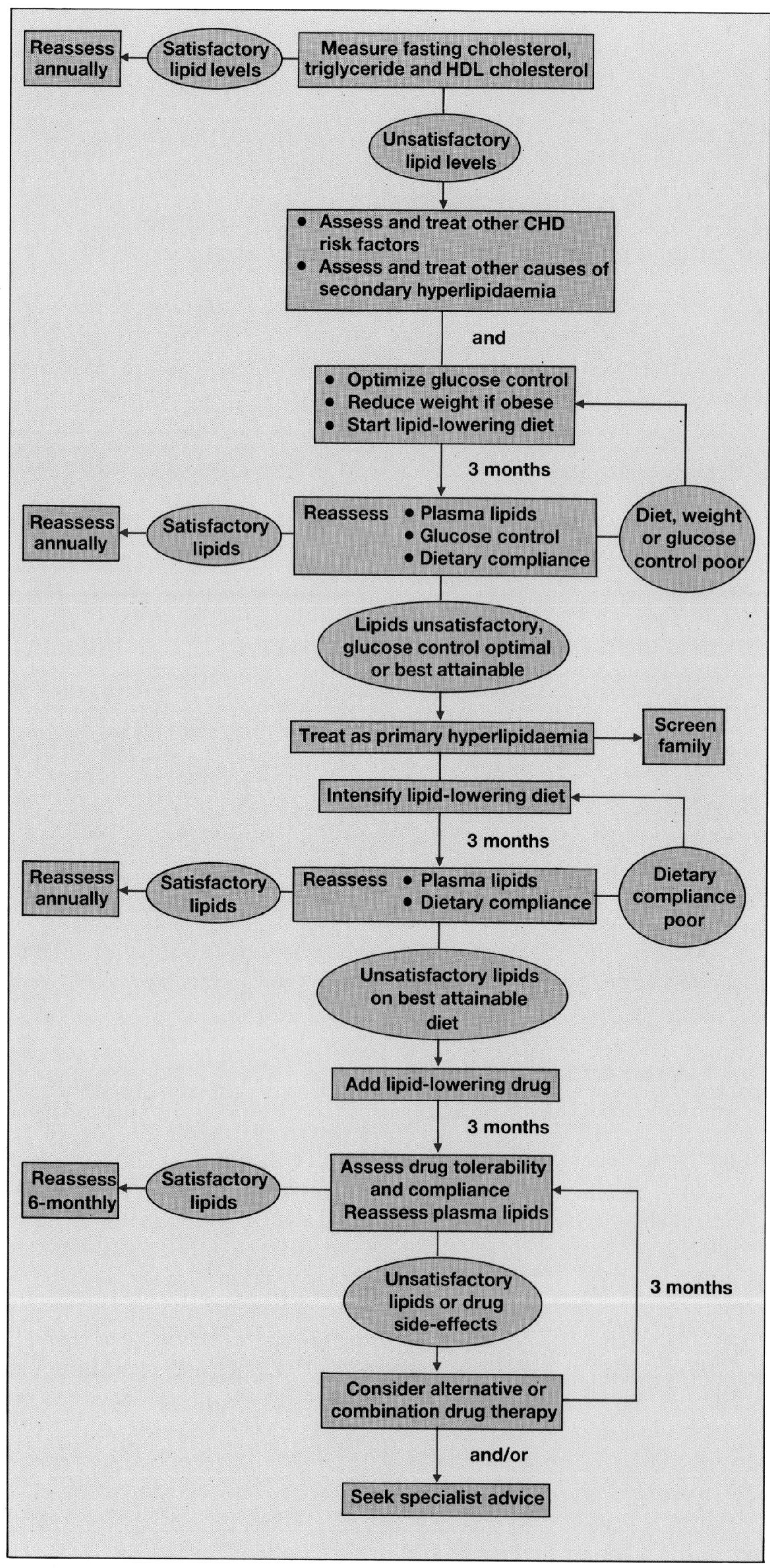


**Fig. 17.4.** Management of hyperlipidaemia.

betic heart, collagen and periodic acid–Schiff (PAS)-positive staining material are deposited around blood vessels and between the muscle fibres [44], a process accelerated by coexisting hypertension, both in humans [45] and in animal models [46]. The microvascular abnormalities seen in the diabetic heart are similar to those described elsewhere in the body, with capillary microaneurysms and thickening of the capillary basement membranes. A milder degree of basement membrane thickening has been observed in IGT. There is no evidence for ischaemia at a microvascular level [44], although leakage of protein from abnormally permeable capillaries may stimulate interstitial fibrosis. Abnormal cardiac function after exercise has recently been described in children and adolescents with diabetes [47], and an apparent association with finger contractures may suggest a generalized fibrotic process. Diabetic children have an exaggerated pressor response to exercise [48], which could both affect the pattern of ventricular contraction and also contribute to myocardial damage. Functionally, the fibrosis reduces ventricular compliance, impairing both filling and emptying. The inability of the myocardium to distend may reduce contractility by blunting the Starling reflex, and autonomic neuropathy may further impair the ability of the ventricle to respond to stress.

Metabolic changes associated with diabetes can cause reversible myocardial dysfunction. In NIDDM, improvement of control by diet or insulin therapy may be accompanied by improved ventricular function and exercise tolerance [49]. Diabetic animals show changes in the activity and type of actinomyosin and myosin ATPases [50] which result in defective activation of the contractile proteins. In normal subjects, injection of insulin has a small immediate positive inotropic action which precedes hypoglycaemia and its catecholamine response [51], but the mechanism of this is not known.

### ASSESSMENT AND MANAGEMENT

In any diabetic presenting with breathlessness or exercise intolerance, heart failure should be suspected, and the diagnosis cannot be excluded by a normal ECG and chest X-ray. Non-invasive assessment of myocardial contraction by radionuclide ventriculography or echocardiography will detect resting abnormalities, and the echocardiogram will also give valuable information about the heart valves and pericardium. After exercise, the ejection fraction should increase, and combining an exercise ECG with radionuclide ventriculography may reveal a fall in ejection fraction or regional akinesia due to silent reversible ischaemia.

Optimizing glucose control is important in the treatment of heart failure, first because of the effects on myocardial function described above, and secondly because glucose may contribute to osmotic gradients resulting in pulmonary oedema [52]. Detection and treatment of hypertension may prevent further deterioration as well as reducing the cardiac workload. Similarly, treatment of reversible ischaemia with nitrates and calcium channel antagonists may improve exercise tolerance.

Thiazide diuretics may worsen diabetic control and aggravate hyperlipidaemia (see Chapter 18); loop diuretics are therefore preferred, but hypokalaemia must be avoided as it impairs insulin secretion and predisposes to arrhythmias. The potassium-sparing diuretics, triamterene and amiloride, may also worsen control in poorly controlled diabetic patients and paradoxically increase plasma potassium levels after a glucose load [53]. Plasma potassium and glucose concentrations must therefore be carefully monitored during diuretic therapy.

Angiotensin-converting enzyme (ACE) inhibitors are effective second-line therapy, and have been shown to improve the prognosis in non-diabetic subjects with severe heart failure [54]. They are less effective than diuretics when used alone [55], but as diuretics activate the renin–angiotensin system, the combination of ACE inhibitors and diuretics is particularly effective. Blood pressure should be monitored when starting treatment because of first-dose hypotension (see Chapter 18), and plasma potassium levels monitored during treatment.

## *Myocardial infarction*

The mortality rate following myocardial infarction in diabetic patients is about twice that of the general population, and a review of published figures since 1929 [56] has revealed no sign of improvement with time, although the mortality (both in diabetic and control subjects) has varied widely. A concomitant prospective analysis showed that the proportions of deaths attributable to heart failure, sudden death and arrhythmias were similar to those in non-diabetic subjects, and that the principal cause of death was pump failure.

Infarct size is an important determinant of mortality and correlates with the degree of stress hyperglycaemia in non-diabetic cases [57]. However, most studies have not found larger infarcts in diabetic than in control populations [58]. Ischaemia of the surviving myocardium due to multivessel disease and pre-existing ventricular dysfunction due to cardiomyopathy, hypertension, or previous infarction will reduce the heart's ability to compensate for the loss of infarcted muscle. Compensatory reflexes are also blunted by autonomic neuropathy. Cardiac pain sensation may be impaired in autonomic neuropathy, although a recent study of in-patients revealed no evidence of delayed referral [58].

Ischaemia inhibits both glycolysis and the oxidation of non-esterified fatty acids (NEFA), the principal source of energy in the myocardium [59, 60]. At the same time, the stress hormone response and suppression of insulin secretion raises plasma levels of glucose and NEFA and reduces glucose entry into the myocardium. These metabolic abnormalities are exaggerated in diabetes by insulin deficiency and/or resistance.

NEFA inhibit ATP generation in the mitochondria, and in experimental infarction have been shown to increase infarct size, reduce myocardial contractility and increase oxygen requirements [61]. In man, serum NEFA levels correlate with the risk of postinfarction arrhythmias [62]. They also increase platelet aggregability and reduce the synthesis of prostacyclin in the endothelium [61].

Postinfarct blood glucose levels are of prognostic significance both in diabetic patients [58] and in stress hyperglycaemia [57], but it is not clear whether the raised blood glucose contributes to the increased mortality or is simply consequent upon the stress response and therefore an indicator of poor outcome. Careful metabolic control using an intravenous insulin infusion has not been consistently beneficial [63, 64], but normoglycaemia is only achieved some hours after admission when the damage is probably already complete. In dogs with experimental infarction, glucose–insulin–potassium infusions have been shown to reduce infarct size and to improve the metabolic derangement around the infarct zone [65], but trials in humans have produced conflicting results, and their use has not been accepted.

Diabetic ketoacidosis complicates only some 3% of myocardial infarcts in diabetic patients but is obviously important in affected individuals [56].

### MANAGEMENT OF MYOCARDIAL INFARCTION

Several points specific to diabetes should supplement normal coronary care. First, blood glucose levels should be carefully controlled, where necessary by intravenous insulin infusion. A successfully used regimen is given in Table 17.7 [66]. Hypokalaemia should be avoided, since this predisposes to ventricular arrhythmias, and the plasma potassium level should be kept above 4 mmol/l. Secondly, heart failure should be sought and treated aggressively; there is an argument for early invasive monitoring by Swan–Ganz catheter to allow optimal therapy, since cardiovascular reflexes may be impaired. Thirdly, in view of the increased numbers of diabetic patients presenting with reinfarction, secondary prevention is important, and risk factor management, β-blockade and suitability for bypass surgery should all be considered.

The treatment of myocardial infarction has recently undergone major changes, with the widespread use of intravenous thrombolytic therapy and aspirin [67]. If myocardium is to be salvaged in diabetic patients, the early correction of metabolic control may become especially important. Reperfusion arrhythmias have not been a problem in general, but separate studies in diabetic patients are needed. In view of their hypercoagulable state, diabetic subjects may respond differently to thrombolysis, and more information is required before they can gain maximum benefit from this treatment. Thrombolysis is contraindicated by proliferative retinopathy because of the risk of haemorrhage.

**Table 17.7.** Intravenous insulin infusion and glycaemic monitoring schedule suggested for diabetic patients with acute myocardial infarction. (Adapted from [66] with permission from the *British Medical Journal*.)

| (a) Infusion regimen<br>Blood glucose (mmol/l) | Infusion rate (U/h) |
|---|---|
| <4 | 0 |
| 4–8 | 1 |
| 8–12 | 2 |
| >12 | 4 |
| **(b) Monitoring regimen**<br>**Time (h)** | **Monitor glucose** |
| 0–4 | Hourly |
| 4–24 | 4-hourly |
| >24 | Before meals |

### *Angina pectoris*

Symptoms of angina may be masked in diabetes by autonomic neuropathy, and breathlessness may be the only symptom of silent reversible ischaemia. Non-invasive techniques to confirm the diagnosis include exercise ECG, $^{201}$Thallium ventricular perfusion scanning and exercise radionuclide ventriculography.

The sensitivity and specificity of these techniques depends on the study population and there is little information on their reliability as compared with coronary angiography in diabetic patients. The effects of hypertension and cardiomyopathy may produce non-specific changes, and glucose ingestion can cause both ST depression and T-wave inversion [68]. The specificity of the exercise ECG may be increased, with some loss of sensitivity, by choosing 1.5- or 2-mm ST depression as the criterion for a positive test [69]. The diagnosis must be made after consideration of all the available information rather than relying on a single result.

Nitrates, calcium antagonists and β-blockers may be used in the normal way in the treatment of angina, but certain features of diabetes may influence the choice. Nitrates can cause postural hypotension in patients whose baroreceptor reflexes are impaired by autonomic neuropathy; this problem can be minimized by advising patients to spit out the sublingual tablet as soon as pain is relieved.

Non-selective β-blockade impairs insulin release and hence may worsen diabetic control in NIDDM. It can mask the warning symptoms of hypoglycaemia, and also impairs catecholamine-mediated glycogenolysis and gluconeogenesis, slowing recovery from hypoglycaemia. In addition, β-blockers may adversely affect plasma lipids, exacerbate heart failure and ischaemia of the lower limb and cause impotence. In spite of all this, they are used successfully in many diabetic patients, and one long-term study [70] failed to demonstrate an increase in severe hypoglycaemic episodes with β-blockade in IDDM. Cardioselective agents such as atenolol, metoprolol and acebutolol should be used to minimize non-cardiac side-effects, and these points should be considered when selecting treatment and monitoring response.

Calcium channel antagonists have also been reported to worsen blood glucose control in large doses and in acute studies, but this does not seem to be a problem in NIDDM patients with hypertension [71]. There are significant differences between the available drugs in their suppression of sinoatrial node function, atrioventricular conduction and myocardial contractility. Verapamil has the most pronounced effects on the heart and may exacerbate heart failure, whereas the cardiac effects of nifedipine are slight, although reflex tachycardia may result. The effects of diltiazem are intermediate and it is a useful single agent for angina prophylaxis.

### *Coronary artery surgery and angioplasty*

Surgical treatment of coronary disease should be considered either when medical treatment has failed to relieve symptoms adequately or when the prognosis may be improved by surgery. Coronary angiography is normally only undertaken when this is considered.

There has been debate as to whether the pattern of coronary atherosclerosis in diabetes is more diffuse, or simply more severe than in non-diabetic patients. This point is clearly important when coronary surgery or angioplasty are contemplated. In one angiographic study, diabetic patients had more severe and extensive disease than carefully matched non-diabetic controls [72]. The number of stenosed segments per vessel was significantly greater in the diabetic group, but did not affect operability, the number of inoperable vessels being similar in the two groups.

The exercise ECG is a valuable prognostic indicator in selecting patients for angiography. In non-diabetic subjects, poor prognosis is associated with ST depression at a low workload or heart rate (stage 3 of the Bruce protocol or 120 beats/min), failure of the systolic pressure to rise above 130 mmHg or a fall in blood pressure indicating impaired ventricular function [69]. There is no evidence that the absence of chest pain confers a better prognosis than symptomatic ischaemia of equivalent severity.

In non-diabetic subjects, prognosis is improved by surgery in patients with disease affecting the left main coronary artery, three-vessel disease or two-vessel disease in which the left anterior descending artery is involved [73]. The use of internal mammary grafts improves long-term results. The effect of percutaneous transluminal coronary angioplasty (PTCA) on prognosis is not known, but its success and safety are increasing with a mortality rate of around 1% in spite of its increasing use in multivessel disease [74].

The in-hospital mortality of diabetic patients

undergoing coronary artery bypass grafting (CABG) has been about twice that of controls. In a review of long-term results of surgery, initial symptomatic relief was similar in diabetic and non-diabetic subjects, but 15-year survival was 53% in non-diabetics, 43% in diabetic patients treated by diet alone, 33% in those on oral hypoglycaemic agents and 19% in those on insulin [75]. Late graft patency was similar in all groups. With improved technique and postoperative care, a more recently operated series [76] showed no significant excess in perioperative morbidity or mortality in diabetic patients, even though they had twice the control rate of previous infarction and hypertension. Survival and symptomatic relief in the medium term were also comparable. There are no longer any grounds for denying the benefit of this treatment to people with diabetes.

PTCA is suited mainly to localized stenoses and may therefore be less appropriate for diabetic patients in whom widespread disease is common, although PTCA is increasingly used in multivessel disease [74]. In one large series, the slightly higher mortality seen in diabetic patients was attributable to the worse pattern of their disease [77], and patients should be selected with this in mind. The long-term results in diabetes are uncertain, but one small series [78] has reported that restenosis is more frequent; further information is clearly needed.

Given the poor prognosis of CHD in diabetes and the demonstrable prognostic benefits of surgery in selected non-diabetic cases, it seems reasonable to pursue an active policy to detect those diabetic patients who may benefit from surgery in the same way. Until the situation has been clarified, angioplasty should be reserved for symptomatic relief or for localized disease in diabetes. A suggested scheme of selection is given in Fig. 17.5.

## Peripheral arterial disease

Intermittent claudication may present as numbness or weakness, especially if the limb is already affected by neuropathy. As ischaemia worsens, it may progress to pain or discomfort at rest, especially at night, and finally to necrosis. Surgery is directed either to the symptoms of claudication and rest pain, or to the jeopardized limb which may otherwise require amputation; its prophylactic use in mild claudication is not justified.

Clinical assessment involves palpation of the aorta and iliac vessels in the abdomen as well as

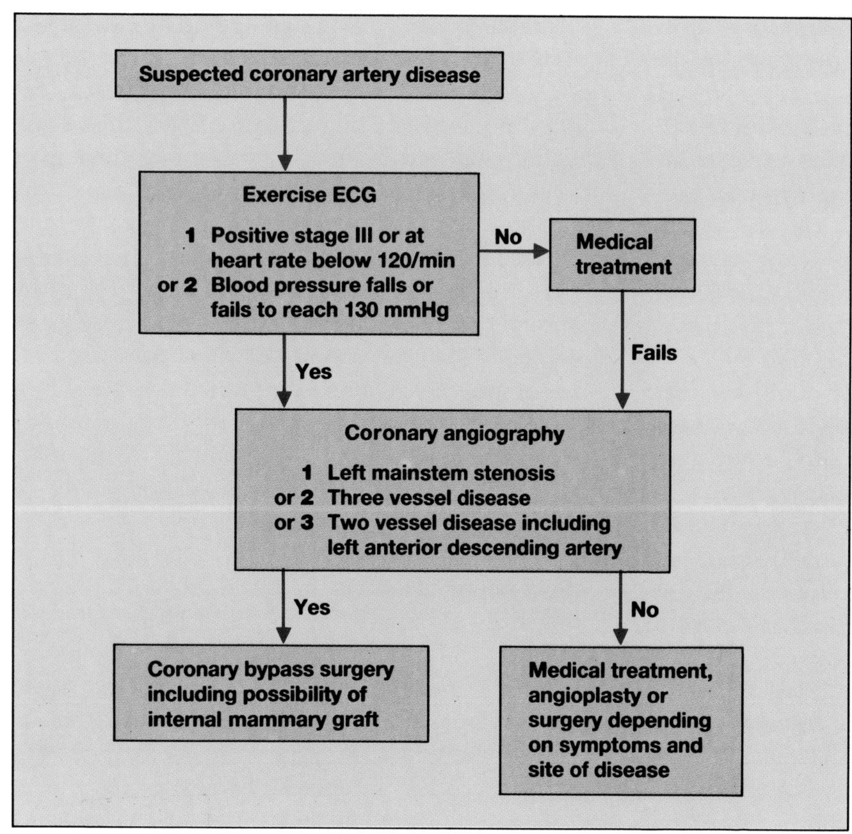


**Fig. 17.5.** Management of coronary artery disease.

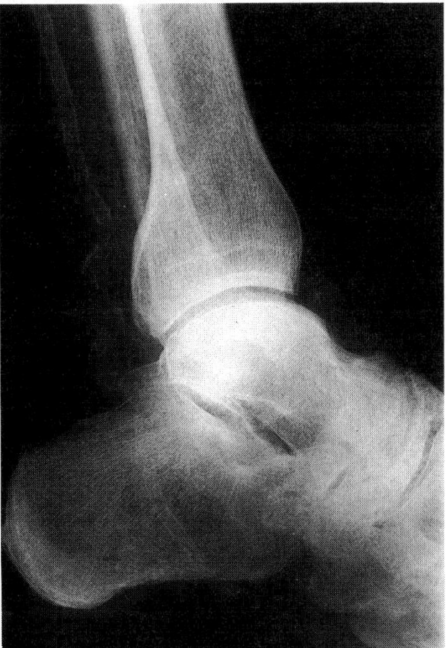
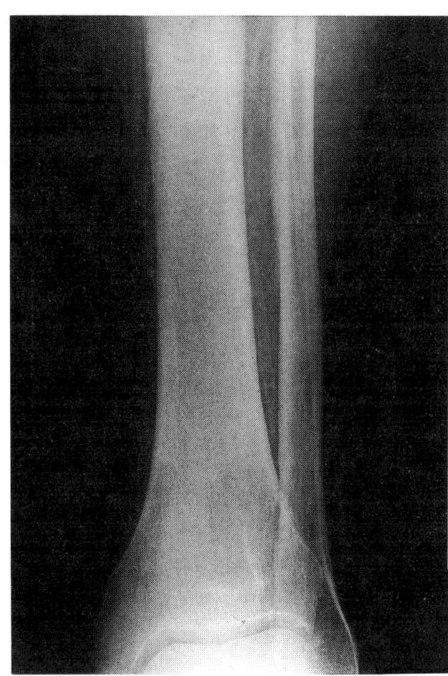

**Fig. 17.6.** Radiographic calcification accompanying medial sclerosis involving the distal lower limb arteries.

the limb pulses, and auscultation for bruits. The skin must also be examined for signs of poor nutrition, sites of possible trauma and disordered sweating. The latter is useful in assessing the potential value of sympathectomy, since loss of sweating indicates that the sympathetic nerves are already affected by neuropathy [79].

Conservative treatment involves careful diabetic control, prohibition of smoking, weight reduction where necessary and meticulous foot care. Drugs designed to improve blood flow are disappointing, but venesection to reduce blood viscosity has been shown to improve walking distance in selected patients [80] and merits further evaluation in diabetic patients, whose blood viscosity is raised.

When reconstruction is contemplated, arteriographic assessment must include the distal vessels which are often affected by both atheroma and medial sclerosis with calcification (see Figs 16.8 and 17.6) in diabetes. Aorto-iliac and aorto-femoral grafts are technically as successful as in non-diabetic cases. In one series, all patients survived with patent grafts, and patency at 5 years was 94% in both groups. However, at 4 years one-third of the diabetic patients were dead and the diabetic survivors showed more progression of distal arterial disease [79]. Comparable good results have been obtained with femoro-popliteal grafts.

Distal arterial surgery is only indicated for rest pain or limb salvage. Grafts from the femoral or popliteal vessels to arteries at ankle level are technically demanding, but can save limbs. In one recent report of 26 patients (25 diabetic) undergoing distal grafts using the saphenous vein *in situ* [81], only one major amputation was required, but three patients died in the first month from myocardial infarction and seven required minor amputations. This reflects the severity of disease in this group of patients.

Percutaneous transluminal balloon angioplasty is best suited to dilating discrete stenoses in proximal vessels, which may sometimes improve perfusion in the difficult problem of distal disease. The initial success rate of angioplasty is reduced in diabetic patients but, as with PTCA, this is due to the pattern of disease encountered rather than the presence of diabetes itself [82]. The restenosis rate after angioplasty in diabetes is not certain. Ankle systolic pressures have been observed to fall during the first year following successful angioplasty of iliac or superficial femoral artery stenoses in diabetic patients, although there was no concomitant deterioration in symptoms [83].

ROGER H. JAY
D. JOHN BETTERIDGE

## References

1 Borch-Johnsen K, Kreiner S. Proteinuria: value as a predictor of cardiovascular mortality in insulin dependent diabetes mellitus. *Br Med J* 1987; **294**: 1651–4.
2 Marks HH, Krall LP. Onset, course, prognosis and mortality in diabetes mellitus. In: Marble A, White P, Bradley RF, Krall LP, eds. *Joslin's Diabetes Mellitus* 11th edn. Philadelphia: Lea & Febiger, 1971: 209–54.
3 Jarrett RJ. The epidemiology of coronary heart disease and related factors in the context of diabetes mellitus and

impaired glucose tolerance. In: Jarrett RJ, ed. *Diabetes and Heart Disease*. Amsterdam: Elsevier Science Publishers BV, 1984: 1–23.

4 Fuller JH, Shipley MJ, Rose G, Jarrett RJ, Keen H. Coronary heart disease risk and impaired glucose tolerance: the Whitehall study. *Lancet* 1980; **i**: 1373–6.

5 Sasaki A, Kamado K, Horiuchi N. A changing pattern of causes of death in Japanese diabetics. Observations over fifteen years. *J Chron Dis* 1978; **31**: 433–44.

6 Kawate R, Yamakido M, Nishimoto Y, Bennett PH, Hamman RF, Knowler WC. Diabetes mellitus and its vascular complications in Japanese migrants on the island of Hawaii. *Diabetes Care* 1979; **2**: 161–70.

7 Seftel HC, Walker ARP. Vascular disease in South African Bantu diabetics. *Diabetologia* 1966; **2**: 286–90.

8 Krut LH, Dubb A, Mangera C. Serum lipid levels in black diabetics in Baragwaneth Hospital. *S Afr Med J* 1980; **57**: 350–4.

9 Pyörälä K, Laakso M, Uusitupa M. Diabetes and atherosclerosis: an epidemiologic view. *Diabetes/Metab Rev* 1987; **3**: 464–524.

10 Fuller JH, Shipley MJ, Rose G, Jarrett RJ, Keen H. Mortality from coronary heart disease and stroke in relation to the degree of hyperglycaemia: the Whitehall study. *Br Med J* 1983; **287**: 867–70.

11 Most RS, Sinnock P. The epidemiology of lower extremity amputations in diabetic individuals. *Diabetes Care* 1983; **6**: 87–91.

12 Kannel WB, McGee DL. Diabetes and glucose tolerance as risk factors for cardiovascular disease: the Framingham Study. *Diabetes Care* 1979; **2**: 120–6.

13 Kannel WB, McGee DL. Diabetes and cardiovascular risk factors: the Framingham study. *Circulation* 1979; **59**: 8–13.

14 Kesson CM, Slater SD. Smoking in diabetics. *Lancet* 1979; **i**: 504–5.

15 Hayward RE, Lucena BC. An investigation into the mortality of diabetics. *J Inst Actuaries* 1965; **91**: 286–315.

16 Meade TW, Brozovic M, Chakrabarti RR *et al*. Haemostatic function and ischaemic heart disease: principal results of the Northwick Park Heart Study. *Lancet* 1986; **ii**: 533–7.

17 Fuller JH. The haemocoagulation system and macroangiopathy in insulin dependent diabetes. *Ann Clin Res* 1984; **16**: 137–41.

18 Betteridge DJ. Platelets and diabetes mellitus. In: Taylor KG, ed. *Diabetes and the Heart*. Tunbridge Wells: Castle House Publications, 1987: 79–119.

19 Bedi HK, Vyas BR, Bomb BS, Agarival ML, Bedi T. Fibrinogen content and fibrinolytic activity of blood in diabetics before and after antidiabetic drugs. *J Ass Phys India* 1977; **25**: 181–5.

20 Stout RW. Insulin and atheroma — an update. *Lancet* 1987; **i**: 1077–9.

21 Jarrett RJ. Is insulin atherogenic? (editorial). *Diabetologia* 1988; **31**: 71–5.

22 West KM, Ahuja MMS, Bennett PH *et al*. The role of circulating glucose and triglyceride concentrations and their interactions with other 'risk factors' as determinants of arterial disease in nine diabetic population samples from the WHO multinational study. *Diabetes Care* 1983; **6**: 361–9.

23 Brownlee M, Cerami A, Vlassara H. Advanced products of nonenzymatic glycosylation in the pathogenesis of diabetic vascular disease. *Diabetes Metab Rev* 1988; **4**: 437–51.

24 Brownlee M, Vlassara H, Cerami A. Nonenzymatic glycosylation products on collagen covalently trap low-density lipoprotein. *Diabetes* 1985; **34**: 938–41.

25 Vlassara H, Brownlee M, Manogue K *et al*. Cachectin/TNF and IL-1 induced by glucose-modified proteins: role in normal tissue remodelling. *Science* 1988; **240**: 1546–8.

26 University Group Diabetes Program. A study of the effects of hypoglycemic agents on vascular complications in patients with adult-onset diabetes: V. Evaluation of phenformin therapy. *Diabetes* 1975; **24** (suppl 1): 65–184.

27 Lipid Research Clinics Program. The Lipid Research Clinics Coronary Primary Prevention Trial results I. Reduction in the incidence of coronary heart disease. *J Am Med Ass* 1984; **251**: 351–64.

28 Lipid Research Clinics Program. The Lipid Research Clinics Coronary Primary Prevention Trial results. II. The relationship of reduction in incidence of coronary heart disease to cholesterol lowering. *J Am Med Ass* 1984; **251**: 365–74.

29 Frick MH, Elo O, Haapa K *et al*. Helsinki Heart Study: primary-prevention trial with gemfibrozil in middle-aged men with dyslipidemia; safety of treatment, changes in risk factors and incidence of coronary heart disease. *N Engl J Med* 1987; **317**: 1237–45.

30 Albrink MJ. Dietary and drug treatment of hyperlipidaemia in diabetics. *Diabetes* 1974; **23**: 913–18.

31 Pietri A, Dunn FL, Raskin P. The effect of improved diabetic control on plasma lipid and lipoprotein levels. A comparison of conventional therapy and continuous subcutaneous insulin. *Diabetes* 1980; **29**: 1001–5.

32 Chait A, Bierman EL, Albers JJ. Low density lipoprotein receptor activity in cultured fibroblasts: mechanism of insulin-induced stimulation. *J Clin Invest* 1979; **64**: 1309–19.

33 Steinbrecher UP, Witztum JL. Glucosylation of low density lipoproteins to an extent comparable to that seen in diabetes slows their catabolism. *Diabetes* 1984; **33**: 130–4.

34 Witztum JL, Fischer M, Pietro T, Steinbrecher UP, Elam RL. Non-enzymatic glycosylation of high density lipoprotein accelerates its catabolism in guinea pigs. *Diabetes* 1982; **31**: 1029–32.

35 Friedewald WT, Levy RI, Fredrickson DS. Estimation of the concentration of low-density lipoprotein cholesterol ion plasma without use of the preparative ultracentrifuge. *Clin Chem* 1972; **18**: 499–502.

36 Study Group of the European Atherosclerosis Society. The recognition and management of hyperlipidaemia in adults: a policy statement of the European Atherosclerosis Society. *Eur Heart J* 1988; **9**: 571–600.

37 Stone DB, Connor WE. The prolonged effects of a low cholesterol, high carbohydrate diet upon the serum lipids in diabetic patients. *Diabetes* 1963; **12**: 127–35.

38 British Diabetic Association. Dietary recommendations for diabetics in the 1980s — a policy statement by the British Diabetic Association. *Hum Nutr Appl Nutr* 1982; **36A**: 378–94.

39 Ad Hoc Committee to Design a Dietary Treatment of Hyperlipoproteinemia. Recommendations for treatment of hyperlipidemia in adults. A joint statement of the nutrition committee and the council on arteriosclerosis. *Circulation* 1984; **69**: 1065A–90A.

40 Wahl P, Hasslacher CL, Lang PD *et al*. Lipid-lowering effect of bezafibrate in patients with diabetes mellitus and hyperlipidaemia. In: Greten H, Lang PD, Schettler G, eds. *Lipoproteins and Coronary Heart Disease: New Aspects in the Diagnosis and Therapy of Disorders of Lipid Metabolism*. Baden-Baden: Gerhard Witztrock, 1980: 154–8.

41 Garg A, Grundy SM. Lovastatin for lowering cholesterol levels in non-insulin-dependent diabetes mellitus. *N Engl J Med* 1988; **318**: 81–6.

42 Boucher CA, Fallon JT, Johnson RA, Yurchak PM. Cardiomyopathic syndrome caused by coronary artery disease. III: prospective clinicopathological study of its prevalence among patients with clinically unexplained chronic heart failure. *Br Heart J* 1979; **41**: 613–20.

43 Shapiro LM. A prospective study of heart disease in diabetes mellitus. *Q J Med* 1984; **209**: 55–68.

44 Regan TJ, Lyons MM, Levinson GE *et al.* Evidence for cardiomyopathy in familial diabetes mellitus. *J Clin Invest* 1977; **60**: 885–99.

45 Factor SM, Minase T, Sonnenblick EH. Clinical and morphological features of human hypertensive diabetic cardiomyopathy. *Am Heart J* 1980; **99**: 446–58.

46 Fein FS, Capasso JM, Aronson RS *et al.* Combined renovascular hypertension and diabetes in rats: a new preparation of congestive cardiomyopathy. *Circulation* 1984; **80**: 318–30.

47 Baum VC, Levitsky LL, Englander RM. Abnormal cardiac function after exercise in insulin-dependent diabetic children and adolescents. *Diabetes Care* 1987; **10**: 319–23.

48 Karlefors T. Circulatory studies during exercise with particular reference to diabetics. *Acta Med Scand* 1966; **180** (suppl 449).

49 Uusitupa M, Mustonen J, Laakso M, Pyörälä K. Left ventricular dysfunction in diabetes: evidence for the impact of metabolic factors. *Diabetologia* 1987; **30**: 193–4.

50 Dillman WH. Diabetes mellitus induces changes in cardiac myosin in the rat. *Diabetes* 1980; **29**: 579–82.

51 Fisher BM, Gillen G, Dargie HJ, Inglis GC, Frier BM. The effects of insulin-induced hypoglycaemia on cardiovascular function in normal man: studies using radionuclide ventriculography. *Diabetologia* 1987; **30**: 841–5.

52 Axelrod L. Response of congestive heart failure to correction of hyperglycemia in the presence of diabetic nephropathy. *N Engl J Med* 1975; **293**: 1243–5.

53 Walker BR, Capuzzi DM, Alexander F *et al.* Hyperkalaemia after triamterene therapy in diabetic patients. *Clin Pharmacol Ther* 1972; **13**: 643–51.

54 The CONSENSUS Trial Study Group. Effects of enalapril on mortality in severe congestive heart failure. Results of the Cooperative North Scandinavian Enalapril Survival Study (CONSENSUS). *N Engl J Med* 1987; **316**: 1429–35.

55 Richardson A, Bayliss J, Scriven AJ, Parameshwar J, Poole-Wilson PA, Sutton GC. Double-blind comparison of captopril alone against frusemide plus amiloride in mild heart failure. *Lancet* 1987; **ii**: 709–11.

56 Gwilt DJ. Why do diabetics die after myocardial infarction? *Practical Diabetes* 1984; **1**: 36–9.

57 Oswald GA, Smith CCT, Betteridge DJ, Yudkin JS. Determinants and importance of stress hyperglycaemia in non-diabetic patients with myocardial infarction. *Br Med J* 1986; **293**: 917–22.

58 Yudkin JS, Oswald GA. Determinants of hospital admission and case fatality in diabetic patients with myocardial infarction. *Diabetes Care* 1988; **11**: 351–8.

59 Opie LH. Metabolism of free fatty acids, glucose, and catecholamines in acute myocardial infarction. *Am J Cardiol* 1975; **36**: 938–53.

60 Liedtke AJ. Alterations of carbohydrate and lipid metabolism in the acutely ischaemic heart. *Prog Cardiovasc Dis* 1981; **23**: 321–6.

61 Gwilt DJ, Pentecost BL. The heart in diabetes. In: Nattrass M, ed. *Recent Advances in Diabetes* 2. Edinburgh: Churchill Livingstone, 1986: 177–94.

62 Oliver MF, Kurien VA, Greenwood TW. Relation between serum free fatty acids and arrhythmias and death after myocardial infarction. *Lancet* 1968; **i**: 710–15.

63 Gwilt DJ, Petri M, Lamb P, Nattrass M, Pentecost BL. Effect of intravenous insulin infusion on mortality among diabetic patients after myocardial infarction. *Br Heart J* 1984; **51**: 626–31.

64 Clark RS, English M, McNeill GP, Newton RW. Effect of intravenous infusion of insulin in diabetics with acute myocardial infarction. *Br Med J* 1985; **291**: 303–5.

65 Dalby AJ, Bricknell OL, Opie LH. Effect of glucose-insulin-potassium infusions on epicardial ECG changes and on myocardial metabolic changes after coronary artery ligation in dogs. *Cardiovasc Res* 1981; **15**: 588–98.

66 Gwilt DJ, Nattrass M, Pentecost BL. Use of low-dose insulin infusions in diabetics after myocardial infarction. *Br Med J* 1982; **285**: 1402–4.

67 ISIS-2 (Second International Study of Infarct Survival) Collaborative Group. Randomised trial of intravenous streptokinase, oral aspirin, both or neither among 17,187 cases of suspected acute myocardial infarction. *Lancet* 1988; **ii**: 349–60.

68 Riley CG, Oberman A, Sheffield LT. Electrocardiographic effects of glucose ingestion. *Arch Intern Med* 1972; **130**: 703–7.

69 Crean PA, Fox KM. Exercise electrocardiography in coronary artery disease. *Q J Med* 1987; **237**: 7–13.

70 Barnett AH, Leslie D, Watkins PJ. Can insulin-treated diabetics be given beta-adrenergic blocking drugs? *Br Med J* 1980; **280**: 976–8.

71 Whitcroft I, Thomas J, Davies IB, Wilkinson N, Rawthorne A. Calcium antagonists do not impair long term glucose control in hypertensive non-insulin diabetics (NIDDs). *Br J Clin Pharmacol* 1986; **22**: 208P.

72 Dortimer AC, Shenoy PN, Shiroff RA *et al.* Diffuse coronary artery disease in diabetic patients. Fact or fiction? *Circulation* 1978; **57**: 133–6.

73 Oakley CM. Surgery and prognosis in coronary heart disease. *Q J Med* 1986; **231**: 637–41.

74 Detre K, Holubkov R, Kelsey S *et al.* Percutaneous transluminal coronary angioplasty in 1985–1986 and 1977–1981. The National Heart, Lung and Blood Institute Registry. *N Engl J Med* 1988; **318**: 265–70.

75 Lawrie GM, Morris GC, Glaeser DH. Influence of diabetes mellitus on the results of coronary bypass surgery. Follow-up of 212 diabetic patients ten to 15 years after surgery. *J Am Med Ass* 1986; **256**: 2967–71.

76 Devineni R, McKenzie FN. Surgery for coronary artery disease in patients with diabetes mellitus. *Can J Surg* 1985; **28**: 367–70.

77 Ellis SG, Roubin GS, King SB *et al.* In-hospital cardiac mortality after acute closure after coronary angioplasty: analysis of risk factors from 8207 procedures. *J Am Coll Cardiol* 1988; **11**: 211–16.

78 Margolis JL, Krieger J, Glemser E. Coronary angioplasty: increased restenosis rate in insulin-dependent diabetics. Circulation 1984; **70** (suppl 2): 175.

79 Wheelock FC, Gibbons GW, Marble A. Surgery in diabetes. In: Marble A, Krall LP, Bradley RF, Christlieb AR, Soeldner JS, eds. *Joslin's Diabetes Mellitus*, 12th edn. Philadelphia: Lea & Febiger, 1985: 712–32.

80 Ernst E, Matrai A, Kollar L. Placebo-controlled, double-blind study of haemodilution in peripheral arterial disease. *Lancet* 1987; **i**: 1449–51.

81 Rhodes GR, Rollins D, Sidawy AN, Skudder P, Buchbinder D. Popliteal-to-tibial *in situ* saphenous vein bypasses for

limb salvage in diabetic patients. *Am J Surg* 1987; **154**: 245–7.
82 Johnston KW, Rae M, Hogg-Johnston SA *et al*. 5-year results of a prospective study of percutaneous transluminal angioplasty. *Ann Surg* 1987; **206**: 403–13.
83 Burnett JR, Walshe JA, Howard PR *et al*. Transluminal balloon angioplasty in diabetic peripheral vascular disease. *Aust NZ J Surg* 1987; **57**: 307–9.

# 18 Hypertension in Diabetes Mellitus


## Summary

- Hypertension affects over 30% of European diabetic patients and is twice as common as in the non-diabetic population.
- Diabetes may predispose to hypertension by promoting sodium retention, increasing vascular tone and by contributing to nephropathy. Hypertension in NIDDM may, like the commonly associated hyperlipidaemia, be partly a consequence of insulin resistance and hyperinsulinaemia.
- The presence of hypertension in diabetic patients increases mortality four- to fivefold, largely through coronary heart disease and stroke. Women and Afro-Caribbean patients are particularly at risk.
- Hypertension may also be an aetiological factor in diabetic nephropathy (to which it may determine susceptibility) and in retinopathy.
- Initial investigations of the hypertensive diabetic patient must exclude rare causes of secondary hypertension, assess vascular and renal damage, and identify other cardiovascular risk factors.
- General measures such as dietary advice and reducing alcohol intake may themselves normalize blood pressure. Other cardiovascular risk factors — particularly smoking and hyperlipidaemia — must be treated energetically.
- First-line antihypertensive drugs in diabetic patients include: diuretics at low dosage, to avoid adverse metabolic effects due to potassium depletion; cardioselective β-blockers, which may worsen metabolic control; calcium channel blockers, which do not affect metabolic control and have useful anti-anginal and anti-arrhythmic effects; and ACE inhibitors, which have few metabolic side-effects and can reduce albumin excretion in diabetic nephropathy. Second-line drugs include vasodilators and centrally-acting agents.
- Patients failing to respond to general measures should receive a single suitable first-line drug. Treatment failures should be given, in sequence: another suitable first-line drug; a logical combination of two first-line drugs; and then triple therapy with another first-line drug or a vasodilator.
- Only 5% of patients will fail to respond to triple therapy; possible underlying causes of hypertension should be investigated and addition of a fourth drug (e.g. clonidine) may be helpful.


Hypertension in diabetes represents an important health problem as the combination of the two diseases is common, carries significant morbidity and mortality, and is frequently difficult to treat.

## Epidemiology

These two common conditions will frequently be associated by chance alone, but diabetes apparently predisposes to hypertension and, conversely, hypertensive people are more likely to develop diabetes.

The reported prevalence of hypertension in diabetic people varies widely, but is probably 1.5–2 times higher than in the general population. As many as 30–50% of the European diabetic population aged 35–54 years may be hypertensive, with even higher frequencies in women and Afro-

Caribbean patients [1–3]. Many newly diagnosed NIDDM patients are found to be hypertensive, whereas hypertension generally appears later in IDDM, predominantly associated with nephropathy: after 30 years of IDDM, 50% of patients have hypertension and most of these have nephropathy [4] (see Fig. 18.1).

Hypertensive patients show an increased prevalence of impaired glucose tolerance and diabetes, predominantly NIDDM. This is sometimes present when hypertension is diagnosed but more often appears subsequently, possibly in part because certain antihypertensive drugs are diabetogenic [5]. This is discussed further in recent developments at the end of this chapter.

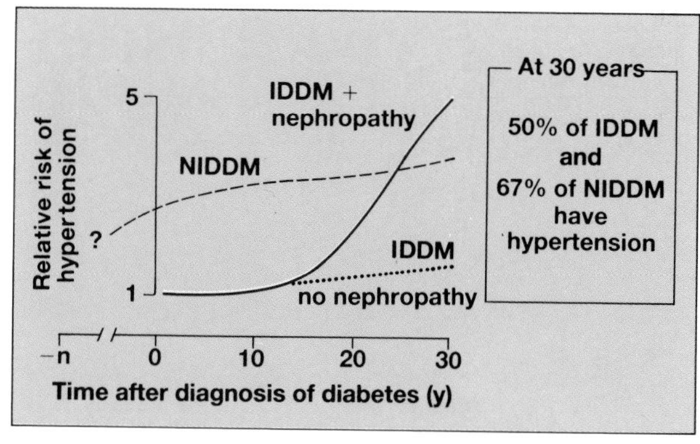


**Fig. 18.1.** Schematic time-course of development of hypertension in NIDDM patients, and in IDDM patients with and without nephropathy. The majority of hypertensive IDDM subjects are those with nephropathy.

## Aetiology of hypertension in diabetes

As shown in Table 18.1, diabetes and hypertension are occasionally associated in specific endocrine syndromes (acromegaly, Cushing's and Conn's syndromes, phaeochromocytoma) or as a result of treatment with the oral contraceptive pill or glucocorticoids. These rare possibilities must always be considered, as both hypertension and diabetes may be cured by treating the underlying problem. Hypertension in diabetes may also be due to nephropathy, renal scarring following repeated urinary tract infections, or coincidental renal disease.

Diabetes in general predisposes to hypertension. Postulated mechanisms are shown in Fig. 18.2. Hyperglycaemia promotes reabsorption of glucose in the proximal convoluted tubule, causing obligatory sodium reabsorption, increased total body sodium content (usually by about 10%) and expansion of the extracellular fluid (ECF) volume; however, this occurs in normotensive as well as hypertensive diabetic subjects [6–9]. The activity of the renin–angiotensin–aldosterone system in diabetic man and animals is generally decreased or normal [9, 10]; as a decrease would be expected with ECF expansion, 'normal' levels may in fact be inappropriately increased. Circulating renin activity may, however, be increased in volume-depleted patients with ketoacidosis [11]. Circulating catecholamine levels are increased in poorly controlled diabetes [12] but essentially normal in most patients [13]. Peripheral resistance may be increased through enhanced vascular sensitivity to various vasoconstrictor agents, including noradrenaline and angiotensin II [7, 8, 14].

Hypertension and diabetic nephropathy are

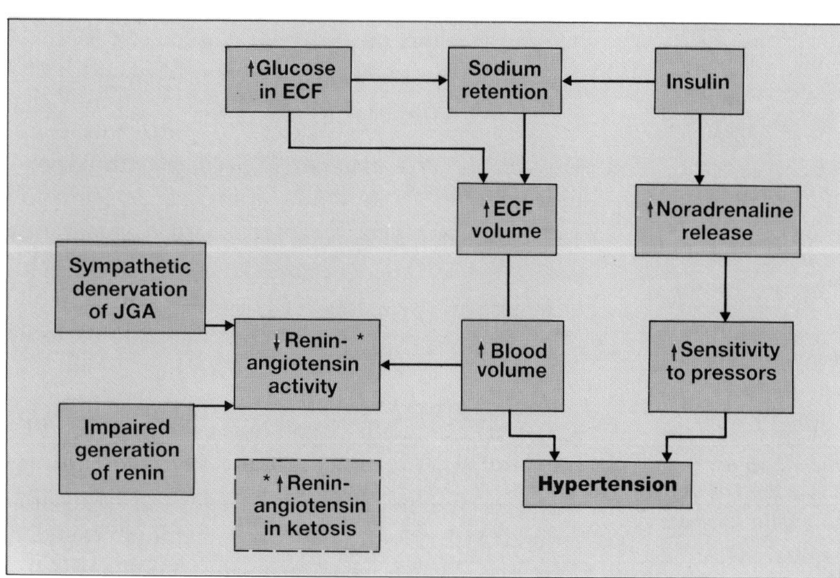


**Fig. 18.2.** Metabolic factors which may contribute to hypertension in diabetes. Sodium retention (due to both hyperglycaemia and high insulin levels) increases extracellular fluid (ECF) volume. Hyperinsulinaemia (in NIDDM, or during insulin treatment) also stimulates noradrenaline release, which together with enhanced vascular sensitivity to pressors, may increase peripheral resistance. Renin–angiotensin–aldosterone axis activity is generally suppressed by increased ECF volume and sodium load but is increased by volume depletion in ketoacidosis. Renin biosynthesis and release from the juxtaglomerular apparatus (JGA) may also be impaired in diabetes (see [4] for review).

**Table 18.1.** Possible associations of diabetes with hypertension.

| |
|---|
| *Endocrine diseases causing both hypertension and diabetes* |
| Acromegaly |
| Cushing's syndrome |
| Conn's syndrome |
| Phaeochromocytoma |
| *Drugs causing both hypertension and diabetes* |
| Oral contraceptives (combined preparations) |
| Glucocorticoids |
| *Antihypertensive drugs causing diabetes* |
| Potassium-losing diuretics (especially chlorthalidone) |
| β-blockers |
| Diazoxide |
| *Hypertension secondary to diabetic complications* |
| Nephropathy |
| Renal scarring following recurrent urinary tract infections |
| Isolated systolic hypertension due to atherosclerosis |
| *Hypertension associated with NIDDM, insulin resistance and hyperlipidaemia ('syndrome X')* [24] |
| *Hypertension associated with intensified insulin treatment* |
| *Coincidental hypertension in diabetic patients* |
| Essential hypertension |
| Isolated systolic hypertension |

intimately interrelated (see Chapters 13 and 14). Advanced nephropathy occurs more often in IDDM than in NIDDM, perhaps because the latter appears later in life and many NIDDM patients die from other causes before renal failure can develop. None the less, some two-thirds of North American diabetic patients with end-stage nephropathy have NIDDM [4]. The risk of NIDDM patients progressing to renal failure appears to be greater in Afro-Caribbean and Asian people than in Caucasians [15]. Blood pressure is already slightly but significantly elevated at the early stage of microalbuminuria, although there is debate as to whether blood pressure or urinary albumin excretion rises first [16, 17]. Almost all IDDM patients with macroproteinuria are hypertensive by WHO criteria (see below) and blood pressure rises further as renal function deteriorates. Hypertension is a major determinant of the rate of fall of glomerular filtration rate (GFR), and effective antihypertensive treatment is one of the few factors known to delay the otherwise inexorable decline towards renal failure, as illustrated in Fig. 18.3 [18–20] (see Chapters 13 and 14). There is growing evidence that treatment with angiotensin-converting enzyme (ACE) inhibitors during the microalbuminuric stage [21–23], even in normotensive individuals [23], may slow the progression to macroproteinuria. It is not yet clear whether this action is due to a fall in systemic blood pressure or to a selective reduction in intraglomerular hypertension [19] (see Chapter 14).

NIDDM is commonly associated with hypertension, obesity, hyperinsulinaemia, insulin resistance and hyperlipidaemia. Insulin resistance may play a central role in causing this constellation of interdependent factors [24], which act in concert to increase the risks of large-vessel atheroma and death from coronary heart disease or stroke. Obesity and hyperinsulinaemia may both contribute to hypertension, but hyperinsulinaemia is apparently the more important. Circulating insulin concentrations correlate closely with blood pressure across a broad population spectrum [25] and acute fasting — which reduces plasma insulin levels but not weight — significantly lowers blood pressure [26]. Hyperinsulinaemia may raise blood pressure by stimulating proximal tubular sodium reabsorption [27] and by activating the sympathetic nervous system, causing a rise in plasma noradrenaline [28] which is also reversed by fasting [26]. Exogenous insulin may exert similar effects and intensifying insulin treatment may significantly raise blood pressure [29].

A further causal link between hypertension and diabetes is that several antihypertensive drugs — notably the potassium-losing diuretics — may worsen glucose tolerance [30]. Thiazide diuretics are among the drugs most widely prescribed in the elderly and an important iatrogenic cause of diabetes, which may be cured by stopping unnecessary diuretic treatment, using lower dosages or changing to alternative medication.

## Morbidity and mortality of hypertension in diabetes

The major threat posed by the combination of hypertension and diabetes (especially with hyperlipidaemia) is accelerated, severe atherosclerosis of the large arteries. Coronary heart disease and peripheral vascular disease are commoner in diabetes and even more so when associated with hypertension [31]. Myocardial infarction and stroke are the major excess causes of death in NIDDM [32], and the overall mortality in diabetic patients with hypertension (systolic BP >160 mmHg) is 4 times greater in males and 5 times greater in females than in matched normotensive diabetic people [3, 33]. Diabetic hypertensive women also lose the protection against

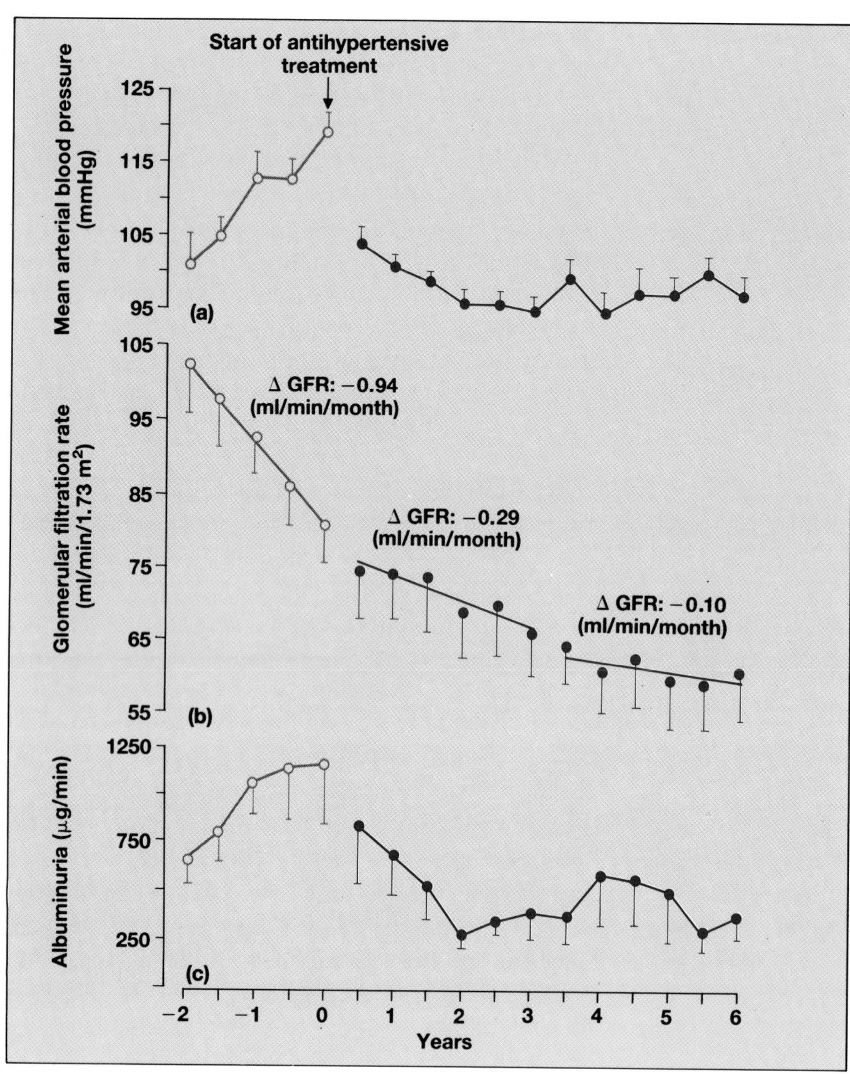


**Fig. 18.3.** Effects of antihypertensive therapy on blood pressure (a), GFR (b) and urinary albumin excretion (c), in hypertensive patients with diabetic nephropathy. Various combinations of β-blockers, diuretics, vasodilators and centrally acting agents were used. (Redrawn from [18], with kind permission of the Editor of the *British Medical Journal*.)

atheroma which they usually enjoy before the menopause [3, 33]. Mortality is particularly high in Afro-Caribbean populations [34].

As well as its incontrovertible role in *macro*-vascular disease, hypertension has also been implicated in the pathogenesis of the *micro*vascular diabetic complications. Epidemiological studies have reported significant associations between hypertension and nephropathy [17–20] and retinopathy [35]. The beneficial effects of anti-hypertensive treatment in nephropathy have already been mentioned, and some preliminary evidence suggests that this may also delay the development of retinopathy [35].

It has been suggested that susceptibility to nephropathy in IDDM is determined by an inherited predisposition to hypertension, as manifested by two putative markers for essential hypertension — having parents with hypertension, and increased lithium–sodium counter-transport activity in red blood cells [36, 37]. The latter abnormality may reflect abnormal renal tubular cation exchange which could lead to sodium retention. However, the significance of these findings has been debated [17].

## Screening and diagnosis of hypertension in diabetes

Because the two conditions coexist so commonly, patients known to have diabetes must be screened regularly for hypertension and vice versa. Hypertensive patients, especially if obese or treated with potentially diabetogenic drugs (see below), should be tested for diabetes at diagnosis and during follow-up. In this event, treatment should be changed to drugs which do not impair glucose tolerance (e.g. ACE inhibitors or calcium entry blockers), when normoglycaemia may be restored.

All diabetic patients must have their blood pressure checked at diagnosis and at least annually thereafter. This is vitally important in patients with other cardiovascular risk factors, nephropathy (especially macroproteinuria, which is associated with a several-fold increase in cardiovascular mortality [38]), or poor diabetic control.

Blood pressure must be measured using an accurate sphygmomanometer and a cuff of an appropriate size (i.e. wider for NIDDM patients with fat arms). The WHO criteria in general use define hypertension as a blood pressure exceeding 160/95 and borderline hypertension as being below these limits but above 140/90 mmHg [1]. Hypertension is diagnosed when readings consistently exceed 160/95 mmHg for several weeks, or when the pressure is very high (diastolic pressure >110 mmHg), or when there is clinical evidence of tissue damage due to long-standing hypertension. The WHO thresholds may be too high in diabetic patients because of their additional risk of vascular disease [39]; this argument may be supported by the apparent benefits of treating 'normotensive', microalbuminuric patients [23]. Age-related centile charts of systolic and diastolic blood pressure in different populations have been produced (Fig. 18.4 [40]) but there are not yet any clear guidelines for their use in diagnosing hypertension in clinical practice.

### *Investigation of hypertension in diabetes*

The initial investigation of the hypertensive diabetic patient (Table 18.2) must aim to exclude the rare causes of secondary hypertension; to assess the extent of tissue damage due to hypertension and diabetes; and to identify other potentially treatable risk factors of vascular disease.

The major points in the history and examination are shown in Table 18.2. The urine must be tested for protein, using 'Albustix' dip-sticks for macroproteinuria or preferably the simple screening procedures now available for microalbuminuria (see Chapter 14). A fresh sample should be examined microscopically for red and white blood cells, casts and other signs of renal disease; microscopic haematuria can occasionally occur in IDDM patients, particularly children, in the apparent absence of significant renal dysfunction but coexistent renal disease must always be excluded [41]. Blood urea, creatinine, electrolytes (especially potassium) and fasting lipid concentrations should be checked. If the serum creatinine concentration is raised, glomerular filtration rate should be measured, ideally by a formal clearance method.

Secondary hypertension may be indicated by clinical findings of endocrine or renal disease, significant hypokalaemia (plasma potassium <3.5 mmol/l, without previous diuretic treatment), failure of hypertension to respond to standard treatment, or a sudden decline in renal function after starting treatment with ACE inhibitors (suggestive of renal artery stenosis).

## Management of hypertension in diabetes

### *Treatment targets*

Treatment should lower blood pressure to a level where the additional morbidity and mortality attributable to hypertension are eliminated. This threshold in diabetic people is unknown, but reduction of *severe* hypertension (diastolic pressure >115 mmHg, or that accompanied by hypertensive tissue damage) to below 140/90 significantly diminishes cardiovascular mortality in non-diabetic populations [42]. The criteria for treating *mild* hypertension (diastolic pressures, 90–110 mmHg) are less clear-cut: the British Medical Research Council study (in non-diabetic patients) showed that the incidence of stroke was halved but that mortality due to coronary heart disease — the main cause of death in NIDDM — was unaffected [43].

While awaiting more precise information, and given the increased hazards of diabetes at all grades of hypertension [32], it seems reasonable to treat mild hypertension (>160/95 mmHg) in diabetic patients and probably to aim for the WHO target pressures (140/90 mmHg). Reducing blood pressure to 'normal' levels may theoretically increase mortality from coronary artery disease, especially in the elderly with pre-existing myocardial ischaemia. However, patients with nephropathy, and perhaps other significant micro- or macrovascular complications, should probably be treated to normalize their blood pressure as far as possible [18–22]. Appropriate target levels in these cases may be the age-related population mean values (see the centile charts in Fig. 18.4).

### *General measures*

Modification of the patient's lifestyle often

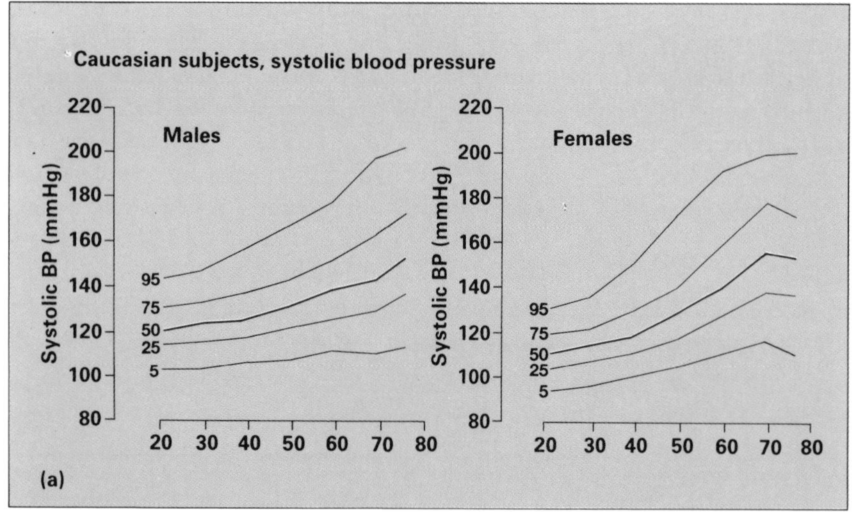


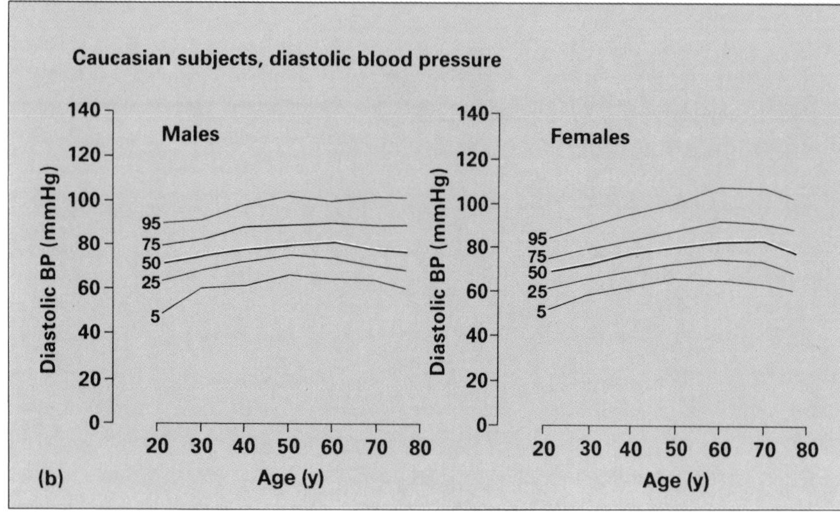


Fig. 18.4. Centile charts showing age-related distribution of systolic and diastolic blood pressures in healthy American Caucasian (a) and (b), and (opposite) Negro (c) and (d) populations.

markedly reduces blood pressure, and may avoid the need for drug treatment.

EDUCATION

Hypertension is almost always asymptomatic and yet another burden for a person with diabetes. Its significance and the need for treatment must therefore be fully explained, without using 'threats' to try to win co-operation. Overall compliance with antihypertensive medication is probably less than 50% but may be improved by involving the patient in making decisions about his own treatment [44].

DIET, DRINK AND EXERCISE

Current dietary guidelines for diabetes should generally be followed. Overweight patients should have a formal weight-reducing diet prescribed and reviewed periodically by a dietitian. Moderate sodium restriction (i.e. not adding salt to food) has a definite hypotensive action [45] and a high-fibre, low-fat, low-sodium diet can lower blood pressure as much as antihypertensive drugs and also improves $HbA_1$ and triglyceride concentrations [46]. Nephropathic patients should probably be given a moderately low-protein diet, which may slow the rate of decline in renal function [17] (see Chapter 16).

Alcohol, a potent cause of 'refractory' hypertension, should be restricted to 20 units/week in men and 12 units/week in women, and excluded altogether if the blood pressure is difficult to control. Regular exercise is probably beneficial, and a gradually increasing programme within the patient's capacity should be encouraged.

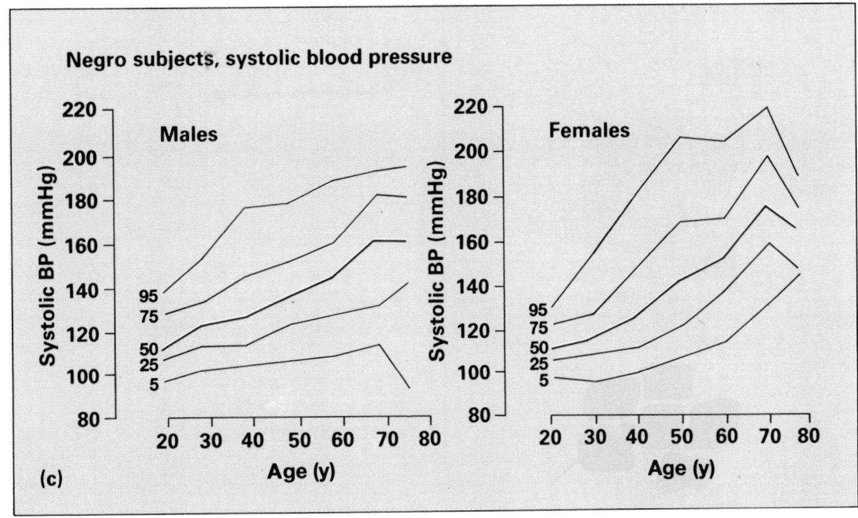


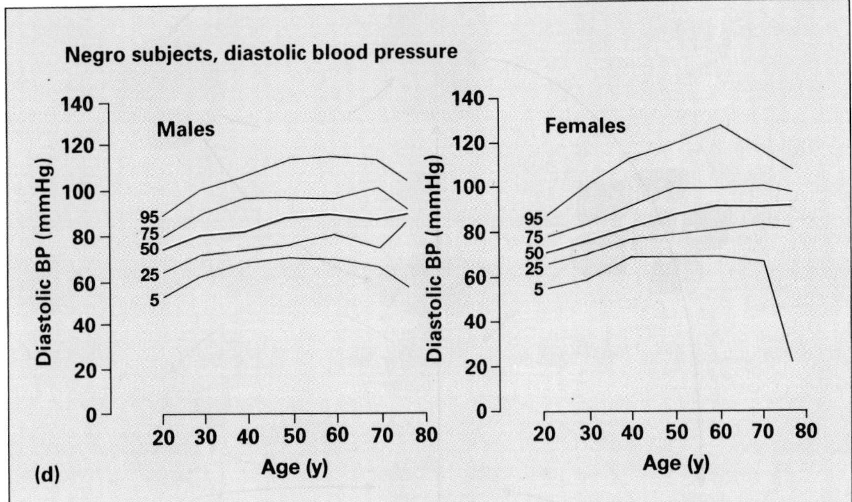


**Fig. 18.4.** (continued) (Redrawn from Acheson RM. [40], with kind permission from the Editor.)

SMOKING

Smoking is one of the most important risk factors for macrovascular disease, increasing 10-year mortality by 20% in non-diabetic people but by a staggering 120% in diabetic subjects [47] (Fig. 18.5). Smoking has also been implicated in the pathogenesis of retinopathy [48] and nephropathy [49]. All diabetic patients must therefore be questioned about smoking and strongly urged to stop. They may be encouraged by the information that stopping smoking has a greater effect on reducing mortality in hypertension than antihypertensive drugs.

HYPERLIPIDAEMIA

Well-controlled IDDM patients are generally normolipidaemic but NIDDM patients, particularly those with hypertension, have an atherogenic lipidaemic profile (see Chapter 17) which may be exacerbated by antihypertensive treatment [50]. Hyperlipidaemia may respond to weight loss, stopping smoking, reducing alcohol intake, improved glycaemic control or a change in antihypertensive drugs (avoiding thiazide diuretics and β-blockers). Some patients may require specific lipid-lowering drugs such as a fibrate, cholestyramine or a statin (see Chapter 17). Omega-3 fish oils improve the lipaemic profile in NIDDM, but aggravate glycaemic control and are therefore not currently recommended [51].

### *Antihypertensive drugs*

Many antihypertensive drugs present particular problems in diabetes; there is no 'ideal' drug for diabetic hypertension and no general agreement about treatment regimens [52]. The current

Table 18.2. Investigation of the diabetic patient with hypertension.

| | Questions to be answered |
|---|---|
| *History*<br>Cardiovascular symptoms<br>Previous urinary disease<br>Smoking and alcohol use<br>Medication<br>Family history of hypertension or cardiovascular disease | *Is hypertension significant?*<br><br>*Does hypertension have an underlying cause?*<br>• Renal<br>• Endocrine<br>• Drug-induced |
| *Examination*<br>Blood pressure erect and supine<br>Left ventricular hypertrophy?<br>Cardiac failure?<br>Peripheral pulses (including renal bruits and radio-femoral delay)<br>Fundal changes<br>Evidence of underlying endocrine or renal disease | *Has hypertension caused tissue damage?*<br>• Left ventricular hypertrophy<br>• Ischaemic heart disease<br>• Cardiac failure<br>• Peripheral vascular disease<br>• Renal impairment<br>• Fundal changes |
| *ECG*<br>Left ventricular hypertrophy<br>Ischaemic changes<br>Rhythm | *Are other cardiovascular risk factors present?*<br>• Smoking<br>• Hyperlipidaemia<br>• Poor glycaemic control<br>• Positive family history |
| *Chest radiograph*<br>Cardiac shadow size<br>Left ventricular failure | |
| *Blood tests*<br>Urea, creatinine, electrolytes<br>Fasting lipids | |

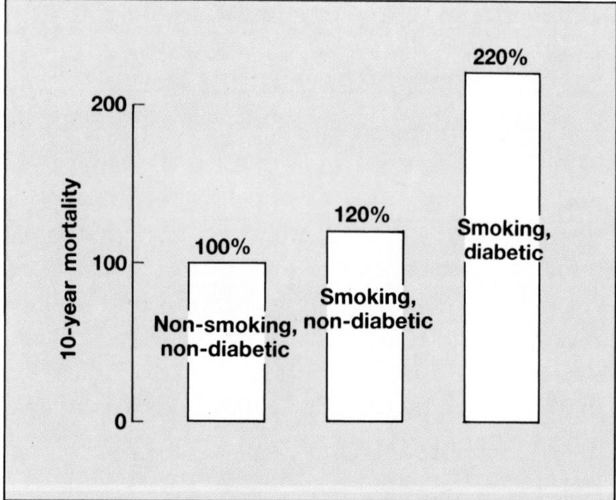


Fig. 18.5. Risks of smoking in non-diabetic and diabetic populations. Smoking more than doubles the 10-year mortality in diabetic people. (Adapted from [46].)

first-line drugs are diuretics, cardioselective β-adrenergic blockers, calcium channel blockers and ACE inhibitors (see Table 18.3).

#### DIURETICS

Diuretics are often effective antihypertensive agents in diabetes, in which the total body sodium load is increased and the extracellular fluid volume expanded [7–9]. However, diuretics which increase urinary potassium losses can worsen glucose tolerance, as insulin secretion is impaired by potassium depletion: the use of thiazide diuretics may increase the risk of non-diabetic hypertensive patients developing diabetes by up to 3 times [30]. Potassium depletion is particularly severe with chlorthalidone (which should therefore be avoided), less with frusemide and bendrofluazide and apparently trivial with indapamide [53]. This mechanism is irrelevant to C-peptide-negative IDDM patients who are totally dependent on exogenous insulin. Diuretics may precipitate hyperosmolar, non-ketotic coma and should be avoided or used at the lowest effective dose in patients with a history of this complication.

Thiazides may aggravate hyperlipidaemia [54], although low dosages probably carry a small risk [49, 55]. Thiazides have also been associated with impotence and may be best avoided in diabetic men with erectile failure.

**Table 18.3.** Antihypertensive drugs used in diabetes.

| Group | Examples | Dosage | Relative indications | Relative contraindications | Precautions |
|---|---|---|---|---|---|
| Diuretics | Bendrofluazide<br>Hydrochlorothiazide<br>Indapamide<br>Frusemide | 1.25–2.5 mg o.d.<br>25 mg o.d.<br>2.5–5 mg o.d.<br>40–80 mg o.d. | Cardiac failure<br>Renal failure (frusemide) | Hyperosmolar coma<br>Impotence<br>Gout<br>Hyperlipidaemia | Give with potassium supplements or ACE inhibitors<br>Monitor blood potassium<br>Check blood glucose and lipids |
| β-blockers (cardioselective) | Atenolol<br>Metoprolol | 50–100 mg o.d.<br>50–100 mg b.d. | Angina<br>Previous myocardial infarction | Cardiac failure<br>Heart block<br>Peripheral vascular disease<br>Impotence<br>Asthma, chronic airflow obstruction<br>Hyperlipidaemia | Warn about loss of hypoglycaemic awareness<br>Monitor blood glucose and lipids |
| ACE inhibitors | Captopril<br>Enalapril | 12.5–50 mg b.d. (6.25 mg initially)<br>10–40 mg o.d. (2.5–5 mg initially) | Cardiac failure<br>Proteinuria | Renal artery stenosis<br>Renal impairment | First-dose hypotension (use small starting dose at night)<br>Monitor renal function<br>Monitor plasma potassium (risk of hyperkalaemia) |
| Calcium entry blockers | Nifedipine<br>Diltiazem<br>Verapamil | 20 mg b.d. (sustained release)<br>60–120 mg t.d.s.<br>120–240 mg b.d. (sustained release) | Angina<br>Arrhythmias | Significant cardiac failure<br>Treatment with digoxin + β-blocker (verapamil) | |
| Other agents | Labetolol<br>Prazosin<br>Hydralazine<br>Clonidine | 50–1200 mg b.d.<br>0.5–5 mg t.d.s.<br>25–50 mg b.d.<br>50–400 mg t.d.s. | Hypertensive crisis<br>Impotence<br>Renal failure<br>Migraine | | First-dose hypotension (prazosin)<br>Use with diuretics and β-blockers |

Dosage schedules: o.d., one daily; b.d., twice daily; t.d.s., thrice daily.

**Table 18.4.** 'Logical' double-drug antihypertensive therapy.

| Combination | Specific benefits | Disadvantages |
|---|---|---|
| Diuretic + ACE inhibitor | ACE inhibitors prevent activation of angiotensin–aldosterone system due to diuretic-induced ECF volume contraction, and help to retain potassium | High risk of 'first-dose' hypotension with ACE-inhibitor in patients overtreated with diuretics |
| Diuretic + atenolol | – | Possibly aggravate hyperglycaemia in NIDDM |
| Diuretic + nifedipine | Diuretic reduces mild ankle swelling due to nifedipine | – |
| Atenolol + nifedipine | Atenolol counteracts tachycardia due to nifedipine's vasodilator action: effective anti-anginal therapy | May aggravate or provoke cardiac failure (both are negative inotropes) |

Diuretics should be used in the lowest possible dose and combined with potassium supplements (or an ACE inhibitor) to minimize potassium depletion. Atenolol and nifedipine are used as examples of a β-blocker and a calcium channel blocker suitable for use in diabetic patients.

Diuretics suitable for use in diabetic hypertension include bendrofluazide, hydrochlorothiazide and indapamide. Low dosages (Table 18.3) should be used, in combination with potassium supplements (or an ACE inhibitor). If ineffective, diuretics should be combined with another first-line drug (e.g. an ACE inhibitor), rather than given at increased dosage. Frusemide can be used instead in patients with renal impairment or stubborn oedema. Plasma urea, creatinine and potassium should be checked initially and 3- to 6-monthly thereafter, dangerous hyperkalaemia can develop in diabetic patients with renal impairment.

### β-ADRENERGIC BLOCKING AGENTS

β-blockers may significantly lower blood pressure in diabetic hypertension, even though renin release (one of these agents' major targets) is generally already reduced in diabetes. These drugs are often ineffective in Afro-Caribbean patients, who have a particular tendency to low-renin hypertension [34].

Like diuretics, β-blockers may aggravate both hyperglycaemia and hyperlipidaemia [30, 54]. Their hyperglycaemic effect is attributed to inhibition of $\beta_2$-adrenergic-mediated insulin release [56], and has been estimated to increase the risks of a non-diabetic person developing the disease by 6-fold and by 15-fold if given together with thiazides [30]. However, recent studies suggest that the hazards of both hyperglycaemia and hyperlipidaemia have been exaggerated [34, 57]. The metabolic side-effects of β-blockers can be reduced by using low dosages combined with other agents, particularly the calcium entry blockers.

β-blockers have other side-effects relevant to diabetes. They may interfere with the counter-regulatory effects of catecholamines secreted during hypoglycaemia, blunting perception of anxiety, tachycardia and tremor and delaying recovery from hypoglycaemia. In clinical practice, however, this rarely presents a serious problem, especially when cardioselective $\beta_1$-blockers are used [58]. β-blockers may also aggravate impotence, and are generally contraindicated in significant cardiac failure, second- or third-degree heart block, peripheral vascular disease, asthma or chronic airflow obstruction.

Atenolol is a useful drug as it is cardioselective, water-soluble (which reduces central nervous system side-effects and renders its metabolism and dosage more predictable) and effective as a single daily dose, which probably encourages compliance.

### CALCIUM ENTRY (SLOW VOLTAGE-DEPENDENT CHANNEL) BLOCKERS

These useful vasodilator agents do not worsen metabolic control when used at currently accepted dosages [34, 59]. Calcium entry blockers have a slight negative inotropic effect and are contraindicated in significant cardiac failure, although the mild ankle oedema often associated with their use is probably due to relaxation of the precapillary sphincter rather than to right ventricular failure.

Because of their other cardiac actions, they are particularly indicated in hypertensive patients who also have angina (nifedipine and diltiazem especially) or supraventricular tachycardia (verapamil). Their vasodilator properties may also be beneficial in peripheral vascular disease. Calcium entry blockers may usefully be combined with diuretics or β-blockers, but the specific combination of verapamil and β-blockers (especially with digoxin) must be avoided because of the risk of conduction block and asystole.

Sustained-release nifedipine, given twice daily, is a convenient preparation for general use.

#### ACE INHIBITORS

ACE inhibitors are useful in diabetic hypertension, even though renin–angiotensin–aldosterone axis activity is not generally increased [10]. When used alone, however, these agents have a limited hypotensive action in many Afro-Caribbean patients [60]. They have no adverse metabolic effects, and may be particularly beneficial in diabetic nephropathy, by reducing albuminuria and possibly the progression of the condition [21–23, 61, 62]. Their antiproteinuric effect may be due specifically to relaxation of the efferent arteriole in the glomerulus (which is highly sensitive to vasoconstriction by angiotensin II), so reducing the intraglomerular hypertension which has been postulated to favour albumin filtration [17, 19], although the importance of this mechanism remains controversial [63]. This selective effect may not be shared by other antihypertensive drugs, such as the calcium channel blockers [62]. ACE inhibitors are also indicated in cardiac failure, in combination with relatively low dosages of diuretics (see Chapter 17).

ACE inhibitors may occasionally precipitate acute renal failure, particularly in the elderly, those taking non-steroidal anti-inflammatory agents and patients with renal artery stenosis. Other side-effects (rashes, neutropenia, taste disturbance) are unusual with the low dosages currently recommended but are more prominent in renal failure. Because of their tendency to potassium retention, potassium-sparing diuretics or potassium supplements should not be taken concurrently. Blood creatinine and potassium levels should be monitored regularly, especially in patients with renal failure, in whom hyperkalaemia may occasionally reach dangerous levels.

Captopril, enalapril and lisinopril are all suitable for use in diabetic patients; enalapril and lisinopril are given once daily for hypertension. The first dose of an ACE inhibitor should be small (e.g. 6.25 mg of captopril) and given just before bedtime to minimize postural hypotension, which may be profound in subjects overtreated with diuretics, although rarely symptomatic.

#### SECOND-LINE AGENTS

Should the above drugs be ineffective or contraindicated, others can be used, usually in conjunction with one or more first-line agents.

Direct vasodilators (e.g. the $\alpha_1$-blocker, prazosin, and hydralazine) cause tachycardia and sodium retention and can logically be combined with a β-blocker and/or a diuretic. Hydralazine is useful in renal failure as it does not accumulate to toxic levels. Prazosin has been recommended in diabetic hypertension as it is effective, devoid of metabolic side-effects and not associated with impotence [64].

Labetolol, a racemate which blocks both α- and β-adrenoceptors (properties of its D- and L-isomers respectively), is useful in hypertensive crisis and in phaeochromocytoma.

Clonidine, a central $\alpha_2$-agonist, has obtrusive side-effects (drowsiness, dry mouth, depression and postural hypotension) but it is specifically indicated in patients who also suffer from migraine, in which it has a prophylactic effect.

Alpha-methyldopa and ganglion blockers cause numerous side-effects (including impotence) and are now little used.

### *Treatment strategy*

Antihypertensive treatment is simply one aspect of a multipronged attack on cardiovascular risk factors. Any drugs must be chosen carefully to minimize any adverse effects on the patient's diabetic control, cardiovascular risks or quality of life. A treatment schedule is suggested below and summarized in Fig. 18.6.

**1** *General measures.* When the diagnosis has been confirmed and secondary hypertension excluded, general measures alone can be tried to 2–3 months

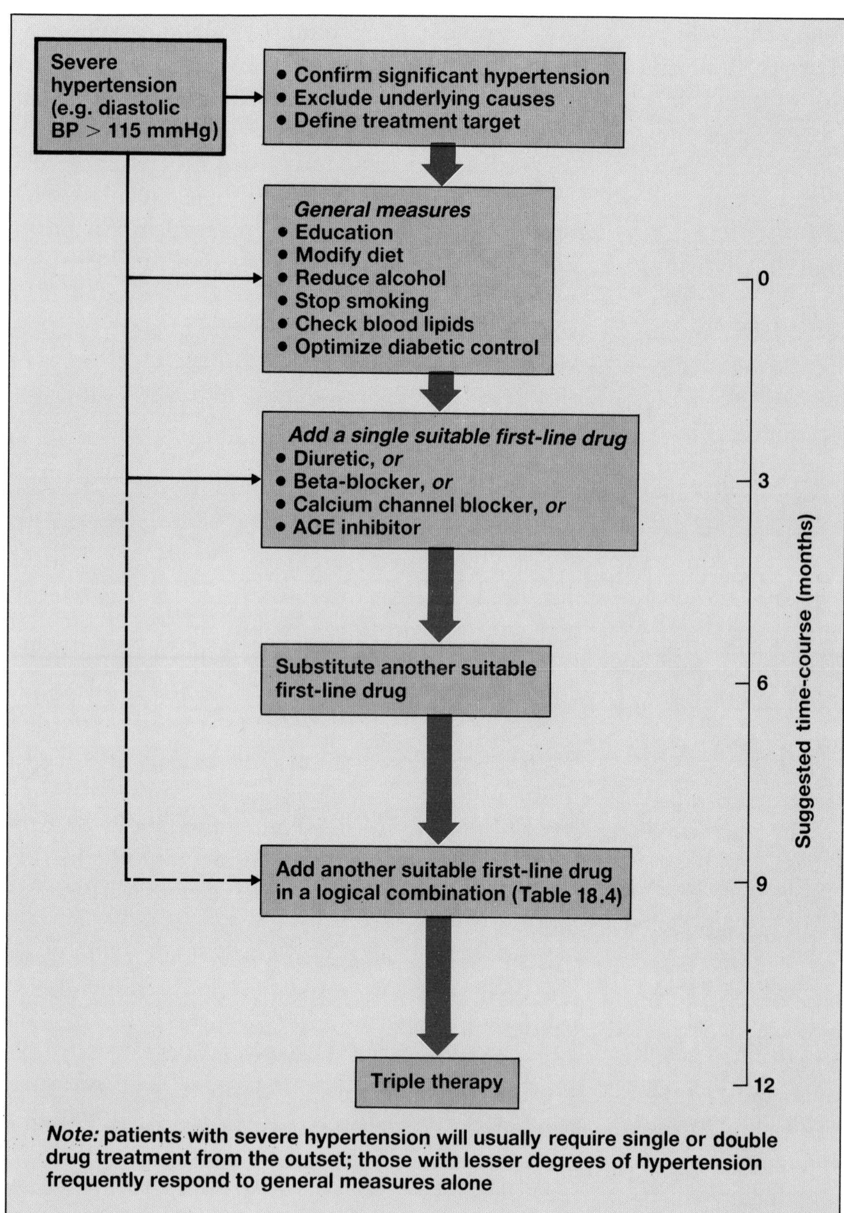


**Fig. 18.6.** Suggested management scheme for diabetic patients with hypertension. Drug treatment should be started as shown if hypertension remains uncontrolled after 3 months of general measures. Patients with severe hypertension will generally need drug treatment from the outset.

in most patients. However, those with severe hypertension (defined as above) are unlikely to respond and will also require antihypertensive drugs from the outset. General measures should be continued indefinitely.

2 *Single-drug therapy*. If general measures alone are ineffective, a single first-choice drug should be selected from Table 18.3, according to the patient's individual needs (angina, cardiac failure, hyperlipidaemia, etc.). The drug's action and possible side-effects must be fully explained. Weight, cardiovascular status, glycaemic control, renal function and blood lipid levels should be monitored.

3 *Alternative single-drug therapy*. If hypertension persists for a further 2–3 months and compliance seems satisfactory, another suitable first-line drug should be substituted.

4 *Double-drug therapy*. If single-drug therapy fails, another first-line drug should be added to give a 'logical' combination (Table 18.4).

5 *Triple-drug therapy*. Should double-drug therapy prove ineffective after 2–3 months, a third drug (e.g. another first-line agent or a vasodilator) should be added.

6 *Management of resistant hypertension*. About 95% of hypertensive patients will respond to triple-drug therapy. In resistant cases, the possibility of

secondary hypertension should be reconsidered and compliance reinforced if possible. All other risk factors must be minimized, although adherence to advice about diet, smoking and alcohol is often poor in this group. The addition of a fourth drug (e.g. clonidine) may be helpful.

The duration of antihypertensive treatment is controversial, as blood pressure may remain normal for some time after stopping effective treatment. Antihypertensive drugs may be withdrawn for a trial period in those patients who have been well-controlled for several months. Those who remain normotensive without treatment should be encouraged to continue the general measures and be reviewed to ensure that hypertension does not recur.

## Recent developments

There have been continuing developments in several scientific and clinical aspects of hypertension in the context of diabetes.

### *How common is the problem?*

Recent studies using ambulatory 24-h blood pressure monitoring have shown that occasional blood pressure measurements may seriously underestimate both the prevalence of hypertension and the burden of hypertension in individual cases [65–67]. This is particularly important for IDDM and NIDDM patients with albuminuria, in whom the early detection and treatment of hypertension is an important priority (see Chapter 16). Many patients with microalbuminuria are not hypertensive by WHO criteria, yet many have a significantly raised blood pressure profile throughout the day and fail to show the fall that normally occurs during the night [65–67]. A recent long-term follow-study [68] has confirmed that mild degrees of hypertension are an important determinant of the rate of progression of diabetic nephropathy. These findings could potentially greatly expand the population of diabetic people who will require antihypertensive treatment.

### *What are the causes of hypertension in diabetes?*

The possible influence of insulin in determining blood pressure continues to attract much attention, in diabetes, essential hypertension and the condition which is now generally termed 'syndrome X' (hypertension, insulin resistance, hyperinsulinaemia, glucose intolerance, dyslipidaemia and truncal obesity; see [24–26, 69]). One theme being pursued is that high insulin concentrations, induced by insensitivity of the 'metabolic' tissues to insulin action, could raise blood pressure in various ways. Recently, the suggested ability of insulin to stimulate the sympathetic nervous system [26, 28] has been elegantly confirmed by direct micro-electrode recordings from sympathetic nerves [70], although interestingly, there was no rise in blood pressure under the conditions of this study (a hyperinsulinaemic, euglycaemic clamp). It is not yet clear whether the vasculature remains sensitive to insulin's various actions in the 'insulin-resistant' conditions of NIDDM, essential hypertension and 'syndrome X' [24–26, 68, 71]. Insulin has vasorelaxant properties [72], and vascular insensitivity to this action could, in theory, tend to raise blood pressure. As in several other areas of diabetes research, the potential role of insulin is having to be re-evaluated following the discovery that circulating 'insulin' (as measured by conventional radioimmunoassay) in NIDDM subjects consists largely of cross-reacting proinsulin derivatives which do not share insulin's metabolic actions [73]. This is particularly relevant to vascular disease in diabetes, as it appears that the proinsulin derivatives may themselves predispose independently to coronary heart disease [74].

Another topic of interest is the vascular responses to various vasoactive agents, which could contribute to the regulation of blood pressure and perhaps the development of certain vascular complications. Previous suggestions that the vasoconstrictor effect of noradrenaline is enhanced in insulin-deficient diabetic rats and humans [7, 8, 14] have been confirmed by some recent *in vitro* studies of isolated rat arteries [75], although this remains a controversial topic as others have not found any significant difference in vascular reactivity from non-diabetic vessels [76] (M.W. Savage *et al.*, unpublished observations). Specific subsets of diabetic patients may have abnormal vascular responses, which may be relevant to hypertension and microvascular disease. IDDM patients with microalbuminuria show exaggerated vasoconstrictor responses to noradrenaline, measured in hand veins *in vivo* [77]. The efferent glomerular arterioles and resistance arterioles are also sensitive to noradrenaline, and increases in the tone of these vessels could tend to raise intraglomerular pressure (and so predispose to increased urinary albumin excretion) and systemic blood pressure. Such abnormalities could be due to intrinsic defects of the α-adrenoceptor or postreceptor transduction, and preliminary evidence points to the $\alpha_2$-adrenoceptor [78].

The possible importance of general cellular disturbances such as intracellular changes in sodium and other electrolytes is still actively debated [79], as are the effects of altered activity of cationic pumps in the cell membrane such as the $Na^+-H^+$ exchanger [80, 81] and the $Na^+-Li^+$ antiport pump which has been used as a surrogate for it (see pp. 157 and 158). The situation remains confused, and many previous studies may be difficult to interpret because of the finding that insulin itself influences $Na^+-Li^+$ transport activity [82].

### *How should hypertension be treated in diabetic patients?*

The choice of 'first-line' drugs is still hotly debated, even in hypertensive patients who do not have diabetes, as is clear from the recent report of the British Hypertension Society [83]. Thiazide diuretics and β-blocking agents continue to lose ground generally, especially in the treatment of hypertension in diabetic patients. This is largely because of wider recognition of their unfavorable metabolic effects (notably hyperglycaemia and dyslipidaemia), although low doses of thiazides may be effective and relatively innocuous (see p. 220). It has been suggested that treatment with thiazides can accelerate the progression of nephropathy in diabetic patients [84], and it has been estimated that a hypertensive, non-diabetic subject treated with a thiazide or a β-blocker is about 8 times more likely to develop NIDDM than a diabetic subject is likely to become hypertensive [5].

ACE inhibitors are becoming more popular, perhaps because of accumulating evidence that ACE itself may play a pathogenic role in coronary heart disease and that ACE inhibitors may have beneficial effects beyond their antihypertensive properties. Newer agents such as enalapril and perindopril are more convenient to take (with once-daily dosages) and may have a lower incidence of certain side-effects such as first-dose hypotension, compared with captopril. Potential problems of all ACE inhibitors include potassium retention, especially in patients with renal impairment, and acute renal failure (which may be largely irreversible) in subjects with renal artery stenosis, including that due to atheroma in diabetic people.

Calcium entry blockers are also used increasingly frequently, and include nifedipine (now available as sustained-release and once-daily preparations), amlodipine and nicardipine. Further studies have confirmed that these drugs do not cause hyperglycaemia or dyslipidaemia, and in contrast to some previous reports [62], the Melbourne study [85] found that nifedipine reduced urinary albumin excretion in IDDM patients to a similar degree as an ACE inhibitor (perindopril).

Alpha-adrenergic blocking agents also seem to be prescribed more often in diabetic patients with hypertension. They do not have adverse metabolic effects and do not apparently cause impotence. Doxazosin seems less likely than the original prazosin to cause severe postural hypotension or a reflex tachycardia, and can be given once daily.

MARK W. SAVAGE
GARETH WILLIAMS

## References

1 World Health Organization Multinational Study. Prevalence of small vessel and large vessel disease in diabetic patients from 14 centres. *Diabetologia* 1985; **28** (suppl): 615–40.
2 Drury PL. Hypertension. In: Nattrass M, Hale PJ, eds. *Non-Insulin Dependent Diabetes. Clin Endocrinol Metab* 1988; **2**: 375–9.
3 Jarrett RJ, ed. *Diabetes and Heart Disease*. Amsterdam: Elsevier, 1984: 1–23.
4 Simonson DC. Etiology and prevalence of hypertension in diabetic patients. *Diabetes Care* 1988; **11**: 821–7.
5 Lundgren H, Björkman L, Keiding P, Lundmark S, Bengtsson C. Diabetes in patients with hypertension receiving pharmacological treatment. *Br Med J* 1988; **297**: 1512–13.
6 Feldt-Rasmussen B, Mathiesen ER, Deckert T *et al*. Central role for sodium in the pathogenesis of blood pressure changes independent of angiotensin, aldosterone and catecholamines in Type 1 (insulin-dependent) diabetes mellitus. *Diabetologia* 1987; **30**: 610–17.
7 Weidmann P, Beretta-Piccoli C, Keusch G, Gluck Z, Mujagic M, Grimm M, Meier A, Ziegler WH. Sodium-volume factor, cardiovascular reactivity and hypotensive mechanism of diuretic therapy in mild hypertension associated with diabetes mellitus. *Am J Med* 1979; **67**: 779–84.
8 Weidmann P, Beretta-Piccoli C, Trost BN. Pressor factors and responsiveness in hypertension accompanying diabetes mellitus. *Hypertension* 1985; **7** (suppl II): 33–42.
9 DeChatel R, Weidmann P, Flammer J, Ziegler WH, Beretta-Piccoli C, Vetter W, Reubin FC. Sodium, renin, aldosterone, catecholamines and blood pressure in diabetes mellitus. *Kidney Int* 1977; **12**: 412–21.
10 Christlieb AR, Kaldany A, D'Elia JA. Plasma renin activity and hypertension in diabetes mellitus. *Diabetes* 1976; **25**: 969–74.
11 Christlieb AR, Assal J-P, Katsilambros N, Williams GH,

Kozak GP, Suzuki T. Plasma renin activity and blood volume in uncontrolled diabetes: ketoacidosis, a state of secondary aldosteronism. *Diabetes* 1975; **24**: 190–3.
12 Christensen NJ. Plasma norepinephrine and epinephrine in untreated diabetes, during fasting and after insulin administration. *Diabetes* 1974; **23**: 1–8.
13 Christensen NJ. Plasma catecholamines in long-term diabetes with and without neuropathy and in hypophysectomized subjects. *J Clin Invest* 1972; **51**: 779–87.
14 Christlieb AR, Janka H-U, Kraus B, Gleason RE, Icasas-Cabral EA, Aiello LM, Cabral BV, Solano A. Vascular reactivity to angiotensin II and to norepinephrine in diabetic subjects. *Diabetes* 1976; **25**: 268–74.
15 Grenfell A, Watkins PJ. Clinical diabetic nephropathy: natural history and complications. In: Watkins PJ, ed. *Long-term Complications of Diabetes. Clin Endocrinol Metab* 1986; **15**: 783–806.
16 Wiseman MJ, Viberti GC, Mackintosh D, Jarrett RJ, Keen H. Glycaemia, arterial pressure and microalbuminuria in Type 1 (insulin-dependent) diabetes mellitus. *Diabetologia* 1984; **26**: 401–5.
17 Deckert T, Feldt-Rasmussen B, Borch-Johnsen K, Jensen T, Kofoed-Enevoldsen A. Albuminuria reflects widespread vascular damage. The Steno hypothesis. *Diabetologia* 1989; **32**: 219–26.
18 Parving H-H, Anderson AR, Smidt UM, Hommel E, Mathiesen ER, Svendsen PAå. Effect of antihypertensive treatment on kidney function in diabetic nephropathy. *Br Med J* 1987; **294**: 1443–52.
19 Anderson S, Brenner BM. Influence of antihypertensive therapy on development and progression of diabetic glomerulopathy. *Diabetes Care* 1988; **11**: 846–9.
20 Parving H-H, Hommel E. Prognosis in diabetic nephropathy. *Br Med J* 1989; **299**: 230–3.
21 Björck S, Nyberg G, Mulec H *et al*. Beneficial effects of angiotensin converting enzyme inhibition on renal function in patients with diabetic nephropathy. *Br Med J* 1986; **293**: 471–4.
22 Parving H-H, Hommel E, Smidt UM. Protection of kidney function and decrease in albuminuria by captopril in insulin dependent diabetics with nephropathy. *Br Med J* 1988; **297**: 1086–91.
23 Marre M, Chatellier G, Leblanc H, Guyene TT, Menard J, Passa P. Prevention of diabetic nephropathy with enalapril in normotensive diabetics with microalbuminuria. *Br Med J* 1988; **297**: 1092–6.
24 Reaven GM. Role of insulin resistance in human disease. *Diabetics* 1988; **37**: 1596–1607.
25 Manicardi V, Camellini L, Bellode G, Coscelli C, Ferranini E. Evidence for an association of high blood pressure and hyperinsulinemia in obese man. *J Clin Endocrinol Metab* 1986; **62**: 1302–4.
26 Landsberg L. Insulin and hypertension: lessons from obesity. *N Engl J Med* 1987; **317**: 378–9.
27 Baum M. Insulin stimulates volume absorption in the rabbit proximal convoluted tubule. *J Clin Invest* 1987; **79**: 1104–9.
28 Rowe JW, Young JB, Minaker KL, Stevens AL, Pallotta J, Landsberg J. Effect of insulin and glucose infusions on sympathetic nervous system activity in normal man. *Diabetes* 1981; **30**: 219–25.
29 Murray DP, Ferriss JB, O'Sullivan DJ. Is good diabetic control bad for blood pressure? *Clin Sci* 1988; **74** (suppl 17): 58.
30 Struthers AD. The choice of anti-hypertensive therapy in the diabetic patient. *Postgrad Med J* 1985; **61**: 563–9.
31 Kannel WB, McGee DL. Diabetes and glucose tolerance as risk factors for cardiovascular disease. The Framingham study. *Diabetes Care* 1979; **2**: 120–6.
32 Fuller JH. Epidemiology of hypertension associated with diabetes mellitus. *Hypertension* 1985; **7** (part II): 3–7.
33 Dupree EA, Meyer MB. Role of risk factors in the complications of diabetes mellitus. *Am J Epidemiol* 1980; **112**: 100–12.
34 Cruikshank JK, Anderson NMcF, Wadsworth J *et al*. Treating hypertension in black compared with white non-insulin-dependent diabetics: a double blind trial of verapamil and metoprolol. *Br Med J* 1988; **297**: 1155–9.
35 Teuscher A, Schnell H, Wilson PWF. Incidence of diabetic retinopathy and relationship to baseline plasma glucose and blood pressure. *Diabetes Care* 1988; **11**: 246–51.
36 Krolewski AS, Canessa M, Warram JH, Laffel LMB, Christlieb AR, Knowler WC, Rand LI. Predisposition to hypertension and susceptibility to renal disease in insulin-dependent diabetes mellitus. *N Engl J Med* 1988; **318**: 140–5.
37 Mangili R, Bending JJ, Scott G, Li LK, Gupta A, Viberti GC. Increased sodium–lithium counter-transport activity in red cells of patients with insulin-dependent diabetes and nephropathy. *N Engl J Med* 1988; **318**: 146–50.
38 Borch-Johnsen K, Kreiner S. Proteinuria — A predictor of cardiovascular mortality in insulin-dependent diabetes mellitus, *Br Med J* 1987; **294**: 1651–4.
39 Drury PL, Tarn AC. Are the WHO criteria for hypertension appropriate in young insulin-dependent diabetics? *Diabetic Med* 1985; **2**: 79–82.
40 Acheson RM. Blood pressure in a national sample of US adults: percentile distribution of age, sex and race. *International Journal of Epidemiology* 1973; **2**: 293–301.
41 Hommel E, Carstensen H, Skøtt P, Larsen S, Parving H-H. Prevalence and causes of microscopic haematuria in Type 1 (insulin-dependent) diabetic patients with persistent proteinuria. *Diabetologia* 1987; **30**: 627–30.
42 World Health Organization. The 1986 guidelines for the treatment of mild hypertension. *Hypertension* 1986; **8**: 957–61.
43 Collins R, Peto R, MacMahon S *et al*. Blood pressure, stroke, and coronary heart disease. Part 2. *Lancet* 1990; **335**: 827–38.
44 Mühlhauser I, Sawicki P, Didjurgeit V, Jörgens V, Berger M. Uncontrolled hypertension in type 1 diabetes: Assessment of patients' disires about treatment and improvement of blood pressure control by a structured treatment and teaching programme. *Diabetic Med* 1988; **5**: 693–8.
45 Dodson PM, Beevers M, Hallworth R, Webberley MJ, Fletcher RF, Taylor KG. Sodium restriction and blood pressure in hypertensive type II diabetics: randomized blind controlled and crossover studies of moderate sodium restriction and sodium supplementation. *Br Med J* 1989; **298**: 227–30.
46 Pacy PJ, Dodson PM, Jubicki AJ, Fletcher RF, Taylor KG. Comparison of the hypotensive and metabolic effects of bendrofluazide therapy with a high fibre, low sodium, low fat diet in diabetic subjects with mild hypertension. *J Hypertens* 1984; **2**: 215–20.
47 Saurez L, Barrett-Connor E. Interaction between cigarette smoking and diabetes mellitus in the prediction of death attributed to cardiovascular disease. *Am J Epidemiol* 1984; **120**: 670–5.
48 Mühlhauser I, Sawicki P, Berger M. Cigarette-smoking as a risk factor for macroproteinuria and proliferative retinopathy in Type 1 (insulin-dependent) diabetes. *Diabetologia* 1986; **29**: 500–3.
49 Telmer S, Christiansen JS, Andersen AR, Nerup J, Deckert T. Smoking habits and prevalence of clinical diabetic micro-

angiopathy in insulin-dependent diabetics. *Acta Med Scand* 1984; **215**: 613–18.

50 Dall'Aglio E, Strata A, Reaven G. Abnormal lipid metabolism in treated hypertensive patients with non-insulin-dependent diabetes mellitus. *Am J Med* 1988; **84**: 899–903.

51 Glauber H, Wallace P, Griver K, Brechtel G. Adverse metabolic effect of omega-3 fatty acids in non-insulin dependent diabetes mellitus. *Ann Intern Med* 1988; **108**: 663–8.

52 Kaplan NM. Critique of recommendations from Working Group on Hypertension in Diabetes. *Am J Kidney Dis* 1989; **13**: 38–40.

53 Osei K, Holland G, Falko JM. Indapamide — effects on apoprotein, lipoprotein, and glucoregulation in ambulatory diabetic patients. *Arch Int Med* 1986; **146**: 1973–7.

54 MacMahon SW, Macdonald GJ. Antihypertensive treatment and plasma lipoprotein levels. The associations in data from a population study. *Am J Med* 1987; **80** (suppl 2A): 40–7.

55 Prince MJ, Stuart CA, Padia M, Bandi Z, Holland OB. Metabolic effects of hydrochlorothiazide and enalapril during treatment of the hypertensive diabetic patient. Enalapril for hypertensive diabetics. *Arch Int Med* 1988; **148**: 2363–8.

56 Wright AD, Barber SG, Kendall MJ, Poole PH. Beta-adrenoceptor-blocking drugs and blood sugar control in diabetes mellitus. *Br Med J* 1979; **1**: 159–64.

57 Marengo C, Marena S, Renzetti A, Mossino M, Pagano G. Beta-blockers in hypertensive non-insulin-dependent diabetes: comparison between penbutolol and propranolol on metabolic control and response to insulin-induced hypoglycaemia. *Acta Diabetol Lat* 1988; **25**: 141–7.

58 Lager I, Blohme G, Smith U. Effect of cardioselective and nonselective beta-blockade on the hypoglycaemic response in insulin-dependent diabetics. *Lancet* 1979; **i**: 458–62.

59 Trost BN, Weidmann P. Effects of calcium antagonists on glucose homeostasis and serum lipids in non-diabetic and diabetic subjects: a review. *J Hypertens* 1987; **5** (suppl 4): 81–104.

60 Burr AJ, Hay J. Captopril and hypertension in black diabetics. *Br Med J* 1989; **299**: 458–9.

61 Taguma Y, Kitamoto Y, Futaki G, Ueda H, Monma H, Ishizaki M, Takahishi H, Sekino H, Sasaki Y. Effect of captopril on heavy proteinuria in azotemic diabetics. *N Engl J Med* 1985; **313**: 1617–20.

62 Mimran A, Insua A, Ribstein J, Monnier L, Bringer J, Mirouze J. Contrasting effects of captopril and nifedipine in normotensive patients with incipient diabetic nephropathy. *J Hypertens* 1988; **6**: 919–23.

63 Bank N, Klose R, Aynedjian HS, Nguyen D. Sablay LB. Evidence against increased glomerular pressure initiating diabetic nephropathy. *Kidney Int* 1987; **31**: 898–905.

64 Lipson LG. Treatment of hypertension in diabetic men: problems with sexual dysfunction. *Am J Cardiol* 1984; **53**: 46A–50A.

65 Hansen KW, Pedersen MM, Marshall SM, Christiansen JS, Mogensen CE. Circadian variation of blood pressure in patients with diabetic nephropathy. *Diabetologia* 1992; **35**: 1074–9.

66 Moore WV, Donaldson DL, Chonko AM, Ideus P, Wiegman TB. Ambulatory blood pressure in Type 1 diabetes mellitus. Comparison to presence of incipient nephropathy in adolescents and young adults. *Diabetes* 1992; **41**: 1035–41.

67 Wiegman TB, Herron KG, Chonko AM, MacDougall ML, Moore WV. Recognition of hypertension and abnormal blood pressure burden with ambulatory blood pressure recordings in type 1 diabetes. *Diabetes* 1990; **39**: 1556–60.

68 Microalbuminuria Collaborative Study Group (UK). Risk factors for development of microalbuminuria in insulin dependent diabetic patients: a cohort study. *Br Med J* 1993; **306**: 1235–9.

69 Reaven GM, Hoffman BB. Hypertension as a disease of carbohydrate metabolism. *Am J Med* 1989; **87** (suppl): 2–6.

70 Berne C, Fagius J, Pollare T, Hjemdahl P. The sympathetic response to euglycaemic hyperinsulinaemia. Evidence from micro-electrode nerve recordings in healthy subjects. *Diabetologia* 1992; **35**: 873–9.

71 Ferrannini E, Buzzigoli G, Bonadonna R *et al*. (1987) Insulin resistance in essential hypertension. *N Engl J Med* 1987; **317**: 350–7.

72 Yamamoto M, Asayama K, Kanai M, Sugimoto T, Yagi S, Takata S, Ikeda T, Hattori N. Effects of insulin on vasoconstrictor responses to alpha agonist and tilting. *Angiology* 1990; **41**: 394–400.

73 Temple RC, Clark PMS, Nagi DK, Schneider AE, Yudkin JS, Hales CN. (1990) Radioimmunoassay may overestimate insulin in non-insulin dependent diabetics. *Clin Endocrinol* 1990; **32**: 689–93.

74 Nagi DK, Hendra TJ, Ryle AJ *et al*. The relationships of concentrations of insulin, intact proinsulin and 32–33 split proinsulin with cardiovascular risk factors in Type 2 (non-insulin-dependent) diabetic subjects. *Diabetologia* 1990; **33**: 532–7.

75 Taylor PD, Thomas C, Poston L. Endothelium-dependent relaxation and noradrenaline sensitivity in mesenteric resistance arteries of streptozotocin-induced diabetic rats. *Br J Pharmacol* 1992; **107**: 393–9.

76 Gebremedhin D, Koltai MZ, Pogatsa G, Magyar K, Hadhazy P. Altered responsiveness of diabetic dog renal arteries to acetylcholine and phenylephrine: role of endothelium. *Pharmacology* 1989; **38**: 177–84.

77 Bodmer CW, Patrick AW, How TV, Williams G. Exaggerated sensitivity to norepinephrine-induced vasoconstriction in insulin-dependent diabetic patients with microalbuminuria: possible etiology and diagnostic implications. *Diabetes* 1992; **41**: 209–14.

78 Janssen M, Bodmer CW, Schaper NC, Lake D, Williams G. Exaggerated alpha-2 adrenoceptor mediated vasoconstriction in IDDM patients with microalbuminuria. *Diabetic Med* 1993; **10** (suppl. 3): 45.

79 Weidmann P, Ferrari P. Central role of sodium in hypertension in diabetic subjects. *Diabetes Care* 1991; **14**: 220–32.

80 Huot SJ, Aronson PS. $Na^+-H^+$ exchanger and its role in essential hypertension and diabetes mellitus. *Diabetes Care* 1991; **14**: 521–35.

81 Doria A, Fioretto P, Avogaro A *et al*. Insulin resistance is associated with high sodium-lithium countertransport in essential hypertension. *Am J Physiol* 1991; **261**: E684–91.

82 Foyle WJ, Drury PL. Reduction of $Li^+-Na^+$ countertransport by physiological levels of insulin *in vitro*. *J Hypertens* 1991; **9**: 713–17.

83 Severe P, Beevers G, Bulpitt C *et al*. Management guidelines in essential hypertension: report of the second working party of the British Hypertension Society. *Br Med J* 1993; **306**: 983–7.

84 Walker WG, Herman J, Yin D, Murphy RP, Patz A. Diuretics accelerate diabetic nephropathy in hypertensive insulin dependent and non-insulin dependent subjects. *Trans Assoc Am Phys* 1987; **00**: C305–15.

85 Melbourne Diabetic Nephropathy Study Group (1991) Comparison between perindopril and nifedipine in hypertensive diabetic patients with microalbuminuria. *Br Med J* **302**, 210–16.

# PART 6
# OTHER DIABETIC COMPLICATIONS

# 19 The Diabetic Foot

**Summary**

- Both neuropathy and ischaemia, frequently acting in combination and often complicated by infection, predispose to ulceration in the diabetic foot.
- The 'neuropathic' foot is numb, warm and dry, with palpable pulses; complications include neuropathic ulcers, Charcot arthropathy and (rarely) neuropathic oedema.
- Neuropathic ulcers occur at points of high pressure loading, especilly on the soles or at sites of deformity; pressure damage leads progressively to callosity formation, autolysis and finally ulceration. Secondary infection is common. Treatment involves removing skin calosities to drain the ulcer, reducing pressure loading by special shoes or total-contact plaster casting, and appropriate antibiotics.
- Charcot arthropathy usually involves the metatarso-tarsal joints, frequently follows minor trauma, and presents as warmth, swelling and redness, sometimes with pain. Bone scans allow early diagnosis and radiographs later show disorganization of the joint and new bone formation. Treatment is by immobilizing and unloading the limb, with non-steroidal anti-inflammatory drugs for pain.
- Neuropathic oedema may be due to microcirculatory disturbances following autonomic denervation; ephedrine treatment is often effective.
- The 'ischaemic' foot is cold and pulseless and subject to rest pain, ulceration and gangrene.
- Ischaemic ulceration usually affects the foot margins. Medical treatment alone is often effective; focal stenoses of the iliac, femoral or even popliteal arteries are often amenable to angioplasty or bypass grafting; amputation must be avoided if at all possible.
- The management of diabetic foot ulceration is best guided by determining the relative contributions of neuropathy, ischaemia and infection. Collaborative teamwork involving the chiropodist, orthotist (shoe fitter), nurse, physician and surgeon is most effective.
- Effective education is essential in the prevention of diabetic foot problems.

Three factors predispose to tissue damage in the diabetic foot, namely neuropathy, peripheral vascular disease and infection. Infection is rarely a sole factor but often complicates neuropathy and ischaemia.

From the practical point of view, the diabetic foot can generally be considered as one of two entities, the 'neuropathic foot' and the 'ischaemic foot'. In the neuropathic foot, somatic and autonomic nerve fibres have been damaged but the circulation is intact and the pulses palpable, resulting in a warm, numb, dry foot [1]. The neuropathic foot has three main complications: the neuropathic ulcer, the neuropathic (Charcot) joint and neuropathic oedema. The ischaemic foot suffers predominantly from its reduced blood supply, but usually also shows a variable degree of neuropathy and so should strictly be termed the 'neuroischaemic' foot. Blood flow is reduced because of atherosclerosis in the major leg arteries, particularly in the calf vessels; the possible role of 'small vessel' (arteriolar) disease has received much attention in the past but there is no strong evidence to show that it plays an important part in tissue necrosis [2]. The neuro-ischaemic foot is usually cold and pulseless and may be complicated by rest pain, ulceration due to localized pressure necrosis, and ultimately gangrene.

Neuropathic and neuro-ischaemic feet are therefore distinguished by characteristic lesions, which need specific management. The following sections will describe the clinical features of diabetic feet, simple bedside investigations (vibration perception threshold and ankle blood pressure measurements) which may help to identify the cause of tissue damage, and the various treatments available. Finally, the organization of diabetic foot care will be discussed.

## The neuropathic foot

### *The neuropathic ulcer*

#### PRESENTATION

This characteristically occurs at sites of high mechanical pressure on the plantar surface of the foot (Fig. 19.1). The presence of neuropathy (even in its earliest stage, with relatively mild sensory defects) may itself disturb the posture of the foot and so predispose to local increases in pressure [3], which are also commonly caused by deformities such as claw or hammer toes, pes cavus, Charcot joints and previous ray amputations [4]. The situation is exacerbated by wearing tight, ill-fitting shoes, especially in the presence of oedema. If the foot is deformed, the high vertical and shear forces under the plantar surface of the metatarsal heads lead to the formation of callosities (Figs 19.1 and 19.2) [5], of which the patient is often unaware. Repetitive mechanical forces lead to inflammatory autolysis and subkeratotic haematomas, which eventually break through to the skin surface, forming an ulcer (Figs 19.2 and 19.3). The pressures to which localized areas of the sole are subjected under normal walking conditions can be measured accurately by pressure transducers worn in the shoes, or by the 'optical paedabarograph' (Fig. 19.4). Pressures over the metatarsal heads in neuropathic feet are often increased several-fold.

Ulcers are often infected by staphylococci streptococci, coliforms or anaerobes [4]. Streptococci and staphylococci may act synergistically, the streptococci producing hyaluronidase which facilitates the spread of the necrotizing toxins released by staphylococci. In severe cases, this can result in thrombotic arterial occlusion and gangrene. In the deep tissues of the foot, aerobic organisms may act synergistically with microaerophilic or anaerobic organisms to produce necrotizing infection, which often generates subcutaneous gas (Fig. 19.5) or spreads to involve the bones (Fig. 19.6). Extensive tissue loss and gangrene may finally result.

#### MANAGEMENT OF THE NEUROPATHIC ULCER

Excess callus tissue should be pared away with a scalpel (but only by a trained chiropodist) to expose and drain the ulcer base [6]. Oral antibi-

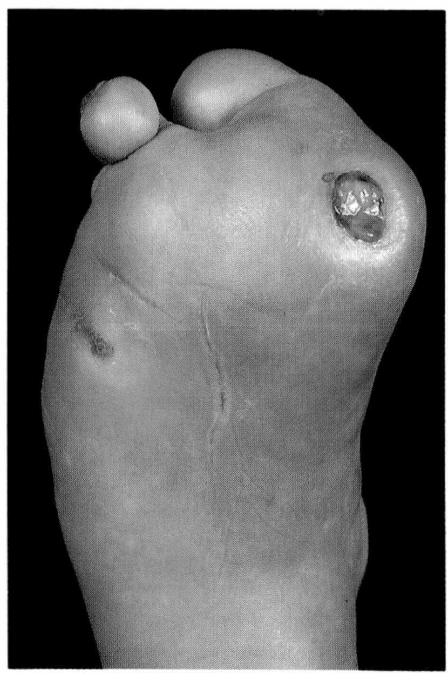

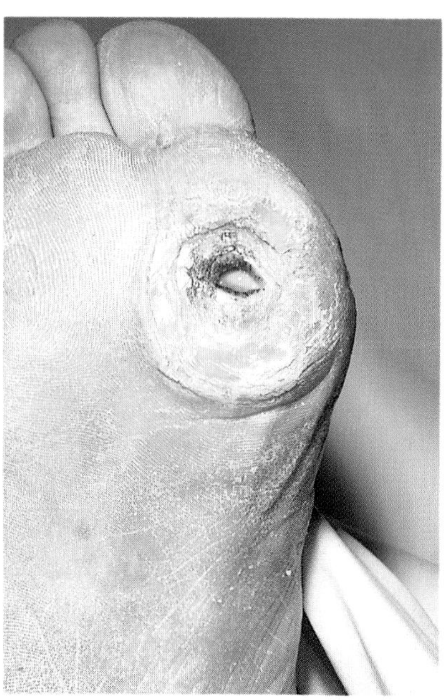

**Fig. 19.1.** Typical 'punched-out' neuropathic ulcers arising in heavily calloused skin underlying the first metatarsal head. Note previous amputations (left) and particularly thick callosities (right). (Left panel reproduced by kind permission of Dr Ian Casson, Broadgreen Hospital, Liverpool.)

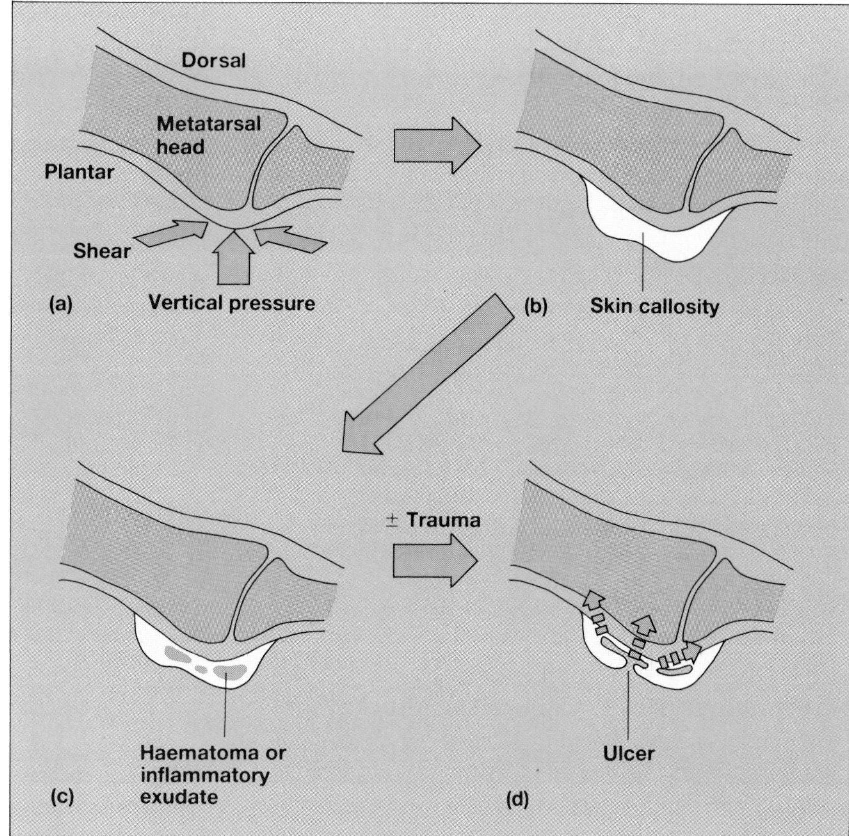


**Fig. 19.2.** Formation of a neuropathic pressure ulcer. (a) Abnormal foot posture and loss of sensation, both due to neuropathy, increased vertical pressure and tangential shear forces applied to vulnerable areas such as the metatarsal heads. (b) Increased pressure and shear forces cause hyperkeratosis and ultimately callosity formation. (c) Haematomas and inflammatory exudate (initially sterile) form within the callosity, finally breaking through to the surface to form an ulcer (d). Trauma accelerates the process. Secondary infection may spread to cause soft-tissue necrosis or osteomyelitis.

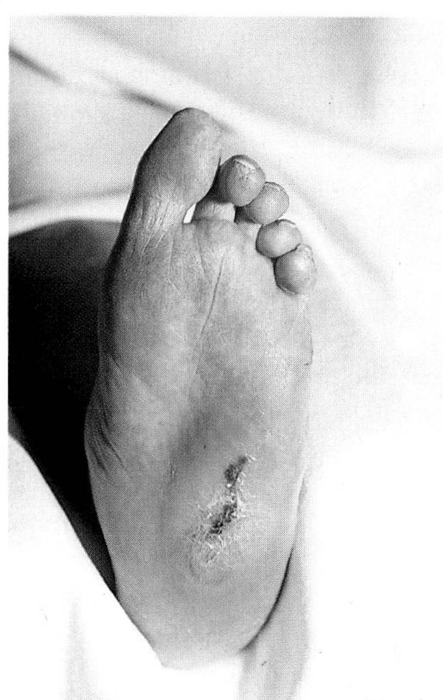

**Fig. 19.3.** Large subcutaneous haematoma following trauma to a neuropathic foot which subsequently broke through the skin to form an ulcer. (Reproduced by kind permission of Mr Patrick Laing, Royal Liverpool Hospital.)

otics, appropriate to the organisms isolated from a swab of the ulcer base, should be given until the ulcer has healed. Suitable antibiotics include phenoxymethyl penicillin (500 mg 6-hourly) for streptococcal infections, flucloxacillin (500 mg 6-hourly) for straphylococci and metronidazole (400 mg 8-hourly) for anaerobic infections. If the ulcer is superficial and there is no cellulitis, out-patient treatment is adequate. If cellulitis is present, however, the limb is potentially threatened and the patient should be hospitalized immediately and treated strictly by the regimen described in Table 19.1.

Reduction of weight-bearing forces is necessary both in the acute phase and also in long-term management. In the presence of sepsis, bedrest is indicated but foam wedges must be used to protect the heels against pressure damage. In the short term, a light-weight, total-contact plaster cast which entirely encases the foot (including the ulcerated area) can be applied to unload pressure from the ulcer and reduce shear forces on vulnerable parts of the foot (Fig. 19.7) [7]. In the long term, weight-bearing forces can be redistributed

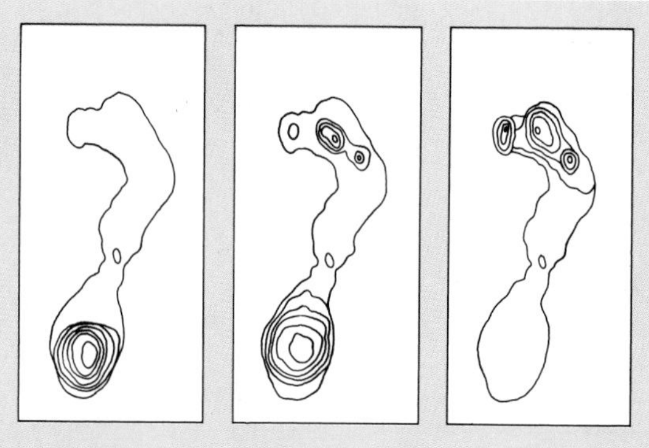

Fig. 19.4. Map of pressure distribution over the sole of a diabetic patient with peripheral neuropathy measured by the optical paedabarograph, at three successive stages during normal walking. Note the high pressures (>10 kg/cm$^2$) generated under the first and second metatarsal heads, which are considerably greater than in subjects without neuropathy and with normal foot posture. (Reproduced by kind permission of Dr Andrew Boulton, Manchester Royal Infirmary.)

more equally over the sole by using special footwear and insoles made of energy-absorbing material such as Plastozote or microcellular rubber [1, 8].

Certain cases may need shoes constructed specifically by the orthotist, but extra-depth stock shoes will be adequate for many patients. These shoes are made in standard sizes but are deeper to allow insertion of either sponge rubber cushions or of purpose-made insoles or foot cradles.

**Table 19.1.** Treatment of sepsis in the neuropathic foot.

- Admit to hospital
- Bedrest
- Antibiotics: 'general cover' regimen or specific, if organisms known:
  cefuroxime 1.5 g 8-hourly i.v.
  flucloxacillin 500 mg 6-hourly i.v.
  metronidazole 1 g 8-hourly rectally
  } 'general cover' regimen
- Urgent surgical drainage of pus and debridement of dead tissue
- Send pus and tissue for culture; adjust antibiotics accordingly
- Consider ray amputation of digit if bone is destroyed
- Ensure tight glycaemic control, using i.v. insulin if necessary

### *Neuropathic (Charcot) arthropathy*

#### PRESENTATION

The precipitating event is often surprisingly minor trauma such as tripping, which results in a swollen, erythematous, hot and sometimes painful foot (Figs 19.8 and 19.9). Initial radiological examination is usually normal, but subsequent films show

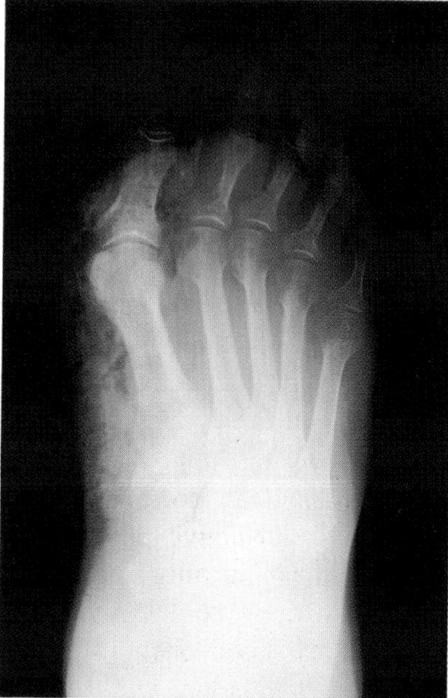

Fig. 19.5. Extensive soft-tissue infection with gas formation arising from a neuropathic ulcer in a diabetic foot. (Reproduced by kind permission of Dr Ian MacFarlane, Walton Hospital, Liverpool.)

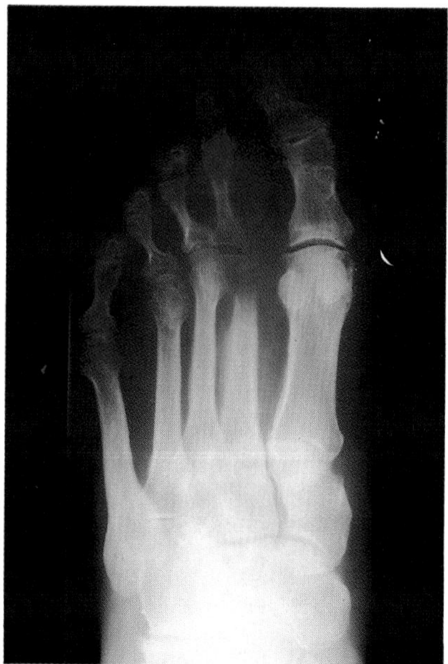

Fig. 19.6. Osteomyelitis destroying the head of the second metatarsal. The infection spread from an underlying neuropathic ulcer. (Reproduced by kind permission of Dr Ian MacFarlane, Walton Hospital, Liverpool.)

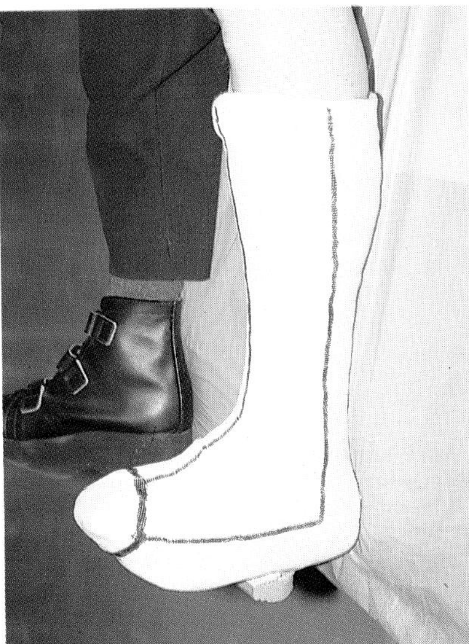

**Fig. 19.7.** Total-contact plaster cast used to treat neuropathic ulcer. Weight is taken by the plastic rocker, off-loading pressure from the ulcerated area. Lines show where the cast is cut for removal. (Reproduced by kind permission of Mr Patrick Laing, Royal Liverpool Hospital.)

evidence of fracture, osteolysis and fragmentation of bone, followed by new bone formation and finally subluxation and disorganization of the joint (Fig. 19.10). Bone scans are more sensitive indicators of new bone formation than radiography and should be used to confirm the diagnosis (Fig. 19.11). This destructive process often takes place over only a few months, and can lead to considerable deformity of the foot. The tarsometatarsal joints are most commonly involved [9].

Early diagnosis is essential and is suggested by three features:

1 A history of trauma, often minor.
2 The presence of unilateral warmth and swelling.
3 Positive radiographic or bone scan findings.

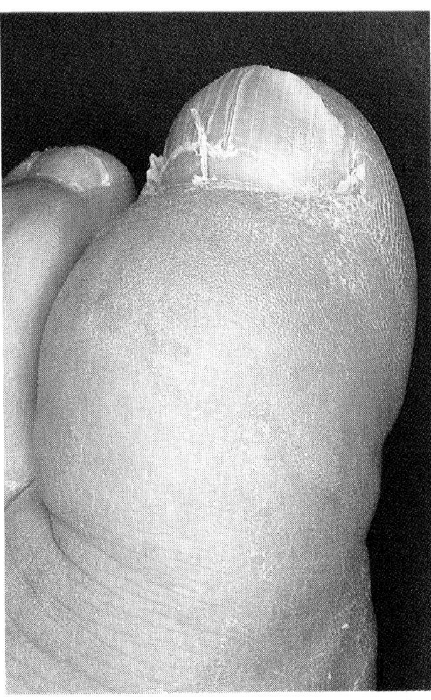

**Fig. 19.8.** Acute Charcot arthropathy affecting the interphalangeal joint of the great toe. Sudden onset of pain, redness and swelling with no obvious preceding trauma initially suggested a diagnosis of acute gout. (Reproduced by kind permission of Dr Geoffrey V. Gill, Walton Hospital, Liverpool.)

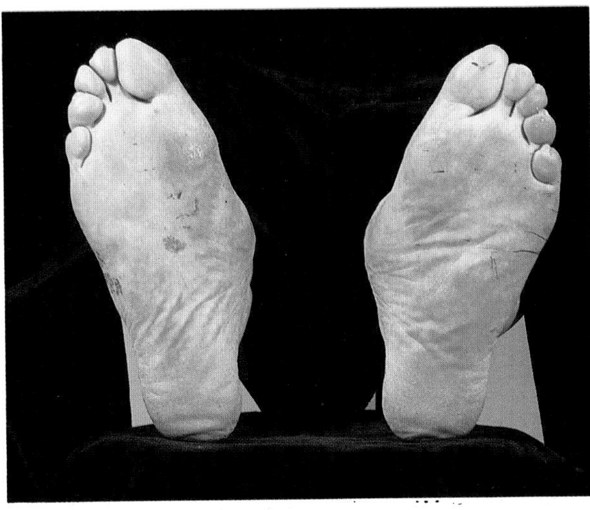

**Fig. 19.9.** Advanced Charcot arthropathy of both feet, showing gross disorganization. (Reproduced by kind permission of Dr Ian Casson, Broadgreen Hospital, Liverpool.)

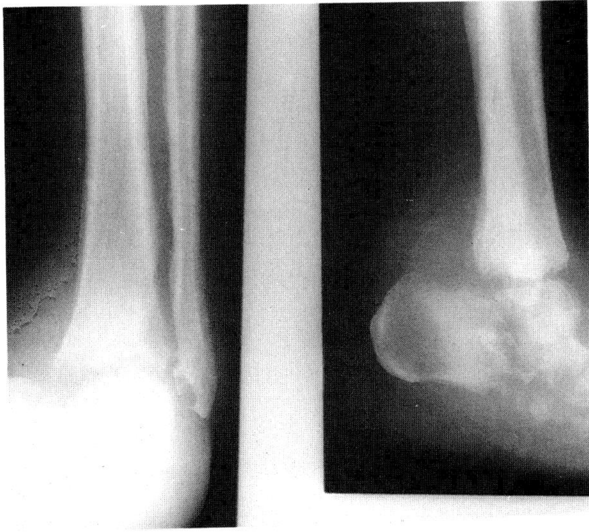

**Fig. 19.10.** Radiograph of advanced Charcot arthropathy, showing destruction of the ankle and foot joints, with widespread bone resorption, soft tissue swelling and a large effusion.

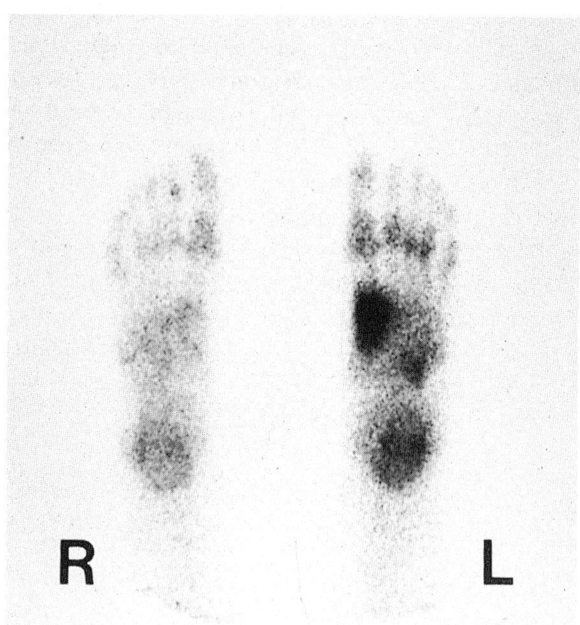


**Fig. 19.11.** $^{99m}$Tc bone scan showing increased uptake in the region of the base of the first metatarsal and the metatarsocuneiform joint, indicating new bone formation in early Charcot arthropathy (L). At this stage, plain radiography showed no definite abnormality.

MANAGEMENT

Initial management comprises immobilization and unloading of the injured limb, such as by non-weight-bearing crutches or a total-contact plaster cast [10]. This is continued until oedema and warmth have subsided, when the foot should be gradually mobilized using a moulded insole in a custom-fitted shoe. Non-steroidal anti-inflammatory drugs may be useful in painful cases.

### *Neuropathic oedema*

PRESENTATION

Neuropathic oedema is fluid accumulation in the feet and lower legs which is associated with severe peripheral neuropathy and is not explicable by other causes such as cardiac failure or hypoalbuminaemia. It is extremely uncommon. Its pathogenesis may be related to abnormal vasomotor function following autonomic denervation, causing arterio-venous shunting and disturbances in hydrostatic pressure in the microcirculation (see Chapter 4).

MANAGEMENT

The sympathomimetic drug, ephedrine (30 mg 8-hourly), has been shown to be useful, probably by reducing peripheral blood flow and by increasing urinary sodium excretion [11].

## The neuro-ischaemic foot

### *Presentation*

REST PAIN

Pain is continuous in the foot, often worse at night and characteristically relieved by dependency; it may be reduced by elevating the head of the bed. At this stage, the foot is often pink because of capillary dilatation in response to hypoxia but, in contrast to the neuropathic foot, it is cold.

ULCERATION

Gangrene and ulcers in the ischaemic foot usually result from continuous excessive pressure on the margins of the foot (Fig. 19.12); ulceration of the plantar surface is rare because its pressure loading is intermittent. The most important precipitating factor is the wearing of tight shoes, which is exacerbated by deformity and oedema [4]. Digital ischaemia and gangrene are also common in patients with diabetic nephropathy, who frequently have extensive medial calcification of the digital and limb arteries (see Figs 16.8 and 16.9). Ulceration is often complicated by secondary infection, commonly with both aerobic and anaerobic bacteria.

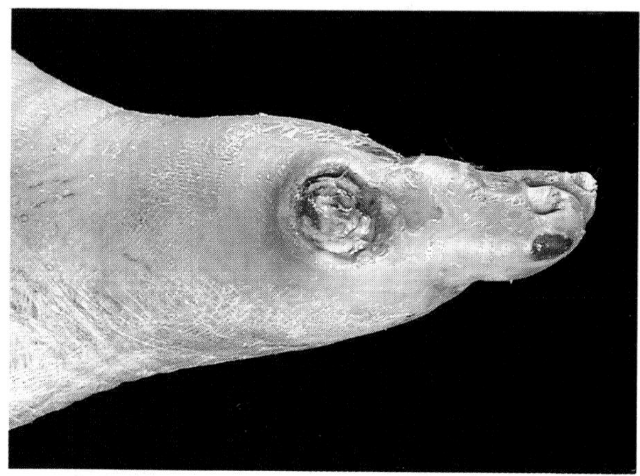

**Fig. 19.12.** Ulceration over the medial margin of the first metatarsal head in a neuro-ischaemic foot.

MANAGEMENT

*Medical management.* This is indicated if the ulcer is small, shallow and of recent onset (within the previous month), and is the mainstay of treatment for patients in whom reconstructive surgery is not feasible because of widespread vascular disease.

It is important to eradicate infection promptly with specific antibiotic therapy. Cardiac failure, which accounted for foot oedema in two-thirds of cases in one series [4], must also be treated, but with care to avoid dehydration. The provision of suitable shoes is simpler than for the purely neuropathic foot. Deep, widely fitting shoes are needed to protect the margins of the foot and accommodate any deformity, and can often be obtained ready-made. Regular chiropody should be performed to debride ulcers and, in the case of subungual ulcers, to cut back the nail to encourage free drainage of pus.

*Surgical treatment.* If the ulcer does not respond to medical management within 4 weeks, angiography should be carried out to identify any stenoses which might be amenable to angioplasty or other reconstructive surgery.

The lesions most suitable for angioplasty are focal stenoses of less than 4 cm long and occlusions shorter than 10 cm long. Angioplasty is indicated for localized stenoses in the iliac or femoral arteries. At present, iliac artery angioplasties have a higher general success rate than those in the femoral or popliteal vessels [12]. Diabetic patients show a predilection to stenosis in the branches of the popliteal artery; experience with popliteal artery dilatation is very limited, but fewer than 50% of reconstructions remain patent after 2 years [13].

The relative roles of angioplasty and bypass surgery are currently being assessed. They are likely to be complementary measures, but angioplasty is particularly useful for patients unfit for major arterial reconstruction. If a block in the femoral artery is not amenable to angioplasty, reversed saphenous-vein grafts may successfully bypass the femoral to the popliteal artery and have resulted in high rates of limb salvage, even in elderly diabetic patients [14]. More distal stenoses in the branches of the popliteal artery are now treated by bypass grafts bridging the femoral to distal tibial or peroneal arteries and by percutaneous transluminal angioplasty [13]. Methods using the saphenous vein *'in situ'* have been developed, thus preserving the vasa vasorum and minimizing endothelial injury [15].

Sympathectomy generally fails to promote ulcer healing but may occasionally ameliorate rest pain [16]. In many cases, neither angioplasty nor arterial reconstruction are possible, when digitial necrosis in the ischaemic foot is often best managed with the conservative methods described above. Amputation of the foot should be avoided if at all possible as rehabilitation is often poor. Limited surgery, such as 'ray' excision of the affected digit may sometimes be successful and the patient's ability to walk and balance may be little impaired if the great toe is preserved (Fig. 19.13) but this option should also only be considered if conservative methods fail [17].

## Assessment of the foot

Neuropathy, ischaemia, deformity and oedema are all important factors which may lead to ulceration in the diabetic foot. When assessing the foot, the relative contribution of each of these factors must be determined in order to plan rational management.

### *Integrated examination of the diabetic foot*

INSPECTION AND PALPATION

The key points are shown in Table 19.2. All areas

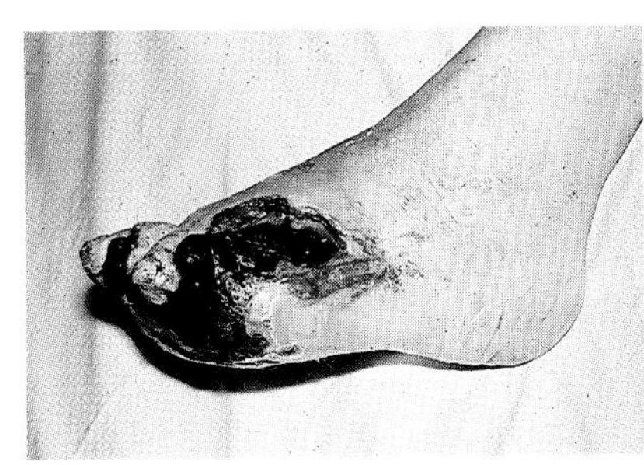

(a)

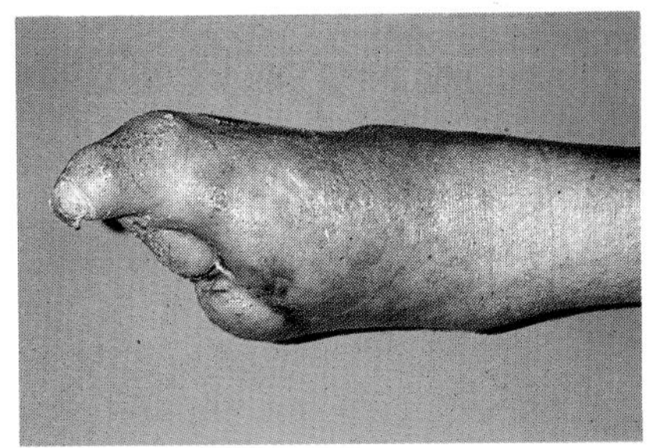

(b)

**Fig. 19.13.** Distal gangrene in a neuro-ischaemic foot (a). After ray excision (b), the great toe is preserved and the foot remains able to maintain balance and walking.

**Table 19.2.** Examination of the foot in a diabetic patient.

*Colour*:
- Red foot (cellulitis or early Charcot arthropathy)
- Pale or cyanotic foot (ischaemia)
- Pink foot associated with pain and absent pulses (severe ischaemia)

*Deformity*:
- Claw toe, hammer toe, hallux valgus, hallux varus
- Pes cavus, prominent metatarsal heads
- Charcot arthropathy

*Oedema*:
- Bilateral may be due to cardiac failure, fluid overload or neuropathy
- Unilateral may indicate sepsis or Charcot arthropathy

*Nails*:
- Atrophic in neuropathy and ischaemia
- Discoloured in fungal infection and subungual ulceration

*Skin callosities*:
- In the neuropathic foot, found on the plantar surface of the metatarsal heads and apices of toes

*Tissue breakdown — ulcers*:
- Neuropathic typically on soles
- Neuro-ischaemic typically on foot margins

*Tissue breakdown*:
- Fissures
- Blisters

*Foot pulses*:
- Posterior tibial and dorsalis pedis are weak or absent in ischaemic feet, often strong in neuropathic feet

*Skin temperature*:
- Neuropathic feet are usually warm, ischaemic feet are cold

*Skin moisture*:
- Neuropathic feet are dry

*Signs of infection*:
- Crepitus, fluctuation, deep tenderness

of the foot, including the dorsum, sole, back of the heel and between the toes, should be first inspected and then palpated. The pulses and temperature and moisture of the skin should be assessed and the presence of oedema and regions of tenderness noted.

### NEUROLOGICAL EXAMINATION

Perception of pinprick, light touch and vibration should be determined and the knee and ankle tendon reflexes examined, with and without reinforcement.

### BEDSIDE INVESTIGATIONS

Bacteriological swabs should be taken from the base of any ulcers. Physical examination can be complemented by two other simple tests, measurement of vibration perception threshold (VPT) and the determination of the ankle–brachial pressure index.

### VIBRATION PERCEPTION THRESHOLD

VPT can be measured using a hand-held Biothesiometer [18]. The vibrating tactor is applied to the test site (e.g. medial malleolus or tip of the big toe) and the amplitude of vibration increased from zero until the patient first perceives the sensation of vibration. The threshold is usually taken as the mean of three values, expressed in arbitrary voltage units (which are related to the amplitude of vibration). The vibration threshold increases with age, and values must always be compared with age adjusted nomograms. As discussed in Chapter 11, VPT values may vary considerably with time and site.

### ANKLE–BRACHIAL PRESSURE INDEX

The pressure index [19] is calculated by dividing the systolic blood pressure at the ankle by the brachial systolic pressure (measured in the conventional way). The ankle systolic pressure is measured by applying a 12-cm sphygmomanometer cuff just above the ankle. The cuff is inflated to obliterate the posterior tibial pulse and is then slowly released. The systolic pressure is indicated by the return of flow.

In normal subjects, the pressure index is usually greater than 1.0. Some 5–10% of diabetic patients have stiff, non-compressible peripheral vessel walls (probably due to medial calcification), which artificially elevate the systolic pressure. Nonetheless, the pressure index can be a useful guide to the state of the peripheral arteries: values below 0.6 in diabetic patients indicate a severely compromised circulation.

The results of the clinical examination and bedside investigation should lead to a rational management plan, based on the treatment approaches outlined above.

## Organization of foot care for diabetic patients

No single individual can handle every diabetic foot problem. The care of the diabetic foot depends crucially on close liaison between chiropodist, shoe-fitter, nurse, physician and surgeon, ideally in the forum of the diabetic foot clinic [4]. This

**Table 19.3.** Simple foot care advice for the diabetic patient.

**Do**
- Wash feet daily with mild soap and warm water
- Check feet daily
- Seek urgent treatment of any problems
- See a chiropodist regularly
- Wear sensible shoes

**Don't**
- Use corn cures
- Use hot water bottles
- Walk barefoot (except children and adolescents)
- Cut corns or callosities
- Treat foot problems yourself

**Table 19.4.** Danger signs in the diabetic foot.

Check your feet every morning
Come to the clinic *immediately* if you notice:
- swelling
- colour change of a nail, toe or part of a foot
- pain or throbbing
- thick hard skin or corns
- breaks in the skin, including cracks, blisters or sores

**Table 19.5.** Simple footwear advice for diabetic patients.

For everyday use, especially when on the feet for long periods:
- wear a lace-up shoe, with plenty of room for the toes, and either flat or low heeled
- never wear slip-on or court shoes, except for special occasions
- don't wear slippers at home

should provide routine chiropodial care, specific treatment for ulcers and an open access service for emergencies, with the ultimate goal of preventing diabetic foot problems.

This aim will only be achieved through education of the patient in practical aspects of foot care. It is important to emphasize simple advice (Table 19.3). The early recognition of danger signs is important (Table 19.4) and special advice should be given about selection of shoes (Table 19.5). Tissue damage is always potentially serious in the diabetic foot and provision of an emergency service which allows rapid self-referral of the patient, even for apparently trivial lesions, is an important part of preventative care [20].

Many disasters can still befall the diabetic foot but fortunately, most are preventable with adequate education, routine foot care and attention to footwear. Early detection followed rapidly by specific treatment of neuropathic and neuro-ischaemic lesions provide the best opportunity for a favourable outcome.

MICHAEL E. EDMONDS
ALI V.M. FOSTER

## References

1 Edmonds ME. The diabetic foot: pathophysiology and treatment. In: Watkins PJ, ed. *Long-term Complications of Diabetes. Clin Endocrinol Metab*. London: WB Saunders 1986; **15**: 889–916.
2 Logerfo FW, Coffman JD. Vascular and microvascular disease of the foot in diabetes. *N Engl J Med* 1984; **311**: 1615–19.
3 Boulton AJM. The importance of abnormal foot pressures and gait in the causation of foot ulcers. In: Connor H, Boulton AJM, Ward JD, eds. *The Foot in Diabetes*. Chichester: John Wiley & Sons, 1987; 11–21.
4 Edmonds ME, Blundell MP, Morris HE, Thomas EM, Cotton LT, Watkins PJ. Improved survival of the diabetic foot: the role of a specialised foot clinic. *Q J Med* 1986; **232**: 736–71.
5 Delbridge L, Ctercteko G, Fowler C, Reeve TS, Le Quesne LP. The aetiology of diabetic neuropathic foot ulceration. *Br J Surg* 1985; **72**: 1–6.
6 Edmonds ME. The diabetic foot. *Med Int* 1985; **13**: 551–3.
7 Coleman WC, Brand PW, Burke JA. The total contact cast. *J Am Podiatry Ass* 1984; **74**: 548–51.
8 Tovey FI. Establishing a diabetic shoe service. *Practical Diabetes* 1985; **2**: 5–8.
9 Sinha S, Munichoodappa CS, Kozak GP. Neuroarthropathy (Charcot joints) in diabetes mellitus. *Medicine (Baltimore)* 1972; **51**: 191–210.
10 Frykberg RG, Kozak GP. The diabetic Charcot foot. In: Kozak GP, Hoar SC, Rowbotham JL *et al.*, eds. *Management of Diabetic Foot Problems*. Philadelphia: WB Saunders, 1984; 103–12.
11 Edmonds ME, Archer AG, Watkins PJ. Ephedrine: A new treatment for diabetic neuropathic oedema. *Lancet* 1983; **i**: 548–51.
12 Nieman HL, Brabdt TD, Greenberg M. Percutaneous transluminal angioplasty: an angiographer's viewpoint. *Arch Surg* 1981; **116**: 821–8.
13 Sprayregen S, Sniderman KW, Sos TA *et al.* Popliteal artery branches: percutaneous transluminal angioplasty. *Am J Roentgenol* 1980; **135**: 945–50.
14 Reinhold RB, Gibbons GW, Wheelock FC, Hoar CS. Femoral–popliteal bypass in elderly diabetic patients. *Am J Surg* 1979; **137**: 549–55.
15 Leather RP, Shah DM, Karmody AM. Infrapopliteal bypass for limb salvage: increased patency and utilization of the saphenous vein used '*in situ*'. *Surgery* 1981; **90**: 1000–8.
16 Cotton LT, Cross FW. Lumbar sympathectomy for arterial disease. *Br J Surg* 1985; **72**: 678–83.
17 Foster AVM, Gibby D, Nelson M, Nash C, Edmonds ME. Successful management of digital necrosis by autoamputation: avoidance of surgery in the diabetic ischaemic foot. *Diabetic Med* 1988; **5** (suppl): 5.
18 Guy RJC, Clark CA, Malcolm PN, Watkins PJ. Evaluation of thermal and vibration sensation in diabetic neuropathy. *Diabetologia* 1985; **28**: 131–7.
19 Foster AVM, Edmonds ME. Examination of the diabetic foot. Part II. *Practical Diabetes* 1987; **4**: 153–4.
20 Foster AVM, Edmonds ME. Diabetic foot emergencies: A strategy for their care. *Diabetic Med* 1987; **4**: 555A–6A.

# 20 Gastrointestinal Problems in Diabetes Mellitus

**Summary**

- Impaired gut motility, largely attributed to autonomic (especially vagal) neuropathy, is common in diabetic patients.
- Diabetic gastrointestinal involvement is usually asymptomatic; diabetic patients with significant gastrointestinal symptoms must be fully investigated to exclude other pathology.
- Disordered gut motility may be identified by manometry, scintigraphy of isotope-labelled meals or barium studies, but abnormalities often correlate poorly with symptoms.
- Oesophageal dilatation and hypomotility are occasionally associated with heartburn and dysphagia.
- Gastric emptying of both solids and liquids is delayed and uncoordinated. Severe gastroparesis may cause severe vomiting, weight loss and unstable diabetic control.
- Diabetic diarrhoea is often intermittent, worse at night, urgent and watery and does not usually cause malabsorption or weight loss. Incontinence due to anorectal dysfunction may also occur.
- Upper gastrointestinal symptoms may respond to prokinetic drugs such as metoclopramide, domperidone, cisapride or erythromycin derivatives, and diabetic diarrhoea may be helped by $\alpha_2$-adrenergic agonists such as clonidine.

Problems relating to the gastrointestinal system are commonly encountered in patients with diabetes mellitus. Newer techniques of assessment have demonstrated, even in patients who are entirely asymptomatic, impairment of smooth muscle function with decreased motility throughout most of the gut. Symptoms, when present, are usually mild and intermittent but, in a minority of patients, can be severe enough to cause considerable disability and interfere with the patient's usual lifestyle.

The diagnosis of specific diabetic gastrointestinal involvement is usually made by excluding other disorders which commonly affect the gut in diabetic and non-diabetic patients alike. The typical gastrointestinal symptom complexes usually occur in long-standing IDDM patients and are associated with clinical neuropathy, but can sometimes develop shortly after diagnosis and may affect NIDDM patients.

Because of the often vague and non-specific nature of the symptoms, together with a lack of suitable screening methods, the prevalence of gastrointestinal problems in diabetic patients remains uncertain. However, this may be much higher than previously suspected. When a careful history was taken, 76% of 136 unselected diabetic out-patients had one or more gastrointestinal symptoms [1]. Recent reports emphasize the high proportion of asymptomatic diabetic patients in whom abnormal gut motility can be demonstrated. In a scintigraphic study of unselected IDDM patients, the transit of a solid bolus through the oesophagus was delayed in 42% of patients and gastric emptying was delayed in 56% [2]. Another study, also using scintigraphy, found abnormal oesophageal motility in 38% of 40 asymptomatic IDDM patients [3].

## Pathophysiology

Gastrointestinal motility is a complex, highly-coordinated neuromuscular process responsible for antegrade progression of luminal contents through the alimentary tract. Smooth muscle cells of the muscle propria (circular and longitudinal) represent the final effectors of motility having innate electrical pacemaker potentials. These are under continuous regulation by extrinsic autonomic nerves and intrinsic (myenteric) nerve plexuses which are largely autonomous, as well as by circulating peptide hormones and locally-produced chemical mediators.

The pathophysiology of the gut motility disturbance in diabetes is probably multifactorial but considerable evidence suggests that autonomic neuropathy plays a dominant role [4]. Several studies have found that disturbed gastrointestinal motility is associated with abnormal cardiac autonomic function tests [3–6]. Damage to the efferent nerve supply impairs the tone and contractility of gut smooth muscle. Autonomic nerve morphology in human diabetes has been little studied and the precise extent of involvement of the extrinsic and intrinsic nerve supply and the relative contributions of parasympathetic and sympathetic damage at the various levels of the gut have not yet been determined. The possible effects of afferent sensory denervation on gut reflex activity and awareness of symptoms are also largely unknown.

A recent study has shown that diabetic patients with gastrointestinal motility disorders had visceral afferent neuropathy as manifested by raised thresholds to cerebral evoked potentials following oesophageal stimulation [7].

Other factors may contribute to the abnormal gut motility in diabetes. A primary disturbance of smooth muscle function is unlikely, since the hypotonic gut muscle still responds when adequately stimulated by prokinetic drugs [8]. The possible role of disturbances in the secretion of the various gut regulatory peptides, which influence gut motility, digestion and absorption and whose secretion is partly modulated by the autonomic nervous system [9], has not yet been systematically studied.

In recent years, a variety of techniques including manometry and radionuclide scintigraphy (Table 20.1) have helped to clarify the defects in gut motility in diabetes and other disorders. Manometry is more sensitive than traditional radiographic methods but requires intubation and is time-consuming. On the other hand, scintigraphic imaging of fluid and solid markers labelled with gamma-emitting radioisotopes is simple, quick, non-invasive, as sensitive as manometry and involves less radiation dosage than radiography. Evaluation of gut motility using such techniques is, however, generally restricted to specialist centres. The evaluation of prokinetic drugs such as metoclopramide and domperidone has also added impetus to the understanding of gastrointestinal disorders in diabetes.

Abnormalities in specific parts of the gut (Table 20.2) will now be described in greater detail.

**Table 20.1.** Methods for evaluation of gastrointestinal motility.

| Method | Technique | Remarks |
|---|---|---|
| Radiography | Barium contrast with video recording | Measures propulsion<br>Non-quantitative information |
| Manometry | Gut intubation with strain-gauge device | Invasive<br>Measures mainly pressure |
| Radionuclide scintigraphy | Radioisotope-labelled fluid and solid markers with gamma camera | Simple and non-invasive<br>Measures propulsion<br>Quantitative information |

**Table 20.2.** Gut denervation problems in diabetes.

| Level | Clinical features |
|---|---|
| Oesophageal hypomotility | Occasional heartburn and dysphagia |
| Gastric hypomotility | Gastroparesis symptoms: fullness, vomiting, weight loss, poor diabetic control |
| Pyloro-jejunal hypertonia | Intermittent nausea and vomiting? |
| Gall-bladder hypomotility | Enlargement and poor contractions<br>No symptoms |
| Small-intestinal hypomotility | High bacterial overgrowth<br>Intermittent diarrhoea |
| Ileo-colonic denervation | Impaired water absorption<br>Watery diarrhoea |
| Colonic hypomotility | Chronic constipation<br>Occasional megacolon |
| Anorectal dysfunction | Faecal incontinence |

## Clinical features of gastrointestinal involvement

### *Oesophageal dysfunction*

Impaired oesophageal smooth muscle function can be frequently demonstrated in asymptomatic patients, but symptoms — consisting of heartburn and dysphagia for solids — are uncommon. Diabetic patients who develop significant oesophageal symptoms therefore require a barium swallow or endoscopy to exclude alternative causes, especially hiatus hernia, reflux oesophagitis, moniliasis and malignancy. Oesophageal symptoms may also indicate an underlying psychiatric illness such as anxiety or an affective disorder [10].

Barium swallow studies in diabetic patients may show a variety of abnormalities, including mild dilatation, decreased or absent primary peristaltic waves, sporadic tertiary contractions, prolonged transit and delayed emptying of the contrast, together with gastro-oesophageal reflux. The most characteristic manometric features are those of hypomotility with decreased amplitude, frequency and velocity of the peristaltic waves in the distal oesophagus following swallowing. Reduced resting pressure and uncoordinated function of the lower sphincter are also seen. Multiphasic, multipeaked oesophageal peristaltic pressure waves in diabetic patients with neuropathy have been regarded as pathognomonic of the disease [11], but other changes are now considered non-specific. Certain oesophageal contraction abnormalities, such as increased distal wave amplitude and triple-peaked waves, are independent of diabetic neuropathy and correlate more with the psychiatric state of the patient [10].

Radionuclide scintigraphy allows quantification of the delayed oesophageal transit of liquid and solid food boluses [5, 12] and time–activity curves in the different segments of the oesophagus [3]. A solid food bolus is probably more useful than liquid in detecting abnormal oesophageal emptying [13].

Oesophageal motor dysfunction probably results from vagal neuropathy. The motility changes are similar to those following surgical vagotomy and scintigraphic abnormalities correlate with the results of vagally mediated cardiovascular tests of autonomic function [3, 5].

### *Diabetic gastroparesis*

Diabetic gastroparesis with delayed gastric emptying is a well-recognized complication of diabetes and is characterized by hypomotility of gastric smooth muscle. When present, symptoms are non-specific and include early satiety and upper abdominal fullness during or immediately after eating. Patients who are more severely affected may complain of anorexia or may lose weight, symptoms which, in young diabetic women, must be distinguished from anorexia nervosa. Diabetic control may become difficult, with frequent and severe hypoglycaemic episodes because insulin injections and carbohydrate absorption are no longer in phase. Such patients may be erroneously labelled as 'brittle diabetics'. Less commonly, some patients develop intermittent bouts of nausea and vomiting lasting for a few days, and rarely, vomiting may become persistent and intractable. The vomitus may contain material ingested several hours previously and occasionally altered blood ('coffee grounds') from Mallory–Weiss tears. A gastric splash may be elicited, or noticed by the patient, several hours after taking fluids. Diabetic gastroparesis, like surgical vagotomy, can predispose to the formation of bezoars, which can obstruct gastric outflow and also give rise to nausea, vomiting and abdominal distension [14]. Patients with symptomatic gastroparesis invariably have other clinical features of autonomic neuropathy such as postural hypotension, abnormal sweating and bladder dysfunction. They require frequent hospital admissions, become malnourished and are often depressed, and generally have a poor prognosis [15].

Diabetic patients complaining of gastric symptoms should always undergo routine investigation including upper gastrointestinal radiography and endoscopy to exclude an ulcer, pyloric stenosis or malignancy. In gastroparesis, barium meal examination characteristically shows a dilated stomach with food and fluid residues still present in the fasting state (Fig. 20.1). Following the meal, absent or ineffective peristalsis, delayed gastric emptying and atony of the duodenal bulb are seen. Radionuclide scintigraphy can demonstrate the individual progress of the liquid and solid components labelled by two different isotopes of the test meal and this method remains the gold standard for measurement of gastric emptying. The normal stomach empties solids and liquids by different mechanisms, at different rates and in different patterns. Several distinctive abnormal emptying patterns have been observed in patients with gastroparesis. Gastric emptying of both liquid and solid tends to be slower in diabetic patients (either symptomatic or asymptomatic), with loss of the normal differentiation between the two components [1, 16]. This abnormality is in keeping with impaired distal stomach (antral) motor function in diabetic patients. Gastric motility

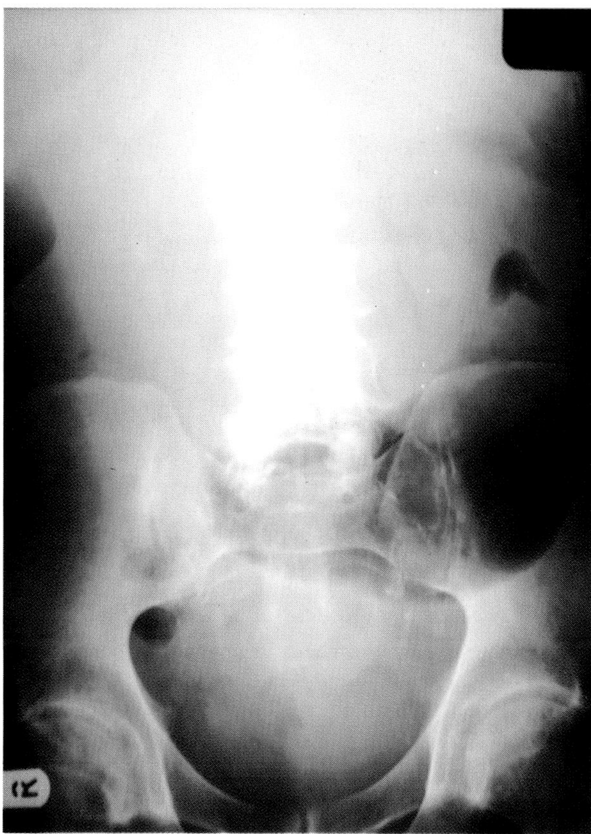


**Fig. 20.1.** Plain abdominal radiograph showing gastric dilatation.

abnormalities correlate poorly with upper gastro-intestinal symptoms and some severely symptomatic patients unexpectedly show nearly normal emptying of liquids and digestible solids [17]. Moreover, some patients display rapid early gastric emptying [18], which may result from impaired receptive relaxation of the proximal stomach (fundus) and may represent a milder degree of neuropathy before gastric stasis has supervened. The use of solid radiopaque markers as a measure of the progress of indigestible substances may be a more sensitive indicator of gastric motor dysfunction than radionuclide scintigraphy [17]. In the normal stomach, digestible solids empty during the postprandial period whereas indigestible material empties later during the interdigestive (fasting) period. Patients with symptomatic gastroparesis will usually show delayed gastric transit of indigestible solid markers as a result of the decreased antral motor activity. The delayed emptying of indigestible solids may contribute to nausea and vomiting and also encourage bezoar formation.

The underlying cause of gastroparesis is probably vagal neuropathy, as is suggested by these patients' impaired acid secretion in response to insulin-induced hypoglycaemia [19] or sham feeding [20]. Furthermore, the gastric motility changes in diabetic patients are similar to those following truncal vagotomy. In diabetic patients with abnormal parasympathetic tests of cardiac function, the mean gastric emptying rate (assessed by scintigraphy) is significantly impaired [6]. There have been few histological studies of the vagus nerve from patients with gastroparesis [21, 22]. These have shown losses of both unmyelinated and myelinated axons, supporting vagal neuropathy as a causal factor in diabetic gastroparesis.

The underlying mechanism of gastroparesis is still unclear. Manometric pressure measurements show diminished smooth muscle activity in both fundus and antrum. In symptomatic patients, myo-electric activity is especially reduced in the antral smooth muscle, with decreased phase II and absent interdigestive phase III motor complexes [8, 23, 24]. Similar myo-electric abnormalities are found in patients with postvagotomy gastroparesis [8]. The interdigestive motor complexes are considered to play an integral role in the clearing of undigestible debris from the stomach and upper small intestine. Somewhat paradoxically, it has been observed, using quantitative manometry, that diabetic patients with nausea and vomiting have increased tonic activity of the pyloric smooth muscle [25]. This interesting observation has now been extended in diabetic patients with gastroparesis. For instance, in a recent manometric study, although all patients with gastroparesis showed postprandial antral hypomotility, most of these same patients had in addition periods of non-propagated, high-amplitude contractile activity ('bursts') involving the jejunum [26]. This hyperactivity distal to the stomach is somewhat unexpected in view of the generalized hypomotility of the gut, but may explain the difficulty often encountered in passing a Crosby capsule into the duodenum in patients with gastroparesis. It may also explain in part the symptoms and perhaps their intermittency in 'gastroparetic' patients, and clearly further studies are indicated.

The possible role of gut hormone disturbances in gastroparesis remains unclear. Diabetic patients with gastroparesis have higher than normal plasma concentrations of motilin, a 22 amino-acid peptide which is widely distributed throughout the upper gut and whose experimental administration causes contraction of the stomach and duodenum. However, this association may be merely coincidental, since metoclopramide can improve gastric motor activity without normalizing plasma motilin levels [24]. It has been speculated that hyperglycaemia, by a mechanism as yet undetermined, may also be a contributory factor [24, 27] and may account for the intermittency of abnormal gastric emptying [28].

### *Gall-bladder dysfunction*

Enlargement and poor contraction of the gall-bladder following a fatty meal, so-called 'diabetic cholecystopathy', is sometimes observed in diabetic patients. The finding is usually made by chance during ultrasonography or, more frequently, cholecystography [29]. There are no symptoms and there does not appear to be a higher frequency of associated gallstones. A similar abnormality of gall-bladder function can be seen following bilateral vagotomy.

### *Diabetic diarrhoea*

Diabetic diarrhoea is a well-recognized complication of diabetes but remains poorly understood. Those affected usually have long-standing, poorly controlled IDDM and clinical evidence of somatic and autonomic neuropathy. The typical symptoms are intermittent bouts of diarrhoea, with the passage of upwards of 20 stools daily, often preceded by urgency. Although characteristically frequent at night, diarrhoea also continues during the day, occurring especially shortly after meals which may suggest, perhaps surprisingly, an exaggerated gastrocolic reflex. The bouts may persist for a few days or weeks and are then followed by spontaneous remission for a variable period. The stools vary in consistency but are frequently watery. Between episodes, the bowel habit often returns to normal and the patient may even complain of constipation. Fortunately, the symptoms are usually only mildly troublesome but a few patients suffer severely disabling diarrhoea which may force them to become housebound. Body weight and nutrition are usually maintained, even in those severely affected. Weight loss in a patient with diabetic diarrhoea is more likely to be due to associated gastroparesis.

There are no pathognomonic tests for diabetic diarrhoea and it is important to remember that the diagnosis must be made by exclusion. Diarrhoea associated with steatorrhoea may be the result of chronic pancreatic disease, which should respond to exocrine pancreatic replacement treatment. A further possibility is coeliac disease, which may resemble diabetic diarrhoea in its intermittency and nocturnal predilection. Coeliac disease will usually cause weight loss with clinical and biochemical features of malabsorption; an abnormal jejunal biopsy will support the diagnosis and the symptoms should respond to a gluten-free diet.

Diabetic diarrhoea is suggested by the typical clinical features, the lack of other positive findings and the almost invariable presence of diabetic peripheral neuropathy. Cardiovascular autonomic function tests are usually, but not always, abnormal at the time of onset of the symptoms. Routine assessment of small intestinal absorption (including serum iron, folate and vitamin $B_{12}$ concentrations, the D-xylose tolerance and Shilling tests) should be entirely normal. There are no characteristic abnormalities in the barium meal follow-through examination and the jejunal biopsy in patients with diabetic diarrhoea shows normal histology.

The pathogenesis of diabetic diarrhoea is unclear and may be multifactorial. In some patients, the small intestinal motility disturbance which leads to stasis of gut contents may allow abnormal bacterial overgrowth. Excess bacterial activity has been demonstrated in a few patients with diarrhoea by the $^{14}C$–glycocholate test. This might explain the prompt improvement in the diarrhoea which sometimes follows treatment with a broad-spectrum antibiotic.

Manometric pressure studies of gut motility in patients with diabetic diarrhoea are lacking. However, a disturbance of small intestinal motility involving both parasympathetic and sympathetic innervation can be demonstrated in patients with autonomic neuropathy [1] and with gastroparesis [23]. A possible role of autonomic neuropathy is supported by the observations that both truncal vagotomy and sympathectomy in non-diabetic patients may cause diarrhoea. The streptozotocin-diabetic rat frequently displays lower gut dysmotility associated with both parasympathetic and sympathetic denervation [30]. Chronic streptozotocin-diabetic rats develop impaired ileal and colonic absorption of fluid and electrolytes which results from denervation of $\alpha_2$-adrenergic receptors on enterocytes [31]. There are as yet only preliminary reports of the $\alpha_2$-adrenergic agonists, limidine [32] and clonidine [33], being effective in some patients with diabetic diarrhoea.

Impaired bile acid absorption, which could lead to increased fluid and electrolyte load in the colon and so to watery diarrhoea, has been implicated in the pathogenesis of both postvagotomy and diabetic diarrhoea [34]. However, the failure of bile acid-binding agents such as cholestyramine to improve symptoms argues against bile acid malabsorption as an important factor in diabetic diarrhoea.

### *Colonic dysfunction*

Constipation is a common gastrointestinal symptom in diabetic patients and results from large intestinal hypomotility. The prevalence of this complaint rises with increasing severity of symptomatic neuropathy, reaching 88% in one series [1]. The constipation may vary from mild to severe, the latter patients having two or fewer bowel actions per week. In some patients, constipation may be intermittent and can alternate with diabetic diarrhoea. Routine investigation of constipation in diabetic patients should include rectal examination, procto-sigmoidoscopy and testing for occult blood. It is usually necessary, especially in older patients, to exclude colonic carcinoma by performing a barium enema, which may show marked colonic dilatation (megacolon or megasigmoid).

Colonic dysfunction is associated with other clinical features of autonomic neuropathy but its precise pathogenesis remains poorly understood. Diabetic patients with severe constipation have an absent gastrocolic response to eating as assessed by measurements of distal colonic myo-electrical and motor activity. These motility abnormalities can be improved by intramuscular neostigmine or intravenous metoclopramide [35].

### *Anorectal dysfunction*

In its milder, but nevertheless still troublesome form, symptoms of anorectal dysfunction include mucus leakage and faecal staining without the need to wear a pad. More severe loss of anal sphincter control with faecal incontinence is a distressing symptom usually associated with autonomic neuropathy and often, but not always, associated with diabetic diarrhoea. The symptom is liable to occur not only during sleep but also during the day. Faecal incontinence may develop in up to 20% of diabetic patients [1], who are usually slow to volunteer this embarrassing complaint.

Anorectal manometry in patients with faecal incontinence has shown reduced internal sphincter tone but with preservation of voluntary sphincter contraction, suggesting that external sphincter tone remains relatively normal [36]. However, another study in similar patients demonstrated impaired external sphincter function [37]. Some patients with faecal incontinence also have an increased threshold for conscious rectal sensation which suggests impaired afferent nerve function as another contributory factor [38]. The latter has been supported by the finding of increased sensory thresholds, as measured by electrical stimulation, in the upper anal canal in patients with minimal symptoms and regarded as an early abnormality in the development of incontinence [39]. Diabetic patients with faecal incontinence also have longer pudental nerve latency times, again suggesting that somatic neuropathy is a contributory factor [40].

## **Treatment of gastrointestinal problems**

To date, there is no convincing evidence that intensified glycaemic control with either conventional insulin injections or continuous subcutaneous insulin infusion can reverse the clinical features of established diabetic gastrointestinal involvement. Likewise, several carefully-conducted trials have failed to show any clear beneficial effect of aldose reductase inhibitors such as sorbinil on clinical autonomic neuropathy or the gut manifestations [4]. Once the various gastrointestinal symptom complexes have become apparent clinically, the treatment is primarily symptomatic.

Prokinetic agents, which are drugs enhancing the transit of material through the gastrointestinal tract, represent the main line of treatment for gut hypomotility disorders in diabetes. This class of pharmaceutical agent consists of different subclasses of drugs (Table 20.3) with distinct, although not completely understood, mechanisms of action. These agents have been recently reviewed [41] and their actions include: (1) increased cholinergic activity, (2) antagonism of inhibitory neurotransmitter substances (e.g. dopamine, serotonin), and (3) mimicking noncholinergic nonadrenergic compounds such as motilin.

Metoclopramide is both a cholinergic agonist and dopamine antogonist which increases smooth muscle tone and contractility by enhancing the

Table 20.3. Prokinetic drugs.

| Subclass | Increased cholinergic activity | Dopamine antagonist | Serotonin antagonist | Increased motilin activity |
|---|---|---|---|---|
| *Substituted benzamides* | | | | |
| Metoclopramide | + | + | | |
| Cisapride | + | | + | |
| *Antidopaminergic agents* | | | | |
| Domperidone | | + | | |
| *Macrolide agents* | | | | |
| Erythromycin | | | | + |
| EM 523 | | | | + |
| EM 523L | | | | + |

local effect of acetylcholine in the myenteric plexus and also has a central action as an anti-emetic. Domperidone, like metoclopramide, is a potent dopamine antagonist but lacks cholinergic activity. Cisapride promotes acetylcholine release in the myenteric plexus and is also a serotonin antagonist. Unlike metoclopramide and domperidone, cisapride has no dopamine antagonist properties. Recent studies have shown that erythromycin and other macrolide derivatives (e.g. EM 523, EM 523L), the so-called motilides, stimulate the onset of migrating motor complexes. These agents probably bind to, and act through, motilin receptors [41, 42].

### *Oesophageal dysfunction*

Oesophageal motor dysfunction is usually asymptomatic and treatment is seldom required. If heartburn or dysphagia are troublesome and other causes have been excluded, the patient should be given a trial of treatment with a prokinetic drug such as cisapride in an attempt to increase oesophageal contractions. The oesophagus may, however, be more resistant to treatment with prokinetic drugs than delayed gastric emptying [12].

### *Gastroparesis*

Gastric symptoms of nausea and vomiting may respond to metoclopramide. The usual dosage is 10–20 mg taken about 30 min before each meal and at bedtime. Side-effects occasionally limit its use. Domperidone, 10–20 mg 4–8 hourly, may also help symptoms [43]. There is some evidence, however, that long-term administration of metoclopramide or domperidone may reduce their gastrokinetic properties [43, 44]. Cisapride (10 mg three or four times daily) is a more recent prokinetic drug which stimulates oesophageal, gastric and intestinal motility in general [28]. Cisapride can improve the rate of gastric emptying of both solids and liquids [13] but a few patients may develop marked stool frequency as a result of increased small bowel and colonic motility. A recent clinical trial using erythromycin, 250 mg three times daily, showed substantial improved solid and liquid emptying in patients with proven gastroparesis [42]. Further studies with erythromycin and its derivatives are awaited.

Patients experiencing more severe gastric symptoms present a difficult problem. Acute bouts of vomiting may require hospital admission for both intravenous fluid replacement and control of the diabetes. Intranasal gastric suction should be carried out to decompress the stomach and metoclopramide given intravenously. Eating should be re-introduced as frequent, small semi-fluid feeds. In the longer term, patients should probably avoid high-fibre foods. Surgical drainage procedures will need to be considered for the few patients with vomiting which has become refractory to conventional measures. Surgical experience is limited, with only a few reports in the literature, and it may not always relieve symptoms. To reduce the tendency to postoperative biliary reflux vomiting and gastritis, a Roux-en-Y gastrojejunostomy has been recommended [21].

An alternative to gastric surgery for refractory gastroparesis is the use of jejunostomy with direct enteral feeding which has been described in a small number of severely affected patients [45]. Gastric bezoars, when identified, should be treated by endoscopic fragmentation [15].

### *Diabetic diarrhoea*

The treatment of this condition is often unsatisfactory and difficult to evaluate as the episodes of diarrhoea may be self-limiting. Mild symptoms are best managed by opiate derivatives such as codeine phosphate and loperamide hydrochloride. If a disturbance of bowel flora is suspected, tetracycline or other broad-spectrum antibiotics may rapidly abolish symptoms and can then be given intermittently for 1 week in every 4. For more resistant cases, especially where the diarrhoea is watery, a specific $\alpha_2$-adrenergic agonist such as limidine [32] or clonidine [33] may be tried on the basis that adrenergic innervation of intestinal enterocyte receptors has a role in fluid and electrolyte absorption. The use of bile acid-binding agents such as cholestyramine, although helpful in postvagotomy diarrhoea, has proved disappointing in diabetic patients.

### *Diabetic constipation*

The treatment of constipation in diabetic patients is often neglected. If constipation is not improved by routine laxatives, treatment with one of the prokinetic group of drugs may be helpful [46].

### *Faecal incontinence*

This distressing condition is difficult to treat and the patient may have to resort to the use of absorbent pads. Treatment by means of biofeedback has been described in a limited number of patients [38].

## Other gastrointestinal disorders in diabetes mellitus

Diabetic patients may develop the same gastrointestinal disorders that occur in the general population. Although these conditions are not directly related to diabetes, their prevalence and clinical features may in some circumstances be modified by the presence of the disease.

### *Oral disorders*

Both their increased tendency to infection and microangiopathy may make diabetic patients more prone to gingival and periodontal disease [47]. Diabetic patients have a high oral carrier rate of *Candida albicans* [48] and, especially if taking long-term antibiotic treatment such as for foot problems, may be more liable to pharyngeal and oesophageal candidosis. The latter can be confirmed by examination of material recovered at endoscopy. Oropharyngeal and oesophageal candidosis should usually respond to oral nystatin, ketoconazole, amphotericin or fluconazole. Oral disorders associated with diabetes, including sialosis, xerostomia, impairment of taste, as well as infections, have been recently reviewed [49].

### *Atrophic gastritis*

Atrophy of the gastric mucosa and impaired gastric acid secretion following histamine have been reported to be more common in diabetic patients. The diminished gastric acid secretion may result in part from vagal neuropathy but may also be due to autoimmune gastritis. Through its association with other organ-specific autoimmune diseases, the prevalences of gastric parietal cell and intrinsic factor antibodies and of pernicious anaemia are relatively high in IDDM [50].

### *Gastric and duodenal ulceration*

The prevalence of gastric ulcers in diabetic patients is probably similar to that in the general population. Earlier reports of a lower prevalence of duodenal ulceration have remained unconfirmed, although this might be expected in diabetic patients because of the decreased gastric acid secretion. There is some evidence that bleeding from duodenal ulcers may have more severe consequences in diabetic patients because of vascular changes. The clinical features of gastric outlet obstruction due to peptic ulceration and scarring may be accentuated in diabetic patients because of coexistent vagal neuropathy.

### *Gallstones and cholecystitis*

Diabetic patients might be expected to be at increased risk of developing gallstones since many are overweight and have abnormal lipid metabolism which could lead to alterations in bile composition. Moreover, autonomic neuropathy could lead to delayed gall-bladder emptying. There are however only few reports of the prevalence of gallstones and gall-bladder disease in diabetic patients. A recent study concluded that the risk of gallstones in diabetes is only increased in the elderly [51].

Diabetic patients who develop cholecystitis suffer higher morbidity and mortality following both emergency and elective biliary tract surgery [52]. Diabetic patients must therefore be monitored very closely for complications, especially infection, in the postoperative period. Careful bacteriological examination, including culture of the bile duct during surgery and of the T-tube postoperatively, is recommended and it is probably best to continue antibiotic treatment after surgery. Prophylactic cholecystectomy was previously recommended in asymptomatic diabetic patients but this policy has recently been questioned [53].

### *Steatorrhoea*

Chronic pancreatitis may be associated with secondary diabetes. Where pancreatic exocrine function is insufficient, steatorrhoea will result and may resemble diabetic diarrhoea. Although coeliac disease was considered to occur more frequently in IDDM, it has been claimed that this condition is no more common than in the general population [54]. As described above, coeliac disease may resemble diabetic diarrhoea clinically but the two conditions can be easily distinguished.

BASIL F. CLARKE

## References


1 Feldman M, Schiller LR. Disorders of gastrointestinal motility associated with diabetes mellitus. *Ann Intern Med* 1983; **98**: 378–84.

2 Horowitz M, Harding PE, Maddox A, Madden GJ, Collins PJ, Chatterton BE, Wishart J, Shearman DJC. Gastric and oesophageal emptying in insulin-dependent diabetes mellitus. *J Gastroenterol Hepatol* 1986; **1**: 97–113.

3 Westin L, Lilja B, Sundkvist G. Oesophagus scinitgraphy in patients with diabetes mellitus. *Scand J Gastroenterol* 1986; **21**: 1200–4.

4 Ewing DJ, Clarke BF. Diabetic autonomic neuropathy: present insights and future prospects. *Diabetes Care* 1986; **9**: 648–65.

5 Channer KS, Jackson PC, O'Brien I, Corrall RJM, Coles DR, Davies ER, Virjee JP. Oesophageal function in diabetes mellitus and its association with autonomic neuropathy. *Diabetic Med* 1985; **2**: 378–82.

6 Buysschaert M, Moulart M, Urbain JL, Pauwels S, Roy LD, Ketelslegers JM, Lambert AE. Impaired gastric emptying in diabetic patients with cardiac autonomic neuropathy. *Diabetes Care* 1987; **10**: 448–52.

7 Rathmann W, Enck P, Frieling T, Gries FA. Visceral afferent neuropathy in diabetic gastroparesis. *Diabetes Care* 1991; **14**: 1086–89.

8 Malagelada JR, Rees WDW, Mazzotta L, Gu VLW. Gastric motor abnormalities in diabetic and post-vagotomy gastroparesis: effect of metoclopramide and bethanicol. *Gastroenterology* 1980; **78**: 286–93.

9 Smith PH, Madson KL. Interactions between autonomic nerves and endocrine cells of the gastroenteropancreatic system. *Diabetologia* 1981; **20**: 314–24.

10 Clouse RE, Lustman PJ, Reidel WL. Correlation of esophageal motility abnormalities with neuropsychiatric status in diabetics. *Gastroenterology* 1986; **90**: 1146–54.

11 Loo FD, Dodds WJ, Soergel KH, Arndorfer RC, Helm JF, Hogan WJ. Multipeaked esophageal peristaltic pressure waves in patients with diabetic neuropathy. *Gastroenterology* 1985; **88**: 485–91.

12 Maddern GJ, Horowitz M, Jamieson GG. The effect of domperidone on oesophageal emptying in diabetic autonomic neuropathy. *Br J Clin Pharmacol* 1985; **19**: 441–4.

13 Horowitz M, Maddox A, Harding PE, Maddern GJ, Chatterton BE, Wishart J, Shearman DJC. Effect of cisapride on gastric and oesophageal emptying in insulin-dependent diabetes mellitus. *Gastroenterology* 1987; **92**: 1899–1907.

14 Brady PG, Richardson R. Gastric bezoar formation secondary to gastroparesis diabeticorum. *Arch Int Med* 1977; **137**: 1729.

15 Ewing DJ, Campbell IW, Clarke BF. The natural history of diabetic autonomic neuropathy. *Q J Med* 1980; **49**: 95–108.

16 Campbell IW, Heading RC, Tothill PH, Buist AS, Ewing DJ, Clarke BF. Gastric emptying in diabetic autonomic neuropathy. *Gut* 1977; **18**: 462–7.

17 Feldman M, Smith HJ, Simon TR. Gastric emptying of solid radiopaque markers: studies in healthy subjects and diabetic patients. *Gastroenterology* 1984; **87**: 895–902.

18 Loo FD, Palmer DW, Soergel KH, Kalbfleisch JH, Wood CM. Gastric emptying in patients with diabetes mellitus. *Gastroenterology* 1984; **86**: 485–94.

19 Hosking DJ, Moony F, Stewart IM, Atkinson M. Vagal impairment of gastric secretion in diabetic autonomic neuropathy. *Br Med J* 1975; **2**: 588–90.

20 Feldman M, Corbett DB, Ramsey EJ, Walsh JH, Richardson CT. Abnormal gastric function in longstanding insulin dependent diabetic patients. *Gastroenterology* 1979; **77**: 12–17.

21 Guy RJC, Dawson JL, Garrett JR, Laws JW, Thomas PK, Sharma AK, Watkins PJ. Diabetic gastroparesis from autonomic neuropathy: surgical considerations and changes in vagus nerve morphology. *J Neurol Psychiatr* 1984; **47**: 686–91.

22 Britland ST, Young RJ, Sharma AK, Lee D, Ah-See AK, Clarke BF. Vagus nerve morphology in diabetic gastropathy. *Diabetic Medicine* 1990; **7**: 780–87.

23 Camilleri M, Malagelada JR. Abnormal intestinal motility in diabetics with the gastroparesis syndrome. *Eur J Clin Invest* 1984; **14**: 420–7.

24 Achem-Karam SR, Funakoshi A, Vinik AI, Owyang C. Plasma motilin concentration and interdigestive migrating motor complexes in diabetic gastroparesis; effect of metoclopramide. *Gastroenterology* 1985; **88**: 492–9.

25 Mearin F, Camilleri M, Malagelada JR. Pyloric dysfunction in diabetics with recurrent nausea and vomiting. *Gastroenterology* 1986; **90**: 1919–25.

26 Jebbink HJA, Smout AJPM, Bravenboer B, Van Berge Henegouwen GP, Fone DR, Akkermans LMA. Abnormal gastrointestinal motility in Type 1 diabetics with autonomic neuropathy and the gastroparesis syndrome. *Diabetologia* 1991; **34** (suppl 2): A155.

27 Fraser RJ, Horowitz M, Maddox AF, Harding PE, Chatterton BE, Dent J. Hyperglycaemia slows gastric emptying in Type 1 (insulin-dependent) diabetes mellitus. *Diabetologia* 1990; **33**: 675–80.

28 Feldman M, Smith JH. Effect of cisapride on gastric emptying of indigestible solids in patients with gastroparesis diabeticorum. *Gastroenterology* 1987; **92**: 171–4.

29 Marumo K, Fujii S, Seki J, Wada M. Studies on gallbladder dysfunction in patients with diabetes mellitus. In: Goto Y, Horiuchi A, Kogurie K, eds. *Diabetic Neuropathy*, International Congress Series No 581. Amsterdam: Excerpta Medica, 1982: 284–9.

30 Schmidt RE, Nelson JS, Johnson EM. Experimental diabetic autonomic neuropathy. *Am J Pathol* 1981; **103**: 210–25.

31 Chang EB, Bergenstal RM, Field M. Diarrhea in streptozotocin treated rats. *J Clin Invest* 1985; **75**: 1666–70.

32 Goff JS. Diabetic diarrhea and limidine. *Ann Intern Med* 1984; **101**: 874–5.

33 Fedorak RN, Field M, Chang EB. Treatment of diabetic diarrhea with clonidine. *Ann Intern Med* 1985; **102**: 179–9.

34 Molloy AM, Tomkin GH. Altered bile in diabetic diarrhoea. *Br Med J* 1978; **2**: 1462–3.

35 Battle WM, Snape WJ, Alavi A, Cohen S, Braunstein S. Colonic dysfunction in diabetes mellitus. *Gastroenterology* 1980; **79**: 1217–21.

36 Schiller LR, Santa Ana CA, Schmulen AC, Hendler RS, Harford WV, Fordtran JS. Pathogenesis of fecal incontinence in diabetes mellitus: evidence for internal anal sphincter dysfunction. *N Engl J Med* 1982; **307**: 1666–71.

37 Tunuguntla AK, Wald A. Comparison of anorectal function in diabetics and non-diabetics with fecal incontinence. *Gastroenterology* 1984; **86**: 1285.

38 Wald A, Tunuguntla AK. Anorectal sensorimotor dysfunction in fecal incontinence and diabetes mellitus. Modification with biofeedback therapy. *N Engl J Med* 1984; **310**: 1282–7.

39 Aitchison M, Fisher BM, Carter K, McKee R MacCuish AC, Finlay IG. Impaired anal sensation and early diabetic faecal incontinence. *Diabetic Med* 1991; **8**: 960–63.

40 Pinna Pintor M, Zara GP, Falletto E, Maraschiello A, Monge L, Dematteis. Pelvic floor neuropathy in diabetic patients with faecal incontinence. *Gastroenterology* 1990; **98**: (suppl): A381.

41 Reynolds JC, Putnam PE. Prokinetic agents. *Gastroenterology Clin North Amer* 1992; **21**: 567–96.

42 Janssens J, Peeters TL, Vantrappen G, Tack J, Urbain JL, De Roo M, Muls E, Bouillon R. Improvement of gastric emptying in diabetic gastroparesis by erythromycin. *N Engl J Med* 1990; **322**: 1028–31.

43 Horowitz M, Harding PE, Chatterton BE, Collins PJ, Shearman DJC. Acute and chronic effects of domperidone on gastric emptying in diabetic autonomic neuropathy. *Digest Dis Sci* 1985; **30**: 1–9.

44 Schade RR, Dugas MC, Lhotsky DM, Gavaler JS, Van Thiel DH. Effect of metoclopramide on gastric liquid emptying in patients with diabetic gastroparesis. *Digest Dis Sci* 1985; **30**: 10–15.

45 Jacober SI, Narayan A, Stroden WE, Vinik AI. Jejunostomy feeding in the management of gastroparesis diabeticorum. *Diabetes Care* 1986; **9**: 217–19.

46 Snape WJ, Battle WM, Schwartz SS, Braunstein SN, Goldstein HA, Alavi A. Metoclopramide to treat gastroparesis due to diabetes mellitus. A double-blind controlled trial. *Ann Intern Med* 1982; **96**: 444–6.

47 Katz P, Wirthlin MR, Szpunar SM, Selby JV, Sepe SJ, Showstack JA. Epidemiology and prevention of periodontal disease in individuals with diabetes. *Diabetes Care* 1991; **14**: 375–85.

48 Tapper-Jones LM, Aldred MJ, Walker DM, Hayes TM. Candidal infections and populations of candida albicans in mouths of diabetics. *J Clin Pathol* 1981; **34**: 706–11.

49 Lamey P-J, Darwazeh AMG, Frier BM. Oral disorders associated with diabetes mellitus. *Diabetic Med* 1992; **9**: 410–16.

50 Irvine WJ, Clarke BF, Scarth L, Cullen DR, Duncan LJP. Thyroid and gastric autoimmunity in patients with diabetes. *Lancet* 1970; **ii**: 163–8.

51 Hayes PC, Patrick A, Roulston JE, Murchiston JT, Allan P, Plevris JN, Clarke BF, Bouchier IAD. Gallstones in diabetes: prevalence and risk factors. *Eur J Gastroenterol Heptatol* 1992; **4**: 55–9.

52 Sandler RS, Maule WF, Baltus ME. Factors associated with postoperative complications in diabetics after biliary tract surgery. *Gastroenterology* 1986; **91**: 157–62.

53 Pelligrini CA. Asymptomatic gallstones. Does diabetes mellitus make a difference? *Gastroenterology* 1986; **91**: 245–6.

54 Walsh CH, Cooper BT, Wright AD, Malins JM, Cooke WT. Diabetes mellitus and coeliac disease: a clinical study. *Q J Med* 1978; **47**: 89–100.

# 21 The Skin in Diabetes Mellitus

**Summary**

- Various skin conditions occur frequently in diabetes, although common lesions may be associated by chance.
- Necrobiosis lipoidica diabeticorum consists of non-scaling plaques with atrophic epidermis and thick, degenerating collagen in the dermis, usually in the pretibial region.
- Granuloma annulare is an annular or arciform lesion with a raised papular border and flat centre, usually found on the dorsum of the hands and arms. Histologically, there is mid-dermal collagen degeneration and abundant mucin.
- Diabetic dermopathy consists of bilateral pigmented pretibial patches ('shin spots') which mostly affect older male diabetic patients.
- 'Diabetic thick skin' includes both the rare scleroedema (affecting the neck, upper back and arms) and the common diabetic hand syndrome (Dupuytren's contractures, sclerosing tenosynovitis, knuckle pads and carpal tunnel syndrome).
- Acanthosis nigricans forms brown, velvety hyperkeratotic plaques in the axilla or back of the neck, often associated with insulin resistance. Histologically, the epidermis is extensively folded with increased melanocytes.
- Bullosis diabeticorum usually occurs in patients with long-standing neuropathy and consists of tense blisters on a non-inflamed base which appear suddenly on the feet or hands.
- Cutaneous complications of diabetic treatment include reactions to sulphonylurea drugs (especially first generation), insulin allergy and injection-site lipodystrophy.
- The rare glucagonoma syndrome (associated with an A-cell pancreatic tumour) presents with a migratory erythematous eruption, with peripheral scaling and vesiculation leading to erosions and ulceration. The characteristic sites are perioral, genital and perianal.

Skin disorders affect about 30% of diabetic patients [1]. These conditions fall into four general categories (see Table 21.1). This chapter will concentrate principally on disorders regarded as cutaneous markers of diabetes and the dermatological complications of treatment; other rarer associations are reviewed elsewhere [2].

Certain cutaneous disorders clearly occur commonly in diabetes, but it is often difficult to define the exact nature of their association with the disease. First, the mechanisms responsible for the skin lesions are poorly understood and have no obvious biological links with the disease process of diabetes. Secondly, conclusions drawn from a highly-selected group of patients referred to a dermatological practice may not apply to the general diabetic population. Thirdly, if both conditions are common, they will often be associated by chance alone and not necessarily causally related. Various 'cutaneous manifestations' of diabetes have been described in the older literature, but their relative frequencies in IDDM and NIDDM and precise relationship to glucose metabolism need to be clarified. An example is generalized pruritus, previously widely regarded as a marker of diabetes. A recent study of 300 patients found that although localized vulval pruritus (associated with candidiasis) was three times more common in diabetic than in non-diabetic women,

**Table 21.1.** The skin and diabetes mellitus.

*'Cutaneous markers' of diabetes*
Necrobiosis lipoidica diabeticorum
Granuloma annulare
Diabetic dermopathy ('shin spots')
Diabetic thick skin (including diabetic hand syndrome)
Acanthosis nigricans
Diabetic bullae

*Complications of diabetes*
Neurovascular and ischaemic skin changes and foot ulceration
Digital gangrene (due to atherosclerosis)
Disordered sweating (with autonomic neuropathy)
Increased susceptibility to skin infections:
- bacterial (boils, erythrasma)
- yeasts (candidiasis — intertrigo, perineal infections, balanitis)
- fungal dermatoses

*Complications of diabetic treatment*
Sulphonylureas:
- maculopapular eruptions
- Stevens–Johnson syndrome
- purpura
- photosensitivity
- erythema nodosum
- porphyria cutanea tarda
- alcohol-induced flushing with chlorpropamide ('CPAF')

Insulin:
- localized allergy (late-phase, Arthus or delayed reactions)
- systemic allergy (urticaria, anaphylaxis)
- lipoatrophy
- lipohypertrophy
- idiosyncratic reactions (pigmentation, keloid formation)

*Rare associations with endocrine and other syndromes*
Glucagonoma (migratory necrolytic erythema)
Cushing's syndrome (skin atrophy, striae, hirsutes)
Acromegaly (thickened skin, increased sweating)
Partial and total lipodystrophy (variable loss of subcutaneous fat)
Alaxia telangiectasia

the prevalence of generalized pruritus was the same (3%) in the diabetic as in the general population [3].

## Cutaneous conditions considered as markers of diabetes

### *Necrobiosis lipoidica diabeticorum (NLD)*

This rare condition, first described by Oppenheim in 1929 [4] and named by Urbach in 1932 [5], has an incidence of 3 per 1000 diabetic patients per year. Three-quarters of cases are women, with an average age of onset of 34 years [6].

The appearance of the fully developed lesion is diagnostic: non-scaling plaques with atrophic yellow centres, surface telangiectasia and a violaceous or erythematous border (sometimes raised) are usually seen in the pretibial region (Fig. 21.1). The lesions vary in size, small papules often coalescing to form large irregular plaques, sometimes several centimetres in diameter. One-third of the lesions ulcerate. Multiple or bilateral lesions occur in most cases, and sites other than the pretibial are affected in 15% of patients.

The histological hallmark of the condition — 'necrobiosis' — refers to degeneration and thickening of collagen bundles in the dermis. The necrobiotic foci are acellular, associated with granular debris scattered throughout the dermis and surrounded by a mixed cellular infiltrate of lymphocytes, histiocytes, fibroblasts and epitheloid cells. Granulomata or lymphoid nodules [7] may form in some lesions. The epidermis is normal in early lesions, but later becomes thin and atrophic. Trauma (and in other reports, the Koebner phenomena) can induce lesions of necrobiosis with early microangiopathy associated with ballooning degeneration of isolated endothelial cells and proliferative end arteritis. Late lesions have a paucity of blood vessels and cutaneous nerves [8].

The pathogenesis of the disorder is not known [9] and the nature of the association between necrobiosis and diabetes is uncertain. The much-quoted statistic that 90% of people with NLD are diabetic, will develop diabetes or have a family history of the disease [6] derives from a retrospective review in 1966, in which the selection criteria are unknown and over 50% of the patients had not been seen for over 10 years. Moreover, 'impending diabetes' was presumed on the basis of glucose tolerance testing after prednisone treatment, a procedure since abandoned because it is non-specific and non-reproducible. Other studies of the time (when the diagnostic criteria for diabetes were less rigorous) found that about 60% of patients with necrobiosis had diabetes [10, 11]. A recent study showed normal $HbA_1$ levels in non-diabetic people with necrobiosis lipoidica, demonstrating that significant hyperglycaemia is not necessary for its development [12]. Overall, therefore, the association between NLD and diabetes seems weaker than previously assumed, and NLD may not be a specific marker for diabetes.

Evaluation of treatment of NLD, which must take into account the 20% spontaneous remission rate, has not yet been rigorously undertaken. Active red margins have now been shown to have an inflammatory infiltrate that extends well beyond the clinical margin of the lesion [13]. This region may respond to steroids either injected or applied locally on and beyond the lesional margins. Topical or intralesional steroids are contraindicated once atrophy is apparent; local emollients may then be used instead. Skin grafts of necrobiotic ulcers or lesions are often complicated by recurrence within or around the grafts. Variable success has been reported with oral treatment of NLD with aspirin and dypytidamole [14] or pentoxifylline [15].

*Granuloma annulare (GA)*

Granuloma annulare was described by Fox in 1895 [16]. The most common form consists of one or more annular or arciform lesions with a raised, flesh-coloured papular border and a flat, often hyperpigmented centre (Fig. 21.2). In 63% of a large series, the dorsum of the hands and arms was affected; the feet, legs and trunk were less frequently involved [17]. An uncommon generalized form comprises numerous flesh-coloured papules which are distributed symmetrically, often on sun-exposed areas. GA differs histologically from NLD in that the epidermis is normal and the necrobiotic collagen is localized to the mid-dermis and associated with abundant mucin.

Clinically, it can be difficult to distinguish GA from NLD and this has led to attempts to establish an association between GA and diabetes, as reported for NLD. There are case reports of diabetic patients with GA [18, 19], particularly the disseminated form and an even rarer perforating type. Review of 23 cases of perforating GA identified two subtypes; a papular and an ulcerative form with the ulcerative type strongly associated with diabetes [20]. However, both diabetes and GA are relatively common and chance associations are therefore likely. Several large studies [21, 22] have been unable to show a significant association between the two disorders, although a recent retrospective investigation reported a marginally higher than expected incidence of IDDM in patients with localized GA [23]. Patients with GA showed no increased incidence of glucose intolerance in one study [24] while another showed an increase area under the glucose and insulin curves

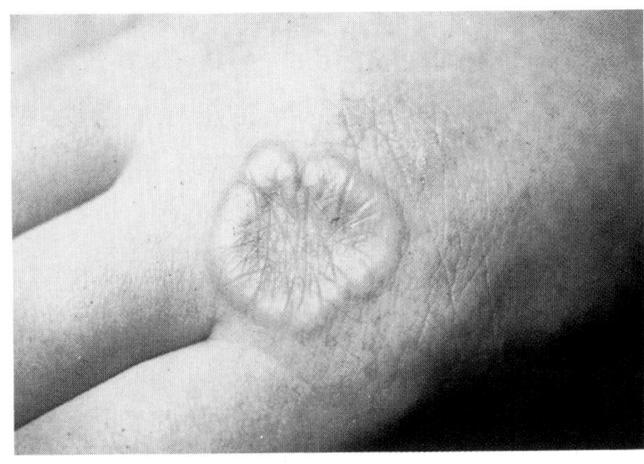

**Fig. 21.2.** Granuloma annulare. (Courtesy of Dr Geoffrey V. Gill, Walton Hospital, Liverpool.)

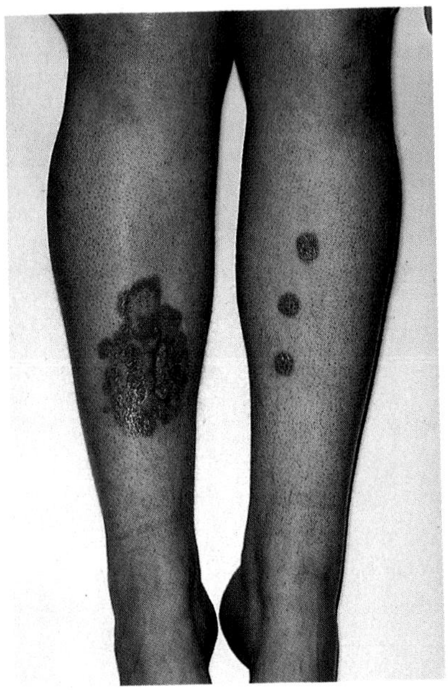

(a)

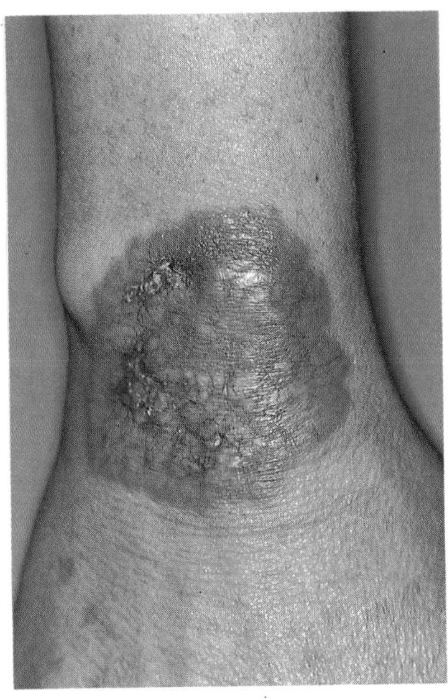

(b)

**Fig. 21.1.** Necrobiosis lipoidica diabeticorum. (a) A typical lesion on the front of the right shin, with three smaller areas on the left shin. (b) An area of necrobiosis with the typical yellow atrophic centre and telangiectases, on the unusual site of the dorsum of the wrist. (Courtesy of Dr Ian A. MacFarlane and Dr Geoffrey V. Gill, Walton Hospital, Liverpool).

compared to 14 age- and weight-matched controls [25]. HLA phenotypes associated with GA are not seen in IDDM [26]. GA is therefore associated with diabetes in a small percentage of cases.

### *Diabetic dermopathy (pigmented pretibial patches)*

This condition, first described by Melin in 1964 [27] and subsequently named 'diabetic dermopathy' by Binkley [28], is also known as 'shin spots' or 'pigmented pretibial patches'. These lesions are not pathognomic of diabetes, having been reported in 1.5% of healthy medical students and in 20% of euglycaemic patients with various endocrine diseases [29]. Absence or reduction in the bulk of extensor digitorum brevis muscle is thought to be a sign of diabetic neuropathy and an increased incidence of pretibial patches was noted in these patients [30]. The incidence of retinopathy has been reported to be statistically significantly higher (39.1%) with dermopathy compared to diabetics without dermopathy (6.9%) [31].

Initially, lesions are round or oval, red or brownish papules which slowly evolve into discrete, sharply circumscribed, atrophic, hyperpigmented or scaly lesions (Fig. 21.3). Sometimes, only depressed areas of normal skin colour are seen. Ulceration is rare. Lesions are bilateral but not perfectly symmetrical. The anterior and lateral aspects of the shin are most commonly affected but other sites have been reported. Men are more often affected: dermopathy occurs in about 60% of male diabetic patients older than 50 years of age and in 29% of similarly aged female patients [27].

Histological features are not diagnostic and the underlying pathophysiology is not understood. Patients often associate the appearance of lesions with some preceding trauma but experimental skin damage has failed to reproduce the lesions [27]. Treatment is not required. Dermopathy may regress spontaneously but new lesions continue to develop.

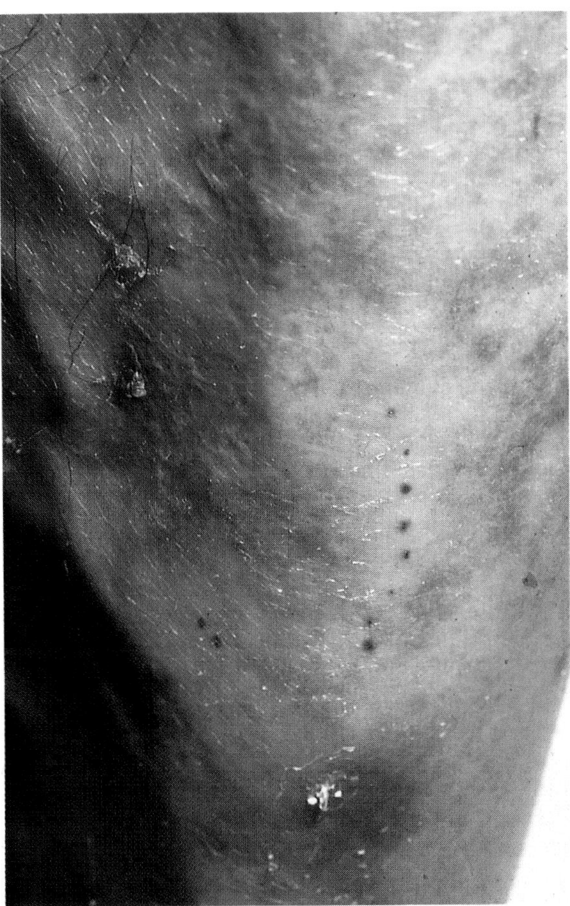

**Fig. 21.3.** Diabetic dermopathy ('shin spots'). (Reproduced by kind permission of Dr Julian Verbov, Royal Liverpool University Hospital.)

### *'Diabetic thick skin' (including scleroedema diabeticorum)*

'Scleroedema' describes a rare condition with marked non-pitting induration and thickening of the skin. Two types have been described. The first is *scleroedema of Bushke*, which is not significantly associated with diabetes and may follow acute viral or streptococcal infection. The second type, *scleroedema diabeticorum*, which tends to be more persistent, is associated with IDDM. Both forms can involve the back of the neck and the upper part of the back, but that associated with diabetes frequently extends to involve the upper limbs and hands and can result in joint contractures [32].

More common 'diabetic thick skin' syndromes (see Chapter 22) may share a similar pathophysiological mechanism with scleroedema [33]. The diabetic thick skin syndrome includes fibroproliferative complications of the diabetic hand, namely Dupuytren's contractures (Fig. 21.4), sclerosing tenosynovitis of the palmar flexor tendons, Garrod's knuckle pads (Fig. 21.5) and carpal tunnel syndrome [34]. Various manifestations of diabetic thick skin syndrome are apparently common in IDDM, occurring in 22–40% of adult patients [32] and in 51% of diabetic children, many of whom have contractures and limited joint mobility of the fingers due to the

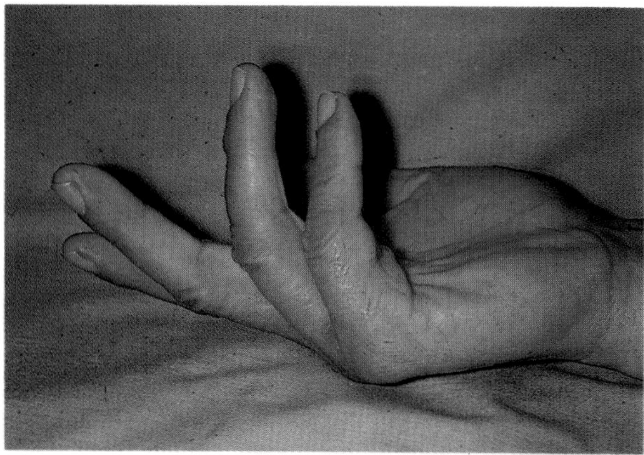

**Fig. 21.4.** Dupuytren's contracture in a diabetic patient with thickened skin and limited joint mobility. (Courtesy of Mr M.H. Matthewson, Addenbrooke's Hospital, Cambridge.)

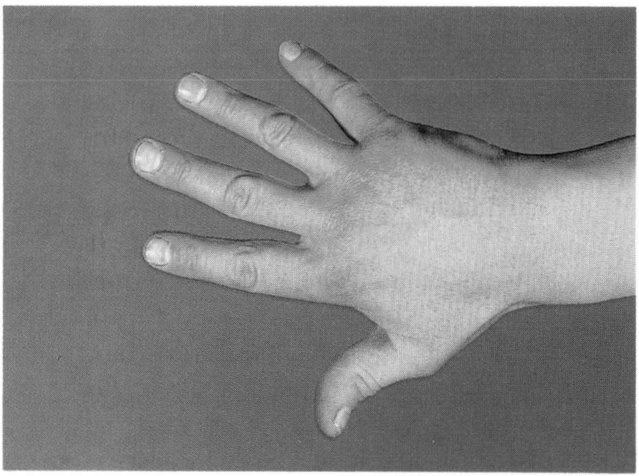

**Fig. 21.5.** Garrod's knuckle pads — thickening of the skin and superficial subcutaneous tissues — overlying the proximal interphalangeal joints in a patient with IDDM. (Courtesy of Mr M.H. Matthewson, Addenbrooke's Hospital, Cambridge.)

condition [35]. The reported prevalence in NIDDM ranges from 4 to 70%.

The thickened skin of diabetic patients can be distinguished both histologically and ultrastructurally from other non-diabetic forms of thick skin such as progressive systemic sclerosis. Diabetic thick skin shows a normal epidermis and thickening of the dermis with hyalinized, disorganized collagen which extends into subcutaneous fat. Small amounts of acid mucopolysaccharide are often deposited in the papillary dermis. On electron microscopy, diabetic thick skin has a predominance of densely packed, large (>60-nm diameter) collagen fibres, distinct from the bimodal distribution in scleroderma. The accumulation of large collagen fibres in diabetic thick skin can be explained by the known effects of hyperglycaemia on collagen metabolism [34, 36].

Most diabetic patients with thickened skin are asymptomatic and require no treatment. Diabetic knuckle pads can be treated by the application of liquid nitrogen, and Dupuytren's contractures by surgery. It is not yet known whether strict diabetic control can prevent or reverse diabetic skin thickening.

### *Acanthosis nigricans*

This uncommon condition is characterized by brown, velvety, hyperkeratotic plaques which most often affect the axillae, back of the neck and other flexural areas. The lesions range in severity from minimal discoloration which spares the skin creases to thicker, more extensive hyperkeratotic areas (Fig. 21.6).

Histologically, the epidermis is extensively folded, slightly thickened and has increased cell density. The dark colour is caused by an increased number of melanocytes [37] (Fig. 21.7).

In 1976, Kahn *et al.* drew attention to the frequent association of acanthosis nigricans with a large heterogeneous group of disorders with the common feature of insulin resistance, ranging from asymptomatic hyperinsulinaemia to overt diabetes [38]. Flier [37] has classified the acanthosis–insulin resistance syndromes into two main groups, type A (genetic defects in the insulin receptor or post-receptor mechanisms) and type B (acquired insulin resistance, due to autoantibodies directed against the insulin receptor).

Endocrine-associated acanthosis nigricans

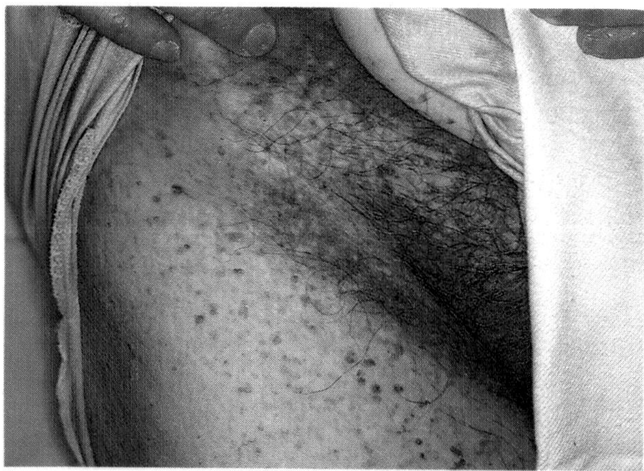

**Fig. 21.6.** Acanthosis nigricans in the groin. (Reproduced by kind permission of Dr Shevaun Mendelsohn, Royal Liverpool Hospital.)

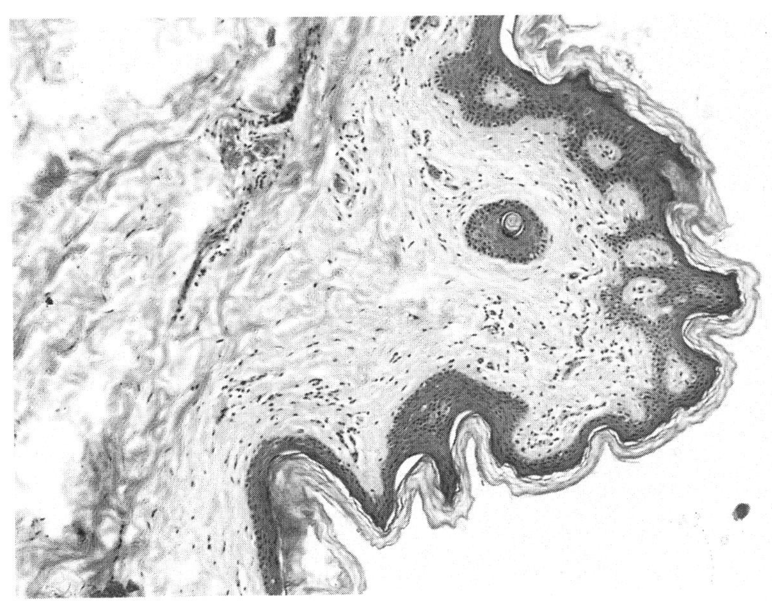

**Fig. 21.7.** Acanthosis nigricans, histological features (see text for explanation). Haematoxylin and eosin stain, ×350. (Reproduced by kind permission of Dr T.W. Stewart, Royal Liverpool Hospital.)

appears to be a true cutaneous marker, if not of overt diabetes, then at least of abnormal carbohydrate metabolism. These patients should be encouraged to maintain an ideal weight and participate in regular exercise. The mechanism responsible for the development of acanthosis nigricans is uncertain, although the high circulating insulin concentrations associated with insulin resistance could promote epidermal growth.

Acanthosis and insulin resistance can also be associated in obesity, where receptor and post-receptor defects have been shown to play a role in the insulin-resistant state, and in various endocrinopathies (recently reviewed in [39]). Acanthosis nigricans can also occur without insulin resistance, as a paraneoplastic syndrome (usually associated with gastrointestinal malignancy), in which epidermal growth may be stimulated by tumour-derived growth factors.

If necessary, the cosmetically disturbing appearance of acanthosis nigricans may be improved by applying mild peeling agents such as 5% salicyclic acid in a bland cream. One report documents improvement with oral fish oil (omega-3-fatty-acid-rich) [40].

### *Bullosis diabeticorum (diabetic bullae)*

This very rare condition, first described by Kramer [41], affects men more than women and has a predilection for patients with long-standing diabetes complicated by neuropathy [42]. One or more tense blisters on a non-inflammatory base appear suddenly, often overnight, with no preceding trauma, and heal during some weeks with or without scarring. The lesions are usually confined to the feet and lower legs but may involve the hands (Fig. 21.8).

Recent electron-microscopical studies [42] have revealed a subepithelial blister with the split occurring at the level of the lamina lucida; the appearance of intra-epithelial splitting reported previously may have resulted from biopsies of older lesions in which the blister floor had re-epithelialized.

The condition can only be diagnosed in diabetic patients in whom other bullous disorders have been excluded by the absence of immunoglobulin deposition (demonstrated by direct immunofluorescence) in the skin. It is not clear how this entity differs from the localized variant of bullous pemphigoid, in which direct immunofluorescence of

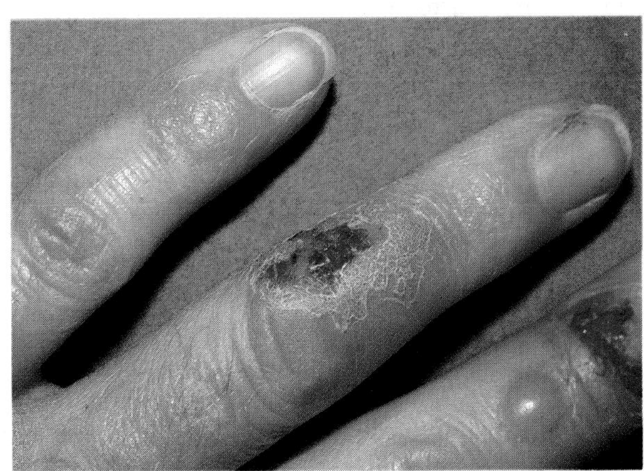

**Fig. 21.8.** Bullosis diabeticorum.

the basement membrane is frequently negative and the split is also in the lamina lucida.

The aetiology is not understood, but a recent study showed a reduced threshold to suction-induced blister formation in diabetic patients [43].

## Cutaneous complications of diabetic treatment

### *Complications of sulphonylureas*

Various cutaneous reactions occur with first-generation sulphonylureas such as chlorpropamide and tolbutamide. These usually develop in the first two months of treatment and may be either toxic or allergic.

Two to three per cent of patients develop maculopapular eruptions [44]. Erythema multiforme major (Stevens–Johnson syndrome; see Fig. 21.9), consisting predominantly of mucous membrane blistering, has been described with chlorpropamide [45]. As with other causes of the Stevens–Johnson syndrome, ocular involvement can be serious and can potentially lead to blindness; an early ophthalmological opinion must therefore be sought. Other rare skin manifestations include purpura (with or without thrombocytopenia), photosensitivity, erythema nodosum, and exacerbations of porphyria cutanea tarda. Generalized hypersensitivity reactions have also been reported. Alcohol-associated facial flushing (the 'chlorpropamide–alcohol flush', or CPAF) often develops with chlorpropamide [46].

Second-generation sulphonylureas are now widely prescribed, but seem to cause fewer cutaneous side-effects: for example, skin reactions have been reported in only 0.2% of patients taking glyburide [47]. Alcohol-induced flushing, does not occur commonly with second-generation sulphonylureas [46].

### *Complications of insulin treatment*

Cutaneous reactions to insulin previously occurred in half of the patients treated, but have become much less frequent since purified pork and human insulins were introduced. The following reactions have been described.

#### INSULIN ALLERGY

This may be local or systemic and develops within 1–4 weeks of starting treatment. Local allergy was

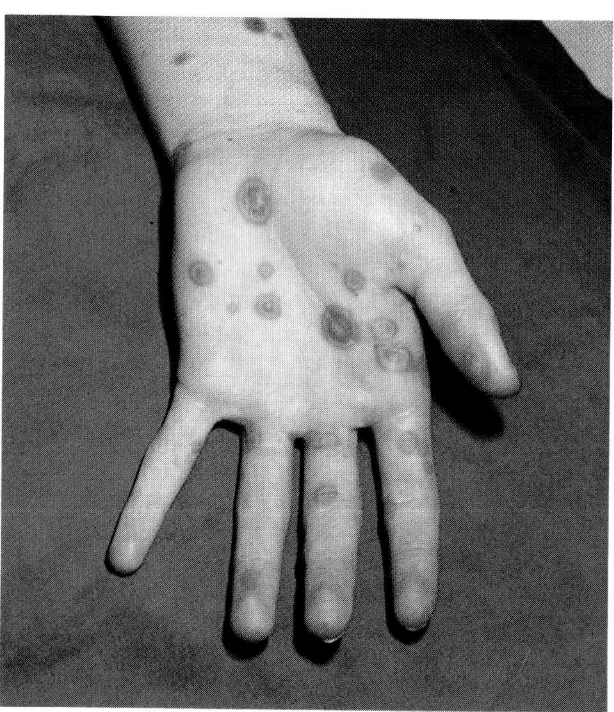

(a)

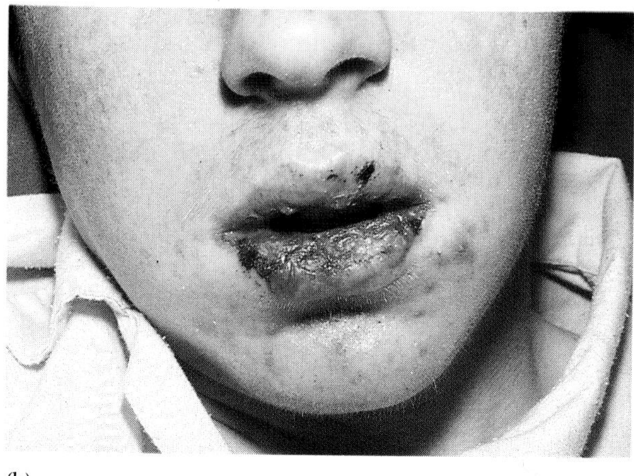

(b)

**Fig. 21.9.** Stevens–Johnson syndrome, showing typical 'target lesions' of erythema multiforme (a), and mouth ulceration (b). This is a rare complication of treatment with sulphonylureas. (Reproduced by kind permission of Dr Shevaun Mendelsohn, Royal Liverpool University Hospital.)

extremely common in the 1960s with the use of 'impure' insulins [48], but the reported prevalence in patients receiving monocomponent porcine insulin was zero in one study [48] and 5% in another [49]. Local reactions are of three types. The commonest is the late-phase reaction, a biphasic IgE reaction characterized by immediate burning and pruritus with a wheal and flare at the injection site. It may resolve or become indurated, with pruritus continuing for hours to days. Two rarer forms are the Arthus-type reaction, producing a pruritic, painful nodule 6–8 h after injection, and the delayed hypersensitivity reaction, which is similar but appears 12–24 h after injection.

Systemic manifestations include generalized urticaria and, rarely, anaphylaxis. Urticarial allergic reactions to newer insulins are uncommon, with an incidence of 0.1–0.2% [50] and anaphylaxis is very rare. Even lower frequencies should be expected with the more widespread use of human insulins, although patients sensitized to animal insulins may continue to suffer anaphylaxis even when changed to human insulin [51].

Insulin allergy has also been described to high molecular weight insulin aggregates [52] and granulomatous insulin reactions to additives such as protamine or serfen used in some depot formulations [53, 54].

#### LIPODYSTROPHY

Lipoatrophy and insulin hypertrophy are complications of insulin injection. Lipoatrophy presents as circumscribed depressed areas of skin at the injection site and occasionally at distant sites as well. Before purified human insulins were available, lipoatrophy occurred in about 25% of insulin-treated patients [55]. Improvement or resolution of lesions has been noted in most patients after changing to purified porcine insulin [49]. Lipoatrophy may be due to a local immune response to injected insulin [56].

Insulin hypertrophy (lipohypertrophy) presents as a soft dermal nodule with normal surface epidermis at the injection site, which has often been used for many years (Fig. 21.10). This reaction may be due to the lipogenic action of insulin.

#### IDIOSYNCRATIC REACTIONS

Pigmentation can occur at the injection site, and rarely, keloids may form. Bilateral symmetrical plaques resembling acanthosis nigricans have also been reported at the site of repeated injections [57].

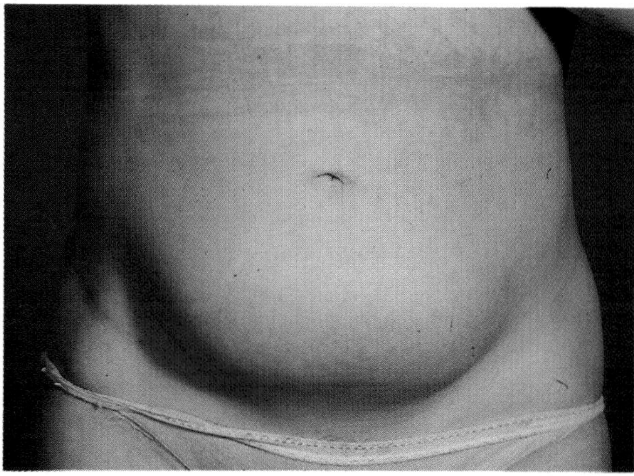

**Fig. 21.10.** Lipohypertrophy at site of habitual insulin injection.

### Glucagonoma syndrome (necrolytic migratory erythema)

This rare syndrome, due to a glucagon-secreting islet-cell neoplasm, was first described by Becker in 1942 [58]. Sixty to seventy per cent of glucagonoma patients develop a polymorphous, erythematous eruption with peripheral scaling which waxes and wanes in cycles of 7–14 days and may remit and relapse spontaneously. Superficial vesiculation can lead to erosions and necrosis. The eruption is usually worst around the mouth, in the groin and perineum and around the genitals. Associated features include painful glossitis, weight loss, relatively mild diabetes (in 80–90%), intermittent diarrhoea, mood changes and venous thrombosis (which commonly causes death).

Similar rashes may occur without glucagonoma or elevated plasma glucagon levels and may also develop in zinc deficiency [59, 60]. The rash may respond to zinc supplementation and treatment with somatostatin or its analogues may be helpful, even when glucagon levels are not greatly suppressed [61]. The tumour and secondary deposits can be treated by chemotherapy (e.g. streptozotocin) or embolization.

SUSAN E. HALL
R. GARY SIBBALD

### References

1 Braverman I. Cutaneous manifestations of diabetes mellitus. *Med Clin North Am* 1971; **55**: 1019–29.

2 Sibbald RG, Schachter RK. The skin and diabetes mellitus. *Int J Dermatol* 1984; **23**: 567–84.

3 Neilly JB, Martin A, Simpson N, MacCuish AG. Pruritus in diabetes mellitus. *Diabetes Care* 1986; **9**: 273–5.

4 Oppenheim M. *Eigentumliche disseminierte Degeneration des Bindegeswebes der Haut bei einem Diabetickes*, Vol 179. 1931: 1929–30.

5 Urbach E. Beiträge zu einer physiologischen und pathologischen Chemie der Haut; eine neue diabetische Stoffwechseldermatose: Nekrobiosis Lipoidica Diabeticorum. *Arch Dermatol Syphilol* 1932; **166**: 273–85.

6 Muller SA, Winkelman RK. Necrobiosis lipoidica diabeticorum. *Arch Dermatol* 1966; **93**: 272–81.

7 Alegre VA, Winkleman RK. A new histological feature of necrobiosis lipoidica diabeticorum: lymphoid nodules. *J Cut Pathol* 1988; **15**: 75–7.

8 Heny MC, Allen SG, Song MK, Heng MK. Focal endothelial cell degeneration and proliferative endarteritis in trauma-induced early lesions of necrobiosis lipoidica diabeticorum. *Am J Dermatopathol* 1991; **13**: 108–114.

9 Jelinek JE. *The Skin in Diabetes*. Philadelphia: Lea & Febiger, 1986: 31–72.

10 Chernowsky ME. Current concepts of necrobiosis lipoidica. *South Med J* 1961; **54**: 25–9.

11 Heite HJ, Scharwenka HX. Erythema elevatum diutium, Granuloma annulare, Necrobiosis lipoidica und Granulomatosis disciformis Gottran-Miesches; eine vergleichende häufigkeitsanalytische Studie. *Arch Klin Exp Dermatol* 1959; **208**: 260–90.

12 Dandona P, Freedman D, Barter D, Majewski BB, Rhodes EL, Watson B. Glycosylated haemoglobin in patients with necrobiosis lipoidica and granuloma annulare. *Clin Exp Dermatol* 1981; **6**: 299–302.

13 Boulton AJ, Cutfield RG, Abouganem D *et al*. Necrobiosis lipoidica diabeticorum: a clinico-pathological study. *J Am Acad Dermatol* 1988; **18**: 530–7.

14 Quimby SR, Muller SA, Schroeter AL *et al*. Necrobiosis lipoidica diabeticorum: platelet survival and response to inhibitors. *Cutis* 1989; **43**: 213–6.

15 Littler CM, Tschen EH. Pentoxifylline for necrobiosis lipoidica diabeticorum (letter). *J Amer Acad Dermatol* 1987; **17**: 314–6.

16 Fox TC. Ringed eruption of the fingers. *Br J Dermatol* 1895; **7**: 91–5.

17 Wells RS, Smith MA. The natural history of granuloma annulare. *Br J Dermatol* 1963; **75**: 199–205.

18 Romaine R, Rudner EJ, Altman J. Papular granuloma annulare and diabetes mellitus. *Arch Dermatol* 1968; **98**: 152–4.

19 Delaney TJ, Gold SC, Leppard B. Disseminated perforating granuloma annulare. *Br J Dermatol* 1973; **89**: 523–6.

20 Shimiza H, Harada T, Baba E *et al*. Perforating granuloma annulare. *Int J Dermatol* 1985; **24**: 581–3.

21 Meier-Ewart H, Allenby CF. Granuloma annulare and diabetes mellitus. *Arch Dermatol Res* 1971; **241**: 194–8.

22 Mobacken H, Gisslen H, Johannison G. Granuloma annulare cortisone-glucose tolerance test in a non-diabetic group. *Acta Derm Veneneol* 1970; **50**: 440–4.

23 Muhlemann MF, Williams DRR. Localized granuloma annulare is associated with insulin dependent diabetes mellitus. *Br J Dermatol* 1984; **111**: 325–9.

24 Andersen BL, Verdich J. Granuloma annulare and diabetes mellitus. *Clin Exp Dermatol* 1979; **4**: 31–7.

25 Kidd GS, Graff GE, Davies BF *et al*. Glucose tolerance in granuloma annulare. *Diabetes Care* 1985; **8**: 380–4.

26 Friedman-Birnbaum R, Haim S, Gideone O, Barzilai A. Histocompatibility antigens in granuloma annulare. *Br J Dermatol* 1978; **98**: 452–8.

27 Melin H. An atrophic circumscribed skin lesion in the lower extremities of diabetics. *Acta Med Scand* 1964; **176** (suppl 423): 1–75.

28 Binkley GW. Dermopathy in the diabetic syndrome. *Arch Dermatol* 1965; **92**: 625–34.

29 Danowski TS, Sabeh G, Sarver MF. Shin spots and diabetes mellitus. *Am J Med Sci* 1966; **251**: 570–5.

30 Lithner F, Bergenheim T, Borssen B. Extensor digitorum brevis in diabetic neuropathy: a controlled evaluation in diabetic patients aged 15–50 years. *J Int Med* 1991; **230**: 449–53.

31 Vijuyusingam SM, Thai AC, Chan HL. Non-infective skin associations of diabetes mellitus. *Ann Acad Med (Singapore)* 1988; **17**: 526–35.

32 Editorial. Diabetic skin, joints and eyes. How are they related? *Lancet* 1987; **ii**: 313–4.

33 Hanna W, Friesen D, Bombardier C, Gladman D, Hanna A. Pathologic features of diabetic thick skin. *J Am Acad Dermatol* 1987; **16**: 546–53.

34 Seibold JR, Uitto J, Dorart BB, Prockop DJ. Collagen synthesis and collagenase activity in dermal fibroblasts from patients with diabetes and digital sclerosis. *J Lab Clin Med* 1985; **105**: 664–7.

35 Buckingham B, Perejda AJ, Sandborg C, Kershnar AK, Uitto J. Skin, joints, and pulmonary changes in type 1 diabetes mellitus. *Am J Dis Child* 1986; **140**: 420–3.

36 Ville DB, Powers ML. Effect of glucose and insulin on collagen secretion by human skin fibroblasts *in vitro*. *Nature* 1977; **268**: 156–8.

37 Flier JS. Metabolic importance of acanthosis nigricans. *Arch Dermatol* 1985; **121**: 193–4.

38 Kahn CR, Flier JS, Bar RS *et al*. The syndromes of insulin resistance and acanthosis nigricans. Insulin receptor disorders in man. *N Engl J Med* 1976; **294**: 739–45.

39 Ober KP. Acanthosis nigricans and insulin resistance associated with hypothyroidism. *Arch Dermatol* 1985; **121**: 229–31.

40 Sherertz EF. Improved acanthosis nigricans with lipodystrophic diabetes during dietary fish oil supplementation. *Arch Dermatol* 1988; **124**: 1094–6.

41 Kramer DW. Early warning signs of impending gangrene in diabetes. *Med J Rec* 1930; **132**: 338–42.

42 Toonstra J. Bullosis diabeticorum: Report of a case with a review of the literature. *J Am Acad Dermatol* 1985; **13**: 799–805.

43 Bernstein JE, Levine LE, Mederican MM *et al*. Reduced threshold to suction-induced blister formation in insulin-dependent diabetes. *J Am Acad Dermatol* 1983; **8**: 790–1.

44 Stowers JM, Borthwick LJ. Oral hypoglycaemic drugs: clinical pharmacology and therapeutic use. *Drugs* 1977; **14**: 41–56.

45 Stewart RC, Piazza EU, Hyman J, Hurwitz D. Chlorpropamide therapy of diabetes. *N Engl J Med* 1959; **26**: 427–30.

46 Skillman TG, Feldman JM. The pharmacology of sulfonylureas. *Am J Med* 1981; **70**: 361–72.

47 Bigby M, Jick S, Jick H *et al*. Drug-induced cutaneous reactions: a report from the Boston Collaborative Drug Surveillance Program on 15 438 consecutive in-patients (1975–1982). *J Am Med Ass* 1986; **250**: 3358–63.

48 Arkins JA, Enghieing NH, Lennon EJ. *Allergy* 1926; **33**: 69.

49 Wright AD, Walsh CH, Fitzgerald MG, Malins JM. Very pure porcine insulin in clinical practice. *Br Med J* 1979; **1**: 25–7.

50 Anderson JA, Adkinson NF. Allergic reactions to drugs and

biologic agents. *J Am Med Ass* 1987; **258**: 2891–9.

51 Fineberg SE, Galloway JA, Fineberg NS *et al*. Immunogenicity of recombinant DNA human insulin. *Diabetologia* 1983; **25**: 465–9.

52 Ratner RE, Philips TM, Steiner M. Persistent cutaneous insulin allergy resulting from high molecular weight insulin aggregates. *Diabetes* 1990; **39**: 728–33.

53 Hulshof MM, Faber WR, Kniestedt WF *et al*. Granulomatous hypersensitivity to protamine as a complication of insulin therapy. *Br J Dermatol* 1992; **127**: 286–8.

54 Jermendy G, Szabo E. Granulomatous dermatitis caused by surfen in diabetics treated with Insulin-depot-s-Richter (Monotard MC, Novo) *Orvosi Hetila* 1989; **130**: 1825–8.

55 Renold AE, Winegard AI, Martin DB. Diabète sucré et tissu adipeux. *Helv Med Acta* 1957; **24**: 322–7.

56 Reeves WG, Allen BR, Tattersall RB. Insulin-induced lipoatrophy: Evidence for an immune pathogenesis. *Br Med J* 1980; **280**: 1500–3.

57 Matthew G, Fleming MD, Stewart IS. Cutaneous insulin reaction resembling acanthosis nigricans. *Arch Dermatol* 1986; **122**: 1054–6.

58 Becker SW, Kahn D, Rothman S. Cutaneous manifestations of internal malignant tumours. *Arch Dermatol Syphilol* 1942; **45**: 1069.

59 Goodenberger DM, Lawley TJ, Strober W *et al*. Necrolytic migratory erythema without glucagonoma: Report of two cases. *Arch Dermatol* 1979; **115**: 1429–32.

60 Tucker SB, Schroeter AL, Brown PW *et al*. Acquired zinc deficiency: Cutaneous manifestations typical of acrodermatitis enteropathica. *J Am Med Ass* 1976; **235**: 2399–402.

61 Sohier J, Jeanmougin M, Lombrail P, Passa P. Rapid improvement of skin lesions in glucagonomas with intravenous somatostatin infusion. *Lancet* 1980; **i**: 40.

# 22 Connective-Tissue and Joint Disease in Diabetes Mellitus

**Summary**

• Joint disease in diabetes is mainly due to either excessive collagen deposition or dysfunction of the autonomic nervous system.
• In the hand, there can be limited joint mobility (LJM), tenosynoviosclerosis (trigger finger), Dupuytren's disease and carpal tunnel syndrome.
• Diabetic collagenosis in the hand, particularly LJM, is associated with an increased prevalence of microvascular complications.
• Frozen shoulder (adhesive capsulitis) with painful restricted shoulder movement has a recurrent relapsing course with eventual recovery of some degree.
• Ankylosing hyperostosis of the spine (symptomless or causing back pain and stiffness) occurs mainly in NIDDM.
• Algodystrophy presents with pain, swelling, autonomic dysfunction and diffuse osteoporosis on X-ray; Charcot's joints and the shoulder–hand syndrome are examples of this disorder.

The first description of a neuropathic joint in diabetes was made in 1936 but it is only in the last two decades that the more subtle articular and periarticular features of diabetes have been clearly defined. The diabetic atherosclerotic plaque and capillary basement membrane thickening are both disorders of extracellular connective tissue and it is, therefore, not surprising that the interstitial connective tissues of bone, joints and periarticular structures are also affected (for reviews see [1–4]).

The disorders involving primarily skin and bone are described elsewhere (Chapters 21 and 22). The diseases of joints and periarticular structures fall into two broad groups:

1 Diseases characterized by an excessive deposition of connective tissue (mainly collagen).
2 Diseases related to autonomic nervous system dysfunction.

Some disorders, for example shoulder–hand syndrome, may include both processes.

## Articular and periarticular disease usually characterized by excessive collagen deposition

### *The hand*

Lundbaeck described hand stiffness in young diabetic patients in 1957 and since then there has been increasing awareness of the link between many hand abnormalities and diabetes [5] (Table 22.1). One or more abnormalities may be present in the same patient: for example, limited joint mobility (LJM), tenosynoviosclerosis and carpal tunnel syndrome comprise a common triad in the adult diabetic hand. In many accounts, diagnosis of the specific abnormality has been imprecise and misleading and has led to unhelpful terms such as 'diabetic hand syndrome' and 'juvenile diabetic cheiro-arthropathy'. These are prejudicial as larger joints such as the elbow or knee may also be affected. In a severe case, the signs of thick, tight, waxy skin, joint restriction (with or without flexion contractures) and tenosynoviosclerosis are highly reminiscent or scleroderma ('pseudoscleroderma'). Occasionally, the dorsal dermal sclerosis can be seen proximal to the metacarpophalangeal (MCP) joints, thereby fulfilling the American Rheumatism Association criteria for frank scleroderma. In one study, 81% of diabetic children with dermal sclerosis of hands

**Table 22.1.** The diabetic hand (after [5]).

| Abnormality | Site | Comments |
|---|---|---|
| Thick, tight, waxy skin | Dorsal surface | Affects one-third of patients with limited joint mobility |
| Limited joint mobility (LJM) | MCP and PIP joints (often beginning at little finger) most commonly. Wrists, elbows, knees, less commonly | Children and adults: painless |
| Stiff hand | All fingers | Adults; associated with skin thickening, calcified vessels and vascular insufficiency |
| Dupuytren's disease (DD) | MCP and PIP joints (especially middle and ring fingers) | Thickened palmar fascia; male : female ratio 6 : 1; 10–15% of patients with this abnormality are diabetic |
| Flexor tenosynoviosclerosis and tenosynovitis | Especially thumb, middle and ring fingers | Female preponderance; 'trigger finger' |
| Carpal tunnel syndrome | Median nerve distribution | 5–16% of patients are diabetic; compression and neural factors |
| Reflex sympathetic dystrophy or algodystrophy | Contractures of finger joints | Usually part of 'shoulder–hand syndrome' with muscle atrophy and bone demineralization; painful |

also had involvement of forefeet and toes [6]. Terminology emphasizing connective tissue disease of the diabetic hand should, therefore, be replaced by less committed terms such as 'diabetic collagenosis'.

### LIMITED JOINT MOBILITY

If the tips of fingers and palms of the normal hand are opposed, the MCP and proximal interphalangeal (PIP) joints can be fully extended. Inability to do this, the 'prayer sign' (Fig. 22.1), has proved a useful clinical screening test for LJM. It may also be positive in the presence of finger flexor tendon sheath disease, but it may be distinguished by the fingers involved (Table 22.1), a history of trigger finger or the palpation of a nodule in the tendon sheath. If the elbows are elevated, the degree of possible wrist extension can also be estimated (normally at least 90°).

The reported prevalence of LJM in young IDDM patients is between 8 and 42%. In the largest study, 30% of 309 patients aged 1–28 years had contractures and one-third of affected children had dermal sclerosis [7]. LJM is not apparently related to sex, insulin dosage or short-term metabolic control (as assessed by glycosylated haemoglobin). However, long-term quality of diabetic control may be relevant, as improvement has been reported if control is optimized. The development of LJM is linked to the duration of diabetes: two-thirds of affected young patients with diabetes for more than 5 years will have moderate or severe limitation of three or more joints and affected patients are 4 times more likely to fall below the 25th percentile for height [5]. LJM is not confined to children and young adults with IDDM, but is also a feature of adult-onset IDDM and of NIDDM, at similar prevalence rates [8, 9]. Although genetic factors have been suggested in the development of LJM, with an increased incidence in first-degree relatives, no HLA associations have been identified [10].

The significance of LJM is not the relatively mild disability which it imposes on some diabetic patients, but its possible role as a marker for more sinister diabetic complications. The relationship between LJM and retinopathy has been amply confirmed: 43% of those with LJM and more than 4 years' duration of diabetes had retinopathy, while only 15% of patients with matched disease duration without LJM had retinopathy [11]. Of 299 patients with retinopathy, 48% had LJM whereas only 24% of patients without retinopathy were affected [12]. The association between LJM and other microvascular complications, such as neuropathy and nephropathy, is less clear [9].

A defective microcirculation is likely to be the common denominator between diabetic patients with LJM, hypertensive subjects with LJM [13] and patients with scleroderma. The capillary loop abnormalities at finger nailfolds have been helpful

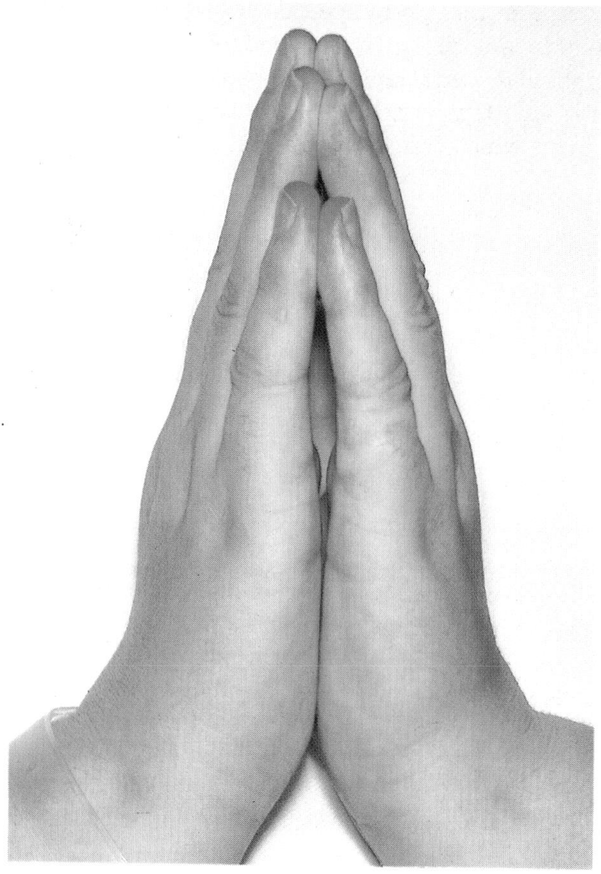

Fig. 22.1. The prayer sign. In normal subjects, finger tips and the palmar surfaces of fingers and palms can be perfectly apposed but in patients with LJM this is impossible. Flexion contractures at the metacarpophalangeal (MCP) and proximal interphalangeal (PIP) joints are demonstrated. Note the swelling of little-finger PIP joints and this patient's inability to extend her wrists fully.

in the assessment of scleroderma, but no abnormalities have been observed in diabetic patients with microvascular disease and LJM [14].

## DUPUYTREN'S DISEASE (DD)

DD is diagnosed by observing or palpating thickened palmar fascia, a palmar or digital nodule (as opposed to a nodule in a tendon sheath), skin tethering and, in late cases, digital contracture. The reported prevalence of DD in diabetes varies from 1.6 to 63% but is probably about 40% [2, 15]. About 10–15% of patients with DD are likely to have diabetes [5, 15]. The male : female ratio is about 6 : 1 [5]. It is linked to the duration of disease but may also be present in up to 16% of adult patients at the time of diagnosis of diabetes [2]. In non-diabetic DD, the lesions are mainly in the little and ring finger rays, but the middle and ring fingers are most affected in diabetes [15].

DD, like LJM, is a marker of microvascular disease [12, 13]. Thirty-six per cent of 299 patients with retinopathy had DD, as opposed to only 16% of diabetic subjects without retinopathy [12].

Increased amounts of type III collagen have been identified in the diseased palmar fascia and especially in the nodular tissue. The increased proportions of type III collagen and type I trimer are typical of embryonic collagen and increased amounts of sulphated glycosaminoglycans present in DD are characteristic of immature tendinous structures [16]. The active deposition of connective tissue in DD is by contractile 'myofibroblasts' and it is also worth noting that these cells have also been reported in the nodules of Ledderhose's disease of the plantar fascia and Peyronie's disease of the penis, both of which are more common in diabetes.

## TENOSYNOVIOSCLEROSIS AND TENOSYNOVITIS

The deposition of excessive connective tissue in flexor tendon sheaths of the hand in diabetes can lead to 'trigger finger' [5, 6]. Palpation of the palm of the hand during passive movement of the fingers can sometimes demonstrate a nodule and finger contractures can occur in chronic involvement. The term 'tenosynoviosclerosis' may be preferred as inflammatory changes in the tendon sheaths are minimal or absent. The index and little fingers are relatively spared and there is a female preponderance [5]. Unlike LJM, trigger finger is often painful.

## CARPAL TUNNEL SYNDROME (CTS)

In a series of 379 patients with CTS, 63 (16.6%) were found to be diabetic [17]. An association with LJM has been proposed, with the suggestion that the median nerve is compressed by excessive collagen deposition in the flexor retinaculum, but the pathogenesis of CTS in diabetes has been inadequately studied. It is certain that a true compression neuropathy can occur but the contribution of diffuse peripheral neuropathy is uncertain. There is some evidence that vitamin B6 (pyridoxine) deficiency may play a part but, although vitamin B6 deficiency has been reported in diabetes, anecdotal reports have failed to demonstrate improvement with vitamin B6 supplements in diabetic CTS; a formal study is awaited.

### *The shoulder*

Adhesive capsulitis (or frozen shoulder) is characterized by painful restriction of all shoulder movements. Episodes of painful restriction of shoulders in diabetic patients are typically recurrent and multifocal. The thickened joint capsule is closely applied and adherent to the head of the humerus and arthrography demonstrates a marked reduction in volume of the glenohumeral joint. There may be increased periarticular uptake of bone-seeking isotopes followed by bone demineralization. A histological study of capsular tissue from a diabetic with frozen shoulder showed microvascular disease and the proliferation of fibroblasts and myofibroblasts as seen in DD. This contrasts with the more inflammatory histology of idiopathic capsulitis.

In one study of 800 diabetic patients, 10% had shoulder capsulitis compared with 2.5% of non-diabetic controls [18]; conversely, up to 28% of unselected patients with shoulder capsulitis have been found to have abnormal glucose tolerance.

By careful matching for age, sex and disease duration, Fisher *et al*. have demonstrated an increased incidence of shoulder capsulitis in diabetic patients who also have LJM of the hands [19]. However, it is unlikely that excessive connective tissue deposition in the shoulder capsule is the only factor in the development of the painful restricted shoulder, as the natural history is one of recurrent relapsing episodes with eventual partial or even complete recovery. Superadded inflammatory or autonomic neuropathic factors may contribute; formal comparison of the idiopathic with the diabetic frozen shoulder should provide further insight.

### *The spine*

The main skeletal abnormality in diabetes, particularly in IDDM, is diabetic osteopenia (see Chapter 23). By contrast, some NIDDM patients display excessive bone deposition in certain sites, most commonly the spine. Ankylosing hyperostosis of the spine (Forestier's disease) occurs in 2–4% of the normal population aged over 40 years; the prevalence of 13% in diabetic patients (rising to 21% in the group aged 60–69 years) suggests that the association is genuine [20]. The condition is often asymptomatic or may cause back pain and stiffness. It is characterized by exuberant osteophytes which form anterior bridges between vertebrae and sclerosis of the underlying vertebral cortex. There is a predilection for the right side of the thoracic spine. The sparing of the posterior spinal joints may account for the preservation of relatively full spinal movements. Ankylosing spondylitis is easily distinguished by its younger age of onset, sacro-iliac joint involvement, its association with HLA B27 and the vertical syndesmophytes between vertebral bodies (rather than curved, beak-like osteophytes of hyperostosis).

### *Lower limbs*

It has been previously noted that patients with LJM of the hands may also have dermal sclerosis of the feet and lack full knee extension. Recently, an association between shoulder capsulitis and capsulitis of the hip in diabetes has been proposed. Of 61 diabetic patients with shoulder disease, 23 had hip restriction, especially of internal rotation, and in 18 this was bilateral [21].

## Articular and periarticular disease related to autonomic dysfunction

Several syndromes of unknown pathogenesis variously described as 'Sudek's atrophy', 'reflex sympathetic dystrophy', 'transient osteoporosis', and 'migratory osteolysis' have been grouped convincingly under the single heading of algodystrophy [22] (Fig. 22.2). They present with pain (often severely disabling), sometimes swelling and invariably features of autonomic dysfunction. There may be a transient hyperaemic phase (which may persist in Charcot's neuroarthropathy) but, more commonly, patients present with a cold, cyanosed, shiny and tender limb. In established disease, X-rays may show a 'spotty' or diffuse osteoporosis. The condition usually resolves spontaneously, occasionally with fibrosis and contracture.

Trauma remains the commonest predisposing cause, but diabetic patients are also more prone. Of 108 consecutive cases, eight had diabetes: two had shoulder–hand syndrome, two had knee involvement, and in four the foot was affected [23]. Few of these patients underwent glucose tolerance testing and the true prevalence may be higher.

### SHOULDER–HAND SYNDROME

This may be considered a rarer, but exaggerated, form of adhesive capsulitis of the shoulder involving the whole upper limb with striking cold, vasomotor changes and distal oedema. Demineralization of the limb, especially the hand, often occurs. Early active mobilization of the limb is essential but regional intravenous guanethidine blockade or stellate ganglion blockade is often required.

### TRANSIENT OSTEOPOROSIS OF THE HIP

In a study of 34 patients with algodystrophy of the hip, five had diabetes [22]. This may represent an advanced or more intense form of capsulitis of the hip.

### NEUROARTHROPATHY OF THE LOWER LIMB (CHARCOT JOINTS)

This may involve, in order of decreasing frequency, the tarso-metatarsal joints, the metatarsophalangeal (MTP) joints, the ankle and the knee. It now seems clear that the initiating event is an increase in blood flow through the lower leg secondary to sympathetic neuropathy. Clinically, the ankle and foot are hot and swollen, often with less pain than might be anticipated. X-rays demonstrate local osteoporosis which may progress to frank osteolysis and fragmentation of bone and cartilage [3, 23] (Figs 22.3 and 22.4). It may progress through a 'coalescence' stage when the bone ends become sclerotic and then a 'reconstitution' stage, when a new joint space appears, but the evolution of a neuropathic joint may be arrested at any stage (see Chapter 19).

Since the decline of neurosyphilis, diabetes is now the commonest cause of neuropathic joints outside lepromatous regions. If there is any doubt about the diagnosis, however, it is essential to exclude septic arthritis, to which diabetic patients are also prone, by aspiration of a hot joint.

### FOREFOOT OSTEOLYSIS

The pathogenesis of forefoot osteolysis is probably shared with Charcot's neuroarthropathy, but it seems to arise directly from the metatarsals themselves rather than the adjacent joints. The metatarsal heads can dissolve, producing a 'sharpened pencil' or 'sucked candy' appearance [3, 23]. Scler-

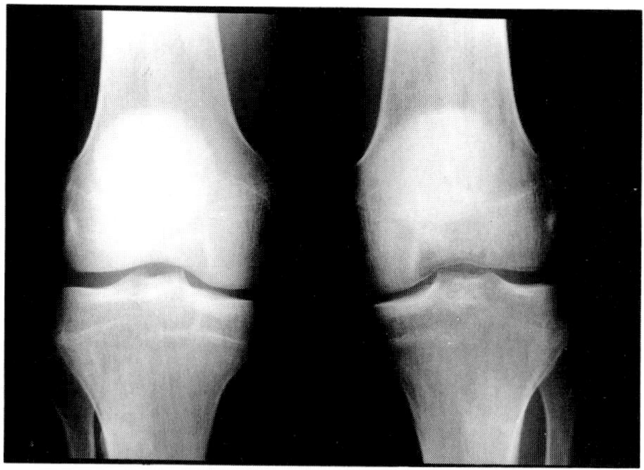

**Fig. 22.2.** Diabetic male aged 26 years. Algodystrophy: minor injury to left knee and increasing pain plus 10° fixed flexion deformity. Left knee was palpably cooler than the right. Normal arthroscopy. The X-ray shows normal right knee. There is demineralization of left femur and tibia. The intercondylar subcortical bone loss of the distal femur is very characteristic. Definite bone loss is seen extending above the patellar level and in the proximal tibia.

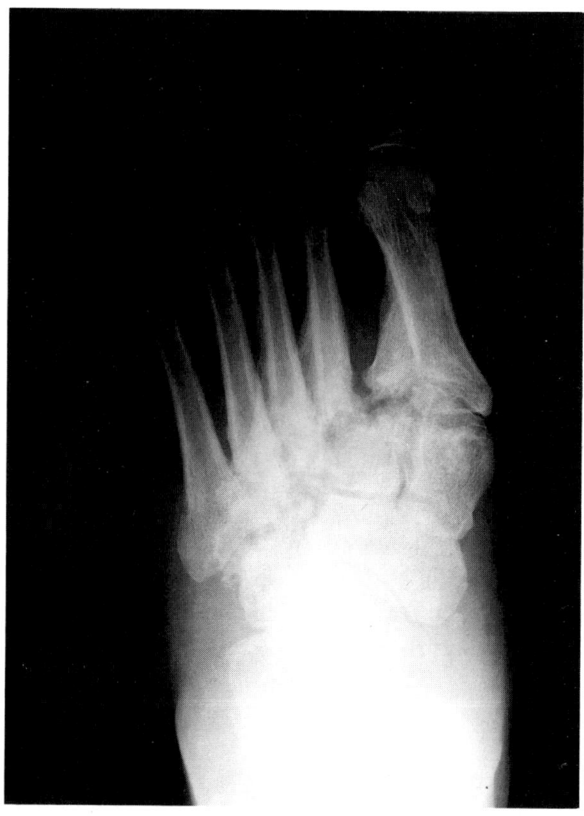

**Fig. 22.3.** Diabetic female aged 24 years. This shows typical Charcot-like changes in tarsometatarsal joints with bone destruction and formation in a thoroughly disorganized fashion. (See also Figs 19.8–19.11.)

osis of bone cortex and reformation of the metatarsal heads often occurs.

## Other joint diseases which may be associated with diabetes

### *Osteoarthritis (OA)*

It is obviously difficult to establish a relationship between such common diseases as OA and diabetes, but a positive correlation has been proposed by controlled studies [24]. The prevalence of OA was higher in young and middle-aged diabetic subjects, and joint damage started at an earlier age and was more severe than in controls. Clinical evidence is scanty but the evidence from studies *in vitro* is impressive (for reviews, see [2, 3]). Cartilage growth is depressed in diabetes and there is reduced synthesis of sulphated proteoglycans, with a reduction in the size of high molecular-weight aggregates. Articular chondrocytes from diabetic hamsters undergo morphological changes and release more collagen-degrading enzymes. Insulin has been shown to stimulate cartilage growth activity and proteoglycan synthesis.

However, OA is more than a simple depletion of proteoglycan from cartilage, also being characterized by bone osteophyte formation and periarticular osteosclerosis. The increased prevalence of ankylosing hyperostosis, a proliferative form of OA affecting the spine (see above), suggests that diabetic patients are at increased risk of generalized OA.

### *Rheumatoid arthritis (RA)*

Thirty-nine out of 295 patients (13%) with RA had a first- or second-degree relative with IDDM [25] and Rudolf *et al.* described seven IDDM children with juvenile RA [26]. As both diseases are associated with HLA DR4, this is not surprising. However, a specific DQβ genotypic marker associated with DR4 has been identified, which is highly associated with diabetes but not with juvenile RA [27]. Payami *et al.* have proposed that IDDM is predisposed to by two HLA-linked alleles, one of which also confers susceptibility to RA [28].

### *Crystal arthropathy (gout and pyrophosphate arthropathy)*

The triad of hyperglycaemia, hyperlipidaemia and hyperuricaemia is well recognized, but obesity is likely to be the linking factor. Although there have been reports of an increased prevalence of diabetes in gouty subjects, a study of glucose tolerance in weight-matched gouty and non-gouty subjects failed to demonstrate any difference [29]. Chronic glucose loading actually promotes uric acid excretion, and the onset of diabetes in patients with established gout is accompanied by a fall in serum urate levels and in the frequency and severity of attacks. However, diabetic ketoacidosis may be complicated by hyperuricaemia, as ketone bodies inhibit renal tubular secretion of uric acid (for review, see [2]). The critical role of renal function in the handling of uric acid in the presence of diabetes was emphasized in a recent study. The lowest uric acid levels were found in male diabetics but the strongest predictor of blood uric acid was plasma creatinine [30]. In conclusion, non-obese diabetics with normal renal function are less likely to develop gout than normal subjects and it is probable that non-obese gouty patients do not have an increased risk of diabetes.

Early descriptions of pyrophosphate arthropathy — characterized by the radiographic appearance of chondrocalcinosis and the clinical syndrome of acute pseudogout — reported an apparent association with diabetes, which has not been confirmed in a large controlled study [31]. However, diabetes and chondrocalcinosis are both associated with haemochromatosis.

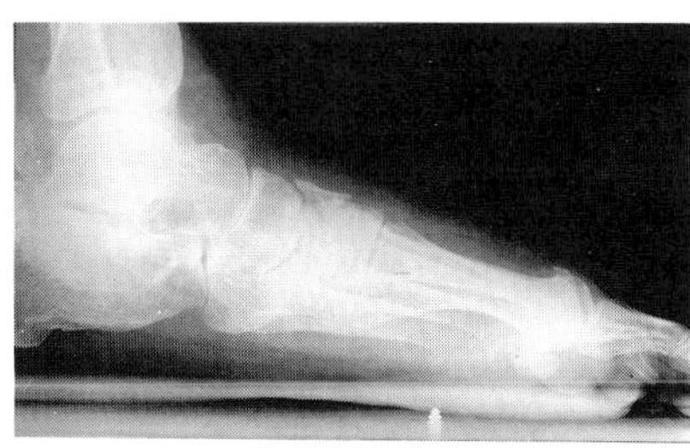

**Fig. 22.4.** Same patient as in Fig. 22.3. Very painful ankle. Bone destruction/osteolysis of talus and calcaneum with greatly increased uptake on bone scan (right). This is evolving into a Charcot arthropathy.

### Pathophysiology of connective-tissue changes in diabetes

Insulin deficiency is probably responsible for two processes highly dependent on insulin as a tissue growth factor: the reduced bone mass of the young diabetic at diagnosis of the disease and the depletion of cartilage proteoglycan in premature OA (see above). With these exceptions, the hallmark of diabetic connective tissue is the excessive deposition of collagen at many periarticular sites and in the skin. It is possible that the increased permeability of diabetic capillaries may trigger proliferation of vessel wall and extravascular connective tissue. The excessive new bone formation found in ankylosing hyperostosis, hyperostosis frontalis interna and osteitis condensans ilii (all more common in diabetes) may be attributable to overactivity of bone growth factors, either through increased tissue concentrations (for example, of insulin-like growth factors [32]) or changes in receptor function. Such growth factors may also stimulate excess collagen deposition in the soft tissues of skin and periarticular structures.

The molecular basis of diabetic collagen deposition remains unclear, but could result from increased synthesis or reduced degradation of collagen. There is little evidence to support increased synthesis *in vivo*, although skin fibroblasts from IDDM patients may synthesize increased amounts of collagen *in vitro* [33]. Resistance of collagen to breakdown may be more important, and could result from biochemical modifications, such as non-enzymatic glycosylation of collagen and increased collagen cross-linking mediated by lysyl oxidase.

Hyperglycaemia *per se* increases non-enzymatic glycosylation of collagen, keratin and haemoglobin A, and the decreased solubility of glycosylated collagen in acetic acid suggests intermolecular cross-linking [34]. However, it now seems less likely that collagen glycosylation is the critical factor. Guitton *et al.* claimed that glycosylation actually *inhibits* cross-linking and maturation of collagen fibres [35]. Moreover, studies of forearm skin biopsies have confirmed increased tissue glycosylation in diabetic as compared with normal subjects, but found no differences in glycosylation between diabetic subjects with LJM and those without [36].

Chang *et al.* [37] concluded that the reduced solubility of collagen in diabetic rats was attributable to an increase in lysine-derived cross-links, as it could be inhibited by β-aminopropionitrile, an inhibitor of lysyl oxidase. Increased lysyl oxidase activity has been reported in diabetes [38] and may be crucial to the excess collagen deposition of LJM, tenosynoviosclerosis, carpal tunnel syndrome, DD, adhesive capsulitis of the shoulder and dermal sclerosis.

### Treatment

#### *General*

Tight control of blood glucose may ultimately reduce skin thickness and improve joint mobility [39, 40] and must obviously underpin all treatment.

Anecdotal reports, yet to be confirmed, have suggested that sorbinil, an aldose reductase inhibitor, may improve the range of movement in patients with painful LJM and some peripheral nerve abnormalities [41]. It is unlikely to have a beneficial effect on painless LJM as defined by Rosenbloom [5]. Cyclo-oxygenase inhibitors prevent an increase in the thermal rupture time of rat-tail collagen (a measure of collagen stability) and may be useful in diabetic collagenosis [42] but no clinical evidence is available.

#### *Specific*

Simple active and passive stretching exercises may help to limit joint contractures, and an active daily programme of shoulder exercises is mandatory in patients with adhesive capsulitis. Glucocorticoids are commonly injected locally into tendon sheaths, the carpal tunnel and the capsulitic shoulder, but seem to be less effective in diabetes than in traumatic or idiopathic cases. This is compatible with the minor, if any, inflammatory component in diabetic patients. Surgical decompression of tendon sheaths and the carpal tunnel, or arthrolysis of the shoulder, may be necessary. Excision of palmar fascia in DD is not worthwhile but surgery may be indicated if severe finger contractures develop.

Treatment of the autonomic disorders is very difficult. Early active mobilization of the capsulitic shoulder will help to prevent the development of shoulder–hand syndrome but if this does occur, regional intravenous guanethidine or stellate ganglion block is necessary. Calcitonin may be helpful in some cases of algodystrophy. The management of the neuropathic ankle and foot depends on providing appropriate protective footwear and on a strict non-weight-bearing policy during periods of active osteolysis (Chapter 19).

Finally, the hot swollen joint (which may not always be painful in diabetic patients) must always be assumed to be infected until this has been actively excluded by aspiration and culture.

ADRIAN J. CRISP

## References


1 Gray RG, Gottlieb NL. Rheumatic disorders associated with diabetes mellitus. *Sem Arthr Rheum* 1976; **6**: 19–34.

2 Crisp AJ, Heathcote JG. Connective tissue abnormalities in diabetes mellitus. *J R Coll Physicians Lond* 1984; **18**: 132–41.

3 Johanson NA. Endocrine arthropathies. *Clin Rheum Dis* 1985; **11**: 297–323.

4 Crisp AJ. Diabetes mellitus and the rheumatologist. *Br J Rheum* 1986; **25**: 135–7.

5 Rosenbloom AL. Skeletal and joint manifestations of childhood diabetes. *Pediatr Clin North Am* 1984; **31**: 569–89.

6 Seibold JR. Digital sclerosis in children with insulin-dependent diabetes mellitus. *Arthr Rheum* 1982; **25**: 1357–61.

7 Rosenbloom AL, Silverstein JH, Lesotte DC, Richardson K, McCallum M. Limited joint mobility of childhood diabetes mellitus indicates increased risk for microvascular disease. *N Engl J Med* 1981; **305**: 191–4.

8 Fitzcharles MA, Duby S, Waddell RW, Banks E, Karsch J. Limitation of joint mobility in adult non-insulin dependent diabetic patients. *Ann Rheum Dis* 1984; **43**: 251–7.

9 Starkman HS, Gleason RE, Rand LI, Miller DE, Soeldner JS. Limited joint mobility of the hand in patients with diabetes mellitus: relation to chronic complications. *Ann Rheum Dis* 1986; **45**: 130–5.

10 Beacom R, Gillespie EL, Middleton D, Sawhney B, Kennedy L. Limited joint mobility in insulin-dependent diabetics: relationship to nephropathy, peripheral nerve function and HLA status. *Q J Med* 1985; **219**: 337–44.

11 Rosenbloom AL, Malone JI, Yucha J, Van Cader TC. Limited joint mobility and diabetic retinopathy demonstrated by fluorescein angiography. *Eur J Paediatr* 1984; **141**: 163–4.

12 Lawson PM, Maneschi F, Kohner EM. The relationship of hand abnormalities to diabetes and diabetic retinopathy. *Diabetes Care* 1983; **6**: 140–3.

13 Larkin JG, Frier BM. Limited joint mobility and Dupuytren's contracture in diabetic, hypertensive and normal populations. *Br Med J* 1986; **292**: 1494.

14 Trapp RG, Soler NG, Spencer-Green G. Nailford capillaroscopy in type I diabetics with vasculopathy and limited joint mobility. *J Rheum* 1986; **13**: 917–20.

15 Noble J, Heathcote JG, Cohen H. Diabetes mellitus in the aetiology of Dupuytren's disease. *J Bone Jt Surg* 1984; **66B**: 322–5.

16 Brickley-Parsons D, Glimcher MJ, Smith RJ, Albin R, Adams JP. Biochemical changes in the collagen of the palmar fascia in patients with Dupuytren's disease. *J Bone Jt Surg* 1981; **63A**: 787–97.

17 Phalen GS. Reflections on 21 years' experience with the carpal tunnel syndrome. *J Am Med Ass* 1970; **212**: 1365–7.

18 Bridgeman JF. Periarthritis of the shoulder and diabetes mellitus. *Ann Rheum Dis* 1972; **31**: 69–71.

19 Fisher L, Kurtz A, Shipley M. Association between cheiroarthropathy and frozen shoulder in patients with insulin-dependent diabetes. *Br J Rheum* 1986; **25**: 141–6.

20 Julkunen H, Heinonen OP, Knekt P, Maatela J. The epidemiology of hyperostosis of the spine together with its symptoms and related mortality in a general population. *Scand J Rheum* 1975; **4**: 23–7.

21 Moren-Hybinette I, Moritz U, Schersten B. The clinical picture of the painful diabetic shoulder — natural history, social consequences and analysis of concomitant hand syndrome. *Acta Med Scand* 1987; **221**: 73–82.

22 Doury P, Dirheimer Y, Pattin S. *Algodystrophy*. Berlin Springer-Verlag, 1981.

23 Brooks AP. The neuropathic foot in diabetes: Part II. Charcot's neuroarthropathy. *Diabetic Med* 1986; **3**: 116–18.

24 Waine H, Nevinny D, Rosenthal J, Jaffe IB. Association of osteoarthritis and diabetes mellitus. *Tufts Fol Med* 1961; **7**: 13–19.

25 Thomas DJB, Young A, Gorsuch AN, Bottazzo GF, Cudworth AG. Evidence for an association between rheumatoid arthritis and autoimmune endocrine disease. *Ann Rheum Dis* 1983; **42**: 297–300.

26 Rudolf MCJ, Genel M, Tamborlane WV, Dwyer JM, Juvenile rheumatoid arthritis in children with diabetes mellitus. *J Pediatr* 1981; **99**: 519–24.

27 Nepom BS, Palmer J, Kim SJ, Hansen JA, Holbeck SL, Nepom GT. Specific genomic markers for the HLA-DQ subregion discriminate between $DR4^+$ insulin-dependent diabetes mellitus and $DR4^+$ seropositive juvenile rheumatoid arthritis. *J Exp Med* 1986; **164**: 345–50.

28 Payami H, Khan MH, Grennan DM, Sanders PA, Dyer PA, Thomson G. Analysis of genetic inter-relationship among HLA associated diseases. *Am J Hum Genet* 1987; **41**: 331–45.

29 Boyle JA, McKiddie M, Buchanan KD, Jasani MK, Gray HW, Jackson IMD, Buchanan WW. Diabetes mellitus and gout. *Ann Rheum Dis* 1969; **28**: 374–8.

30 Tuomilehto J, Zimmet P, Wolf E, Taylor R, Ram P, King H. Plasma uric acid level and its association with diabetes mellitus and some biologic parameters in a biracial population of Fiji. *Am J Epidemiol* 1988; **127**: 321–36.

31 Alexander GM, Dieppe PA, Doherty M, Scott DGI. Pyrophosphate arthropathy: a study of metabolic association and laboratory data. *Ann Rheum Dis* 1982; **41**: 377–81.

32 Press M, Tamborlane WV, Sherwin RS. Importance of raised growth hormone levels in mediating the metabolic derangements of diabetes. *N Engl J Med* 1984; **310**: 810–5.

33 Smith BD, Silbert CK. Fibronectin and collagen of cultured skin fibroblasts in diabetes mellitus. *Biochem Biophys Res Commun* 1981; **100**: 275–82.

34 Buckingham BA, Uitto J, Sandborg C, Keens T, Kaufman F, Landing B. Scleroderma-like syndrome and non-enzymatic glycosylation of collagen in children with poorly controlled insulin-dependent diabetes mellitus. *Pediatr Res* 1981; **15**: 626.

35 Guitton JD, LePape A, Sizaret PY, Muh JP. Effects of *in vitro N*-glucosylation on type I collagen fibrillogenesis. *Biosci Repts* 1981; **1**: 945–54.

36 Lyons TJ, Kennedy L. Non-enzymatic glycosylation of skin collagen in patients with Type I (insulin-dependent) diabetes mellitus and limited joint mobility. *Diabetologia* 1985; **28**: 2–5.

37 Chang K, Uitto J, Rowold EA, Grant GA, Kilo C, Williamson JR. Increased collagen cross-linkages in experimental diabetes: reversal by β-aminopropionitrile and D-penicillamine. *Diabetes* 1980; **29**: 778–81.

38 Madia AM, Rozovski SJ, Kagan HM. Changes in lung lysyl oxidase activity in streptozotocin-diabetes and in starvation. *Biochim Biophys Acta* 1979; **585**: 481–7.

39 Sherry DD, Rothstein RRL, Petty RE. Joint contractures preceding insulin-dependent diabetes mellitus. *Arthr Rheum* 1982; **11**: 1362–4.

40 Lister DM, Graham-Brown RAC, Burden AC. Resolution of diabetic cheiroarthropathy. *Br Med J* 1986; **293**: 1537.

41 Eaton RP, Sibbitt WL, Harsh A. The effect of an aldose reductase inhibiting agent on limited joint mobility in diabetic patients. *J Am Med Ass* 1985; **253**: 1437–40.

42 Yue DK, McLennan S, Handelsman DJ, Delbridge L, Reeve T, Turtle JR. The effects of cyclo-oxygenase and lipooxygenase inhibitors on the collagen abnormalities of diabetic rats. *Diabetes* 1985; **34**: 74–8

# 23 Bone and Mineral Metabolism in Diabetes

**Summary**

- Diabetic osteopenia (reduced bone density) affects many IDDM patients and probably increases their susceptibility to fractures. NIDDM patients may be less affected.
- Bone loss is rapid in the first 2 years after diagnosis, declining to a steady value by 5 years.
- Diabetic osteopenia is a low turnover state, with reduced bone formation and continuing resorption.
- Diabetes has little effect on the mineral content of bone, or on serum calcium levels, although ketoacidosis and hyperglycaemia may cause magnesium and phosphate depletion.
- Hypercalciuria (due to predominant bone resorption) is common in diabetes and is reduced by improving metabolic control.

Diabetes has been associated both with localized changes in bone density (such as those affecting the diabetic foot: see Chapters 19 and 22) and with generalized disturbances of bone and mineral metabolism. The latter, particularly the diffuse reduction in bone density termed 'diabetic osteopenia', will be discussed here.

## Diabetic osteopenia

Reports of the prevalence, extent and natural history of diabetic osteopenia vary widely, probably because of the different methods and study populations employed. Many clinical studies have measured bone density at a single site (commonly the forearm), either with non-invasive methods such as X-ray or photon absorptiometry or by histological examination of bone biopsies. Recently, non-invasive absorptiometric techniques and computerized tomography have been applied to investigate bone density in the axial skeleton, which includes the clinically relevant sites of the spine (Fig. 23.1) and proximal femur where significant osteoporosis leading to fractures is most likely to occur.

### *Prevalence*

In IDDM, it is generally agreed that bone density (measured in the forearm in most studies) is significantly reduced below age-adjusted control values, over 50% of IDDM patients showing a reduction of >10% [1–3]. Significant bone loss may be present at the time of diagnosis (perhaps related to the preceding decline in insulin secretion) and is relatively rapid in the following 2 years, declining gradually thereafter to a steady-state value at about 5 years [3]. Poorly controlled IDDM patients probably suffer proportionately greater bone loss than those enjoying good metabolic control.

The situation in NIDDM is less clear-cut, possibly because of confounding variables such as age, race, obesity, menopausal status and the unknown duration of the disease before diagnosis. One study has reported a reduction in density of around 10% in as many as 60% of NIDDM patients [1], whereas others have found a decrease of this magnitude in only 20% [4]. The available data do not allow the time-course of these changes to be defined. One study has described a subgroup of NIDDM patients who show an *increase* in bone density [4]. This curious and unexpected finding is not apparently explicable by obesity but could

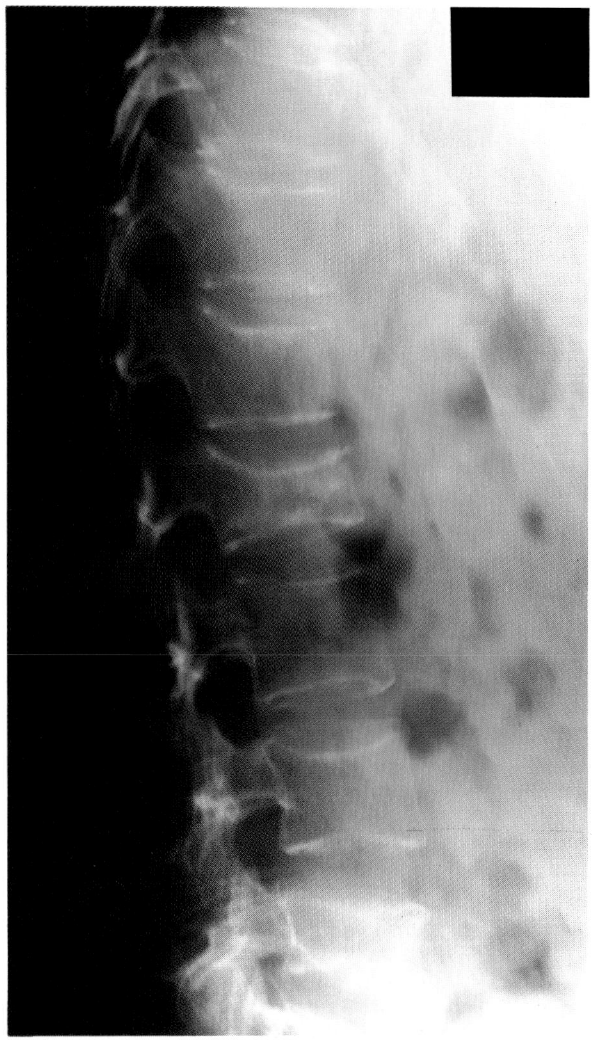

**Fig. 23.1.** Lateral radiograph of thoracic spine in a 23-year-old woman with IDDM, showing reduced bone density and collapse of vertebral bodies due to diabetic osteopenia. (Reproduced by kind permission of Dr Ian MacFarlane, Walton Hospital, Liverpool.)

be related to hyperinsulinaemia, which has been associated with elevated insulin-like growth factor 1 (IGF-1) levels and as such could exert an anabolic effect on bone (see below; [5]).

*Mechanisms of bone loss*

Bone mass is normally maintained by close matching of bone resorption (osteoclastic activity) to bone formation (osteoblastic activity). Bone density can be reduced when these two opposing influences are uncoupled. Diabetic osteopenia appears to be a 'low turnover' state, with reduced bone formation rather than a primary increase in resorption [6] (Fig. 23.2). Bone formation is slowed in diabetes, the osteons taking 2–8 times longer to develop than in non-diabetic subjects [7]. Histomorphometric analyses of iliac crest biopsies have demonstrated increased surface areas, but normal volumes of trabecular and osteoid elements, indicating that resorption of bone is proportionately greater than its formation [8]. Levels of osteocalcin (a protein synthesized by osteoblasts) are reduced, consistent with decreased osteoblastic activity. The fact that the increase in bone resorption is relative and not absolute is confirmed by the urinary excretion of hydroxyproline (an indirect measure of total bone resorption), which is not increased in diabetes.

The factors mediating this uncoupling are unknown, but might involve the effects of insulin deficiency on the cytokines which are increasingly implicated in the local regulation of bone metabolism. In particular, insulin-like growth factors, IGF-1 [9] and probably IGF-2 [10] can stimulate osteoblastic precursors to replicate and differentiate into osteoblasts. In poorly controlled diabetes, growth hormone secretion is increased but circulating levels of IGF may be reduced [5], which could impede bone formation.

The calcium and phosphorus contents of bone are not significantly altered in diabetes; a minor reduction of magnesium levels in IDDM patients [12] does not seem to have any important effect on the degree of bone mineralization.

Bone loss does not appear to be related to other chronic diabetic complications, in that its time-course and prevalence do not match those of retinopathy or other microvascular complications [12].

*Clinical implications*

The tendency to reduced bone density in diabetes might be expected to increase diabetic patients' susceptibility to fracture. This is probably true, although the additional risk may not be great: a review of six studies showed the relative risk of fractures to vary between 1.16 and 2.86 times that of the non-diabetic population [12], although another study has found no excess risk. The risk may be higher in specific subgroups of subjects such as poorly controlled IDDM patients or those with additional risk factors for osteoporosis, notably perimenopausal women. The increasing availability of sensitive, non-invasive measurements of bone density will not only help to clarify the natural history of the condition, but should

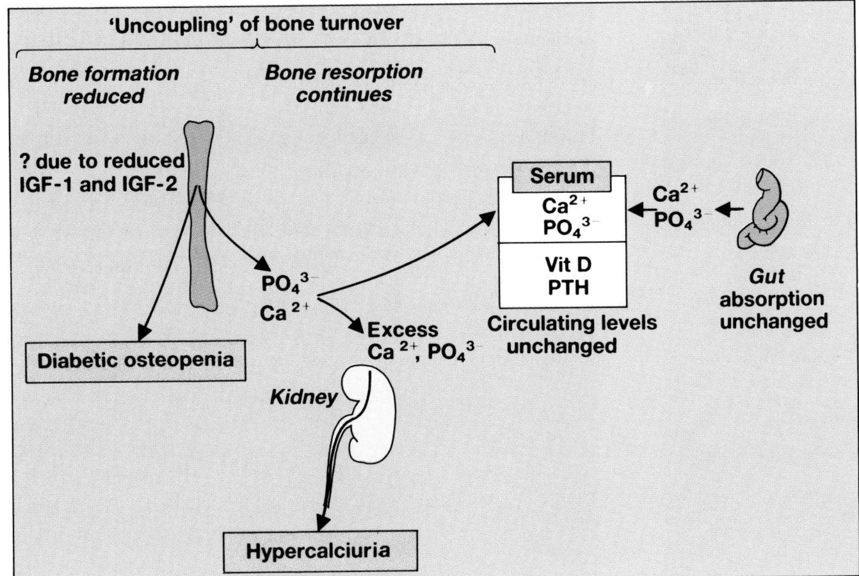


**Fig. 23.2.** Bone and mineral metabolism in diabetes. Bone formation is reduced while resorption continues at its normal pace; this 'uncoupling' liberates calcium from the skeleton (which is eliminated through the kidneys) and leads ultimately to diabetic osteopenia. Gut absorption of calcium and phosphate is normal. Serum levels of calcium and phosphate, and of parathyroid hormone (PTH) and 1,25-dihydroxycholecalciferol (vitamin D) are unchanged in most diabetic patients. IGF-1, 2 = insulin-like growth factors 1 and 2.

also allow at-risk patients to be screened. At present, the only rational measures to protect the skeleton in diabetic patients are probably the maintenance of as good metabolic control as possible, and the possible use of hormonal replacement in postmenopausal women.

## Effects of diabetes on calcium, phosphate and magnesium balance

Insulin is thought to have several effects on the turnover of calcium, magnesium and phosphate. It has complex actions on proximal and distal renal tubular handling of electrocytes, including enhanced phosphate reabsorption [16]. Insulin may also have a permissive effect on the 1-α-hydroxylase in the kidney which converts 25-hydroxycholecalciferol to its active metabolite, 1,25-dihydroxycholecalciferol [16].

The major disturbance in diabetes is hypercalciuria, which tends to fall but is not completely abolished by improved metabolic control [17]. Although the cause of hypercalciuria is unknown, the kidneys seem effectively to act to eliminate any excess calcium mobilized by the relatively increased bone resorption, and serum calcium concentrations generally remain within the normal range. Circulating levels of parathyroid hormone and of 1,25-dihydroxycholecalciferol are also unchanged, although other vitamin D metabolites may show alterations in diabetes [18, 19].

IDDM patients with ketoacidosis and hyperglycaemia may show variable total body depletion of both magnesium and phosphate, although serum levels only rarely fall to the point where clinical problems occur or treatment become necessary [21, 22].

RAYMOND BRUCE
JOHN C. STEVENSON

## References


1 Levin ME, Boisseau VC, Avioli LV. Effects of diabetes mellitus on bone mass in juvenile and adult-onset diabetes *N Engl J Med* 1976; **294**: 241–5.
2 Hui SL, Epstein S, Johnston CC. A prospective study of bone mass in patients with type 1 diabetes. *J Clin Endocrinol Metab* 1985; **60**: 74–80.
3 McNair P, Madsbad S, Christensen MS, Christiansen C, Faber OK, Binder C, Transbol I. Bone mineral loss in insulin treated diabetes mellitus: studies on pathogenesis. *Acta Endocrinol* 1976; **90**: 463–72.
4 De Leeuw I, Abs R. Bone mass and bone density in maturity-type diabetics measured by the $^{125}$I photon absorption technique. *Diabetes* 1977; **26**: 1130–5.
5 Holly JMP, Amiel SA, Sandhu RR, Rees LH, Wass JAH. The role of growth hormone in diabetes mellitus. *J Endocrinol* 1988; **118**: 353–64.
6 Silberberg R. The skeleton in diabetes mellitus: a review of the literature. *Diabetes Res* 1986; **3**: 329–38.
7 Takahashi H, Frost HM. The kinetics of the resorption process in osteonal remodeling of diabetic rib. *Henry Ford Med Bull* 1964; **12**: 537–45.
8 De Leeuw I, Mulkens N, Vertommen J, Abs R. A histomorphometric study of the trabecular bone of diabetic subjects *Diabetologia* 1976; **12**: 385–6.
9 Canalis E. Bone related growth factors. *Triangle* 1988; **27**: 11–19.
10 Strong DD, Beacher AL, Mohan S, Wegerdal JE, Linkhart TA, Baylink DJ. Multiple major skeletal growth factor (SGF) mRNA transcripts expressed in human bone cells. *J Bone Min Res* 1988; **3** (suppl 1): 294.

11 De Leeuw I, Vertommen J, Abs R. The mineral content of the trabecular bone of diabetic subjects (abstract). *Diabetologia* 1976; **12**: 386.

12 McNair P, Christensen MS, Christiansen C, Madsbad S, Transbol I. Is diabetic osteoporosis due to microangiopathy? (letter) *Lancet* 1981; **i**: 1271.

13 Selby PL. Osteopenia and diabetes. *Diabetic Med* 1988; **5**: 423–8.

14 Heath H, Melton LJ, Chu C-P. Diabetes mellitus and risk of skeletal fracture. *N Engl J Med* 1980; **303**: 567–70.

15 DeFronzo RA, Goldberg M, Agus ZS. The effects of glucose and insulin on renal electrolyte transport. *J Clin Invest* 1976; **58**: 83–90.

16 Henry HL. Insulin permits parathormone stimulation of 1,25 dihydroxy Vit D3 in cultured kidney cells. *Endocrinology* 1981; **108**: 733–5.

17 Gertner JM, Tamborlane WV, Horst RL, Sherwin RS, Felig P, Genel M. Mineral metabolism in diabetes mellitus: changes accompanying treatment with a portable subcutaneous insulin infusion system. *J Clin Endocrinol Metab* 1980; **50**: 862–6.

18 Frazer TE, White NH, Hough S, Santiago JV, McGee BR, Bryce G, Mallon J, Avioli LV. Alterations in circulating vitamin D metabolites in the young insulin-dependent diabetic. *J Clin Endocrinol Metab* 1981; **53**: 1154–9.

19 Ishida H, Seino Y, Matsukura S, Ikeda M, Yawata M, Yamashita G, Ishizuka S, Imura H. Diabetic osteopenia and circulating levels of Vitamin D metabolites in type 2 (non-insulin dependent) diabetes. *Metabolism* 1985; **34**: 797–801.

20 Martin HE, Smith K, Wilson ML. The fluid and electrolyte therapy of severe diabetic acidosis and ketosis. *Am J Med* 1958; **24**: 376–89.

21 Guest GM. Organic phosphates of the blood and mineral metabolism in diabetic acidosis. *Am J Dis Child* 1942; **64**: 401–12.

# 24 Sexual Function in Diabetic Women

**Summary**

• Some diabetic women enter menarche later and have less regular cycles than non-diabetic women. Insulin requirements change (usually with an increase) in about 40% of diabetic women around the time of menstruation; the mechanism is unknown.

• Psychosexual development may be delayed in diabetic women, especially when diabetes presents at a young age.

• Fertility is essentially normal in most well-controlled diabetic women, unless serious complications (e.g. nephropathy) are present; contraception is therefore essential if pregnancy is not desired.

• Genito-urinary infections — especially candidiasis and perhaps genital herpes — are relatively common in diabetic women and often interfere with sexual intercourse. Good glycaemic control and specific anti-microbial treatment (e.g. fluconazole for candidiasis) are essential.

• Sexual responsiveness does not seem to be impaired in diabetic women, even though severe autonomic neuropathy might interfere with vaginal lubrication and other genital arousal responses.

• Diabetes in women does not appear to damage their relationship with their partner.

Most studies on sexuality in diabetes have concentrated on men. This section will review the limited work relating to sexuality in diabetic women.

**Menstruation in diabetic women**

Compared with their non-diabetic counterparts, diabetic women show a slight delay in physical maturation. They tend to reach the menarche a little later and to have less regular cycles [1, 2].

About 40% of diabetic women show some change in insulin requirements around the time of menstruation. Patterns vary from one individual to another, the commonest (occurring in about 20% of patients) being a modest increase in insulin requirement for the first two days of menstruation [3–5]. This can be covered by raising the insulin dose by a few units, although occasional patients need much greater increases. The older literature contains several reports of ketoacidosis recurring at the time of menstruation [6, 7]. This is unusual and probably has no true physiological basis; it seems more likely that the young girls with this problem are behaving in a manipulative way, perhaps omitting their insulin during episodes of premenstrual tension. About 10% of diabetic women experience a decrease in insulin requirement just before menstruation and this can be difficult to manage, particularly if cycles are irregular. Other less common patterns also occur.

These changes are not usually due to variation in diet or exercise and are likely to have a hormonal basis. Some diabetic women feel nauseated and eat less premenstrually, whereas others have cravings for carbohydrate, sometimes including sweet foods, at that time. Although major endocrine changes occur during the menstrual cycle, measurements of hormone levels have not so far shown any difference between those patients who show changes in their insulin requirements and those who do not. An interesting study by Walsh [8] demonstrated that glucose tolerance in *non-*

diabetic women was impaired at the time of menstruation in some cases, but there was considerable individual variation [8]. On the other hand, Scott has shown that insulin sensitivity as measured by the artificial pancreas is unaffected by the phase of the menstrual cycle [9].

### Psychosexual development

A high incidence of delay in psychosexual development has been described in insulin-dependent diabetic women. The younger the patient at diagnosis, the greater is the reported delay and it has been suggested that this phenomenon could be a factor in some cases of the adolescent turmoil so frequently noted in juvenile diabetic girls [10].

### Genito-urinary infections

Pruritus vulvae is a well-known presenting symptom of diabetes. Vaginal infections, particularly candidiasis, continue to be common, especially in poorly controlled diabetic patients as the yeasts thrive in glucose-containing media. Severe infections can be very irritating and painful, and may interfere with sexual intercourse. Treatment should aim to improve diabetic control in order to minimize the glycosuria, and the usual antifungal creams and pessaries should be used. In resistant cases, a single dose of the antifungal drug fluconazole may be very effective against candida. Vaginal warts may also be particularly common in diabetic women. Vaginal herpes also appears to be common and the accompanying systemic upset can lead to ketoacidosis. We do not yet know if HIV infection is more common or severe in diabetic patients.

Urinary tract infections are frequent in patients with poorly controlled diabetes and in those with autonomic neuropathy and bladder distension. These infections should be treated in the usual way, together with optimization of diabetic control [11].

### Fertility

In the early days of insulin therapy, many women with IDDM were poorly controlled and suffered amenorrhoea and subfertility as a consequence of debility and general ill-health. Fortunately, most diabetic patients nowadays are very fit, and yet the belief persists in some quarters that diabetic women are infertile. One might expect that diabetic women would be slightly less fertile than the general population because of the high incidence of irregular cycles and perhaps an increased risk of pelvic infection. There is some evidence that this may be the case [12, 13]. Those with renal failure also have generally reduced fertility, but even some of these patients can and do conceive.

In practical terms, however, fertility is not significantly less than that of non-diabetics. It is important to explain this to diabetic girls and women because they often worry that they may be unable to conceive. Conversely, there can be unfortunate consequences for patients who think they do not need to use contraception because they have heard that diabetic women are infertile.

### Sexual responsiveness

The problems of pregnancy in diabetes are well appreciated and documented but, unlike men, women rarely complain of sexual problems [14]. In 1971, Kolodny [15] reported a reduction in orgasm in diabetic women but the patients they studied were all in hospital. Ellenberg [16] found no difference in diabetic women with and without clinical evidence of autonomic neuropathy. Jensen [17] described very minor differences between diabetic and non-diabetic women, which were rather more marked in those with peripheral neuropathy.

The most comprehensive study is that of Tyrer [18], who examined 82 insulin-dependent diabetic women who had been married or cohabitating with their partners for at least a year. Fourteen had symptomatic autonomic neuropathy, 16 had abnormal autonomic function tests but no symptoms and 50 had normal autonomic function. They were compared with a control group of 47 healthy women attending a family planning clinic. During an interview with a psychologist, spontaneous sexual interest, the frequency and speed of vaginal lubrication, non-genital arousal, orgasm and vaginismus were rated on a 4–6 point scale. The only one of these ratings in which the diabetic group differed significantly from the controls was vaginal lubrication, the diabetic group having more individuals at the two extremes, i.e. 'inadequate lubrication' or 'always adequate'. The female psycho-physiological change most directly comparable to penile erection is vasocongestion of the vulva and vagina with associated vaginal lubrication. Abnormalities of lubrication might therefore be expected in diabetic women, particularly in those with autonomic neuropathy. However, this was not demonstrated. Two of the most severely affected patients, who died a few months after the study from sudden cardiorespiratory arrest (presumably due to autonomic neuropathy) appeared to lubricate normally. One had no sexual problems, although the other was troubled with diarrhoea during intercourse.

As might be anticipated from the disturbance of cardiovascular reflexes, patients with autonomic neuropathy reported slightly less non-genital arousal during sexual activity than the non-neuropathic diabetic and non-diabetic controls. In a further assessment, each woman rated the concepts of 'myself' and 'my partner' on a series of seven-point scales to give ratings of sexual attractiveness, sexual arousability, lovingness, calmness, potency and a general evaluation. The only finding of note was that diabetic women rated their partners significantly less potent than did the control group. A marriage–relationship questionnaire showed no difference between diabetic and control groups but, on direct questioning about the effect of diabetes on their marital relationship, 9% felt diabetes had a detrimental effect whereas 21% thought it had a beneficial effect because their husbands were more concerned.

Most studies have looked at IDDM women. Schreiner-Engel [19] studied 35 IDDM subjects and found no difference between them and a control group but also studied 23 NIDDM subjects and found reduced sexual desire, orgasmic capacity, lubrication and sexual activity. She also found a poorer relationship with the sexual partner as compared with a control group but surprisingly, the problems were not correlated with duration of diabetes. It is difficult to find an explanation for these interesting findings. The group studied was small and comprised volunteers; they were heavier, had more vaginitis and more of them were postmenopausal than the controls. The authors suggest that the neurovascular processes which regulate genital vasoconstriction may be important, but if this were the case, we should expect it to be commoner in long-standing diabetes. Autonomic nerve function was not evaluated in this study. The authors also suggest that NIDDM subjects have a poor sexual body image. This could be due to obesity, although details of weight are not given. This area merits further investigation in a larger number of patients.

Thus, there seem to be only minor disturbances in sexual function in diabetic women in contrast to the major problems seen in men. There may be sex-related differences in the way the autonomic nervous system controls genital responses. Another likely factor is that erection in the male is an all-or-nothing phenomenon; any impairment may therefore generate anxiety which can further inhibit the erectile mechanisms, whereas women focus on the subjective quality of their sexual relationship. At any sexual problem clinic, men tend to complain of difficulties with erection or ejaculation, whereas most women complain of inadequate enjoyment and only very few describe inadequate lubrication or orgasmic difficulties.

There is a tendency to become excessively preoccupied with the physiology of sexuality and to forget that, in human terms, a sexual encounter is a much more complicated phenomenon than mere spinal reflex activity. The central nervous system exerts its control, facilitating and inhibiting responses while adding its own special ingredients of fantasy, expectations, memories and emotions. Nocturnal sex dreams in men develop spontaneously in the teens, but in women only with a degree of conditioning based upon exposure and experience. Tenderness and security provided by the feeling of being loved are necessary requirements for the woman's response [20]. It seems likely that a more caring relationship in diabetic marriages can counteract any modest physiological deficit.

### Recent developments

Dunger *et al.* [21] have suggested that the increased incidence of menstrual irregularities in adolescents with IDDM may be related to low concentrations of sex-binding globulin and to abnormalities in gonadotrophin secretion.

Widom *et al.* [22] have recently reported euglycaemic, hyperinsulinaemic 'clamp' studies in diabetic women. Seven IDDM women who experienced worsening glucose control during the luteal phase of the cycle showed a fall in glucose uptake and a raised oestradiol level, which did not occur in women showing no variation in glucose control during the menstrual cycle.

Premenstrual craving for sweet foods may also be a factor influencing blood glucose levels in some patients around the time of menstruation [23].

JUDITH M. STEEL

## References


1 Bergquist N. The gonadal function in female diabetics. *Acta Endocrinol Suppl* (Copenhagen) 1954; **19**: 3–20.

2 Djursing H, Nyholm HC, Hagen C, Carstensen L, Pedersen LM. Clinical and hormonal characteristics in women with anovulation and insulin-treated diabetes mellitus. *Am J Obstet Gynecol* 1982; **143**: 876–82.

3 Steel JM. Sexual function in diabetic women. *Practical Diabetes* 1985; **2**: 10–11.

4 Walsh CM, Malins JM. Menstruation and control of diabetes. *Br Med J* 1977; **2**: 177–9.

5 Steel JM, Duncan LJP. The effects of oral contraceptives on insulin requirements in diabetics. *Br J Fam Plan* 1978; **3**: 77–8.

6 Hubble D. Insulin resistance. *Br Med J* 1954; **2**: 1022–4.

7 Sandstrom R. Diabetes mellitus and menstruation. *Nordic Med* 1969; **81**: 727–8.

8 Walsh CH, O'Sullivan DJ. Carbohydrate tolerance during the menstrual cycle in diabetics. *Lancet* 1973; **ii**: 413–15.

9 Scott AR, McDonald IA, Savage M, Bowman C, Jeffcoate WJ. Insulin sensitivity is unaffected by phase of menstrual cycle in women with insulin dependent diabetes. *Diabetic Med* 1987; **4**: 572A.

10 Surridge DHC, Erdahl DL, Lawson JS, Donald MW, Monga TN, Bird CE, Letemendia FJ. Psychiatric aspects of diabetes mellitus. *Br J Psychiatr* 1984; **145**: 169–76.

11 Sawers JS, Todd WA, Kellet HA, Mills RS, Allan PL, Ewing DJ, Clarke BF. Bacteriura and autonomic nerve function in diabetic women. *Diabetes Care* 1986; **9**: 460–3.

12 Steel JM, Johnstone FD, Smith AF, Duncan LJP. The pre-pregnancy clinic approach. In: Sutherland HW, Stowers JM, eds. *Carbohydrate Metabolism in Pregnancy and the Newborn*. Edinburgh: Churchill Livingstone, 1984: 75–86.

13 Randall J. Fertility and conception. In: Stowers JM, ed. *Carbohydrate Metabolism in Pregnancy and the Newborn*. Berlin: Springer Verlag 1989: 31–40.

14 Jensen SB. Emotional aspects of diabetes mellitus. A study of somatopsychological reactions in 51 couples in which one partner has insulin-treated diabetes. *J Psychosomat Res* 1985; **29**: 353–9.

15 Kolodny RC. Sexual dysfunction in diabetic females. *Diabetes* 1971; **20**: 557–9.

16 Ellenberg M. Sexual aspects of the female diabetic. *Mt Sinai J Med* 1977; **44**: 495–500.

17 Jensen SB. Diabetic sexual dysfunction, a comparative study of 160 insulin treated diabetic men and women and an age matched control group. *Arch Sexual Behav* 1981; **10**: 493–504.

18 Tyrer G, Steel JM, Clarke BF, Ewing DJ, Bancroft J. Sexual responsiveness in diabetic women. *Diabetologia* 1983; **24**: 166–71.

19 Schreiner-Engel P, Schiavi RC, Vietovisz D, Smith H. The differential impact of diabetes type on female sexuality. *J Psychosomat Res* 1987; **31**: 22–33.

20 Kant F. Factors in female sexuality. *Med Aspects Human Sexual* 1973; **7**: 31.

21 Dunger DB. Diabetes in puberty. *Arch Dis Child* 1992; **67**: 569–73.

22 Widom B, Diamond M, Simonsen DC. Alterations in glucose metabolism during menstrual cycle in women with IDDM. *Diabetes Care* 1992; **15**: 213–20.

23 Cawood EHH, Bancroft H, Steel JM. Perimenstrual symptoms in women with diabetes mellitus and the relationship to diabetic control. *Diabetic Med* 1993, in press.

# 25 Sexual Function in Diabetic Men

**Summary**

- Impotence affects about one-third of diabetic men.
- Psychogenic causes, often associated with anxiety and/or depression, are common; nocturnal erections are maintained and patients may respond to expert counselling.
- Autonomic neuropathy may interrupt the parasympathetic outflow which normally produces vasodilatation and engorgement of the penile corpora.
- Vascular causes of impotence include both reduced arterial inflow (through obstruction of iliac or internal pudendal arteries) and venous leakage from the corpora.
- Impotence may also be due to alcohol or cannabis abuse, to antihypertensive or psychotropic drugs, or to hypogonadism.
- Treatments available for 'organic' causes of impotence include suction devices causing passive erection, intracorporeal injection of vasodilators, and surgical implantation of rigid or inflatable prostheses.

Impotence is the inability to achieve or sustain an erection satisfactory for sexual intercourse. It is one of the saddest complications of diabetes and is relatively common in diabetic men. However, in the UK at least, it is probably the least discussed problem related to the disease. Even though the ultimate prognosis in many cases is poor, patients will often appreciate the opportunity to discuss this once-taboo subject with their physician.

The prevalence of impotence in diabetic men is high — up to 35%, according to McCullough [1]. Associated factors at presentation in this study were increasing age and the presence of retinopathy and peripheral and autonomic neuropathy. There was no apparent relationship with the duration of the disease, but poor glycaemic control and excessive alcohol intake at presentation seemed to be important. In a follow-up study of the same population 5 years later, 28% of those originally potent had developed impotence and 9% of the impotent had become potent [2].

It is important to differentiate 'impotence in diabetic men' from 'diabetic impotence', as the latter term implies organic disease which is essentially irreversible and untreatable. The possible causes of impotence must therefore be carefully considered in each individual case.

## Physiology of normal erection and ejaculation

The physiological complexity of the male sexual response (Fig. 25.1) underlines the many ways in which various organic and psychological factors may cause impotence.

Erection is a parasympathetic response to psychic, visual and other stimuli acting on higher cortical centres and to reflex tactile stimulation of the genitalia [3]. The sacral parasympathetic outflow (carried via the pudendal nerves) causes dilatation of the corporeal arteries (end-branches of the internal pudendal artery), leading to engorgement of the corpora cavernosa and corpus spongiosum. Sustained erection depends not only on increased arterial inflow but also on restriction of venous outflow from the corpora.

Ejaculation is a sympathetic response, mediated by the presacral nerves arising from the lower part of the thoraco-lumbar sympathetic outflow, which causes contraction of the vas deferens and seminal vesicles.

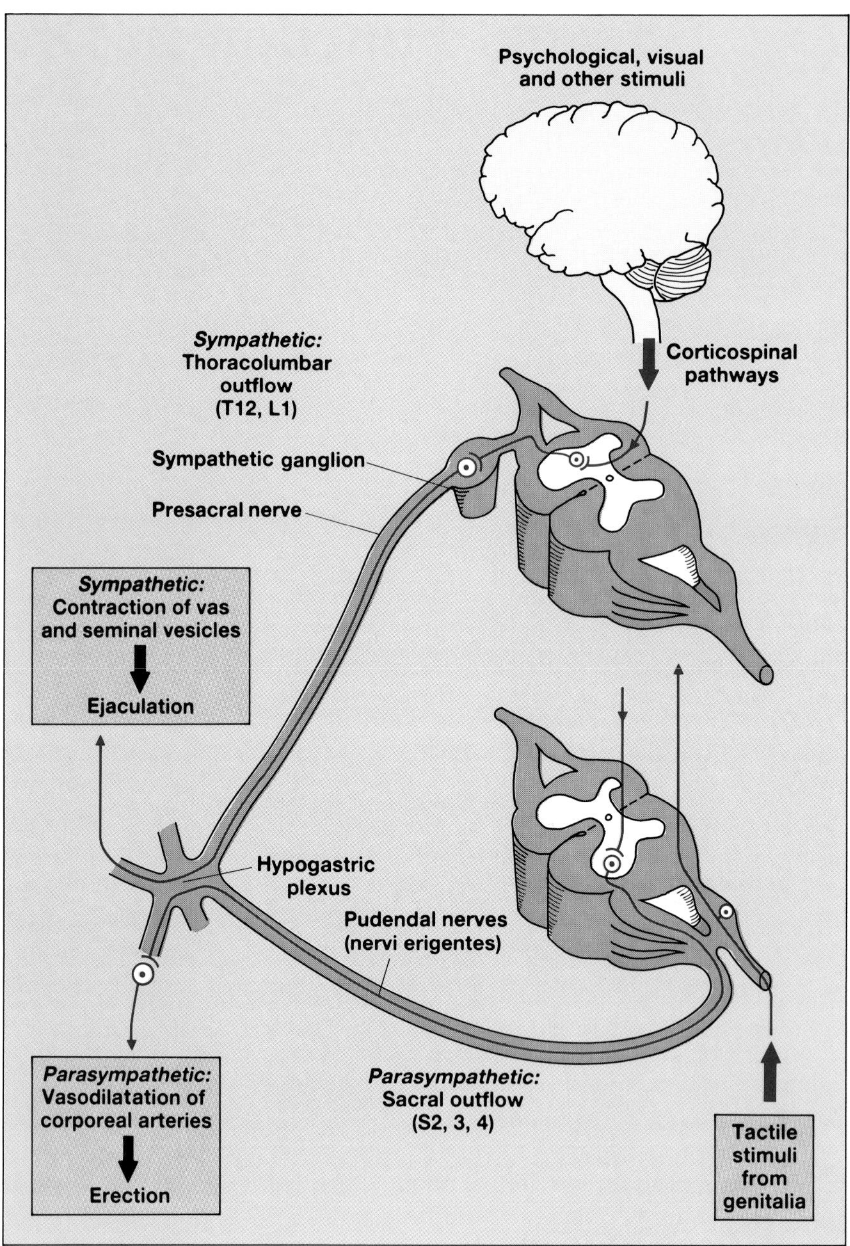


**Fig. 25.1.** Physiological basis of erection and ejaculation.

## Causes of impotence in diabetes

These are summarized in Table 25.1, which shows the level at which various factors can interfere with the male sexual response to produce impotence and/or failure of ejaculation. Although a proportion of diabetic men will have irreversible organic impotence, other potentially treatable causes must be excluded. The development of impotence in any man will depend on many interrelated influences, including his marital relationship; basic personality and upbringing; cultural and personal attitudes to life and sex; tendency to anxiety or depression; presence of and response to pressure at work or at home; and the use of drugs and alcohol. The particular pathophysiological complications and psychosocial pressures of diabetes itself will be superimposed upon and will interact with this complex and delicate background.

*Psychological factors* must also be considered in cases of impotence in diabetic men, as in the population at large [4]. Anxiety and depression are common in diabetic patients and may be fuelled by the very knowledge that diabetes itself can cause impotence.

*Advanced autonomic neuropathy* is almost invariably accompanied by impotence but the

| Component | Interfering factors causing impotence |
|---|---|
| Psychological arousal | Depression, anxiety (including that about diabetes)<br>Psychotropic drugs<br>Alcohol, cannabis |
| Tactile input from genitalia | Peripheral neuropathy |
| Parasympathetic outflow | Autonomic neuropathy<br>Various antihypertensive and other drugs |
| Increased arterial inflow to corpora | Atheroma of iliac or pudendal arteries |
| Reduced venous outflow from corpora | Venous leakage |
| Adequate testosterone levels | Hypogonadism |

**Table 25.1** Factors necessary for erection, and causes of impotence.

relationship of the latter to abnormal electrophysiological tests (see Chapter 12) is not so clear. Invasive research techniques have demonstrated a reduced conduction velocity in the dorsal nerve of the penis in patients with autonomic neuropathy, which was generally correlated with the presence of impotence [5].

*Vascular problems*, either by impeding arterial inflow or allowing excessive venous drainage, may also cause impotence. Atheroma in the common iliac arteries or more distally in the internal pudendal artery may reduce inflow. Arterial disease is difficult to assess non-invasively; in the latter case, the femoral pulses are frequently preserved. Doppler ultrasound may be used to assess penile blood flow: one study has found impaired blood flow in 65% of impotent patients as opposed to only 26% of potent patients with abnormal electrophysiological tests [6]. Abnormal leakage from the corpora into their draining veins can be demonstrated in some impotent patients by selective arteriography and infusion cavernosography [7] and probably contributes to detumescence.

*Endocrine abnormalities* remain a controversial cause of impotence in diabetic men. Although prolactin levels tend to be elevated in diabetes, there is no firm association with impotence [8] However, serum free testosterone levels are apparently reduced in some impotent diabetic men [9].

*Drugs*, particularly antihypertensive and psychotropic agents, *alcohol* and *cannabis* are also associated with impotence.

From the above, it is obvious that many neurological, vascular and endocrine factors may potentially be involved and may be aggravated by coexisting psychogenic problems.

## Investigation of the diabetic man with impotence

This is outlined in Table 25.2. The first step is to elicit an adequate history, concentrating on the above factors, during a free and open discussion with the patient and, ideally, with his partner. The subject is rarely mentioned spontaneously, but it is wrong for the clinician to assume that if it is not brought up, then it is not a problem. The patient should therefore be questioned directly, but it must be stressed that adequate assessment of an impotent man is a skilled task requiring special consideration and training, and is not a topic for a brief chat in a busy clinic.

The patient will also need a full physical examination, particularly to seek evidence of autonomic and peripheral neuropathy, peripheral vascular disease (with the above reservation regarding atheroma restricted to small distal arteries), hypogonadism and alcohol abuse.

**Table 25.2.** Assessment of the diabetic man with impotence.

| |
|---|
| *History and examination for evidence of:* |
| Anxiety, depression |
| Impact of impotence |
| Drug and alcohol use |
| Autonomic neuropathy (especially involving bladder) |
| Peripheral neuropathy |
| Peripheral vascular disease (NB: poor correlation of femoral pulses with pudendal artery patency) |
| Hypogonadism |
| *Further investigations* |
| Formal psychological assessment of patient (and partner) |
| Autonomic function tests |
| Assessment of nocturnal erections (snap-gauge) |
| *Specialist-centre investigations* |
| Penile blood flow |
| Electrophysiological tests) |

The most important need is perhaps to identify the presence of psychogenic factors. Premature ejaculation, as distinct from failure of erection, is almost always psychogenic rather than organic in origin and the presence of nocturnal or early morning erection or emissions (even if erection cannot be maintained during full intercourse) again points to a psychogenic cause. The presence of nocturnal erections may be confirmed by measuring penile tumescence using a strain gauge [4] or maximal penile diameter using a snap-gauge fastener [10]. Although nocturnal erections are generally regarded as proof of organic normality, the erection may still not be rigid enough for satisfactory intercourse. The prevalence of psychogenic problems may be indicated by the finding by Hosking [11] of totally absent nocturnal tumescence in only six out of 30 impotent diabetic men. Other methods for detecting psychogenic problems include formal psychological assessments: the Minnesota multiphasic personality inventory has apparently been able to differentiate those more likely to have psychogenic impotence [12]. The viewing of erotic films to assess psychological state and induce erection does not completely separate organic from psychogenic causes, although responses were undoubtedly blunted in diabetic patients with autonomic dysfunction [13].

In routine clinic practice, basic tests of neurological and autonomic function can be performed and nocturnal penile tumescence assessed with a commercially available disposable snap-gauge. If serious organic disease is present, the possibility of psychological factors being reversible is greatly reduced. On the other hand, it should not be assumed that the presence of relatively minor physical abnormalities precludes a psychogenic component.

### Management plan for the impotent diabetic man

Ideally, there should be close collaboration between the diabetologist, psychologist or psychiatrist, and urologist; all diabetic clinics should have a working relationship with expert marital and sexual therapists [14]. Much help and support can be provided, even if only to reassure the patient that he is not strangely abnormal.

General measures include exclusion of alcohol, withdrawal or substitution of any drugs which may be responsible, and improvement in metabolic control (which alone may help in some cases). Thereafter, the following scheme is suggested:

**1** Establish whether there is a major problem causing personal or marital disharmony, and also whether his spouse or partner is willing to discuss the matter with the appropriate professionals. Many men or their partners will prefer to leave matters at this stage, but if possible, at least two interviews should be allowed initially so that thought and discussion can take place between the partners.
**2** If there is a serious problem causing concern, the offer should be made of detailed assessment of the couple's sexual and psychological condition by a trained therapist or psychologist. The diabetologist should explain the likely treatment plan without giving too much graphic and possibly daunting detail about invasive procedures.
**3** If an important psychogenic element appears likely, sexual counselling should be offered and may have a successful result.
**4** If the problem is organic, then the patient should be offered the choice of the treatments listed below. No order of priority should be suggested, as the subject will no doubt wish to consider possible treatments and discuss them with his partner.

The treatments currently available are:

**1** A non-invasive condom device (Erecaid, Fig. 25.2) applies suction to the penis to cause blood to flow into the erectile tissue where it is trapped by a constricting band placed around the base of the penis [15]. Satisfactory erection can be maintained for intercourse. The device is popular with those who have taken part in clinical studies of this device [15], but it is very expensive.
**2** Intracavernous injections of vasodilators, such as $\alpha_1$-blockers (phentolamine, phenoxybenzamine) or smooth muscle relaxants such as papaverine (5–30 mg). Although apparently an alarming procedure, patients readily learn to inject themselves and many report successful erection and intercourse [16]. Erections may last for 2 h, and priapism is a rare complication. Where available, this treatment should probably precede more invasive surgical procedures.
**3** Surgical implantation of permanently rigid or 'inflatable' prostheses into the corpora cavernosa is a well-established technique. Some sophisticated devices are inflated by a pump which is activated by pressing a button placed subcutaneously in the perineum. These devices are in use by only a relatively small number of diabetic subjects around the world, probably reflecting the attitudes of diabetologists and their patients. This approach may well not appeal to many people, but

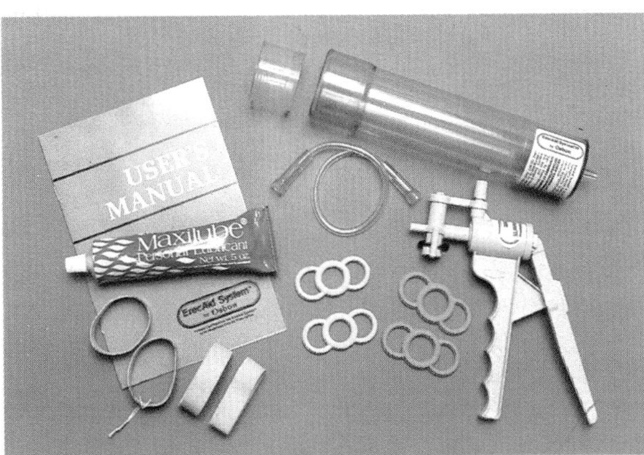


**Fig. 25.2.** The Erecaid Suction Tumescence System. Engorgement is induced by a simple suction device and the erection-like state is maintained using a constriction band. (Reproduced with permission from [15].) For further information contact Cory Bros. Co. Ltd. (Hospital Contracts), 4 Dollis Park, London N3 1HG, UK.

most treated patients are satisfied with its results [17].

Unfortunately, hormone treatment or vascular surgery seems to be of no benefit.

JOHN D. WARD

## References

1 McCulloch DK, Campbell IW, Wu FC, Prescott RJ, Clarke BF. The prevalence of diabetic impotence. *Diabetologia* 1980; **18**: 279–83.

2 McCulloch DK, Young RJ, Prescott RJ, Clarke BF. The natural history of impotence in diabetic men. *Diabetologia* 1984; **26**: 437–40.

3 de Groat WC, Booth AM. Physiology of male sexual function. *Ann Intern Med* 1980; **92**: 329–31.

4 El-Bayoumi M, El Sherbini O, Mosrafa M. Impotence in diabetics: organic versus psychogenic factors. *Urology* 1984; **24**: 459–63.

5 Lin JT, Bradley WE. Penile neuropathy in insulin dependent diabetes mellitus. *J Urol* 1985; **133**: 213–19.

6 Jevitch MJ, Edson M, Jarman WD, Herrera HH. Vascular factors in erectile failure among diabetics. *Urology* 1982; **19**: 163–8.

7 Wagner G, Green R. *Impotence*. New York: Plenum Press, 1981.

8 Jensen SB, Hagen C, Froland A, Pederson PB. Sexual function and the pituitary axis in insulin treated diabetic men. *Acta Med Scand* 1979; **624** (suppl): 65–8.

9 Murray FT, Wyss HU, Thomas RG, Spevack M, Glaros AG. Gonadal dysfunction in diabetic men with organic impotence. *J Clin Endocrinol Metab* 1987; **65**: 127–31.

10 Bradley WE, Lin JT. Assessment of diabetic sexual dysfunction and cystopathy. *Diabetic Neuropath* 1987; **15**: 146–54.

11 Hosking DJ, Bennet T, Hampton JR, Evans DF, Clark AJ, Robertson G. Diabetic impotence: studies of nocturnal erection during REM sleep. *Br Med J* 1979; **2**: 1394–6.

12 Buvat J, Lemaire A, Buvat-Herbaut M *et al*. Comparative investigations in 26 impotent and 26 non-impotent diabetic patients. *J Urol* 1985; **133**: 34–40.

13 Bancroft J, Bell C. Simultaneous recording of penile diameter and penile arterial pulse during laboratory based erotic stimulation in normal subjects. *J Psychosom Res* 1985; **29**: 303.

14 McCulloch DK, Hosking DJ, Tobart A. A pragmatic approach to sexual dysfunction in diabetic men: psychosexual counselling. *Diabetic Med* 1986; **3**: 485–9.

15 Wiles PG. Successful non-invasive management of erectile impotence in diabetic men. *Br Med J* 1988; **296**: 161–2.

16 Brindley GS. Pilot experiments on the actions of drugs injected into the human corpus cavernosum penis. *Br J Pharmacol* 1986; **87**: 495–500.

17 Pfeifer M, Reenan A, Berger R, Best J. Penile prosthesis and quality of life. *Diabetes* 1983; **32**: 77A.

# 26 Infections and Diabetes Mellitus

**Summary**

- Infection impairs glycaemic control in diabetic patients and is one of the commoner identified precipitating factors for diabetic ketoacidosis.
- The presence of diabetes impairs several aspects of phagocyte function, including cell movement, phagocytosis and intracellular killing of microorganisms; hyperglycaemia reduces oxidative killing capacity because increased glucose metabolism through the polyol pathway consumes NADPH, which is necessary to generate superoxide radicals.
- Although diabetic patients are strikingly prone to unusual infections with rare organisms (e.g. mucormycosis, enterococcal meningitis, osteomyelitis), to tuberculosis and to complicated urinary tract infections, it is not clear whether their general susceptibility to infection is increased or not.

It is widely believed that patients with diabetes are more prone to infection than their non-diabetic peers. This assumption is often based on personal experience of a few patients with difficult and protracted episodes of infection. There is no doubt that diabetic patients have higher carriage rates of staphylococci on the skin and of candida on the oral and genital mucosae. Therefore, it is not surprising that when these surfaces are breached by surgery or instrumentation, there is a higher incidence of wound infections and genital or oral candidiasis. However, it is still unclear whether diabetic people have a general increase in the rate of infection. Indirect evidence from a study of American factory workers showed that 28% of the diabetic employees were absent for 10 days or more in one year due to infections as compared with 15% of the controls; however, this difference was not statistically significant [1].

Infection undoubtedly disturbs blood glucose control [2] and infection is one of the commonest precipitating causes of diabetic ketoacidosis [3]. Studies have shown a relationship between the level of blood glucose and carriage rates of staphylococci [4] and, further, the rates of infection [5]. The effect of glucose control is multifactorial and related to defects in the cellular and humoral immune systems.

## Cellular defects

Abnormalities of all aspects of phagocyte function have been described in diabetes, namely adherence [6], cell movement [7], phagocytosis [8] and intracellular killing [9].

### *Cell movement*

Cell movement (cytotaxis, chemotaxis or leucotaxis) is difficult to measure and its relevance to the clinical situation is dubious (except in the rare inherited disorder of Job's syndrome or the 'lazy leucocyte disorder' of poor cell movement). However, movement does appear to be generally depressed in diabetes, with no additive effects of poor glycaemic control. Poor cell movement may, in fact, be inherited, as defects have been reported in the first-degree relatives of patients with IDDM [7].

### *Phagocytosis*

This is the process of ingestion of a target particle,

and encompasses recognition, adherence and engulfment. The phagocyte (neutrophil or macrophage) must first recognize the target as foreign, which it does via receptors on the cell membrane for immunoglobulin (IgG), complement (C3b) and lectins (simple sugars). Immunoglobulin IgA and IgG levels in patients with diabetes may be reduced in those subjects bearing HLA B8/DR3 [10, 11]. However, the levels of antibodies against specific microorganisms (e.g. *Pneumococcus* [12]) have shown no differences between diabetic subjects and controls. Complement deficiency is common in IDDM, with 25% of subjects having low C4 levels [13]. The genes encoding C4 are in linkage disequilibrium with HLA B8/DR3 [14]. It is not clear what effect these abnormalities might have on recognition in general.

Various techniques have been employed to measure phagocytosis. Many of the methods are relatively imprecise and involve visual evaluation of target engulfment or plating techniques which measure phagocytosis by counting the remaining viable colonies of target bacteria. These differing techniques may partly explain the divergent reports relating to defects in phagocytosis. In the author's experience, phagocytosis is a very robust process, unaffected by hyperglycaemia of up to 50 mmol/l [15]. Subtle improvements in phagocytosis have been reported during improvements in diabetic control: treatment of patients with intravenous insulin to reduce the blood glucose concentration from 18 to 5 mmol/l resulted in enhanced phagocytosis [16].

### *Killing*

Following ingestion of the target organism into the phagocyte, lysosomal granules are discharged into the phagocytic vacuole and killing proceeds by both oxidative and non-oxidative means. Oxidative killing occurs at an earlier stage than non-oxidative [17], and employs active oxygen products, e.g. superoxide, hydrogen peroxide and hypochlorite. The energy for this process is provided by the hexose monophosphate shunt (HMPS). Oxidative killing is initiated by a membrane oxidase which utilizes the electron donor, NADPH, and produces superoxide radicals. The neutrophil membrane is permeable to glucose, high intracellular levels of which greatly reduce the availability of NADPH. Under normal circumstances, glucose enters the HMPS and generates NADPH but in hyperglycaemia, high glucose levels swamp the HMPS and are metabolized by aldose reductase through the polyol pathway [18]. Aldose reductase is an NADPH-requiring enzyme and competes for this, thereby reducing the cell's ability to mount an oxidative attack and thereby inhibiting killing. Aldose reductase inhibitors have been shown to reverse these abnormalities, and these agents can restore both superoxide levels and impaired killing capacity to normal [18].

There are several methods for measuring organism-killing ability. Neutrophils can be simply incubated with test organisms and subsequently lysed, when viable bacteria are counted. More reliable and reproducible are the radiometric assays, based on the principle that only viable organisms can take up a radio-labelled marker [19]. Such assays, using specific test strains of *Candida albicans* (which should be obtained from a centre experienced in the technique), can be used for both research and clinical screening of neutrophil function.

## Unusual infections

Patients with diabetes are prone to unusual infections with rare organisms, such as rhinocerebral mucormycosis, Gram-negative enterococcal meningitis, malignant external otitis and emphysematous cystitis or cholecystitis. It is important to recognize these infections, as prompt antimicrobial therapy — sometimes combined with surgery — greatly increases the chances of cure.

### *Rhinocerebral mucormycosis*

This is a fungal infection, usually with *Mucor* (Figs 26.1 and 26.2) or *Rhizopus* spp., which may infect diabetic patients (whether well-controlled or in diabetic ketoacidosis), and especially those who abuse alcohol. It most commonly affects the lungs but may involve the paranasal air sinuses, and in diabetic or immunosuppressed subjects, may invade the skull, orbit or even brain (Fig. 26.3). Even with aggressive treatment, the established infection still carries a mortality of up to 50%. The clinical picture is often that of severe sinusitis with a bloody nasal discharge, but features such as proptosis, limitation of eye movements and failing vision (suggestive of orbital involvement) or of pain and discoloration of the tip of the nose should alert the physician, even in the UK [20]. The patient is also likely to have a severe, persistent acidaemia. Diagnosis is by

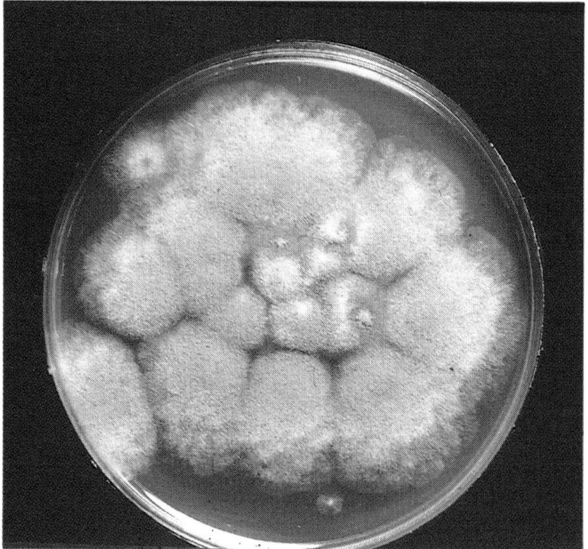

**Fig. 26.1.** Culture plate showing growth of *Mucor*. (Reproduced by kind permission of Dr R.C. Spencer, Royal Hallamshire Hospital, Sheffield.)

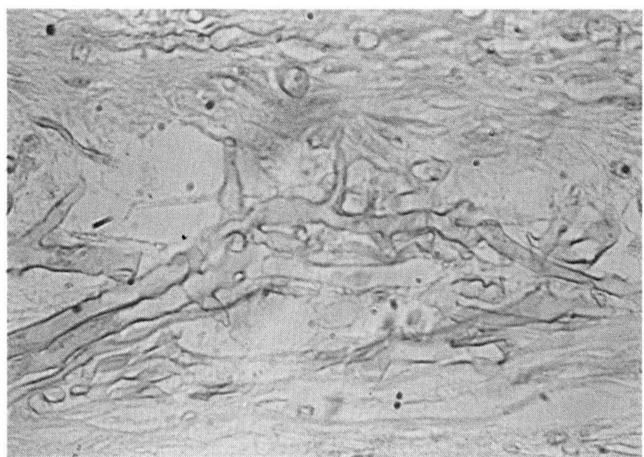

**Fig. 26.2.** Histological section of nasal submucosa, showing invasion by hyphae of *Mucor* (×400). (Reproduced by kind permission of Dr R.C. Spencer, Royal Hallamshire Hospital, Sheffield.)

histology and culture of biopsies of affected mucosae (Figs 26.1 and 26.2). Intravenous amphotericin-B is the drug of choice, and extensive surgical debridement may be necessary.

### *Malignant external otitis*

This infection can be extremely serious, hence its description as 'malignant'. It is almost always due to *Pseudomonas* spp. and may follow syringing of the external auditory canal. It should be suspected in a patient with otalgia and otorrhoea, and poor diabetic control. Standard antipseudomonal agents should be used and a surgical opinion sought.

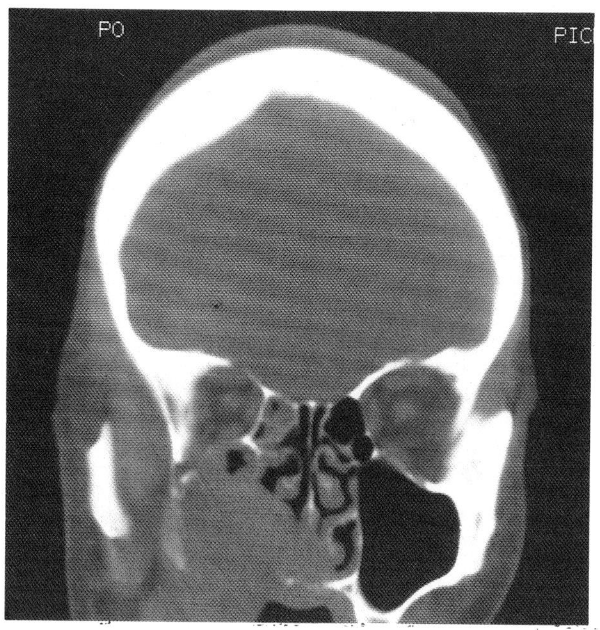


**Fig. 26.3.** CT scan showing rhinocerebral mucormycosis in a diabetic patient. The right maxillary sinus is filled and there is invasion of the floor of the orbit and the turbinates. (Reproduced by kind permission of Dr R. Nakielny, Royal Hallamshire Hospital, Sheffield.)

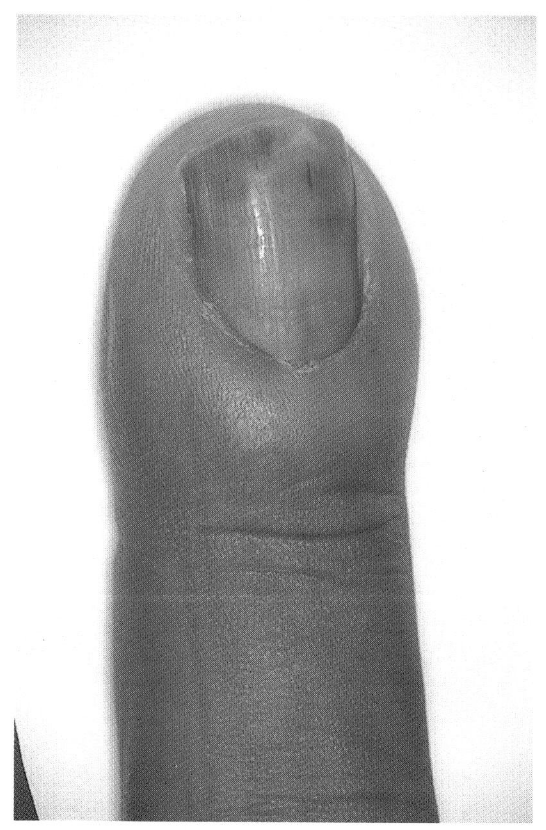

**Fig. 26.4.** Bolstering of the nail-fold due to chronic paronychia involving candida. (Reproduced by kind permission of Dr Ian MacFarlane, Walton Hospital, Liverpool.)

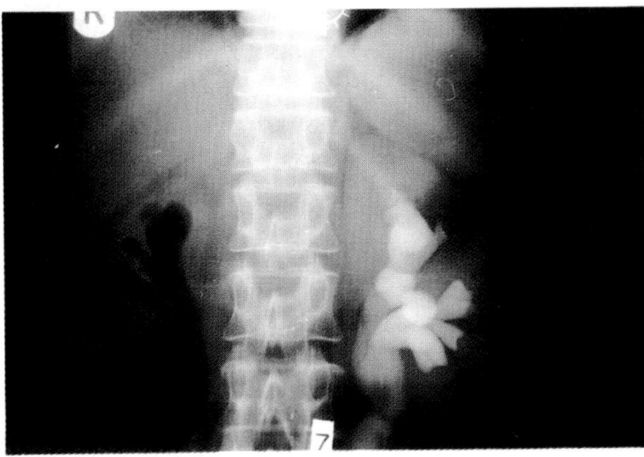

**Fig. 26.5.** Emphysematous pyelonephritis. Intravenous pyelogram showing gas filling the pelvicalyceal system of the right kidney. (Reproduced by kind permission of Dr Ian MacFarlane, Walton Hospital, Liverpool.)

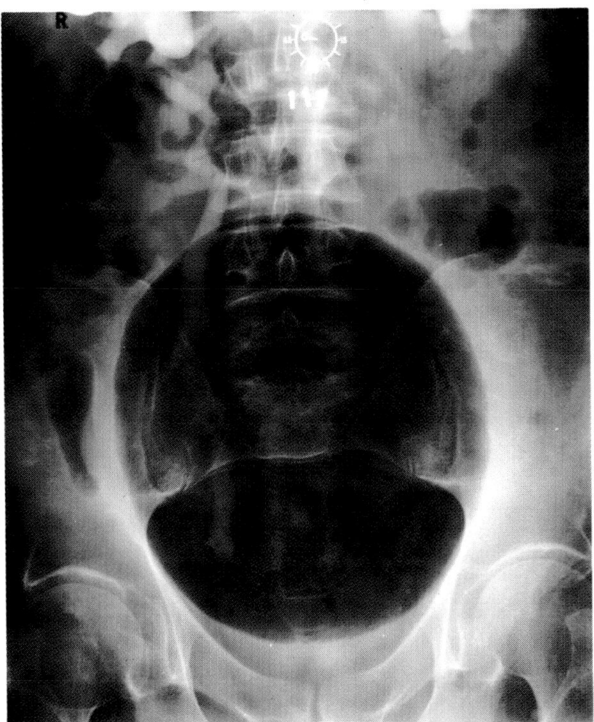

**Fig. 26.6.** Emphysematous cystitis. The bladder is grossly distended with gas. (Reproduced by kind permission of Dr Ian MacFarlane, Walton Hospital, Liverpool.)

### *Enterococcal meningitis*

The classical physical signs of meningitis may be absent in this infection. The patient is likely to be ketoacidotic and the Gram-negative organisms should be obtainable from blood cultures.

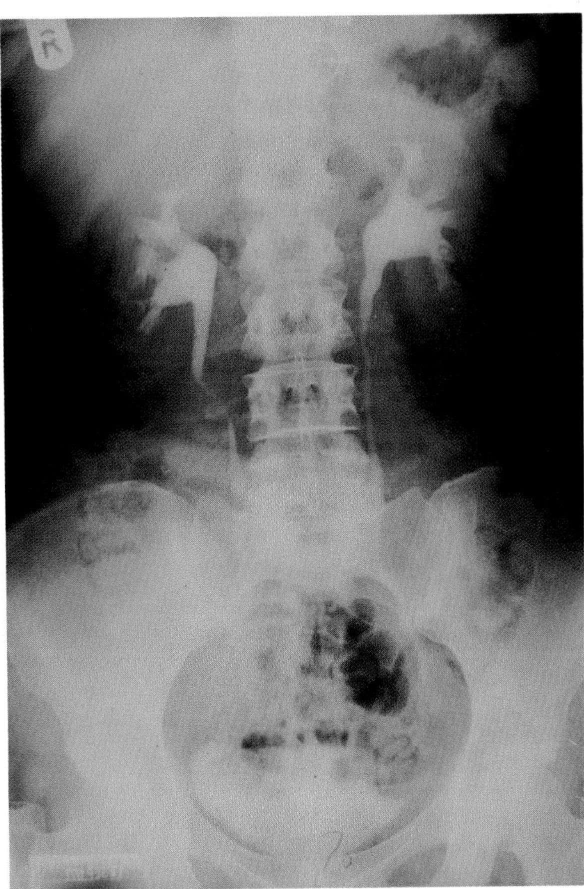

**Fig. 26.7.** Acute papillary necrosis, showing loss of a papilla and a calyceal ring shadow in the left kidney. (Reproduced by kind permission of Dr Ian MacFarlane, Walton Hospital, Liverpool.)

### *Infections of the skin and subcutaneous tissues*

These seem to be common in newly presenting or poorly controlled diabetic patients, and may significantly worsen metabolic control. Acute and chronic paronychia, often involving candida (Fig. 26.4) may occur. *Necrotizing cellulitis* (progressive synergistic gangrene) is usually a combined infection involving streptococci and staphylococci or Gram-negative organisms; this often spreads rapidly under the skin, which can be of deceptively normal appearance. It is rare and tends to affect older and debilitated patients. It demands immediate treatment with high-dose intravenous antibiotics and often requires surgical debridement or even amputation. Mortality is high, as with *Fournier's gangrene* which involves the scrotum and perineum. Diabetic foot ulcers frequently have an infective component and are usually colonized by multiple organisms, aerobic or anaerobic and sometimes gas-forming, often

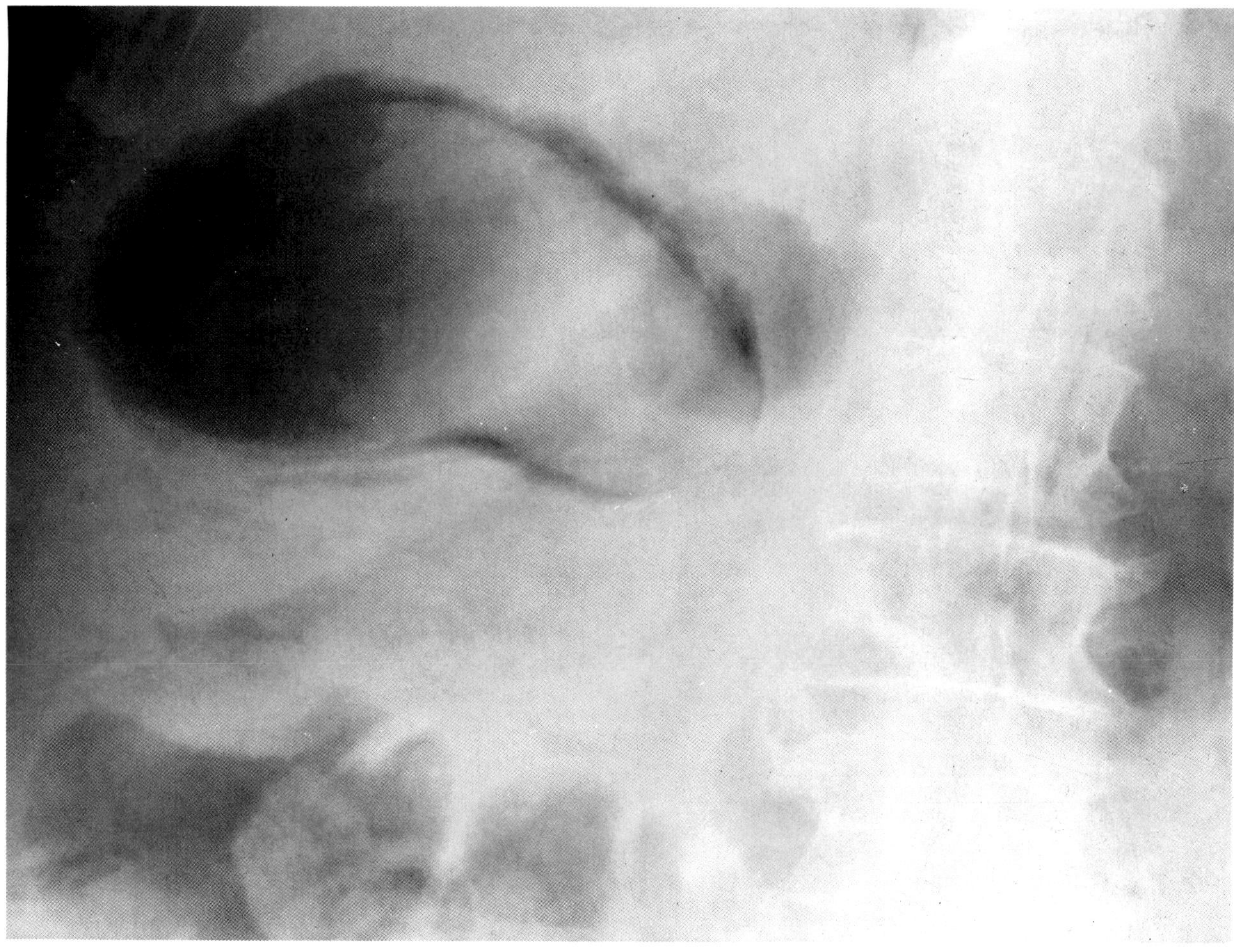

**Fig. 26.8.** Plain abdominal radiograph showing emphysematous cholecystitis. (Reproduced by kind permission of Dr R. Nakielny Royal Hallamshire Hospital, Sheffield.)

acting synergistically [21]. Infection may spread into the surrounding soft tissues, fascial spaces and bones of the feet (see Figs 19.5 and 19.6). Because infection with several organisms is so common, both aerobic and anaerobic cultures should be set up from material taken from the deeper parts of the wound. Fastidious organisms (e.g. *Eikenella* spp.) should be sought on repeated culture in patients who fail to respond to initial antibiotic therapy.

### Infections of the urinary tract

*Cystitis* is common in diabetic women and relatively often is complicated by ascending infection: renal scarring due to *pyelonephritis* is several times commoner in diabetic than in non-diabetic subjects. Renal infections may rarely be complicated by *emphysematous pyelonephritis*, in which Gram-negative rods or other organisms generate gas within the substance of the kidney [22]; the radiographic appearances may be diagnostic (Fig. 26.5). *Emphysematous cystitis* (Fig. 26.6) is another severe and fortunately rare sequel of lower urinary tract infection. Other complications include *perinephric abscess* and *papillary necrosis*, in which fragments of sloughed medullary tissue can be identified histologically in the urine and retrograde pyelography may demonstrate loss of papillae and 'ring shadows' lying in the calyces or pelvis (Fig. 26.7). It must be remembered that intravenous pyelography may precipitate acute renal failure in papillary necrosis and should not be performed if the diagnosis is suspected. All these conditions have a high mortality and must be treated rapidly and energetically.

### Infections of the lung, gut and other sites

*Tuberculosis* was previously common in diabetic patients but now, as in the general population, is relatively rare. Asian and Afro-Caribbean diabetic

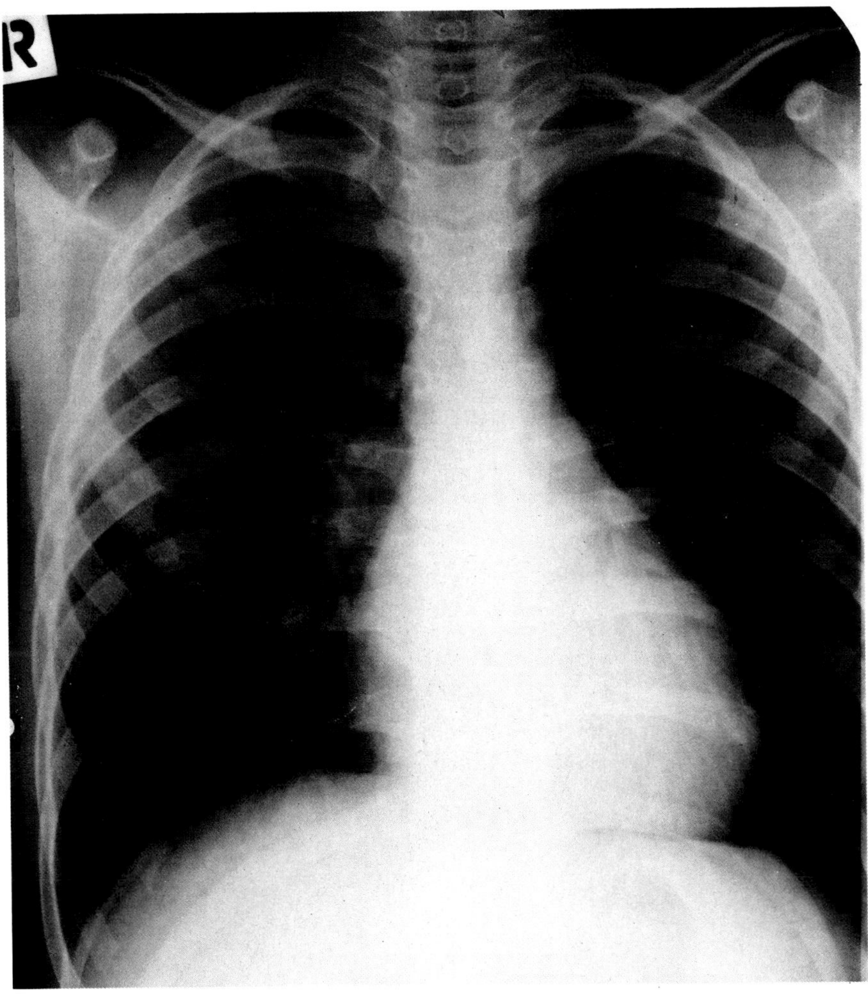


**Fig. 26.9.** Chest radiograph showing osteomyelitis in the left fourth rib of a diabetic child. (Reproduced by kind permission of Dr A. Barringdon, Royal Hallamshire Hospital, Sheffield.)

patients (in the UK) are still at increased risk of developing tuberculosis. Infection is usually due to reactivation of an old focus rather than through fresh contact.

*Emphysematous cholecystitis* (Fig. 26.8) is another rare infection, relatively commoner in diabetic patients, in which clostridia and other gas-forming organisms cause inflammation and often necrosis of the gall-bladder. *Ascending cholangitis*, with gas formation in the biliary system and liver, may ensue and mortality is very high. *Gingivitis* and *periodontal disease* are common in diabetic patients, particularly if poorly controlled.

*Osteomyelitis* in the diabetic foot (see Fig. 19.6) is discussed fully in Chapter 19. *Vertebral osteomyelitis* sometimes associated with epidural abscess formation, may present with backache. Other sites may occasionally be involved (Fig. 26.9). Diagnosis of osteomyelitis may be difficult, especially in the foot, where rarefaction of the bones and periosteal reactions (localized thickening of cortical bone) and non-specific radiographic findings are common (see Chapter 22). Three-phase radionuclide bone scans may demonstrate abnormalities in early blood flow which are apparently more specific [23].

R. MALCOLM WILSON

## References


1 Pell D, D'Alonzo CA. Sickness absenteeism in employed diabetics. *Am J Public Health* 1967; **57**: 253–60.

2 Colwell AR. Clinical use of insulin. In: Ellenberg M, Rifkin H, eds. *Diabetes Mellitus, Theory and Practice*. New York: McGraw-Hill, 1970: 624–37.

3 Nabarro JDN. Diabetic acidosis. In: Leibel BS, Wrenshall, eds. *Nature and Treatment of Diabetes*. New York: Excerpta Medica, 1965: 545–63.

4 Lipsky BA, Pecoraro BE, Chen MS, Koepsell MD. Factors affecting staphylococcal colonisation among NIDDM outpatients. *Diabetes Care* 1987; **10**: 483–6.

5 Rayfield EJ, Ault MJ, Kensch GT, Brothers MJ, Nechemias C, Smith H. Infection and diabetes: the case for glucose control. *Am J Med* 1982; **72**: 439–50.

6 Wilson RM, Galvin AM, Robins RA, Reeves WG. A flow cytometric method for the measurement of phagocytosis of candida by polymorphonuclear leucocytes. *J Immunol Methods* 1985; **76**: 247–53.
7 Molenaar DM, Palumbo PJ, Wilson WR, Rims RE. Leucocyte chemotaxis in diabetic patients and their non-diabetic first degree relatives. *Diabetes* 1976; **25** (suppl 2): 880–3.
8 Bybee JD, Rogers DE. The phagocytic activity of polymorphonuclear leucocytes obtained from patients with diabetes mellitus. *J Lab Clin Med* 1964; **64**: 1–13.
9 Wilson RM, Reeves WG. Neutrophil function in diabetes. In: Nattrass M, ed. *Recent Advances in Diabetes*, Vol 2. Edinburgh: Churchill Livingstone, 1986: 127–39.
10 Smith WI, Rabin BS, Huellmontel A, Van Thiel DH, Drash A. Immunopathology of juvenile-onset diabetes mellitus. I. IgA deficiency and juvenile diabetes. *Diabetes* 1978; **27**: 1092–7.
11 Hoddinott S, Dornan J, Bear JC, Farid NR. Immunoglobulin levels, immunodeficiency and HLA in Type 1 (insulin-dependent) diabetes mellitus. *Diabetologia* 1982; **23**: 326–9.
12 Lederman MM, Rodman HM, Schacter BZ, Jones PK, Schiffman G. Antibody response to pneumonococcal polysaccharides in insulin-dependent diabetes mellitus. *Diabetes Care* 1982; **5**: 36–9.
13 Vergani D, Johnston C, B-Abdullah N, Barnett AH. Low serum C4 concentrations: an inherited predisposition to insulin dependent diabetes. *Br Med J* 1983; **286**: 923–8.
14 Charlesworth JA, Timmermans V, Golding J. The complement system in Type 1 (insulin-dependent) diabetes. *Diabetologia* 1987; **30**: 372–9.
15 Wilson RM, Reeves WG. Neutrophil phagocytosis and killing in insulin-dependent diabetes. *Clin Exp Immunol* 1986; **63**: 478–84.
16 Kjersem H, Hilsted J, Madsbad S, Wandall JH, Johansen KS, Borregaard N. Polymorphonuclear leucocyte dysfunction during short term metabolic changes from normo- to hyperglycaemia in Type 1 (insulin-dependent) diabetic patients. *Infection* 1988; **16**: 215–21.
17 Nathan CF. Secretion of oxygen intermediates: Role in effector functions of activated macrophages. *Federation Proc* 1982; **41**: 2206–11.
18 Wilson RM, Tomlinson DR, Reeves WG. Neutrophil sorbitol production impairs oxidative killing in diabetes. *Diabetic Med* 1987; **4**: 37–40.
19 Bridges CG, Da Silva GL, Yamamura M, Valdimarsson H. A radiometric assay for the combined measurement of phagocytes and intracellular killing of *Candida albicans*. *Clin Exp Immunol* 1980; **42**: 226–33.
20 Larkin JG, Butcher IG, Frier BM, Brebner H. Fatal rhinocerebral mucormycosis in a newly-diagnosed diabetic. *Diabetic Med* 1986; **3**: 266–8.
21 Wheat LJ, Allen SD, Henry M *et al*. Diabetic foot infections. Bacteriologic analysis. *Arch Int Med* 1986; **146**: 1935–40.
22 Zabbo A, Montie JE, Popowniak KL, Weinstein AJ. Bilateral emphysematous pyelonephritis. *Urology* 1985; **25**: 293–6.
23 Seldin DW, Heikin JP, Feldman F, Alderson PO. Effect of soft-tissue pathology on detection of pedal osteomyelitis in diabetics. *J Nucl Med* 1985; **26**: 988–93.

# 27 Diabetes and the Fetus: Mechanisms of Teratogenesis


## Summary

- The common abnormalities caused by diabetes during embryogenesis are cardiac malformations, neural tube defects, impaired ossification (especially caudal regression) and malformations of the gut and urogenital system.
- The identity of the teratogen(s) in diabetes has not been proven.
- In experimental animals, hyperglycaemia has a dose-related effect in inducing malformations but hypoglycaemia may also be teratogenic; the precise dependence of malformations on glycaemic control in man is unknown.
- Hyperglycaemia and hyperketonaemia may impair the activities of important cellular enzymes through glycosylation and alterations in osmolarity and pH.
- Insulin deficiency may reduce availability of cations (zinc, magnesium, calcium); this could interfere with the function of certain enzymes and with ossification.
- Reduced placental blood flow in diabetes may compromise yolk-sac perfusion and metabolism, and so lead to both growth retardation and malformations.
- Later effects of diabetes on the fetus include macrosomia (due to fetal hyperinsulinaemia, stimulated by maternal hyperglycaemia), delayed lung maturation and neonatal hypoglycaemia and hypocalcaemia.


It is hardly surprising that maternal diabetes can have serious consequences for the infant, as a major aspect of pregnancy is to ensure adequate fetal nutrition, and as the levels of all major nutrients and several minerals are often disturbed in diabetes. Until recently, the most common abnormality in the infants of diabetic mothers was macrosomia, but careful observation has now demonstrated a range of anomalies including growth retardation and malformations (for review see [1, 2]). Many of these have been reproduced experimentally in animals with chemically induced or genetically inbred diabetes, or *in vitro* (for review see [3]). In the search for a unifying mechanism for the teratogenic effects of diabetes, several separate but physiologically related putative teratogens need to be considered.

### Pre-embryonic and placental development

The first 18 days of human gestation (5–6 days in the rat) can be regarded as the pre-embryonic period. Diabetes may impair the earlier processes of ovulation, fertilization, movement along the oviduct and implantation [3] but these effects are not strictly considered as teratogenesis.

The fertilized egg in the oviduct is virtually independent of maternal physiology, deriving metabolic energy from cytoplasmic stores of pyruvate and lactate. By 7 days, the morula has become a hollow blastocyst and has begun to implant in the uterus. Yolk-sac development may be disrupted by diabetes, and impaired vessel formation and reduced numbers of mitochondria [4] may inhibit cellular metabolism, especially glycolysis. As anaerobic glycolysis is the major source of metabolic energy during early development, this may partly explain the association between fetal growth retardation and congenital malformations in general [5] and in infants of diabetic mothers in particular [1–3].

In diabetic pregnancy, there is often an increase

in placental weight despite a reduction in blood flow [6]. The increased weight reflects excess stores of glycogen and lipid, together with deposits of fibrin and mucopolysaccharides [7]. An increase in villous surface area has been observed in some, but not all, studies [8]. Recently, Thomas *et al.* [9] found that, despite an elevated maternal–fetal glucose gradient, net glucose transfer to the fetus was reduced. However, Herrera *et al.* [10] found a linear relationship between maternal glucose and placental glucose transfer. Thus, the effect of glycaemia on facilitated glucose transport remains to be clarified.

## Embryogenesis

Teratogenesis strictly refers to disruptions during organ formation, i.e. the period spanning 2.5–8 weeks in human gestation or days 6–11 in rats. The wide variety of abnormalities observed in infants of diabetic mothers suggests that the mechanism(s) of teratogenesis must operate across a range of systems. The common problems include neural tube defects, impaired ossification, gut and urogenital malformation and congenital heart disease.

Between days 18–25 in humans (8.5–10.5 days in rodents), the neural plate folds and closes to form the neural tube. This critical stage is susceptible to various teratogens [11] and the malformation rate is increased at least tenfold in infants of diabetic mothers [3]. Exencephaly, anencephaly (Fig. 27.1), and hydrocephaly all occur both in humans [1, 2], and experimentally in rats *in vivo* [12] and *in vitro* [13].

Hyperglycaemia *per se* has a dose-dependent effect and improved glycaemic control consistently improves malformation rates in experimental animals [3, 12, 13]. High glucose concentrations apparently induce cytoarchitectural changes in the neuroepithelium, including a reduction in cell mitosis and premature differentiation [13]. On the other hand, Sadler and Hunter [11] recently demonstrated a failure of neural development in mouse embryos as a result of *low* glucose levels in the culture medium for as little as 12 h. Growth retardation only accompanied the malformation if the glucose deprivation was more severe or prolonged. A common mechanism by which hypo- and hyperglycaemia give rise to the same malformation has not been described, but pH and osmolarity may be implicated, as acid conditions contribute to neural tube defects [14] and as glucose is weakly ionized under physiological conditions. The caudal regression syndrome (causing sacral agenesis in man) is almost exclusive to infants of diabetic mothers [15] and comparable rat models [12, 16] and arises early in embryogenesis [16]. The defect is probably in the midposterior axis of the mesoderm but the mechanism has not been clarified (Fig. 27.2).

Ossification may be delayed or defective in infants of diabetic mothers and in various animal models, giving rise to micrognathia, cleft palate, malformed ribs and femoral hypoplasia [12, 16–18]. Disturbed enzyme function may be involved. Renal β-glucuronidase shows severely reduced activity, in parallel with delayed ossification [17]. This enzyme may be involved in breakdown of cartilage during ossification, or it may merely reflect a group of enzymes specifically affected by hyperglycaemia or some other disturbance of diabetes. The fact that β-glucuronidase is a glycoprotein and therefore liable to excessive glycosylation may be relevant to its susceptibility to inhibition by maternal diabetes.

In a study of diabetic rats by Eriksson [19], in which micrognathia was the most common abnormality, a significant decrease in total fetal body zinc was observed. This was accompanied by excessive accumulation of zinc, copper and manganese in maternal liver; dietary zinc supplements to the diabetic mothers did not increase fetal zinc levels. Since zinc deficiency *per se* is teratogenic and may inhibit DNA synthesis via decreased activity of zinc-dependent enzymes [20], this may be an important mechanism for some teratogenic effects of diabetes, especially as many other zinc-dependent enzymes have important

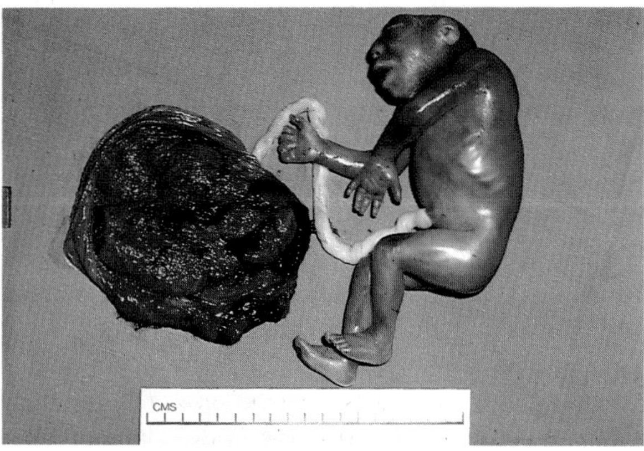


**Fig. 27.1.** Anencephaly in the stillborn child of a diabetic mother. (Reproduced with permission from Mr R.B. Fraser, University of Sheffield.)

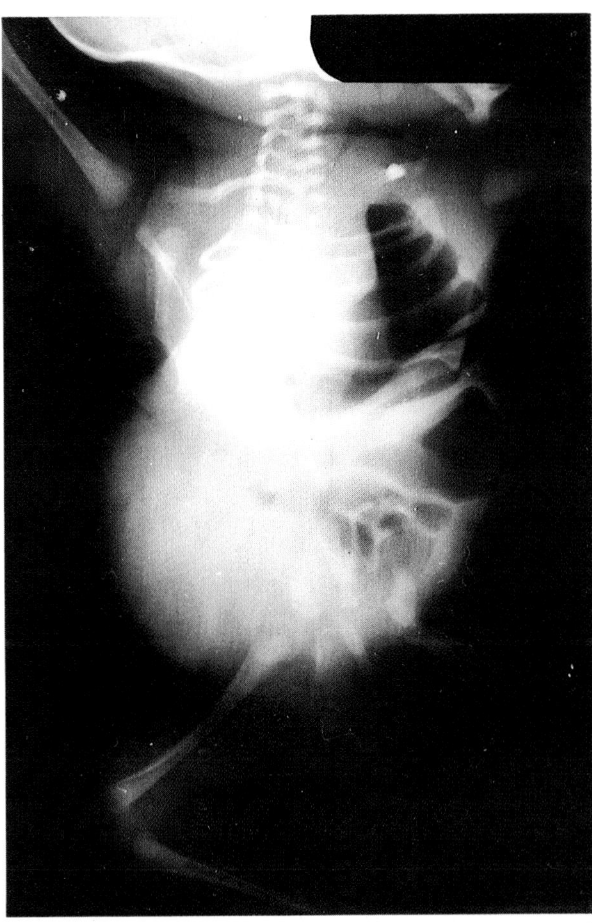

**Fig. 27.2.** Radiograph of the fetus of a diabetic mother, showing sacral agenesis (the 'caudal regression syndrome'). (Reproduced by kind permission of Dr Ian MacFarlane, Walton Hospital, Liverpool.)

roles in cellular function. It is also possible that bone mineral constituents are reduced; hypocalcaemia is observed in up to 50% of infants of diabetic mothers within 72 h of birth [21] but embryonic levels have not been determined. Serum levels of magnesium, a mainly intracellular cation whose metabolism is partly linked with calcium and is partly insulin-dependent, are lower than normal in both diabetic mothers [22] and neonatal infants of diabetic mothers [21], but again embryonic data are not available.

During weeks 5–8 in humans, the gut, urogenital system, cardiovascular system and limbs develop and abnormalities may appear. Anomalies particularly associated with maternal diabetes include gastroschisis, renal agenesis, duodenal and anorectal atresia, and, most commonly, congenital heart disease, especially transposition of the great vessels [2, 12]; many of these are fatal *in utero* or in the neonatal period.

### *Identity of the teratogen in diabetes*

As hyperglycaemia is the most obvious metabolic derangement in diabetes, it has been considered the most likely teratogen in infants of diabetic mothers, and many studies, especially those *in vitro*, support this conclusion. Nonetheless, Mills *et al.* have recently observed a lack of correlation between maternal glycaemia during weeks 5–12 and malformation rate in infants of diabetic mothers [23]. Experiments with other sugars have demonstrated, however, that some of the effects attributable to glucose may be due to changes in osmolarity [24] and/or pH [14].

In very poorly controlled diabetes, ketone bodies are present in the maternal circulation and freely cross the placenta. High levels of 3-hydroxybutyrate *in vitro* caused growth retardation and malformations, and synergism has been demonstrated between subteratogenic doses of 3-hydroxybutyrate and glucose in rat embryos [25]. It has also been suggested that hyperketonaemia during pregnancy may lower intellectual capacity in the offspring, although this is disputed [2].

There has been concern that hypoglycaemia, which is common during the tight control recommended during pregnancy, may also be teratogenic. Whereas Sadler and Hunter [11] found that hypoglycaemia impaired neural development, another study [26] which induced severe hypoglycaemic shock in pregnant rats found no evidence of abnormalities. The excess placental glycogen laid down during the diabetic pregnancy may protect the fetus against maternal hypoglycaemia by releasing glucose into the fetal circulation.

The possible role of insulin — which promotes growth — as a teratogen is unresolved, although it can cause malformations in chick embryos [27]. The human placenta is not permeable to insulin, so periods of maternal hyperinsulinaemia probably do not affect the embryo, although abnormal nutrient levels and particularly hyperglycaemia are likely to influence fetal insulin production. Insulin and primitive B cells have been detected in fetuses from day 14 in rats or week 9 in humans; insulin secretion may be raised in the fetus of the diabetic mother, and probably contributes to macrosomia.

Figure 27.3 summarizes the possible mechanisms of diabetic teratogenesis. The major maternal disruptions are hypoinsulinaemia leading to hyperglycaemia and disturbed intermediary metabolite levels, which lead to alterations in pH

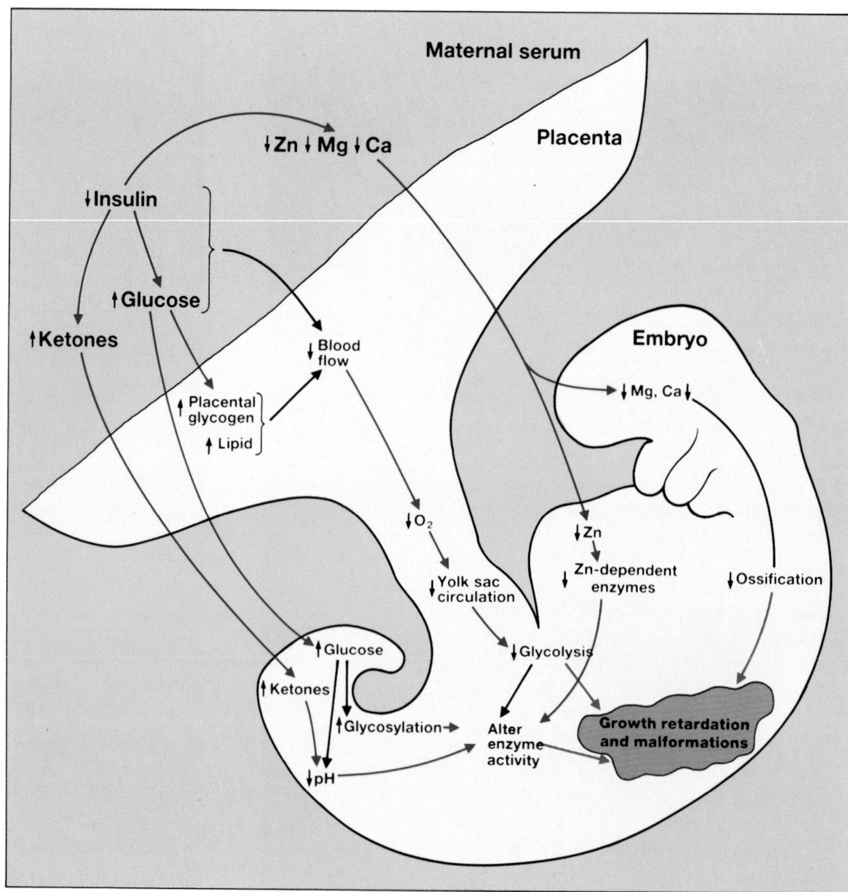


Fig. 27.3. Possible mechanisms for teratogenic effects of maternal diabetes during embryogenesis. Red arrows represent observed effects; black arrows represent speculative or unconfirmed mechanisms; blue arrows indicate that these processes may influence outcomes but mechanisms are not clarified.

and osmolarity in the embryo and impaired metabolism. Altered cation and mineral availability may impair ossification. The activity of a wide variety of enzymes is probably altered. These defects, and others as yet unknown, may lead to the specific malformations associated with diabetes.

Further disturbances of development occur during fetal development due to altered nutrient and hormone levels.

## Fetal development

From week 8 onwards, the human conceptus has recognizable limbs, digits, face and internal organs and is described as a fetus. Subsequent development involves an increase in size from 30 to 500 mm, the appearance and maturation of endocrine and neural systems, and preparation for breathing and feeding. Maternal diabetes may have serious effects on various aspects of this maturation, particularly on total growth, adipose stores, pulmonary maturation and pancreatic development [1, 2]. A combination of abnormal nutrient levels, insulin, insulin-like growth factors (IGF), placental lactogen and IGF inhibitors interact to disrupt normal development. Insulin is certainly required for fetal survival and growth, and fetal hyperinsulinaemia (stimulated by maternal hyperglycaemia) may be responsible for overgrowth of adipose tissue, leading to macrosomia, as postulated by Pedersen [28].

Alterations at this stage can be serious, but do not result in malformations. For further details of effects of diabetes on fetal development see [29, 30].

CAROLINE J. CRACE

## References


1 Freinkel N. Of pregnancy and progeny. Banting Lecture 1980. *Diabetes* 1980; **29**: 1023–35.

2 Reece EA, Hobbins JC. Diabetic embryopathy: pathogenesis, prenatal diagnosis and prevention. *Obstet Gynecol Surv* 1986; **41**: 325–35.

3 Eriksson U. Congenital malformations in diabetic animal models: a review. *Diabetes Res* 1984; **1**: 57–66.

4 Pinter E, Reece EA, Leranth C. Yolk sac failure in embryopathy due to hyperglycaemia. Ultrastructural analysis of yolk sac differentiation in rat conceptuses under hyper-

glycaemic culture conditions. *Teratology* 1986; **33**: 363–8.
5 Van den Berg BJ, Yerushalmy J. The relationship of the rate of intrauterine growth of infants of low birthweight to mortality, morbidity and congenital abnormalities. *J Pediatr* 1966; **69**: 531–45.
6 Eriksson U, Janssen L. Diabetes in pregnancy: decreased placental blood flow and disturbed fetal development in the rat. *Pediatr Res* 1984; **18**: 735–8.
7 Diamant YZ, Metzger BE, Freinkel N, Shafrir E. Placental lipid and glycogen content in human and experimental diabetes mellitus. *Am J Obstet Gynecol* 1982; **144**: 5–11.
8 Boyd PA, Scott A, Keeling JW. Quantitative structural studies on placentas from pregnancies complicated by diabetes mellitus. *Br J Obstet Gynaecol* 1986; **93**: 31–5.
9 Thomas CR, Eriksson GL, Kihlstrom I, Eriksson UJ. The effects of diabetes on placental glucose metabolism and transport in the rat (abstract). *Diabetologia* 1987; **30**: 588A.
10 Herrera E, Palacin M, Martin A, Lasuncion A. Relationship between maternal and fetal fuels and placental glucose transfer in rats with maternal diabetes of varying severity. *Diabetes* 1985; **34** (suppl 2): 42–6.
11 Sadler TW, Hunter ES. Hypoglycemia: how little is too much for the embryo? *Am J Obstet Gynecol* 1987, **157**: 190–3.
12 Brownscheidle CM, Wootten V, Mathieu MH, Davis DL, Hofmann IA. The effects of maternal diabetes on fetal maturation and neonatal health. *Metabolism* 1983; **32** (suppl 1): 148–55.
13 Reece EA, Pinter E, Leranth CZ *et al*. Ultrastructural analysis of malformation of the embryonic neural axis by *in vitro* hyperglycaemia. *Teratology* 1985; **32**: 363–73.
14 Nau H, Scott WJ. Weak acids may act as teratogens by accumulating in the basic milieu of the early mammalian embryo. *Nature* 1986; **323**: 276–8.
15 Mills JL, Baker L, Goldman AS. Malformations in infants of diabetic mothers occur before the seventh gestational week: implications for treatment. *Diabetes* 1979; **28**: 292–3.
16 Eriksson UJ, Styrud J. Congenital malformations in diabetic pregnancy: the clinical relevance of experimental animal studies. *Acta Paediatr Scand Suppl* 1985; **320**: 72–8.
17 Wilson GN, Howe M, Stover JM. Delayed developmental sequences in rodent diabetic embryopathy. *Pediatr Res* 1985; **19**: 1337–40.
18 Johnson JP, Carey JC, Gooch WM, Petersen JP, Beattie JF. Femoral hypoplasia–unusual facies syndrome in infants of diabetic mothers. *J Pediatr* 1983; **102**: 866–72.
19 Eriksson UJ. Diabetes in pregnancy: retarded fetal growth, congenital malformations and feto-maternal concentrations of Zn, Cu, Mn in the rat. *J Nutr* 1984; **114**: 477–84.
20 Duncan JR, Hurley LS. Thymidine kinase and DNA polymerase activity in normal and zinc deficient developing rat embryos. *Proc Soc Exp Biol Med* 1978; **159**: 39–43.
21 Mimouni F, Tsang RC, Hertzberg VS, Miodovnik M. Polycythemia, hypomagnesemia, and hypocalcemia in infants of diabetic mothers. *Am J Dis Child* 1986; **140**: 798–800.
22 Wibell L, Gebbre-Medhin M, Lindmark G. Magnesium and zinc in diabetic pregnancy. *Acta Paediatr Scand Suppl* 1985; **320**: 100–6.
23 Mills JL, Knopp RH, Simpson JL *et al*. Lack of relation of increased malformation rates in infants of diabetic mothers to glycemic control during organogenesis. *N Engl J Med* 1988; **318**: 671–6.
24 Cockroft DL, Coppola DT. Teratogenic effects of excess glucose on head-fold rat embryos in culture. *Teratology* 1977; **16**: 141–6.
25 Lewis NJ, Akazawa S, Freinkel N. Teratogenesis from B-hydroxybutyrate during organogenesis in rat embryo organ culture and enhancement by subteratogenic glucose (abstract). *Diabetes* 1983; **32** (suppl 1): 11A.
26 Ream JR, Weingarten PL, Pappas AM. Evaluation of the prenatal effects of massive doses of insulin in rats. *Teratology* 1970; **3**: 29–32.
27 Landauer W. Rumplessness of chicken embryos produced by the injection of insulin and other chemicals. *J Exp Zool* 1945; **98**: 65.
28 Pedersen JF, Bojsen-Moller B, Poulsen H. Blood sugar in newborn infants of diabetic mothers. *Acta Endocrinol* 1954; **15**: 33–52.
29 Hill DJ, Milner RDG. The role of peptide growth factors and hormones in the control of fetal growth. In: Chiswick ML, ed. *Recent Advances in Perinatal Medicine*, Vol 2. Edinburgh: Churchill Livingstone, 1985: 79–102.
30 Crace CJ, Hill DJ, Milner RDG. Mitogenic actions of insulin on fetal and neonatal rat cells *in vitro*. *J Endocrinol* 1985; **104**: 61–8.

# 28 Psychological Problems and Psychiatric Disorders in Diabetes Mellitus

**Summary**

• Psychological disturbances and psychiatric disorders, mostly mild, are common in diabetic patients but are often missed in the routine diabetic clinic.

• All diabetic care teams should have easy and immediate access to a psychiatrist and/or a clinical psychologist who should have specialist knowledge of diabetes and its management.

• Patients learn to cope with the psychological stress induced by diabetes through a process of adaptation which may be complicated by reactions of denial, anger or depression. Failure to cope, or 'maladaptation', is manifested by emotional, physical and behavioural signs of psychological stress. Management is by 'self-help' measures and relaxation exercises as well as through social support and medical advice.

• A few animal studies and anecdotal case reports in man suggest that psychological stress may directly precipitate diabetes or aggravate diabetic control but there is no firm evidence that such a mechanism operates in human diabetes. Poor diabetic control in patients under psychosocial stress may be due to poor compliance or other factors.

• The commonest psychiatric disorder in diabetic patients is depression with or without anxiety, usually with sleep disturbance. Patients with visual impairment or other complications are particularly at risk.

• Depression frequently responds to general measures such as sympathetic discussion and advice to improve sleep. Moderate or severe depression requires antidepressants, of which tricyclic agents are the first choice. Patients at risk of suicide or antisocial behaviour need urgent psychiatric referral and possibly hospital admission.

• Other psychiatric problems encountered in diabetic patients include anorexia nervosa and other appetite disturbances, injection and needle phobias, obsessional disorders and factitious hyper- or hypoglycaemia.

Strictly defined, *psychology* is the study of normal and abnormal mental functioning and behaviour, and *psychiatry* the diagnosis and treatment of mental disorders. The purpose of this chapter is to discuss the psychological and psychiatric disorders occurring in diabetic patients, their possible causes and impact on diabetes, and their diagnosis, treatment and prognosis. Most of these observations apply equally to IDDM and NIDDM.

## Psychological problems: stress, adaptation and coping

In common with other illnesses and traumatic life-events, diabetes and its sequelae impose a considerable burden of psychological stress. The term 'stress' is in many respects unsatisfactory, mainly because 'stress' cannot be readily defined or measured, but is convenient in that it is widely understood and is acceptable to patients. Moreover, the identification of those factors which cause 'stress' can suggest practical educational and behavioural tactics which may help to overcome them.

Patients attempt to come to terms with diabetes and its attendant psychological stress through a process of *adaptation*, which comprises two phases: first, the realization that certain attitudes and behaviours will have to change and secondly, the exploration of new ways of coping until satisfactory solutions are found. During adaptation, some patients may experience disagreeable emotional reactions, superficially resembling grief, over their potential loss of health and lifestyle. These reactions are usually transient and may include the following:

*Disbelief and denial* of the diagnosis, its implications or even the need for treatment may follow the initial shock of being diagnosed diabetic. These reactions are often accentuated by lack of knowledge and imperfect 'first-aid' education.

*Anger* is another common response, often directed at the illness but sometimes at patients themselves, their parents or the medical or nursing staff; the latter, if inexperienced, may unfortunately tend to neglect the angry patient, to the detriment of his or her diabetic care.

*Depression* often follows the realization that diabetes and the need for treatment and self-monitoring are in most cases lifelong, or that the disease carries the risk of long-term complications. Self-blame and withdrawal may be prominent and frequently accompany feelings of worthlessness and hopelessness. As discussed below, depression with or without anxiety may persist in the long term and represents the commonest psychiatric disorder in diabetic patients.

These reactions are usually short-lived but may be protracted and affect the patient's ability to cope with diabetes and life in general. It is not clear why some individuals cope with diabetes whereas others do not; possible determinants have been investigated in several studies [1] but the tests used to measure 'coping ability' may have little relevance to the diabetic patient's struggle to regain control over his life [2]. *Maladaptation*, where the process of learning to cope is incomplete or prolonged, may be commoner in young patients or those with complications and is often signalled by 'warning signs' indicating psychological stress. These include emotional, physical and social or behavioural reactions (Tables 28.1–28.3), which must be actively sought and recognized early so that specialist advice and help can be provided if necessary. The commonest *emotional reactions* are increases in tension, irritability and moodiness which signify mounting depression and/or anxiety (Table 28.1). *Physical reactions* result from autonomic or endocrine responses to psychological stress and may need to be carefully distinguished from the symptoms of diabetes, its complications or treatment (Table 28.2). *Social and behavioural reactions* of people under stress may be striking, although more subtle features may be difficult to recognize (Table 28.3).

**Table 28.1.** Maladaptation: emotional reactions signifying depression and/or anxiety.

| |
|---|
| Feeling under pressure, threatened or frightened |
| Restlessness, inability to relax |
| Irritability, aggression, conflict with others |
| Inability to concentrate, make decisions or complete tasks quickly |
| Feeling tired or mentally drained |
| Feeling moody, pessimistic or a failure |
| Inability to feel pleasure |
| Tearfulness |

**Table 28.2.** Maladaptation: physical reactions suggesting depression and/or anxiety.

| |
|---|
| Altered appetite or nausea |
| Indigestion or altered bowel habit |
| Insomnia, tiredness |
| Palpitations, breathlessness or chest pain |
| Frequent urge to pass urine |
| Paraesthesiae in fingers or toes or around the mouth |
| Sweating |
| Headache |

**Table 28.3.** Maladaptation: social and behavioural reactions suggesting depression and/or anxiety.

| |
|---|
| Constant seeking of company, social support or reassurance |
| Avoidance of company, withdrawal and indifference to others |
| Capriciousness and unpredictability |
| Unreasonable expectations |
| Indecision in social matters |
| Altered sexual behaviour |

### *Management of maladaptation*

Coping and adaptation will be greatly helped by a sympathetic and understanding approach to the patient, combined with effective education and ready availability of advice about diabetes and its management whenever the patient needs this.

All members of the diabetes team must be alert to the features suggesting maladaptation (Tables 28.1–28.3) and should be able to discuss their significance with the patient and to suggest referral to a psychiatrist or psychologist if necessary. Regular supportive discussions and practical advice and reassurance about specific anxieties may be enough to help the patient to cope better. If not, a 'self-help' approach is often beneficial. The patient should be asked to keep a diary of the nature, severity and duration of his own 'warning signs' of stress and to try to identify their possible causes and anything which could help to alleviate them. Any practical solutions which suggest themselves should be tried and their success or failure evaluated; at the same time, the patient should be urged to try to stop worrying about any problems which are completely insoluble. The patient should review his or her diary and progress at regular intervals, either alone or with a diabetic team member, until he or she has reduced as many causes of stress as possible and has begun to feel in control again. Relaxation exercises can be very useful when patients experience acute tension or worry; instructional tapes (which should be played through and practised with a team member before the patient tries the procedure alone) can be obtained from most clinical psychology departments.

Adaptation may be particularly difficult in patients suffering diabetic complications such as loss of sight, amputation, sexual dysfunction, infertility or complications of pregnancy, renal failure or repeated hospital admissions with poor metabolic control. The basic psychological approach should be as above but individual advice and information will be needed. Some practical points are discussed in the relevant chapters of this book, and the series of *Coping with* ... booklets published by the British Diabetic Association provide valuable advice about specific problems. Local specialists or agencies may also be able to provide particular aspects of support and care, such as facilities for the blind and partially sighted (described in Chapter 9).

### *Metabolic effects of psychological stress in diabetic patients*

The 'fight or flight' reaction provoked by acute physiological or psychological stress triggers the secretion of counter-regulatory hormones which antagonize the effect of insulin and tend to cause hyperglycaemia [3–5]. These observations have probably fuelled the popular and long-standing belief that psychological or psychosocial stress may aggravate metabolic control in diabetic patients or even precipitate the disease.

There have been many anecdotal reports of diabetes (especially IDDM) developing suddenly after a traumatic life-event [6]. However, both diabetes and personal catastrophes are relatively common and will occasionally be associated by chance alone; this association may appear to gain strength when viewed retrospectively, which is a major flaw in the design of all such studies. Theoretical consideration of the central and metabolic effect of opioid peptides and other neurotransmitters has led to speculation that chronic stress could act on the autonomic nervous system to induce a metabolic syndrome similar to NIDDM [7]. Recent animal studies have provided more direct and highly intriguing evidence that psychosocial stress (e.g. overcrowding and noise) may accelerate the development of diabetes in rats, either destined to develop an autoimmune IDDM-like condition [8] or treated with repeated subdiabetogenic doses of the B-cell toxin, streptozotocin [9]. It is not clear whether the diabetogenic effect of stress in these models is due to the counter-regulatory effects of the 'stress' hormones, their possible immunomodulatory actions, or some other factor. The relevance of these observations to man is unknown; at present, there are no convincing epidemiological or other data to suggest that psychological stress can precipitate either IDDM or NIDDM in humans.

The possible detrimental effects of psychological stress on metabolic control in people with established diabetes have also been debated for many years. A number of case reports, again anecdotal and retrospective, have claimed that psychological stress can aggravate metabolic control and even precipitate ketoacidosis in IDDM patients [10]. Several uncontrolled studies, often quoted but never repeated, have reported various metabolic disturbances in diabetic patients subjected to acute psychological stress, such as the (invented) threat of having a leg amputated. The metabolic responses described included diuresis and natriuresis and rises in circulating free fatty acid and ketone body levels; curiously, in view of the hyperglycaemic effects of the 'stress' hormones, the blood glucose level generally remained stable or fell slightly and rose only in occasional subjects [11–14]. As mentioned previously, 'stress' is impossible to quantify or administer in standardized 'doses'; currently used stressors — such as mental arithmetic, television games or simulated public speaking — may be ethically more acceptable than inducing the fear of amputation but may be just as remote from the patient's own sources of tension. Various psychological stressors can cause physiological changes which could affect metabolic control in diabetic patients, such as disturbing intestinal motility [15] and therefore perhaps food absorption, or subcutaneous blood flow [16] and therefore possibly insulin absorption. However, recent carefully controlled studies in IDDM patients with various levels of hyperglycaemia have demonstrated that psychological stress sufficient to produce significant physiological responses such as tachycardia, hypertension and increased plasma catecholamine levels had no effect on blood glucose, free fatty acid or ketone body levels [17].

Firm evidence that psychological stress may significantly worsen diabetic control is therefore lacking. Nonetheless, it is obvious that psychological stress and poor metabolic control frequently coexist, as exemplified by patients with 'brittle' diabetes. Numerous workers have reported that poor glycaemic control is associated with increased anxiety [18], mood disturbance [19] and stress scores [20], but may have fallen into the trap of confusing correlation with causation. Some patients under stress may fail to comply with diet or insulin treatment, whereas others may suffer stress through their inability to achieve adequate control. The picture is further clouded by the possibility that hyperglycaemia itself may be the cause rather than the effect of certain features of anxiety [21]. It is obvious that the precise interaction between psychological stress and metabolic control will only be elucidated when improved ways of delivering and measuring 'stress' relevant to the patient have been developed and rigid criteria for monitoring metabolic control applied [15, 22, 23].

## Psychiatric disorders in diabetic patients

### *Prevalence*

There have been no comprehensive epidemiological surveys of psychiatric disorder in the diabetic population. Wilkinson *et al.* [24], using a two-stage screening procedure, found the overall prevalence of psychiatric disorder in IDDM out-patients in Dundee to be 18% in men and 24% in women. These estimates corresponded closely to those in the local general community, as ascertained from general practitioners' records, and are at the lower end of the prevalences reported from hospital-based populations using the same technique. In specific groups of patients, such as those with unsatisfactory glycaemic control or diabetic complications, frank psychiatric illness may be more common. For example, depression and/or anxiety may affect up to 50% of poorly controlled youngsters with IDDM [25, 26] and a few have severe self-destructive tendencies which may end in suicide [27, 28]. The special problems of depression in blind or partially sighted diabetic patients are discussed in Chapter 9.

It must be emphasized that the Dundee prevalence data were derived from a study using strictly applied research criteria with the specific aim of identifying psychiatric disease; significant psychiatric disease will be detected much less frequently in the routine diabetic clinic. The diagnosis of psychiatric disorder depends on recognizing a pattern of mental and behavioural symptoms, which is intrinsically a subjective and uncertain process. It has been estimated that over one-half of cases of psychiatric disorder, diagnosable by research criteria, affecting general medical patients will be missed by their physicians [29]. In the case of diabetes, Wilkinson *et al.* [30] found that diabetologists in one large clinic detected only 28% of the psychiatric disorders identified by psychiatrists using a standardized psychiatric interview in a sample of out-patients. However, the diabetologists were correct in 94% of cases where they diagnosed psychiatric disorder, and were able to identify most of the cases with major psychiatric disorder requiring treatment.

The presence of specific diabetic complications may engender depression or anxiety in individual cases. However, in the general diabetic population overall, there does not seem to be any relationship between psychiatric disorder and the extent of complications, duration of diabetes, quality of glycaemic control (as measured by $HbA_1$) or method of treatment [26].

### *Nature of psychiatric disorder in diabetic patients*

Most psychiatric disorder accompanying general medical conditions, including diabetes, comprises the single broad category of depression with or without anxiety. About one-half of these patients complain of sleep disturbance and various somatic symptoms which may be precipitated, exacerbated or maintained by psychological factors.

Other disorders, less commonly encountered in diabetic patients but usually readily recognized, include anorexia nervosa and other appetite disturbances; phobias about needles, injections and self-monitoring; obsessional disorders which may be fuelled by rigorous education and attention to detail in self-management [31]; alcohol and drug dependence which may masquerade as 'brittle' diabetes [32]; manic disorder; and schizophrenia. A problem which is probably underestimated is that of factitious hypo- or hyperglycaemia, which may be associated with significant psychiatric disorder. In many cases of mild psychiatric disorder, where true illness is difficult to distinguish from distress, a precise diagnosis may not be possible.

### *Diagnosis of psychiatric disorders in diabetic patients*

As mentioned above, psychiatric disorders are commoner than generally suspected in diabetic patients. The busy diabetic clinic is clearly not the best place to elicit and discuss psychiatric symptoms. It is therefore essential for a psychiatrist and/or psychologist to be easily accessible for rapid referral of patients with suspected problems, and ideally part of the diabetic care team. It is best if these specialists have an interest in and a broad understanding of general medical diseases and diabetes in particular.

At the same time, physicians, nurses and other team members must remain alert to the possibility of psychiatric disorder in diabetic patients, particularly depression with or without anxiety, which may present in several ways (Table 28.4) and will frequently respond well to treatment. Some simple principles in interview technique have been suggested to make it easier for the patient to volunteer and for the interviewer to detect the features of depression and/or anxiety [33] (see Table 28.5).

**Table 28.4.** Features of moderate and severe depression suggesting the need for antidepressant drugs.

| |
|---|
| Sleep disturbance, fatigue, loss of energy |
| Loss of appetite, loss of weight |
| Loss of interests, inactivity |
| Loss of libido |
| Inability to concentrate |
| Marked anxiety |
| Suicidal thoughts* |

* Formal psychiatric referral is also indicated.

**Table 28.5.** Suggested interview style to improve detection of psychiatric disorders (from Goldberg & Huxley 1980 [33]).

| |
|---|
| Establish eye contact at the beginning of the consultation |
| Do not read notes while taking the history |
| Clarify the presenting complaint |
| Do not concentrate on the past history |
| Use direct questions for physical complaints |
| Use an emphatic interview style |
| Be sensitive to non-verbal as well as verbal cues |
| Be able to deal with over-talkative patients |

### *Treatment of psychiatric disorders*

Many minor disorders will respond to simple supportive advice and the general measures outlined below but some will require medical treatment and specialist psychiatric referral. This section will deal with the commonest problem of depression with or without anxiety.

#### GENERAL MEASURES TO TREAT DEPRESSION

The diagnosis and the relationship of depression to the patient's symptoms should initially be explained. Specific causes of depression or anxiety (e.g. fear of blindness, renal failure, infertility, impotence) should be sought and discussed sympathetically but realistically. Practical advice for improving diabetic control and any other medical problems should be offered. The patient should be reassured that he can discuss the problem again if he so wishes and must be given a follow-up appointment.

Sleep disorder is common but will often respond to simple advice, such as to take regular exercise and avoid naps during the day and to avoid large meals, tobacco, alcohol or caffeine-containing drinks in the late evening. Relaxation exercises such as those developed by Surwit and colleagues [34, 35] may improve daytime restlessness or tension and may also improve glycaemic control in both IDDM [36] and NIDDM [37]. Benzodiazepines are best avoided because of the severe problems of dependency. Depressed patients should be advised to continue work and social contacts, in order to maintain self-esteem and avoid loneliness. Mustering friends and statutory or voluntary helping agencies to provide company is often beneficial, especially in the elderly.

### ANTIDEPRESSANT DRUGS

Patients failing to respond to general measures or who display features of moderate to severe depression (Table 28.4) should be given a trial of antidepressant drugs. The more pronounced these features are, the greater is the likelihood that they will respond to these drugs; however, the source of the patient's depression and/or anxiety should also be identified and corrected if possible.

First-choice antidepressant drugs are generally the tricyclic or related agents, especially amitryptiline and imipramine. Guidelines for their use are shown in Table 28.6; they may also be useful in the treatment of painful diabetic neuropathy, as described in Chapter 11. Tricyclic drugs generally relieve certain depressive symptoms, often improving sleep and having a calming effect within the first few days. This may persist with a relatively sedative agent such as amitryptiline, whereas most patients treated with imipramine will then become more alert and energetic. Patients must be told that the maximum benefits of antidepressant treatment may not be felt for 4–6 weeks.

Other antidepressant drugs (such as tetracyclics, e.g. mianserin; serotonin reuptake inhibitors, e.g. fluvoxamine; monoamine oxidase inhibitors; lithium salts) are indicated in patients with medical conditions (especially cardiac disease) which preclude the use of tricyclic agents, or when these latter are ineffective or have significant side-effects. In this event, drug treatment is best supervised by a psychiatrist. Initially, only limited supplies of antidepressant drugs should be prescribed, because patients may show suicidal tendencies when they become more active. Most depressive episodes remit within 3–12 months; antidepressant treatment is generally continued at full dosage until the patient has felt well for a month and is then gradually reduced in steps lasting 1–2 weeks. Drugs can be gradually withdrawn in asymptomatic patients, although some patients benefit from continued treatment at half-dosage for several months to prevent recurrence. Treatment must not be stopped abruptly, and patients should be supervised closely in case symptoms recur.

Side-effects of tricyclic drugs (Table 28.6) may be severe but often improve within a few days of starting treatment and are fully reversible on withdrawing the drugs. Older people are particularly sensitive to dizziness and fainting. These drugs have no adverse metabolic effects but their hypotensive action demands caution in patients with symptomatic autonomic neuropathy and their anticholinergic action may rarely precipitate closed-angle glaucoma in patients with rubeosis iridis.

**Table 28.6.** Tricyclic antidepressants.

*Examples*
- Amitryptiline — sedative; use in agitated or anxious patients
- Imipramine — useful in withdrawn or apathetic patients

*Dosages*
- Start at 75 mg/day, increase to 150 mg/day after 1 week
- Use lower dosages in elderly patients
- Higher dosages (300 mg/day) need specialist supervision

*Therapeutic effects*
- Improved sleep and calming effect within few days
- Maximal clinical benefit may take 4–6 weeks

*Duration of treatment*
- Maintain full dosage until symptom-free for 1 month
- Gradually reduce dosage; do not withdraw abruptly
- Some patients require prolonged maintenance treatment (half of full dosage)

*Side-effects (with specific contraindications in parentheses)*
- Dry mouth
- Blurred vision (glaucoma)
- Hesitancy or retention of urine (prostatism)
- Tachycardia (arrhythmia, heart block)

(the four items above: Anticholinergic effects)
- Hypotension (autonomic neuropathy)
- Sweating
- Excessive sedation (with amitryptiline)
- Late effects (after 2 weeks):
  tremor
  weight gain
  sexual dysfunction

### PROGNOSIS AND OUTCOME OF TREATMENT

Mild depressive disorders and those precipitated by upsetting life-events frequently improve spontaneously and may remit within a few days of starting general measures or medical treatment. Patients who fail to respond or who do so only temporarily, and those who are seriously ill and at risk of suicide will require immediate referral to a psychiatrist. Many psychiatrists now have expertise in the care of patients with general medical conditions. Hospital admission, compulsory if necessary, should be considered if there is a risk of suicide, harm to others or antisocial behaviour, or if home circumstances are unsuitable for the effective treatment of either the psychiatric disorder or the diabetes.

The management of the various psychological and psychiatric problems associated with 'brittle' diabetes is complicated and carries a poor record of success.

### Conclusions

Psychological and emotional factors can affect patients with diabetes in many ways but the psychological and psychiatric aspects of diabetic management have largely been overlooked [38–40]. From this perspective, Williams *et al.* have suggested that the time is right for a reappraisal of the impact that psychological factors have on metabolic control [23]. More importantly, there is a need for convincing evidence that the application of psychological techniques to diabetic care actually improves the patient's metabolic state and quality of life. On the other hand, Bradley has argued that we can only understand the patient's preferences for treatment and the factors affecting his motivation and compliance if treatment is evaluated in relation to his individual characteristics [41]. It therefore becomes necessary to measure psychological as well as clinical and metabolic factors in such studies and to recognize that, even if psychological factors are not measured, these may nevertheless influence outcome.

It is now apparent that psychological problems and psychiatric disorders are relatively common in diabetic patients and that all members of the diabetic care team must appreciate their possible impact on diabetic patients' ability to manage their disease. The need to include a psychiatrist and/or psychologist in the diabetic management team has been increasingly recognized in North America but many diabetic clinics in Britain still have only limited and difficult access to these specialists. It is to be hoped that they will play a wider role in the care of diabetic patients in the future.

GREG WILKINSON

### References

1 Koski M-L. The coping process in childhood diabetes. *Acta Paediatr Scand* 1969; **198** (suppl): 1–56.

2 Cohen F, Lazarus RF. Coping with the stresses of illness. In: Stone GC, Cohen F, Adler N, eds. *Health Psychology: a Handbook*. San Francisco: Jossey-Bass, 1979: 217–54.

3 Cannon WB, De la Paz D. Emotional stimulation of adrenal secretion. *Am J Physiol* 1911; **28**: 64–70.

4 Bliss EL, Migeon CJ, Branch CHH, Samuels LT. Reaction of the adrenal cortex to emotional stress. *Psychosom Med* 1956; **18**: 56–76.

5 Miyabo S, Hisada T, Asato T, Muzushima N, Ueno K. Growth hormone and cortisol responses to psychological stress: comparison of normal and neurotic subjects. *J Clin Endocrinol Metab* 1976; **42**: 1158–62.

6 Hinkle LE, Conger GB, Wolf S. Studies on diabetes mellitus: the relation of stressful life situations to the concentration of ketone bodies in the blood of diabetic and non-diabetic humans. *Diabetes* 1952; **1**: 383–92.

7 Surwit RS, Feinglos MN. Stress and the autonomic nervous system in type II diabetes. A hypothesis. *Diabetes Care* 1988; **11**: 83–5.

8 Carter WR, Herman J, Stokes K, Cox DJ. Promotion of diabetes onset by stress in the BB rat. *Diabetologia* 1987; **30**: 674–5.

9 Mazelis G, Albert D, Crisa C *et al*. Relationship of stressful housing conditions to the onset of diabetes mellitus induced by multiple, sub-diabetogenic doses of streptozotocin in mice. *Diabetes Res* 1987; **6**: 195–200.

10 MacGillivray MH, Bruck E, Voorhess ML. Acute diabetic ketoacidosis in children: role of the stress hormones. *Pediatr Res* 1981; **15**: 99–106.

11 Hinkle LE, Wolf S. A summary of experimental evidence relating life stress to diabetes mellitus. *J Mt Sinai Hosp* 1952; **19**: 537–46.

12 Hinkle LE, Edwards CJ, Wolf S. Studies in diabetes mellitus. II. The occurrence of a diuresis in diabetic persons exposed to stressful life situations with experimental observations on its relation to the concentration of glucose in blood and urine. *J Clin Invest* 1951; **30**: 818–26.

13 Vandenburgh RL, Sussman KE, Titus CC. Effects of hypnotically induced acute emotional stress on carbohydrate and lipid metabolism in patients with diabetes mellitus. *Psychosom Med* 1966; **28**: 382–90.

14 Lustman P, Carney R, Amado H. Acute stress and metabolism in diabetes. *Diabetes Care* 1981; **4**: 658–9.

15 Cann PA, Read NW, Cammack J *et al*. Psychological stress and the passage of a standard meal through the stomach and small intestine in man. *Gut* 1983; **24**: 236–40.

16 Hildebrandt P, Mehlsen J, Sestoft L, Nielsen SL. Mild mental stress in diabetes: changes in heart rate and subcutaneous blood flow. *Clin Physiol* 1985; **5**: 371–6.

17 Kemmer FW, Bisping R, Steingruber HJ *et al*. Psychological stress and metabolic control in patients with type 1 diabetes mellitus. *N Engl J Med* 1986; **314**: 1078–84.

18 Anderson BJ, Miller JP, Auslander WF, Santiago JV. Family characteristics of diabetic adolescents: relationship to metabolic control. *Diabetes Care* 1984; **4**: 586–94.

19 Mazze RS, Lucido D, Shamoon H. Psychological and social correlates of glycemic control. *Diabetes Care* 1984; **7**: 360–7.

20 Chase HP, Jackson GC. Stress and sugar control in children with insulin-dependent diabetes mellitus. *J Pediatr* 1981; **98**: 1011–13.

21 Lustman PJ, Skor DA, Carney RM, Santiago JV, Cryer PE. Stress and diabetic control. *Lancet* 1983; **i**: 588.

22 Hauser ST, Pollets D. Psychological aspects of diabetes mellitus: a critical review. *Diabetes Care* 1979; **2**: 227–32.

23 Williams G, Pickup J, Keen H. Psychological factors and metabolic control: time for reappraisal? *Diabetic Med* 1988; **5**: 211–15.

24 Wilkinson G, Borsey DQ, Leslie P, Newton RW, Lind C, Ballinger CB. Psychiatric morbidity and social problems in

patients with insulin-dependent diabetes mellitus. *Br J Psychiatr* 1988; **153**: 38–43.

25 Tattersall R, Walford S. Brittle diabetes in response to life stress: 'cheating and manipulation'. In: Pickup JC, ed. *Brittle Diabetes*. Oxford: Blackwell Scientific Publications, 1985: 76–102.

26 Orr DP, Golden MP, Myers G, Marrero DG. Characteristics of adolescents with poorly-controlled diabetes referred to a tertiary care center. *Diabetes Care* 1983; **6**: 170–5.

27 Flexner CW, Weiner JP, Sandek CD, Dans PE. Repeated hospitalization for diabetic ketoacidosis. The game of Sartoris. *Am J Med* 1984; **76**: 691–5.

28 Stearns S. Self-destructive behaviour in young patients with diabetes mellitus. *Diabetes* 1959; **8**: 379–82.

29 Goldberg D. Identifying psychiatric illness among general medical patients. *Br Med J* 1985; **291**: 161–2.

30 Wilkinson G, Borsey DQ, Leslie P, Newton RW, Lind C, Ballinger CB. Psychiatric disorder in patients with insulin-dependent diabetes mellitus attending a general hospital clinic: (i) two-stage screening; and detection by physicians. *Psychol Med* 1987; **17**: 515–17.

31 Beer SF, Lawson C, Watkins PJ. Neurosis induced by home monitoring of blood glucose concentrations. *Br Med J* 1989; **298**: 362.

32 Schade DS, Drumm DA, Duckworth WC, Eaton RP. The etiology of incapacitating, brittle diabetes. *Diabetes Care* 1985; **8**: 12–20.

33 Goldberg D, Huxley P. *Mental Illness in the Community. The Pathway to Psychiatric Care*. London: Tavistock Publications, 1980.

34 Forgione GA, Surwit RS, Page D. *Fear: Learning to Cope*. New York: Van Nostrand Reinhold, 1978.

35 Surwit RS. *Progressive Relaxation*. Durham, North Carolina: Duke University Medical Center, 1977.

36 Fowler JE, Budzynski TH, Vanderbergh RL. Effects of an EMG biofeedback relaxation program on the control of diabetes. *Biofeedback Self Regul* 1976; **1**: 105–12.

37 Surwit RS, Feinglos MN. The effects of relaxation on glucose tolerance in non-insulin-dependent diabetes. *Diabetes Care* 1983; **6**: 176–9.

38 Wilkinson G. Psychiatric aspects of diabetes mellitus. *Br J Psychiatr* 1981; **138**: 1–9.

39 Tattersall R. Psychiatric aspects of diabetes — a physician's view. *Br J Psychiatr* 1981; **139**: 485–93.

40 Wilkinson G. The influence of psychiatric, psychological and social factors on the control of insulin-dependent diabetes mellitus. *J Psychosom Res* 1987; **31**: 277–86.

41 Bradley C. Clinical trials — time for a paradigm shift? *Diabetic Med* 1988; **5**: 107–9.

# 29 Eating Disorders and Diabetes Mellitus

**Summary**

• Eating disorders — anorexia and bulimia (food bingeing) — are apparently commoner in diabetic patients (particularly young women) than in the general population.
• Inflexible education about 'ideal' diet and weight may be partly responsible; fear of hypoglycaemia may encourage overeating.
• Diabetic patients may also lose weight by deliberately reducing or omitting insulin treatment.
• Life-threatening electrolyte disturbances and acute renal failure may result from induced diarrhoea or vomiting.
• Abnormal eating attitudes can be identified by standard questionnaires ('EAT' and 'EDI'), but diabetes-biased questions should be avoided.
• Eating disorders are frequently accompanied by poor diabetic control and may precipitate or aggravate acute painful neuropathy and other microvascular complications.
• Eating disorders are difficult to treat in diabetic patients, but may respond to psychotherapy or behavioural therapy; expert psychiatric help is needed.

Sir William Gull described anorexia nervosa in 1874 [1]. His patients, predominantly young girls, felt a compulsion to be thin and insisted they were too fat even when cachectic. They avoided fattening foods and many had bizarre and often secretive eating habits; some also abused laxatives, induced vomiting or exercised strenuously to reduce weight.

The diagnostic criteria for anorexia nervosa [2, 3] stipulate weight loss (exceeding 25% of premorbid weight according to some authorities [3]) due to abnormal eating behaviour, amenorrhoea and a morbid fear of becoming fat (Table 29.1).

Bulimia ('the hunger of an ox') described formally by Russell in 1979 [4] also mostly affects young women (Table 29.1). Patients have binges when they eat large quantities of high-calorie foods (often several thousand calories at a time), followed by vomiting or use of laxatives or severe dietary restriction. They are frightened that they cannot stop eating voluntarily and have feelings of depression and self-depreciation after a binge. This condition is much more difficult to recognize than anorexia nervosa as patients may be obese, of normal weight or thin. Clinical examination is

**Table 29.1.** Current diagnostic criteria for anorexia nervosa and bulimia nervosa, as defined in the *Diagnostic and Statistical Manual of Mental Disorders* [3].

| |
|---|
| *Anorexia nervosa* |
| Weight loss and maintenance of body weight 15% below that expected for age and height |
| Disturbance in the way in which one's body weight, size or shape are experienced |
| Intense fear of gaining weight or becoming fat, even though underweight |
| Absence of ≥ three menses when otherwise expected |
| *Bulimia nervosa* |
| Recurrent episodes of binge eating |
| A feeling of lack of control over eating behaviour during the eating binge |
| Regular self-induced vomiting, use of laxatives or diuretics, strict dieting or fasting or vigorous exercise to prevent weight gain |
| ≥ two binges per week for ≥ 3 months |
| Persistent over-concern with body shape and weight |

usually normal, although some will have erosion of the front teeth as a result of repeated vomiting.

Severely affected patients with these eating disorders may develop major electrolyte disturbances, especially profound hypokalaemia and acute renal failure due to vomiting and/or laxative-induced diarrhoea, and can die as a result of their illness.

Eating disorders have become increasingly recognized over the last 20 years, probably in part through enhanced media publicity, although there is also evidence that anorexia and bulimia are becoming commoner [5–7]. In parts of the world where many people do not have enough to eat, obesity is encouraged as a sign of prosperity. In the Western world, it used to be considered beautiful for women to be plump but in recent years it has become increasingly fashionable to be thin, as is witnessed by the diminishing vital statistics of beauty queens and photographic models. There is therefore a great deal of pressure — particularly from women's magazines — on all women of today to be thin, and this may contribute to the increased prevalence of eating disorders.

Psychiatric hospital units with a special interest in eating disorders have found that while initially they saw many patients with anorexia nervosa, more recently they have been increasing numbers of patients with bulimia and now patients with 'multiple impulsive bulimia' — bulimia associated with other self-damaging forms of behaviour, e.g. multiple overdoses, repeated self-mutilation, drug abuse, sexual disinhibition and stealing.

## The association with diabetes

Eating disorders were first associated with diabetes in 1980 by Fairburn and Steel, who reported three cases [8]. There followed several series of case reports suggesting that the association was commoner than would be expected by chance [9, 11]. In a survey of 208 female IDDM patients aged 16–25 years, Steel *et al.* found that 7% had a clinically apparent eating disorder [12]. Even this high prevalence was probably an underestimate, particularly of bulimia, as only known cases were included; patients were not specifically questioned.

In order to try to assess more accurately the size of the problem and attitudes to eating in more detail, several workers have carried out surveys using standard questionnaires such as the EAT (Eating Attitude Test) and EDI (Eating Disorder Inventory) designed by Garner [13]. The EAT has been widely used to screen for cases of anorexia nervosa in groups at high risk for this disorder, for example among college students [14], and the EDI to assess psychological characteristics relevant to anorexia nervosa and bulimia [15]. Results of the original questionnaires may be difficult to interpret, as answers to some questions (e.g. 'Do you avoid foods with sugar in them?') are likely to be affected by diabetes *per se* [16]. Wing and colleagues found higher scores in diabetic patients using the unmodified EAT and Rodin *et al.* [17], applying the original EAT and EDI to 46 female diabetic patients, found an incidence of 19% for clinically significant disorders of eating and weight. Rosmark removed diabetes-related questions and found that 41 female diabetic patients had higher mean EAT scores than either female non-diabetic controls or male diabetic subjects [18]. Steel *et al.* [19] compared cohorts of 152 young IDDM women and 139 young IDDM men with age- and sex-matched controls, using the EAT and EDI. After diabetes-related questions were excluded, female diabetic patients scored significantly higher than their controls, whereas there was no difference between male diabetic and non-diabetic subjects. These studies add to the mounting evidence that clinical and subclinical eating disorders are particularly common in young female diabetic patients.

## The clinical problem

It has become clear from clinical experience that, in addition to the usual artifices used by patients with anorexia nervosa and bulimia, diabetic patients commonly choose to omit insulin injections or reduce the dose of insulin to control their weight [9–11, 19–22]. The relationship between eating disorders and diabetic control is complex (Fig. 29.1). Many patients with diabetes and eating disorders described in the literature have been poorly controlled [20–24] (see Table 29.2) and those with pathologically high EAT and EDI scores tend to have a high $HbA_1$ [18]. Psychiatrists seeing patients referred to them by physicians because of an eating disorder stress that eating disorders cause poor control [24]. There are undoubtedly cases, particularly those with bulimia, where this appears to be the case. On the other hand, diabetologists seeing patients in the context of life-long diabetes suggest that eating disorders tend to occur more frequently in patients who are already

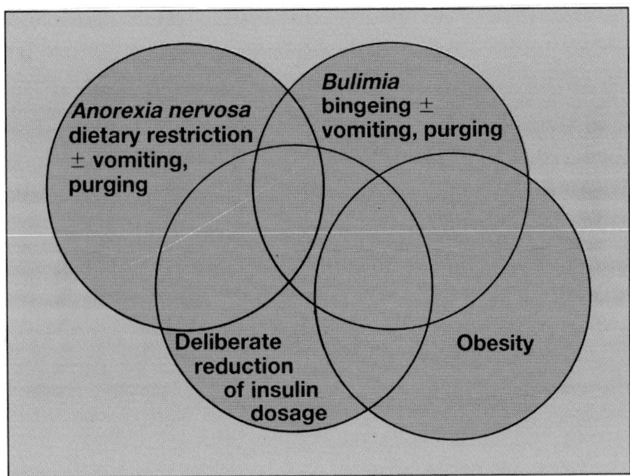


**Fig. 29.1.** The relationship between eating disorders and diabetic control.

**Table 29.2.** Metabolic and microvascular complications in 15 patients with clinically apparent eating disorders, identified from a randomly selected population of 208 female IDDM patients aged 16–25 years. (Adapted from [12].)

| Complication | Number of patients affected |
|---|---|
| Persistent hyperglycaemia | 11 |
| Ketoacidosis | 5 |
| Hypoglycaemia | 3 |
| Retinopathy | 11 |
| (proliferative retinopathy) | (6) |
| Peripheral neuropathy | 6 |
| Nephropathy | 6 |

poorly controlled [11], and that the emergence of an eating disorder in such patients appears to be another facet of long-standing behavioural disturbance. Indeed, eating disorders are a feature of 'brittle' diabetes.

There are, however, small numbers of patients who manage to control their diabetes well despite suffering from an eating disorder. Some with anorexia nervosa manage to reduce their carbohydrate intake and insulin dose in parallel without developing either ketoacidosis or hypoglycaemia. Some with bulimia increase their insulin in an attempt to compensate for a large binge and some try hard to control their eating disorder for fear of upsetting their diabetic control.

In addition to those who fulfil the formal criteria for an eating disorder, there is a large number of diabetic patients who possess the psychological characteristics of an eating disorder and who, as well as the usual tactics used by patients with anorexia nervosa and bulimia, commonly choose to reduce or omit their insulin injections to cause weight loss through diuresis and catabolism [9–11, 19–22]. Many of these patients are overweight, although their weight can be normal or low. This syndrome has been provisionally labelled 'MIDMED' ('manipulation of insulin dose as a manifestation of an eating disorder') [25]. These different clinical situations are summarized in Table 29.2.

### *Relationship to diabetic complications*

There appears to be a high incidence of early-onset microvascular complications — retinopathy, nephropathy, autonomic neuropathy and peripheral neuropathy — in diabetic patients with eating disorders [8, 10, 20] (see Table 29.2). Patients have also been described with acute painful neuropathy coinciding with the development of an eating disorder, becoming very severe at the time of maximum weight loss and remitting as weight was regained [12] (see Fig. 10.7). Poor metabolic control is likely to be of major importance in the aetiology of these microvascular complications but nutritional factors may also contribute.

## Why does diabetes predispose to eating disorders?

The most obvious explanation for the high prevalence of abnormal eating attitudes in diabetic women is that they are constantly educated to focus on diet and food in order to control their diabetes. They are discouraged from eating sweet foods, which they may particularly enjoy, and made to feel guilty if they 'cheat'.

They are also encouraged to control their weight. Many diabetic people rightly associate insulin with weight gain, which often follows the start of treatment through a combination of rehydration and the anabolic effect of insulin, and there may be a marked increase during the first year after diagnosis. Even though many patients do not become overweight according to standard height–weight tables, they may find the rapid change in their body image frightening. Diabetic women tend to score highly on the 'drive for thinness' and 'body dissatisfaction' subscales of the EDI. Insulin-treated diabetic patients tend to be slightly heavier than their peers, probably partly because insulin delivered systemically rather than into the portal circulation over-stimulates adipose tissue formation. Another undoubted factor is that many patients find it easy to eat more than their dietary allowance but difficult to eat less, because of the risk of developing hypoglycaemia; occasionally patients overeat frequently because of a fear of hypoglycaemia.

Diabetes presents a challenge to an adolescent's self-esteem. Young diabetic patients often have low self-esteem and feel ineffective, psychological characteristics which predispose to the development of eating disorders.

It has also been suggested that the conflict between dependence and independence, which is an integral part of adolescent development, is greatly intensified in the diabetic adolescent who is dependent on treatment for survival but who is forced to assume a major role in regulating therapy. Such conflict may also be important in the development of eating disorders [10].

## Treatment of eating disorders in diabetes

Treatment of these conditions is difficult. Patients should be referred for psychiatric help, preferably to a unit specifically interested in eating disorders. These units use behavioural, cognitive and psychotherapy often in combination with family therapy and group therapy. The emphasis may vary depending on the centre. Well-equipped units also have facilities for art and drama therapy, relaxation training, body image work, and may run anxiety management programmes.

Those unwilling to see a psychiatrist may be helped by an experienced, understanding physician preferably working closely with an interested psychiatrist. Patients with bulimia can be helped by discussing their problems and explaining that many others have similar difficulties. Diabetic patients usually already keep a diary in which they record insulin dose, blood glucose levels, hypoglycaemia, etc., and they should be encouraged also to record everything they eat and drink and particularly binges, vomiting and the use of laxatives. They should also be asked to record their feelings at the time of a binge. The diaries should then be discussed and patients encouraged to understand why they binge, to develop strategies to avoid it and to eat regularly (not avoiding meals after a binge), explaining that they may expect to gain weight initially. It is usually necessary to see patients fairly frequently for several months and it is important to involve members of the family.

Antidepressants have a place for those who are depressed and are also helpful in controlling bulimia in some who are not depressed.

Some patients refuse all help because their overwhelming desire to be thin blinds them to the need for a change in their behaviour. In severe cases, in-patient treatment is required and very occasionally it may be necessary to detain a patient compulsorily in a psychiatric unit if his or her life is in danger.

## Conclusions

Eating disorders are particularly disabling in diabetic patients and present special management difficulties. These patients tend to be poorly controlled and often develop serious complications of diabetes. The first step towards more effective treatment is an increased awareness of the problem. Early recognition, sympathetic discussion of the patient's attitude to body weight and to eating and the avoidance of rapid weight gain in the first few months after diagnosis should all help to forestall the more serious manifestations of eating disorders in a substantial proportion of susceptible patients.

## Recent developments

The official diagnostic criteria for these eating disorders have changed over the years and may change again. Many feel that these illnesses represent extremes of a range of behaviour and that cut-off points are artificial. For some purposes, however, it is important to have clear criteria and those defined by the *Diagnostic and Statistical Manual of Mental Disorders (1987)* [3] are shown in Table 29.1. These criteria apply to the general population; it has been proposed that an additional criterion specific to diabetic subjects — namely, the deliberate omission or reduction of insulin dosages — should be included in the next revision of the manual.

The prevalence of eating disorders in the diabetic population remains controversial, possibly because of variations between the groups of patients studied and in the methods used. Clinical interviews are likely to provide greater reliability and validity than self-report questionnaires. Rodin *et al.* [26] conducted clinical interviews and identified present or past history of eating disorders in 13.8% of 58 young diabetic women. Fairburn *et al.* [27] interviewed 54 diabetic women aged 17–25 years, using the previously validated

Eating Disorder Examination; the diabetic women had higher scores of abnormality than non-diabetic controls, but the difference was not significant. Subsequently, the same group [28] diagnosed a clinical eating disorder in 9% of 33 diabetic girls aged 11–18 years, compared with 6% of non-diabetic controls. This difference was also not significant, a finding endorsed by another study [29] which was also based on relatively small numbers of subjects, some of whom were very young (8–18 years). The discrepancy between these negative findings and the studies cited on p. 302 may be explained by age bias and by the low statistical power of some of the recent surveys; for example, Peveler *et al.* [28] estimated that a population 10 times larger than that investigated would have been necessary to show a 2-fold difference in the frequency of eating disorders. The overall balance of evidence suggests strongly that diabetes is a risk factor for eating disorders. There is no doubt that the two conditions commonly coexist, and that eating disorders not sufficiently severe to fulfil the DSM III criteria can have serious psychological and metabolic consequences in people with diabetes.

New forms of therapy are being tried in patients with eating disorders, including family therapy [30] and various drugs which enhance the action of serotonin. These drugs include dexfenfluramine, whose effects include a reduced appetite, especially for carbohydrate-rich foods, and fluoxetine, which is used primarily as an antidepressant but also can reduce food intake and cause weight loss in man and animals. So far, these drugs have been used with limited success to treat bulimia [31, 32] in patients with or without depression (which is relatively common in subjects with eating disorders [30]). Until now, experience with these drugs in diabetic patients with eating disorders has been very limited, although one case of bulimia responded well to fluoxetine [33]. The management of anorexia nervosa remains difficult and the outcome is often unsatisfactory; some approaches are discussed in detail elsewhere [30].

JUDITH M. STEEL

## References


1 Gull WW. Anorexia nervosa (Apepsia hysterica, Anorexia hysterica). *Trans Clin Soc Lond* 1874; **7**: 22.

2 Russell GFM. Anorexia nervosa: its identity as an illness and its treatment. In: Price JH, ed. *Modern Trends in Psychological Medicine*, Vol 2. London: Butterworths, 131–64.

3 *Diagnostic and Statistical Manual of Mental Disorders*, 3rd edn., revised. Washington DC: American Psychiatric Association, 1987.

4 Russell GFM. Bulimia nervosa, an ominous variant of anorexia nervosa. *Psychol Med* 1979; **6**: 429–48.

5 Kendell RE, Hall DJ, Hailey A, Babigian HM. Epidemiology of anorexia nervosa. *Psychol Med* 1976; **3**: 200–3.

6 Crisp AH, Palmer RL, Kalvey RS. How common is anorexia nervosa? A prevalence study. *Br J Psychiatr* 1976; **128**: 549–54.

7 Cooper PJ, Fairburn CG. Binge eating and self-induced vomiting in the community. A preliminary study. *Br J Psychiatr* 1983; **142**: 139–44.

8 Fairburn CG, Steel JM. Anorexia nervosa in diabetes mellitus. *Br Med J* 1980; **280**: 1167–8.

9 Roland OM, Bhanji S. Anorexia nervosa occurring in patients with diabetes mellitus. *Postgrad Med J* 1982; **58**: 354–6.

10 Powers PS, Malone JE, Duncan J. Anorexia nervosa and diabetes mellitus. *J Clin Psychiatr* 1983; **44**: 133–5.

11 Szmukler GI. Anorexia and bulimia in diabetics. *J Psychosomat Res* 1984; **28**: 365–9.

12 Steel JM, Young RJ, Lloyd GG, Clarke BF. Clinically apparent eating disorders in young diabetic women associated with painful neuropathy and other complications. *Br Med J* 1987; **294**: 859–62.

13 Garner DM, Garfinkel PE. The eating attitudes test: an index of the symptoms of anorexia nervosa. *Psychol Med* 1979; **9**: 273–9.

14 Garner DM, Garfinkel PE. Socio-cultural factors in the development of anorexia nervosa. *Psychol Med* 1980; **10**: 647–56.

15 Garner DM, Olmsted MP, Polivy J. Development and validation of a multidimensional eating disorder inventory for anorexia nervosa and bulimia. *Int J Eating Disord* 1983; **2**: 15–34.

16 Wing RA, Nowalk MP, Marcus MD, Koeske R, Finegold D. Subclinical eating disorders and glycemic control in adolescents with type I diabetes. *Diabetes Care* 1986; **9**: 162–7.

17 Rodin GM, Daneman D, Johnson LE, Kenshole A, Garfinkel PE. Anorexia nervosa and bulimia in female adolescents with insulin dependent diabetes mellitus, a systematic study. *J Psychiatr Res* 1985; **19**: 381–4.

18 Rosmark B, Berne C, Holmgren L, Lago C, Renholm G, Schilberg S. Eating disorders in patients with insulin dependent diabetes mellitus. *J Clin Psychiatr* 1986; **47**: 547–50.

19 Steel JM, Young RJ, Lloyd GG, Macintyre CCA. Abnormal eating attitudes in young insulin dependent diabetics. *Br J Psychiatr* 1989; **155**: 515–21.

20 Garner S. Anorexia nervosa in diabetes mellitus. *Br Med J* 1980; **281**: 1144.

21 Hudson MS, Wentworth SM, Hudson J. Bulimia and diabetes. *N Engl J Med* 1983; **309**: 431–2.

22 Szmukler GI, Russell GFM. Diabetes mellitus, anorexia nervosa and bulimia. *Br J Psychiatr* 1983; **142**: 305–8.

23 Hudson JI, Hudson MS, Wentworth SM. Self-induced glycosuria. A novel method of purging in bulimia. *J Am Med Ass* 1983; **249**: 2501.

24 Hillard JR, Hillard PJA. Bulimia, anorexia nervosa and diabetes. Deadly combinations. *Psychiatr Clin North Am* 1984; **7**: 367–79.

25 Steel JM. Eating disorders and diabetes. *Practical Diabetes* 1987; **4**: 256.

26 Rodin GM, Johnson LE, Garfinkel PE, Daneman D,

Kenshole AB. Eating disorders in female adolescents with insulin dependent diabetes mellitus. *Int J Psychiatry Med* 1986; **16**: 49–57.

27 Fairburn CG, Peveler RC, Davies B, Mann J, Mayhou RA. Eating disorders in young adults with insulin dependent diabetes mellitus: a controlled study. *Br Med J* 1991; **303**: 17–20.

28 Peveler RC, Boller I, Fairburn CG, Dunger D. Eating disorders in adolescents with IDDM. *Diabetes Care* 1992; **15**: 1356–60.

29 Striegel-Moore RH, Nicholson TJ, Tamborlane WV. Prevalence of eating disorder symptoms in pre-adolescent and adolescent girls with IDDM. *Diabetes Care* 1992; **15**: 1361–8.

30 Steel JM. Eating disorders in diabetes. In: Kelnar C, ed. *Diabetes in Childhood and Adolescence*. London: Chapman and Hall, in press.

31 Freeman CPA. Practical guide to the treatment of bulimia nervosa. *J Psychosom Res* 1991; **35**: 33–40.

32 Walsh BT. Psychopharmacologic treatment of bulimia nervosa. *J Clin Psychiatry* 1991; **52** (suppl): 34–8.

33 Ramirez LC, Rosenstock J, Stowig S, Cercone S, Raskin P. Effective treatment of bulimia with fluoxetine: a serotonin reuptake inhibitor, in a patient with type 1 diabetes mellitus. *Am J Med* 1990; **88**: 540–1.

# Index

When more than one page reference is given, **bold** print is used to indicate the principal reference.